# Statistical Methods in Healthcare

# Statistical Methods in Healthcare

Edited by

**Frederick W. Faltin**

*Founder and Managing Director, The Faltin Group, Cody, WY, USA*

**Ron S. Kenett**

*Chairman and CEO, The KPA Group, Raanana, Israel*

**Fabrizio Ruggeri**

*Research Director, CNR IMATI, Milan, Italy*

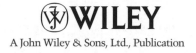

A John Wiley & Sons, Ltd., Publication

This edition first published 2012
© 2012 John Wiley & Sons, Ltd

*Registered office*
John Wiley & Sons Ltd, The Atrium, Southern Gate, Chichester, West Sussex, PO19 8SQ, United Kingdom

For details of our global editorial offices, for customer services and for information about how to apply for permission to reuse the copyright material in this book please see our website at www.wiley.com.

*Library of Congress Cataloging-in-Publication Data*

Statistical methods in healthcare / [edited by] Frederick W. Faltin, Ron S. Kenett, Fabrizio Ruggeri.
      p. ; cm.
   Includes bibliographical references and index.
   ISBN 978-0-470-67015-6 (cloth)
   I. Faltin, Frederick W.   II. Kenett, Ron S.   III. Ruggeri, Fabrizio.
   [DNLM: 1. Statistics as Topic–methods.   2. Data Collection–methods.   3. Delivery of Health Care–statistics & numerical data.   WA 950]
   362.102′1–dc23

                                                                                    2012009921

A catalogue record for this book is available from the British Library.

ISBN: 978-0-470-67015-6

Typeset in 10/12pt Times by Aptara Inc., New Delhi, India
Printed and bound in Malaysia by Vivar Printing Sdn Bhd

1   2012

*To Donna, Erin, Travis and Madeline*
– Frederick W. Faltin

*To Jonathan, Alma, Tomer, Yadin, Aviv and Gili*
– Ron S. Kenett

*To Anna, Giacomo and Lorenzo*
– Fabrizio Ruggeri

# Contents

## Part Three STATISTICAL PROCESS CONTROL IN HEALTHCARE

## Part Four    APPLICATIONS TO HEALTHCARE POLICY AND IMPLEMENTATION

## Part Five    APPLICATIONS TO HEALTHCARE MANAGEMENT

# Foreword

Twenty-five years ago we launched an interesting experiment, 'The National Demonstration Project for Quality Improvement in Healthcare'. It was a modest experiment bringing together twenty-one healthcare providers with twenty-one top industrial companies to explore whether industrial quality methods would work in healthcare settings. The results of this experiment were published as *Curing Health Care: New Strategies for Quality Improvement*. The statistical methods used by most of these healthcare providers were fairly basic tools of quality improvement; yet, many of the improvements were significant.

Looking back this many years later, there was no reason to be surprised by these results. Statistical methods had been used in many areas of healthcare for almost as many years as statistical methods had been used by any organization. Florence Nightingale was one of the first honorary members of the American Statistical Association, an organization that celebrated its 150th anniversary twenty-two years ago. Her pioneering work using clear, simple graphical methods to discover causes of death in hospitals during the Crimean War and alter British barracks was well known and celebrated. Basic, simple statistical methods to explore, understand and present data are as effective in healthcare applications as in any other endeavour.

But somehow, the science of quality control and quality improvement had passed healthcare by. Starting with Shewhart's control chart in 1924, statistical quality control had progressed quickly during the Second World War, and had been widely adopted and used by post-war Japan to become a leading producer of high-quality products. It had been rediscovered in the United States in the 1980s, and widely applied throughout the world in the 1980s and 1990s by companies in almost every competitive industry. Healthcare had evolved many methods of quality assurance, risk management and quality measurement, for the most part independent of what was happening in industry.

In some areas of healthcare, particularly in drug and medical device development and production, sophisticated methods had been created and widely used. Researchers in biostatistics, biometrics and clinical trials had developed and employed some of the most advanced statistical methods, and in turn contributed much to the statistical literature. These methods, however, did not seem to translate easily to the practice of continuous quality improvement in hospital-based care or general clinical practice. There was a considerable gap between what we knew how to do and what we were doing.

The National Demonstration Project evolved into the Institute for Healthcare Improvement, and the growing network of healthcare providers became increasingly adept in learning from sources outside of healthcare, adapting these methods to healthcare applications, and sharing encouraging results with each other. It was not only the statistical tools. The healthcare organizations picked up the methods of putting these tools to use in a scientific approach to improvement using PDSA (Plan-Do-Check/Study-Act), Juran's Quality Improvement Steps, Motorola/General Electric's Define-Measure-Analyse-Improve-Control (Six Sigma Quality), and full-scale implementations of the Toyota Production System (Lean).

Healthcare organizations around the world have formed collaboratives, networks and not-for-profit organizations to share these methods and statistical tools. Thousands of doctors, nurses and other practitioners now routinely attend healthcare quality conferences and daily participate in online courses, web-based sharing and local working groups. Organizations such as the Institute for Healthcare Improvement have tried to structure some of this learning through devices such as IHI's *Improvement Roadmap* and the Open School, but there has not been a simple place to find the statistical tools used in healthcare improvement until now.

Faltin, Kenett and Ruggeri have brought together leading researchers and practitioners in statistical methods to provide a wealth of methods in one place. Starting with some of the most sophisticated methods used in the development of pharmaceutical products and medical devices, and ending with applications to healthcare management, they have managed to cover amazing ground. The chapters on control charts bring together some of the best methods of statistical process control (SPC) in healthcare, and even cover some of the abuses in the use of control charts. The chapter 'Six Sigma in Healthcare' gives a remarkably thorough discussion of both Six Sigma and how it is being applied by many healthcare organizations in Europe and the USA.

But this book goes much further than the typical statistics text and addresses serious policy issues such as kidney allocation and offers advanced statistical methods as an approach to this critical problem. Another critical issue in healthcare, vaccine safety evaluation, is also addressed. In this time of crises in healthcare costs, the economics of healthcare is becoming a major issue. Here too, statistical methods have a large part to play.

The core of healthcare is, of course, clinical outcomes. Statistical methods play a critical role in outcomes analysis. Bias in modelling and monitoring health outcomes are addressed in a chapter by Grigg. Biggeri and Catelan discuss disease tracking. Guglielmi, Ieva, Paganoni and Ruggeri address process indicators and outcome measures in an important area, and Negri gives an excellent discussion of the special tool of meta-analysis.

We no longer need to discuss the value of statistical tools and quality improvement methods in healthcare. The value has been demonstrated thousands of times. What is needed is a comprehensive compilation of these tools in one place written by careful, knowledgeable authors. We should all be grateful to Faltin, Kenett and Ruggeri for providing it.

A. Blanton Godfrey
Dean, College of Textiles and Joseph D. Moore Distinguished University Professor
North Carolina State University
and Chair of the Board of Directors (2009–2012)
Institute for Healthcare Improvement

# Preface

This book has its origins in the confluence of two realizations. First, that the availability and quality of healthcare is the defining issue of our time. And second, that statistics as a discipline pervades every aspect of the healthcare field.

*Statistical Methods in Healthcare* illustrates the spectrum of statistical applications to healthcare. From pharmaceuticals to health economics, drug product development to facilities management, clinical outcomes to electronic medical records, risk assessment to organ allocation, statistics has permeated every corner of healthcare. Accordingly, we have assembled here an array of chapters, prepared by a broadly international group of leading authors, which address all of these topics, and many more. Our objective was not to touch upon every area of statistical application in healthcare – that would be impossible. Rather, our purpose has been to span, as best we can, the diverse domains to which statistics has been applied and, thereby, to contribute to the evolution of statistical methods in healthcare applications.

The book consists of 23 chapters organized in five parts:

**Part One: Statistics in Development of Pharmaceutical Products**

This part consists of chapters dealing with clinical trials, pharmacometrics, risk management in drug product development, statistical aspects in current regulatory guidelines, and future challenges in drug development.

**Part Two: Statistics in Outcomes Analysis**

The second part deals with monitoring healthcare and diseases, a detailed case study on the treatment of acute myocardial infarction patients, and a chapter dedicated to meta-analysis.

**Part Three: Statistical Process Control in Healthcare**

Applications of statistical process control in healthcare are gaining widespread acceptance. In this part we present examples from healthcare, clinical studies and applications of Six Sigma in healthcare.

**Part Four: Applications to Healthcare Policy and Implementation**

This part is focused on aspects of policy and implementation, including healthcare economics, benchmarking, vaccination policy and allocation procedures in kidney transplant surgery.

**Part Five: Applications to Healthcare Management**

This final part covers various aspects of healthcare delivery as a service, including payment procedures, electronic medical records and facilities management.

Not surprisingly, such an effort has been the work of contributors from many fields. *Statistical Methods in Healthcare* integrates contributions from statisticians, economists, physicians, epidemiologists, operations researchers, actuaries and managers, among others. The outcome captures perspectives from all of these disciplines, providing an integrated interdisciplinary view reflecting the richness and complexity of healthcare applications.

Our hope and belief is that this collective effort will prove valuable to those in a wide array of professions which in some way touch upon healthcare. Not only statisticians, but researchers, physicians and administrators will find here statistical applications with detailed examples representing a variety of problems, models and methodologies. Students and practitioners alike will discover opportunities to innovate via the use of statistical methods.

We'd like to acknowledge and thank the many people whose contributions have made this work possible. These include, first and foremost, our esteemed colleagues who have contributed chapters to the work, and the outstanding editorial, production and copy-editing teams at Wiley, who followed up our work together on *The Encyclopedia of Statistics in Quality and Reliability* with another successful outing. And of course, our thanks go especially to our families, for their patience with us while we were preoccupied or otherwise disengaged throughout the duration of this project.

This book includes an accompanying website www.wiley.com/go/statistical_methods_healthcare

# Editors

**Frederick W. Faltin**
Founder and Managing Director
The Faltin Group
25 Casper Drive
Cody, WY 82414, USA

**Ron S. Kenett**
Chairman and CEO, The KPA Group
KPA Ltd, PO Box 2525
Hattaassia Street, 25
Raanana 43100, Israel
and
Research Professor
Università degli Studi di Torino
10134 Turin, Italy

**Fabrizio Ruggeri**
Research Director
CNR IMATI
Via Bassini 15
I-20133 Milano, Italy

# Contributors

**Benjamin M. Adams**
Department of Information Systems
Statistics and Operations Management
University of Alabama
Tuscaloosa, AL
USA

**Zvia Agur**
Optimata Ltd.
Ramat Gan, Israel
and
Institute for Medical Biomathematics
(IMBM)
Bene Ataroth, Israel

**Robert Bauer**
ICON Development Solutions
University Blvd.
Ellicot City, MD
USA

**James C. Benneyan**
Healthcare Systems Engineering Institute
Northeastern University
Boston, MA
USA

**Paola Berchialla**
Department of Public Health and
Microbiology
University of Torino
Turin
Italy

**Annibale Biggeri**
Department of Statistics 'G. Parenti'
University of Florence
Florence, Italy
and
Biostatistics Unit
ISPO Cancer Prevention and Research
Institute
Florence, Italy

**Dolores Catelan**
Department of Statistics 'G. Parenti'
University of Florence
Florence, Italy
and
Biostatistics Unit
ISPO Cancer Prevention and Research
Institute
Florence, Italy

**Shirley Y. Coleman**
Industrial Statistics Research Unit
Newcastle University
Newcastle upon Tyne
UK

**Caterina Conigliani**
Department of Economics
University of Roma Tre
Rome
Italy

**Anja Drescher**
Operations Analytics
Integrated Facilities Management
Jones Lang LaSalle Americas, Inc.
Minnetonka, MN
USA

**Dario Gregori**
Unit of Biostatistics, Epidemiology
and Public Health
Department of Cardiac, Thoracic and
Vascular Sciences
University of Padova
Padua
Italy

**Olivia A. J. Grigg**
CHICAS
School of Health and Medicine
Lancaster University
Lancaster
UK

**Alessandra Guglielmi**
Department of Mathematics
Politecnico di Milano
Milan
Italy

**Serge Guzy**
POPPHARM
Albany, CA
USA

**Francesca Ieva**
Department of Mathematics
Politecnico di Milano
Milan
Italy

**Telba Irony**
General and Surgical Devices Branch
Center for Devices and Radiological Health
US Food and Drug Administration
Silver Spring, MD
USA

**Victoria Jordan**
Office of Performance Improvement
University of Texas MD Anderson Cancer
Center
Houston, TX
USA

**Caiyan Li**
Baxter Healthcare Corporation
Round Lake, IL
USA

**Andrea Manca**
Centre for Health Economics
The University of York, York
UK

**Patrick Musonda**
School of Medicine, Norwich Medical
School
University of East Anglia
Norwich, UK
and
Centre for Infectious Disease Research in
Zambia (CIDRZ)
Lusaka, Zambia

**Eva Negri**
Department of Epidemiology
Istituto di Ricerche Farmacologiche
'Mario Negri'
Milan
Italy

**Daniel P. O'Neill**
Healthcare Solutions
Jones Lang LaSalle Americas, Inc.
Chicago, IL
USA

**Anna Maria Paganoni**
Department of Mathematics
Politecnico di Milano
Milan
Italy

**Melissa Popkoski**
Pharmacy Administrative Services
Horizon Blue Cross Blue Shield of New
Jersey
Newark, NJ
USA

**Allan Sampson**
Department of Statistics
University of Pittsburgh
Pittsburgh, PA
USA

**Anne Shade**
Good Decision Partnership
Ingleneuk, Strathdrynie
Dingwall, Scotland
UK

**Phyllis Silverman**
General and Surgical Devices Branch
Division of Biostatistics
Center for Devices and Radiological Health
US Food and Drug Administration
Silver Spring, MD
USA

**Yafit Stark**
Innovative R&D Division
TEVA Pharmaceutical Industries, Ltd.
Netanya
Israel

**Andrea Tancredi**
Department of Methods and Models for
Economics, Territory and Finance
University of Roma 'La Sapienza'
Rome
Italy

**Rosanna Tarricone**
Department of Policy Analysis and Public
Management
Centre for Research on Health and Social
Care Management – CERGAS
Università Bocconi
Milan
Italy

**Aleksandra Torbica**
Department of Policy Analysis and Public
Management
Centre for Research on Health and Social
Care Management – CERGAS
Università Bocconi
Milan
Italy

**Per Winkel**
The Copenhagen Trial Unit
Centre for Clinical Intervention Research
Rigshospitalet, Copenhagen University
Hospital
Copenhagen
Denmark

**William H. Woodall**
Department of Statistics
Virginia Tech
Blacksburg, VA
USA

**Inbal Yahav**
The Graduate School of Business
Department of Information Systems
Bar Ilan University
Israel

**Shelemyahu Zacks**
Department of Mathematical Sciences
Binghamton University
Binghamton, NY
USA

**Nien Fan Zhang**
Statistical Engineering Division
National Institute of Standards and
Technology
Gaithersburg, MD
USA

# Part One

# STATISTICS IN THE DEVELOPMENT OF PHARMACEUTICAL PRODUCTS

# 1

# Statistical aspects in ICH, FDA and EMA guidelines

## Allan Sampson[1] and Ron S. Kenett[2]

[1]*Department of Statistics, University of Pittsburgh, Pittsburgh, PA, USA*
[2]*KPA Ltd, Raanana, Israel*

## Synopsis

This chapter introduces the regulatory guidelines affecting drug product development and manufacturing that were published by the International Conference on Harmonization of Technical Requirements for Registration of Pharmaceuticals for Human Use (ICH) and other regulatory agencies such as the Food and Drug Administration (FDA) and the European Medicines Authority (EMA). The focus of the chapter is on statistical aspects of these documents, thereby setting the stage for the whole book. These guidelines, collectively, deal with quality, safety and efficacy issues in clinical and pre-clinical research, chemistry, manufacturing and controls (CMC). In essence, they link patient clinical outcomes, drug product critical quality attributes, process parameters and raw material attributes. Establishing the link between patient, product and process is the most important challenge of biopharmaceutical companies and regulatory agencies for ensuring safe, effective and economic healthcare. This challenge is being addressed by the recent Quality by Design (QbD) initiatives of the FDA and ICH, which are also discussed.

## 1.1 Introduction

Healthcare is the treatment and prevention of illness. Healthcare delivery requires both innovators and manufacturers of drug products and medical devices, as well as healthcare providers

*Statistical Methods in Healthcare*, First Edition. Edited by Frederick W. Faltin, Ron S. Kenett and Fabrizio Ruggeri.
© 2012 John Wiley & Sons, Ltd. Published 2012 by John Wiley & Sons, Ltd.

such as hospitals and family medicine. This book, *Statistical Methods in Healthcare*, covers a wide range of activities where statistics impacts on the quality of healthcare, starting with the development of drug products and medical devices, followed by the handling of clinical trials, surveillance and statistical process control of health-related outcomes, economics of healthcare, and healthcare management. The book consists of five parts:

Part One: Statistics in Development of Pharmaceutical Products

Part Two: Statistics in Outcomes Analysis

Part Three: Statistical Process Control in Healthcare

Part Four: Applications to Healthcare Policy and Implementation

Part Five: Applications to Healthcare Management.

This chapter is about the fundamentals in drug development and manufacturing as defined by the regulatory agencies that determine what can be marketed to healthcare consumers. We begin with a general introduction to the organizations that produce such guidelines and regulations.

The pharmaceutical industry became more global in the 1960s and 1970s in parallel with worldwide development of pharmaceutical regulations. Moreover, contemporaneous with these developments, increased societal concerns were voiced for faster development of new biopharmaceutical compounds and for reduction of costs of healthcare and new drug development. One of the perceived roadblocks for expeditiously and efficiently developed new drugs was the fragmentation of pharmaceutical regulations among the United States, Japan and Europe. In the 1980s, the European Community initiated harmonization of European national drug regulations and demonstrated that harmonization of national regulations is possible.

In 1989, under the sponsorship of the United Nations World Health Organization (WHO), a meeting of the International Conference of Drug Regulatory Authorities was held in Paris to plan the harmonization of regulations among Europe, Japan and the USA. In a subsequent 1990 meeting in Brussels, under the auspices of the International Federation of Pharmaceutical Manufacturers and Associations (IFPMA), the steering committee of the International Conference on Harmonization of Technical Requirements for Registration of Pharmaceuticals for Human Use (ICH; http://www.ich.org) was established.

The purpose and terms of reference of the ICH were first declared by the steering committee in 1990, and later revised in 1997and 2000. The terms of reference of the ICH declare its purpose to be (1) to provide a forum for dialogue among industry and regulatory authorities of Europe, Japan and the USA; (2) to contribute to international public health; (3) to monitor and update harmonization documents; (4) to avoid divergent regulations with the development of new therapeutic advances and new technologies; (5) to facilitate adoption of new technologies to safely improve resource utilization; and (6) to foster dissemination and communication about harmonization.

As originally established and currently retained, the steering committee of the ICH consists of two members each from the EU, the European Federation of Pharmaceutical Industries and Associations, the Ministry of Health, Labour and Welfare of Japan, the Japan Pharmaceutical Manufacturers Association, the US Food and Drug Administration (FDA) and the Pharmaceutical Research and Manufacturers of America. The WHO, the European Free Trade Association and Health Canada each contribute one non-voting observer to the Steering Committee. The ICH secretariat, which is housed by the IFPMA, supports the ICH steering committee.

A key decision reached at the first ICH steering committee meeting was to divide the technical topics to be harmonized into three natural groupings: Safety, Quality and Efficacy. A fourth group of Multidisciplinary Topics has since been added. Currently, there are: 9 topics under Safety; 10 topics under Quality; 16 topics under Efficacy; and 5 Multidisciplinary topics. A number of these topics have multiple sub-topics, and several new topics are in their final stages of approval.

The collective impact of these guidelines on the multinational pharmaceutical industry cannot be overstated, particularly in Europe, Japan and the USA. Moreover, any pharmaceutical company that wants to reach these markets needs to pay attention to these guidelines. Individuals working in any aspect of drug development, drug manufacturing or post-marketing monitoring are typically well versed in those guidelines pertinent to their work.

Examples of the guidelines include the Multidisciplinary Guideline M4 and Quality Guideline Q8. Organizations responsible for compiling a new drug application closely follow the format and structure described in M4 concerning the Common Technical Document (CTD). The ICH community recognizes that quality cannot be tested into products and should be built in by design using the information from pharmaceutical development studies as the basis for quality risk management. In that context, the Q8 guideline on 'Pharmaceutical Development' highlights the importance of quality by design (QbD) in pharmaceutical development.

Throughout, statisticians are involved in a variety of drug development, drug manufacturing and healthcare delivery activities. As such, they need to know the statistical aspects of all of those guidelines pertinent to their responsibilities (Peterson et al., 2009a).

This chapter highlights statistical concerns in the four sets of ICH guidelines, and other major regulatory documents with strong statistical focus. The intention is to generate awareness of the breadth and depth of the statistical aspects of these guidelines and not be necessarily fully inclusive.

In addition, we briefly review the guidance documents developed by the FDA and European Medicines Authority (EMA). In general, the FDA and EMA guidance documents are more extensive than the ICH guidelines.

The FDA guidance documents, for example, address some specific statistical concerns not currently covered in the ICH guidelines. For example, the FDA has published a draft guidance on Adaptive Design Clinical Trials for Drugs and Biologics; a topic covered in Chapters 2 and 5 of this book.

However, in addition to these particulars, the FDA has also incorporated the ICH guidelines as guidances. While the role of guidance documents and guidelines in national regulatory policies and procedures is generally overlapping, there are differences among regions. The FDA specifically points out that guidance documents and guidelines 'do not create or confer any rights for or on any person and do not operate to bind FDA or the public'. On the other hand, the Japanese Pharmaceutical Affairs Law includes specifically some of the ICH guidelines (for example, The CTD guideline of M4). The next section provides an overview of the ICH guidelines.

## 1.2   ICH guidelines overview

The list of topics covered by the ICH guidelines is continuously expanding. New topics or revisions of existing documents can be officially proposed by many forums such as scientific societies or ICH regional guideline workshops. Official requests, however, must be channeled through one of the six parties in the steering committee, or by one of the observers on the committee. The next step is the preparation of a short concept paper which may trigger the steering committee to appoint an official Working Group (WG) to proceed with development of the topic. The WG then works to produce a draft guideline with the help of technical experts and the three regions' regulatory authorities (the EMA, the Pharmaceutical and Medical Devices Agency, Japan (JPMDA) and the FDA). The draft is published by the three regulatory authorities for further discussion and broad input. Based on the subsequent regulatory input, the WG then moves to prepare a final document which requires sign off from each of the three regions. With this task completed, the steering committee signs off and thus finalizes the new or revised guideline. Should there be disagreements in any part of this multi-step process, there are established procedures for resolving them.

The four sets of ICH Guidelines cover the development of a new biopharmaceutical product: Quality, Safety, Efficacy and Multidisciplinary. The 10 Quality topics focus on chemical and pharmaceutical quality assurance. The 9 Safety topics relate to *in vitro* and *in vivo* pre-clinical studies, and the 16 Efficacy topics concern clinical studies in human subjects. The Multidisciplinary topics deal with five issues that do not fall clearly into one of the other three sets of topics. Chapters 2–5 in this book provide in-depth studies of statistical and modeling aspects in pre-clinical and clinical research in the spirit of these guidelines.

The Quality guidelines, designated Q1, . . . , Q10 are, respectively: (1) stability; (2) analytic validation; (3) impurities; (4) pharmacopoeias; (5) biotechnology quality; (6) specifications; (7) Good Manufacturing Practice (GMP); (8) pharmaceutical development; (9) quality risk management; and (10) pharmaceutical quality systems.

A number of the quality guidelines are multi-part; for example, Q1 has six sub-guidelines. These guidelines and details of their statistical content are discussed in Section 1.4 of this chapter. Due to their impact, the three guidelines Q8, Q9 and Q10 are our primary focus. Guideline Q8 encourages new drug applications to include a design space and risk-based control strategies. The basic idea of Q8 is that drug product developers should study the behavior of critical quality parameters with an impact on critical quality attributes (CQAs) and determine a control strategy in their proposed new products, under variations in the raw material and process control parameters.

The Safety Guidelines, designated S1, . . . , S9 are, respectively: (1) carcinogenicity studies; (2) genotoxicity studies; (3) toxicokinetics and pharmacokinetics; (4) toxicity testing; (5) reproductive toxicology; (6) biotechnological products; (7) pharmacology studies; and (8) immunotoxicology studies. Topics (1) through (7) correspond to S1 through S7, while topic (8) consists of S8 and S9.

These guidelines are not discussed further in this chapter, and the reader is referred to the ICH website for more details.

The sixteen Efficacy guidelines, designated, E1, . . . , E16 are grouped into sets of related topics. Namely: clinical safety; clinical study reports; dose-response studies; ethnic factors; Good Clinical Practice (GCP); clinical trials; clinical evaluation by therapeutic category; clinical evaluation; and pharmacogenomics. Within some of these groupings there is a single guideline; while in others, there can be as many as four guidelines, and again some of the individual guidelines may be multi-part. For example, Q2 has six sub-topics, one of which has undergone two revisions. Section 1.3 of this chapter delves into the statistical details of many of the Efficacy guidelines.

In addition to these specific ICH guidelines, a substantial literature has developed offering commentary on many of the individual guidelines. As appropriate, some of this literature is noted in this chapter.

The ICH Guidelines are all available on the web at http://www.ich.org/products/guidelines.html, and as such are not individually cited in this chapter.

## 1.3 ICH guidelines for determining efficacy

The efficacy guidelines that are most focused on statistical issues are E9 and E10. The remaining guidelines deal with various statistical concerns, from suggested designs and inference requirements to statistical reporting.

Guideline E1, entitled 'Extent of Population Exposure to Assess Clinical Safety for Drugs Intended for Long-term Treatment of Non-life Threatening Conditions', as its title indicates, discusses the rationale for sample sizes for various studies to characterize adverse drug experience (ADE) rates both in the short term (less than six months from treatment start) and in the longer term. The long-term concern in the guideline is defined to be chronic or repeated intermittent use for longer than six months. Short-term (three to six months) ADE rates of 1% or more are expected to be 'well characterized'; while rates of 0.1% or less are 'not expected' to be characterized. There is a need to examine the time-varying nature of these short-term rates, and E1 notes that 'usually 300–600 patients should be adequate'. This sample size is also adequate for detecting ADEs in the range of 0.5 to 5.0% that occur following short-term delays. In addition, to guard against ADEs that occur after six months, there is a requirement that at least 100 patients be treated and studied for at least one year.

Guideline E1 notes that, with no occurrences of a serious ADE in one year and based on 100 treated patients, there is 'reasonable' assurance that the true incidence is less than 3%. Direct calculation shows that a one-sided exact 95% confidence interval for the probability of a specific serious ADE is less than 0.03 when no events are observed among 100 patients. Overall, E1 expects that at least 1500 patients will be needed during drug development to adequately characterize the ADE concerns.

There are six guidelines that comprise the E2 series, designated E2A, . . . , E2F. They deal with safety issues for drugs under development, as well as for marketed drugs. Guidelines E2A and E2D deal respectively with pre- and post-approval expedited reporting of adverse events and adverse drug reactions; while E2C and E2F deal with pre- and post-approval periodic safety update reports. Electronic formatting issues are discussed in E2B, and requirements for pharmacovigilance planning are discussed in E2E.

The pharmacovigilance planning is designed to aid sponsors in developing post-marketing safety surveillance plans that could be submitted with a new drug license application (NDA). At a minimum, the plan should describe the routine pharmacovigilance that is conducted for all products, with attention to the regional requirements. In terms of product-specific plans, E2E describes a variety of methods in an attached annex. These methods include designs for passive surveillance, stimulated reporting, active surveillance, comparative observational studies, targeted clinical evaluations and descriptive studies. Collectively these methodologies provide a wide range of approaches to monitor the safety of a new compound after approval, and the pharmacovigilance plan included in the NDA is an integral part of the regulatory review process.

Guideline E3, entitled 'Structure and Content of Clinical Study Reports', is a highly detailed guideline. While the context of this guideline is broad, there are several subsections of the report focused on statistics. Section 9.7 of E3 details with planned statistical analyses and justification of the study's sample size, and Section 9.8 addresses changes to the planned analyses that occurred during the study. Interestingly, E3's Section 11.4.2 of the efficacy results presents analytic features that are important for the regulatory statistical review; namely, adjustments for covariates, handling of dropouts and missing data, interim analyses, multiplicity issues and subgroup issues. Annexes III and IV of E3 provide useful approaches to schematically depict study designs and patient disposition.

Guideline E4, entitled 'Dose-Response Information to Support Drug Registration', is a relative short document focusing on the importance of obtaining dose-response information based on the totality of studies comprising the licensing application. Other than presenting several designs, there are few specifics on data analysis. In some sense the most compelling statistical statement is that, beyond the individual study analyses, 'the entire database should be examined intensively for possible dose-response effects'. This suggests that, when a sponsor prepares a clinical plan, there should be focused statistical consideration about how the studies' data will ultimately be integrated to provide accurate dose-response estimates for both efficacy and safety. Moreover, in light of the perceived high failure rate of Phase III trials (Kola and Landis, 2004), planned cumulative integration of dose-response data during drug development may be a helpful tool to improve this situation. Chapters 3 and 4 deal with phenomenological and physiological modeling, and cover dose-response modeling issues. These chapters cover the relatively new domain of pharmacometrics and fundamental biomathematical systems that combine disease progression models with toxicity, pharmacodynamics and pharmacokinetics to determine optimal treatment regimens and uncover mechanisms of action of the drug compound under investigation.

One of the more conceptually challenging guidelines is E5, entitled 'Ethnic Factors in the Acceptability of Foreign Clinical Data'. This guideline's purpose is to facilitate the use of 'foreign' clinical data obtained in one ICH region to gain approval for the study compound in another ICH region where there are differences between regions in characteristics such as genetics, physiology, culture or environment, which E5 terms collectively 'ethnic factors'. A bridging data package consists of the relevant information from the approved package and the necessary bridging studies to allow extrapolation to the new region. The guideline suggests a spectrum of ethnic factors ranging from intrinsic (e.g., genetics, gender) to extrinsic (e.g., medical practice, socioeconomic factors, climate), with a range of factors in between. There are general suggestions about the kinds of bridging studies that might be used depending on the study compound's class and sensitivity to ethnic factors and the kind of ethnic differences between the two ICH regions. There are circumstances where no bridging studies seem to be required. In other cases a pharmacodynamic study or dose-response study is required, and in still other cases a new, controlled clinical trial is required.

The need arising from E5 for statistical development is indicated by phrasing such as 'if the bridging study shows that the dose response, safety and efficacy in the new region are similar, then the study ... is capable of "bridging" the foreign data'. Little is explicitly said about what constitutes similar or equivalent evidence. From a statistical viewpoint, the question arises about how methodology that was developed in other settings to handle equivalence and non-inferiority studies might apply in this context.

The implementation of E5 has raised questions, and the ICH subsequently issued a supplement to E5 entitled 'Ethnic Factors in the Acceptability of Foreign Clinical Data: Questions and Answers'. There have been a number of statistical and design papers written focusing on various aspects of E5; for example, Uyama *et al.* (2005) or Tsou *et al.* (2010), as well as a series of four papers by varying authors in an issue of the *Journal of Biopharmaceutical Statistics* (2002).

Good Clinical Practices are documented in E6 and, as such, have little direct involvement with statistical concerns. The primary sections of this guideline deal with practices for Institutional Review Boards (also called Helsinki Committees), for investigators and for sponsors. Also considered are the structures of the clinical trial protocol and the Investigator's Brochure.

Guidelines for studies in special populations are considered in E7 and in E11. The former deals with geriatric populations and the latter with pediatric populations. Guideline E7 suggests that for compounds prescribed, but not uniquely, to the elderly, a minimum of 100 geriatric patients suffices, and for compounds which are for diseases uncommon in geriatric populations, smaller numbers are sufficient. Clearly for compounds intended for a primarily geriatric population, these patients should be a major portion of the data. Specific studies, such as pharmacokinetic or dose response, can explicitly model the effects of age; while, more broadly, for most compounds the entire clinical database should be examined for age-related effects.

Guideline E11 points out the importance of there being more products available for pediatric populations, and at the same time indicates many of the issues and difficulties in conducting studies in this population. Clearly this is a dynamic population, with substantial physiological, cognitive and developmental differences between the preterm and term newborns and adolescents. Pharmacodynamic and pharmacokinetic studies need to account for age and physiology (e.g., weight) and, if efficacy studies are needed, the sponsor may need to develop and validate endpoint measurements appropriate to the patients' cognitive development. Overlaying all the usual safety concerns, is the concern that the compound might affect growth and development, which may not be seen until a later age in the patient. (For more on this topic see Chapter 3.)

The ICH guideline E8, 'General Considerations for Clinical Trials', is a well-written overview document providing the principles for clinical trials and, more broadly, clinical development plans. While the design and statistical principles described in this guideline are ones many statisticians are aware of, the document as a whole makes excellent reading for a clinician designing a clinical trial or program.

For statisticians, the ICH Efficacy guideline with the most direct impact is E9, 'Statistical Principles for Clinical Trials', completed in 1998. The breadth of topics and the soundness of the material encompass much of what a clinical trials statistician faces in developing new drugs. Moreover, the principles considered are equally applicable to many types of clinical trials beyond those in the biopharmaceutical industry.

The introductory material of E9 (section I) espouses two important principles: one being that all trial statistical work is the responsibility of 'an appropriately qualified and experienced statistician', and the other being how important it is 'to evaluate the robustness of the results' in light of their 'sensitivity ... to various limitations of data assumptions'. This lengthy guideline divides the more technical considerations into five major components: overall clinical development, trial design, trial conduct, data analysis, and safety and tolerability. Due to the extensive nature of the material we can only highlight in this chapter select ideas.

The considerations for clinical development section (II) of E9 focuses on the overall plan, clinical trial purposes, issues concerning and types of response variables, and blinding and randomization. There is a rather complete discussion of the different aspects of handling multiple primary variables when a suitable composite variable cannot be constructed based on them. Guideline E9 notes that 'it should be clear whether an impact on any of the variables, some minimum number of them, or all of them would be necessary', and describes the handling of type I error in each case. Regarding randomization, dynamic allocation of patients to treatments is discussed with the warning that 'the complexity of the logistics and the potential impact should be carefully evaluated when considering dynamic allocation'. The trial designs section (III) of E9, after considering various trial types, discusses fairly comprehensively how to model and analyze multicentre trials. It describes the value of having centers with comparably balanced numbers of patients and also indicates that treatment effect can be obtained from a model without a treatment-by-centre interaction. However, the homogeneity of treatment effect must be examined through, for example, graphical or analytic methods, and, if it is found, the possible causes carefully explained. Equivalence trials and non-inferiority trials are covered, but more complete discussion of many of the statistical issues for these can be found in two later EMA (2000, 2004) Points to Consider documents. The issues concerning switching non-inferiority and superiority objectives in the same trial are not discussed in E9, but in EMA (2000).

The trial conduct section (IV) of E9 considers issues concerning the monitoring of ongoing clinical trials. It basically dichotomizes the types of monitoring that might be considered into those which use only the blinded data and those which use suitably unblinded data. Blinded monitoring may involve modifying the inclusion/exclusion criteria in response to external information or in response to ongoing study results such as accrual rates. Other types of blinded monitoring can lead to adjusting an ongoing trial's sample size based on estimates of a response variance or overall survival rate. As pointed out by E9, blinded adjusted sample size procedures should be documented in the protocol or in an amendment, including a description of what effects there might be on type I error. Unblinded monitoring focuses primarily on group sequential designs, and E9 does not discuss the more recently developed adaptive designs based on unblinded data. The cautions that E9 presents for using group sequential designs equally apply to adaptive designs. The trial conduct section concludes with a discussion of the role of Independent Data Monitoring Committees (IDMCs). Throughout this section is the theme of the importance of preserving the trial's integrity with suitable protection in place if unblinded data are examined during the trial.

Section V of E9 is focused on data analysis and can be seen as a highly abbreviated text of statistical methods for analyzing clinical trials, and only a few of its features are highlighted here. Guideline E9 notes that the main analysis details should be in the study protocol, while the more complete statistical analysis plan may be a separate document (that needs to be completed before the blind is broken). The intention-to-treat and per-protocol analysis sets are discussed and their relative uses compared. Missing data considerations are given with the conclusion that 'unfortunately, no universally applicable methods of handling missing values can be recommended'. Standard advice is given concerning the careful specification of the primary efficacy variable(s) and the corresponding primary analytic model for them. There is also a short discussion of handling covariates, subgroups and interactions.

In E9, section VI deals with evaluation of safety and tolerability and section VII with reporting. The safety population is usually considered as those who received one dose of a trial compound, and there is the strong recommendation that safety data be collected consistently across all the trials in a clinical program, so as to facilitate an integrated summary of safety and tolerability. In many cases, it is suggested that descriptive statistics and graphics suffice to analyze safety where $p$-values and confidence intervals for 'flagging' and aiding interpretation are used as needed. The reporting section of E9 is intrinsically a shortened version of E3 which describes in detail the clinical report.

The ICH E10 is an intriguing and extensive guideline entitled 'Choice of Control Group in Clinical Trials'. It discusses a broad array of designs for clinical trials with an emphasis on the control group(s) in a trial. Guideline E10 classifies trials by five types of control groups: placebo, no-treatment concurrent control, dose-response concurrent control, active control and external control (which includes historical controls). Within each category, there is a detailed presentation of their uses, advantages and disadvantages, ethics, and variations of the designs in that category. For example, in the presentation of the modifications of placebo controls, there are discussions of add-on designs, 'early escape' designs, limited placebo period designs, and randomized withdrawal designs. Guideline E10 also provides two schematics; one indicating design types based upon trial objectives and the other being a flowchart which helps in choosing the concurrent control. While the designs are well described, little is given about methods for analyzing the various designs (for more on this topic see Chapter 2).

The more recent ICH Efficacy documents deal with specific therapeutic classes and modern topics arising from genetic considerations. Document E12 is termed 'Principles for Clinical Evaluation of New Antihypertensive Drugs' and E14 is entitled 'The Clinical Evaluation of QT/QTc Interval Prolongation and Proarrhythmic Potential for Non-Antiarrhythmic Drugs'. Guidelines E15 and E16 are entitled, respectively, 'Definitions for Genomic Biomarkers, Pharmacogenomics, Pharmacogenetics, Genomic Data and Sample Coding Categories' and 'Biomarkers Related to Drug or Biotechnology Product Development: Context, Structure and Format of Qualification Submissions'. Interestingly, the ICH considers E12 a principle document rather than a guideline.

## 1.4   ICH quality guidelines

The ICH Quality guidelines concern designing and ensuring manufacture and delivery of quality drug products. While Q1–Q7 have impact, we focus on the three quality guidelines which are of substantial impact to the healthcare industry – Q8(R2) Pharmaceutical Development, Q9 Quality Risk Management and Q10 Pharmaceutical Quality System – and a concept paper, Q11 Development and Manufacture of Drug Substances.

The key concept behind these three guidelines is that quality of drug products is determined by their underlying design, development, manufacturing and supply processes. Crucially Q8 notes that 'it is important to recognize that quality cannot be tested into products; that is, quality should be built in by design'. A process is well understood when all critical sources of variability are identified and explained, variability is proactively managed by the process, and product quality attributes can be accurately and reliably predicted over the space of design parameters.

Processes must meet current good manufacturing practices to ensure that drug products meet safety and efficacy requirements. In the past, this requirement has been met by performing process validation studies on three batches; however, the ICH Quality guidelines recognize that this approach is unlikely to fully represent routine manufacturing and therefore unlikely to cover all potential sources of variability (e.g., raw materials, operators, shifts, reactor vessels). In addition, the FDA has identified this issue as a challenge to the regulatory process and described the traditional approach as a 'focus on process validation and not process understanding' (Nasr, 2007). Quality by Design is about changing this approach (Kenett and Kenett, 2008).

Quality by Design (QbD) is a systematic approach to development that begins with predefined objectives, that emphasizes product and process understanding and sets up process control based on sound science and quality risk management. In the traditional approach, product quality and performance is achieved by restricting flexibility in the manufacturing process and by end product testing. Under the QbD paradigm, pharmaceutical quality is assured by understanding and controlling manufacturing and formulation variables. End product testing is used to confirm the quality of the product and is not considered part of the ongoing consistency assurance and/or process control (Yu, 2008). A key element in the QbD paradigm is the design space. A design space is defined by Q8 as 'the multidimensional combination and interaction of input variables (e.g., material attributes) and process parameters that have been demonstrated to provide assurance of quality'. Q8 further notes that: 'Working within the design space is not considered as a change. Movement out of the design space is considered to be a change and would normally initiate a regulatory post-approval change process. Design space is proposed by the applicant and is subject to regulatory assessment and approval'.

The determination of a design space requires a combination of experimental data and mechanistic knowledge of chemistry, physics and engineering to model and predict performance. Statistical design of experiments (DOE) is used for setting up a design space. DOE is an efficient method used in industrial statistics for determining impact of multiple parameters and their interactions (Kenett and Zacks, 1998). Setting up a design space also involves scaling up studies to translate operating conditions between different scales or pieces of equipment.

Statistical analysis in product development includes model building. This consists of kinetic models such as rates of reaction or degradation, transport models of movement and mixing of mass or heat, models for manufacturing development including computational fluid dynamics, scale-up correlations and models for process monitoring or control such as chemometric models and control models. Chemometrics is the science of relating measurements made on a chemical system or process to the state of the system via application of mathematical or statistical methods. Measurements are integrated in a process control strategy that involves modeling, multivariate analysis and Statistical Process Control (Kenett and Zacks, 1998; Fuchs and Kenett, 1998). All such models require verification through statistical analysis.

The following provides more details concerning the ICH Q8, Q9 and Q10 Quality guidelines.

Guideline Q8, entitled Pharmaceutical Development, has been revised twice up to August 2009. The guideline describes the suggested contents for the 3.2.P.2 (Pharmaceutical Development) section of a regulatory submission in the ICH M4 CTD format. This section is first produced for the original marketing application and can be updated to support new knowledge gained over the lifecycle of a product. The pharmaceutical development section is intended to provide a comprehensive understanding of the product and manufacturing process for reviewers and inspectors. The guideline also indicates areas where the demonstration of greater understanding of pharmaceutical and manufacturing sciences can create a basis for flexible regulatory approaches. The degree of regulatory flexibility is predicated on the level of relevant scientific knowledge provided.

The Q8 guideline does not apply to contents of submissions for drug products during the clinical research stages of drug development. However, the principles in this guideline are important to consider during those stages as well.

Changes in formulation and manufacturing processes during development and lifecycle management should be looked upon as opportunities to gain additional knowledge and further support the establishment of the design space. Similarly, inclusion of relevant knowledge gained from experiments giving unexpected results can also be useful.

Guideline Q8 notes that 'At a minimum, those aspects of drug substances, excipients, container closure systems, and manufacturing processes that are critical to product quality should be determined and control strategies justified. Critical formulation attributes and process parameters are generally identified through an assessment of the extent to which their variation can have impact on the quality of the drug product.'

The elements of pharmaceutical development consist of a quality target product profile (QTPP), critical quality attributes (CQAs), a risk assessment linking material attributes and critical process parameters (CPPs) to drug product CQAs, a design Space and a control Strategy. The definitions of these terms are given in Q8 as follows. *QTPP*: 'A prospective summary of the quality characteristics of a drug product that ideally will be achieved to ensure the desired quality, taking into account safety and efficacy of the drug product.'; *CQA*: 'A physical, chemical, biological or microbiological property or characteristic that should be within an appropriate limit, range, or distribution to ensure the desired product quality'; and *CPP*: 'A process parameter whose variability has an impact on a critical quality attribute and therefore should be monitored or controlled to ensure the process produces the desired quality'.

Document Q9, entitled Quality Risk Management, is designed to offer a systematic approach to quality risk management. It serves as a foundation or resource document that is independent of, yet supports, other ICH Quality documents, and complements existing quality practices, requirements, standards and guidelines within the pharmaceutical industry and regulatory environment. Quality risk management is a systematic process for the assessment, control, communication and review of risks to the quality of the drug (medicinal) product across the product lifecycle. The basic activities concerning risk management include: *risk assessment*, which consists of the identification of hazards and the analysis and evaluation of risks associated with exposure to those hazards; *risk identification*, which is a systematic use of information to identify hazards referring to the risk question or problem description (information can include historical data, theoretical analysis, informed opinions and the concerns of stakeholders; *risk analysis*, which is the estimation of the risk associated with the identified hazards (it is the qualitative or quantitative process of linking the likelihood of occurrence and severity of harms); *risk evaluation*, which compares the identified and analyzed risk against given risk criteria; *risk control*, which includes decision making to reduce and/or accept risks (the purpose of risk control is to reduce the risk to an acceptable level); and *risk communication*, which is the sharing of information about risk and risk management between the decision makers and others. (See Chapter 6 in this book and Kenett and Raanan, 2010.)

Document Q10, entitled Pharmaceutical Quality System, is a comprehensive model for an effective pharmaceutical quality system that is based on International Organization for Standardization (ISO) quality concepts, includes applicable GMP regulations, and complements Q8 and Q9. The ICH Q10 is a model for a pharmaceutical quality system that can be implemented throughout the different stages of a product lifecycle.

The Q10 guideline promotes a lifecycle approach to product quality by focusing on four elements: (1) process performance and product quality monitoring system; (2) corrective action and preventive action (CAPA) system; (3) change management system; and (4) management review of process performance and product quality.

Specifically, CAPA methodology should result in product and process improvements and enhanced product and process understanding. It applies to pharmaceutical development, technology transfer, commercial manufacturing and product discontinuation. Management review should provide assurance that process performance and product quality are managed over the lifecycle. Depending on the size and complexity of the company, management review can be a series of reviews at various levels of management and should include a timely and effective communication and escalation process to raise appropriate quality issues to senior levels of management for review. The management review system should include: (1) the results of regulatory inspections and findings, audits and other assessments, and commitments made to regulatory authorities; (2) periodic quality reviews (that can include (i) measures of customer satisfaction such as product quality complaints and recalls; (ii) conclusions of process performance and product quality monitoring; and (iii)the effectiveness of process and product changes including those arising from corrective action and preventive actions); (3) any follow-up actions from previous management reviews.

The management review system should identify appropriate actions, such as: (1) improvements to manufacturing processes and products; (2) provision, training and/or realignment of resources; and (3) capture and dissemination of knowledge.

The ICH, in the Q8, Q9 and Q10 guidelines, as well as the FDA, have been strongly promoting QbD in an attempt to curb rising development costs and regulatory barriers to innovation and creativity (FDA, 2006). The introduction of QbD offers to statisticians a level of involvement beyond the traditional role of statisticians in clinical trials (Nasr, 2007, 2009; Kenett and Kenett, 2008; Peterson et al., 2009a). Moreover, QbD will certainly have an impact on modern statistical methodology, bringing forth new and challenging problems that require new statistical methodologies. It is patently clear that, in addition to the key roles that statisticians play in drug discovery and development, abundant opportunities exist for statistical involvement in QbD. With QbD, statisticians can now play a key role throughout the life cycle of drug products. These opportunities are expanded upon in Section 1.6.

## 1.5   Other guidelines

The preceding sections have primarily focused on the ICH Guidelines and in particular their statistical impact and challenges. However, there is an abundance of other guidelines and documents produced by each of the three regulatory regions that deal with design or analysis issues of biopharmaceutical trials, as well as related manufacturing issues. Due to the extent of these guidelines, we only highlight a small fraction of them in this document.

The EMA has published a large number of scientific guidelines categorized in six groupings: quality, biologics, non-clinical, clinical efficacy and safety, multidisciplinary and ICH. To gage a sense of their extensiveness, we note that within the quality topics, there are 11 sub-topics and, for example, in the sub-topic about manufacturing, there are 6 adopted guidelines including process validation, a 2010 concept paper on revisions of process validation, and manufacture of the finished dosage form. Within clinical efficacy, there are 16 sub-topics with multiple guidelines within each of these and all mainly focused on treating specific medical conditions. In addition the EMA has published a number of concept papers in a series called 'Points to Consider'; some of which have later become EMA CHMP (Committee for Medicinal Products for Human Use) Guidelines. Among those of interest to statisticians are 'Points to Consider on Missing Data' (EMA, 2001), which in 2009 has been revised as a draft 'Guideline on Missing Data in Confirmatory Trials' (EMA, 2009); 'Guideline on the Choice of Non-inferiority Margin' (EMA, 2005; an earlier draft document on this topic is 'Points to Consider', EMA, 2004); 'Points to Consider on Applications with 1. Meta-analyses, 2. One Pivotal Study' (EMA, 2001); 'Points to Consider on Switching between Superiority and Non-inferiority' (EMA, 2000); 'Points to Consider on Multiplicity Issues in Clinical Trials' (EMA, 2002); 'Points to Consider on Adjustment for Baseline Covariates' (EMA, 2003); and 'Concept Paper on the Need for a Guideline on the Use of Subgroup Analyses in Randomized Controlled Trials' (EMA, 2010). While the primary EMA statistical documents are highlighted in the preceding, the many other documents in the 'Points to Consider' series and the 'Guideline' series, while focusing on other topics, do contain relevant statistical material. Collectively all these many documents are an excellent resource for those working in quality and efficacy aspects of biopharmaceutical development, although obviously with a focus on EU concerns.

The EMA document on missing data (EMA, 2009) has an extensive review of the possible biases and effects that can be caused by ignoring or not properly taking into account missing data. While not espousing any universal approaches, it does provide rules that 'should be considered' in dealing with missing data. For example, mortality results should have relatively low missingness, but it recognizes that long-term studies in a psychiatric population may have relatively higher amounts of missing data. Methods for handling missing data need to be pre-specified and well documented in the final report. There is a full discussion of various ways to handle missing data based on modeling an understanding of the missing causes, as well as a discussion of multiple imputation and mixed models as approaches. The document concludes with a discussion of sensitivity analyses to assure that the results of the trial are not sensitive to a specific missing data approach. The EMA document on meta-analysis and one pivotal study (EMA, 2001) is really two documents in one with loose connections between the topics. The meta-analysis component discusses the issues about performing a meta-analysis on the studies included in an NDA. The reasons for doing such an analysis can be varied and include, for example, subgroup analyses or evaluating apparently conflicting study results. The document indicates that the meta-analysis should follow a detailed pre-specified protocol completed before any trial results are known; ideally prepared when developing the clinical development program. In those infrequent cases where the meta-analysis is not anticipated, but is carried out to integrate results from conflicting study results, the document addresses how to try to maintain credibility of the meta-analysis.

The FDA has a series of 'Guidances' that represent the FDA's current thinking on a topic. The list of guidance documents is extremely lengthy, with 30 subgroups, again with each subgroup consisting of multiple finalized and draft guidance documents. Three subgroups that directly deal with quality are 'Current Good Manufacturing Practices (CGMPs)/Compliance', 'CMC' (Chemistry, Manufacturing, and Control), and 'CMC – Microbiology'. The guidance on Process Validation: General Principles and Practices (FDA, 2011) outlines the general principles and approaches that FDA considers appropriate elements of process validation for the manufacture of human and animal drug and biological products, including active pharmaceutical ingredients. It incorporates principles and approaches that all manufacturers can use to validate manufacturing processes. Process validation is defined as the collection and evaluation of data, from the process design stage through commercial production, which establishes scientific evidence that a process is capable of consistently delivering quality product. In this context, manufacturers should (1) understand the sources of variation, (2) detect the presence and degree of variation, (3) understand the impact of variation on the process and ultimately on product attributes, and (4) control the variation in a manner commensurate with the risk it represents to the process and product.

Guidances of substantial statistical interest concerning drug development can be found under a variety of topics. Illustrative of these guidance documents are 'Statistical Approaches to Establishing Bioequivalence' (FDA, 2001); 'Exposure-Response Relationships – Study Design, Data Analysis, and Implications for Dosing and Labeling' (FDA, 2003); 'Non-Inferiority Clinical Trials' (FDA, 2010a); and 'Adaptive Design Clinical Trials for Drugs and Biologics' (FDA, 2010b), where the last two are both in draft form.

The FDA draft guidance document concerning non-inferiority clinical trials is pertinent to such trials under the purvey of either the Center for Drug Evaluation and Research (CDER) or the Center for Biologic Evaluation and Research (CBER). This guidance begins with a general discussion of issues concerning non-inferiority trials, and then follows this section with a more detailed discussion of methodology to establish a non-inferiority margin and a comparison of methods, and ends with a section considering practical advice and an appendix providing examples of successful and unsuccessful non-inferiority trials. The first two sections provide a clear conceptual introduction to the rationale of non-inferiority designs, possible designs and methods, and approaches to obtain $M_2$, the largest clinically acceptable difference. Five interesting examples of non-inferiority trials drawn from public sources are given in the appendix.

The adaptive designs FDA draft guidance document is a major document discussing the important issues facing sponsors who are considering adaptive clinical trials to expedite drug development. Adaptive trials allow the change of the design of a clinical trial at interim points in the trial based on accumulating trials data, and are viewed as 'learning' as the trials proceeds. (For a general framework for sample size adaptive designs see Koyama, Sampson and Gleser, 2005a, and for adaptive designs in non-inferiority trials see Koyama, Sampson and Gleser, 2005b). There is a statistical cost for this trial-based gain in knowledge, and this FDA document requires characterizing this cost in a regulatory acceptable way. Besides providing general background and concerns about adaptive designs, the guidance dichotomizes adaptive designs into the two groups 'generally well-understood adaptive designs' and 'adaptive designs whose properties are less well understood'. Examples of the former are designs based on blinded interim analyses and, of the later, designs based on unblinded interim effect size estimates. For the well-understood designs there are valid implementation approaches, and for the less well-understood designs, this draft guidance discusses some relevant statistical considerations. Also discussed are the contents of an adaptive design protocol, as well as an indication of the interactions between a sponsor and the FDA when a sponsor is planning an adaptive design.

The Pharmaceuticals and Medical Devices Agency (PMDA) of Japan has some limited guidance documents in English, especially in terms of manufacturing and quality issues. The most relevant of these are 'Guideline for Descriptions on Application Forms for Marketing Approval of Drugs' (PFSB, 2007), which indicates the manufacturing method details to be included on marketing approval applications, and 'Ministerial Ordinance on Standards for Manufacturing Control and Quality Control for Drugs and Quasi-drugs' (MHLW, 2004).

Other than the ICH Guidelines there are very limited indications about statistical issues in any of the other guidance-type documents.

## 1.6    Statistical challenges in drug products development and manufacturing

This section highlights some key statistical challenges in the modern pharmaceutical industry. Context to these challenges is provided by the 2004 FDA Report 'Innovation or Stagnation: Challenge and Opportunity on the Critical Path to New Medical Products' (FDA, 2004). This report addresses in a clear way the challenges in overcoming the gap between scientific discoveries and their translation into modern medical treatments and also the opportunities to those involved with product development and manufacturing in transforming these processes to overcome this gap. Following the publication of this groundbreaking report, the FDA in 2006 issued a report entitled 'Critical Path Opportunities List'. The report lists specific examples where there are opportunities for innovation in the sciences and technology of product development. Some of the areas where the challenges clearly relate to statistics are in 'streamlining clinical trials', 'harvesting bioinformatics' and 'moving manufacturing into the 21st century'. Illustrative of these areas of statistical opportunities are furthering innovative trial designs concerning which the report focuses on active controlled trials, enrichment designs, integrating prior evidence for designs, adaptive designs, handling missing data, and dealing with multiple endpoints.

The challenges concerning manufacturing described in the 'Critical Path Opportunities List' report are grouped into manufacturing biologics, manufacturing devices, manufacturing drugs and dealing with nanotechnologies.

In 2008 the FDA issued an additional report addressing safety monitoring; in particular, monitoring the safety of a product throughout its entire life cycle. The report entitled 'The Sentinel Initiative: A National Strategy for Monitoring Medical Product Safety' (FDA, 2008) addresses a breadth of concepts focusing on using modern information technology to identify, in a timely fashion, previously unknown risks of medical products, learn about their patterns of use, and assess the outcomes associated with them. The report discusses FDA activities in the context of risk identification, risk assessment and risk minimization. While statistical opportunities in this initiative are not overtly discussed, there are clearly opportunities for innovative statistical methods to detect and describe safety issues in a timely fashion.

Others, outside the regulatory arena, have also identified the challenges for statisticians. For instance, Peterson et al. (2009b) identified a number of factors that are converging to increase the need for sophisticated, statistics-driven approaches to quality and process understanding in the pharmaceutical industry. These include the following.

1. **Regulatory trends:** as clearly described in this chapter, a substantial driver is regulatory agencies that require new, more statistically rigorous and risk-based ways of conducting drug development and manufacturing.

2. **Inherent characteristics of pharmaceutical manufacturing:** in pharmaceuticals it is difficult to tightly connect product specifications to product performance. For example, 'tablet dissolution' rates cannot be clearly linked to drug efficacy and safety over a vast array of potential product users, each with different body size, age, lifestyle, genetics

and drug metabolism chemistries. Furthermore, pharmaceutical companies must maintain quality in a many-step production process that creates a complex molecule that must have the proper molecular structure and be free of serious chemical impurities or biological contaminants. In addition, up to now, there has been a lack of incentive for continuous improvement in pharmaceutical manufacturing after regulatory approval. This is due primarily to the fact that substantial changes in the manufacturing process or recipe required formal regulatory approval. Recently, QbD guidance has been introduced to provide more flexibility with regard to continuous improvement in manufacturing. However, pharmaceutical manufacturers will have to show clear process understanding and prediction ability in order to be granted such flexibility. To meet all these complex challenges, pharmaceutical companies need more, not less, statistical thinking and practice.

3. **Economic pressures:** many companies, faced with thin product pipelines, major patent expirations and downward pressure on pricing, attempt to cut their manufacturing costs, improve yield and productivity, and generate bottom-line savings that can be used to drive growth and innovation. Statistically driven improvement methodologies found in QbD are critical for success in these efforts. The same economic pressures drive the need for more efficient and adaptive designs, better ways of integrating and accumulating product performance during development, and innovative use of simulation and computer modeling.

4. **Increased need for effective technology transfer:** virtually every drug at some stage of its development or manufacture must be transferred from one site to another. Furthermore, mergers, acquisitions, the rise of 'global' generics, the ongoing rationalization of manufacturing and other factors have increased the frequency with which pharmaceutical manufacturing organizations must effectively and efficiently transfer products and manufacturing processes from one location to another. Successful transfer requires a degree of understanding of products and processes that can be greatly improved by statistical techniques.

The effects of multinationalism are also seen in the need for innovations in designing and analyzing multinational clinical trials, as well as developing the designs and statistical methods for bridging studies (as elaborated upon in ICH E5) in order to gain approval of a product in a new region based upon approvals in another region.

Peterson *et al.* (2009a) further note that 'As these trends continue and converge, the role of statistics and statisticians will only grow larger in the industry.'

## 1.7   Summary

This chapter reviewed guidelines and guidance documents regarding safety, efficacy and quality of drug products. These guidelines directly affect drug development, clinical research and drug product manufacturing. The Quality by Design initiative is providing an integrated view linking patients, products and processes in order to achieve safety, efficacy and quality in an economic way.

Section 1.3 described in detail the ICH guidelines concerning efficacy. These guidelines, adopted by the three major regulatory regions, directly impact how biopharmaceutical clinical development is conducted. From a statistician's perspective, E9, 'Statistical Principles for Clinical Trials' provides a clear discussion of the statistical principles and methods for designing and analyzing pharmaceutical clinical trials. Since its completion in 1998, new analytical issues have arisen for clinical trials that present further challenges to regulators and statisticians. Some of these challenges were highlighted in Section 1.5.

In Section 1.4 we mentioned that a design space of a drug product is the multidimensional combination and interaction of input variables (e.g., material attributes) and process parameters that have been demonstrated to provide assurance of quality. Including a design space in a new drug application is a key element of the Quality by Design initiative. Working within the design space is not considered a change requiring regulatory approval. Movement out of the design space is considered to be a change, and requires a regulatory post-approval change process. This difference has significant impact on the bilateral relationships between industry and the regulator. It requires shifting from a paradigm of 'Tell' and 'Do', where no preapproved change is allowed, to 'Do' and 'Tell', where industry has the freedom to improve products and processes, within the boundaries of the knowledge supported by evidence in the drug product application. Statisticians can play a significant role in gaining and documenting such knowledge.

Bayesian methodology is being employed in both development and quality. A Bayesian approach to setting up a design space was proposed by Peterson (2004, 2008). This approach accounts for model parameter uncertainty and correlation among the CQAs. The paper by Stockdale and Cheng (2009) includes examples where this approach is applied to identify a reliable operating range. Fuchs and Kenett (1998, 2007) describe multivariate methods for achieving process control and determining process capability, and Kenett and Kenett (2008) present Bayesian methods for combining information from simulation and physical experiments with expert opinions, in order to derive a comprehensive design space.

Incorporating modern statistical methods in the life cycle of a drug product, from its development to its manufacturing and delivery is what this whole book is about. This first chapter has set the regulatory context that is an essential pillar in the overall system which includes patients, the pharmaceutical industry and regulatory agencies.

# References

EMA (2000) Points to Consider on Switching Between Superiority and Non-inferiority, Committee for Proprietary Medicinal Products, London.

EMA (2001) Points to Consider on Application with 1. Meta-analyses, 2. One Pivotal Study, Committee for Proprietary Medicinal Products, London.

EMA (2002) Points to Consider on Multiplicity Issues in Clinical Trials, Committee for Proprietary Medicinal Products, London.

EMA (2003) Points to Consider on Adjustment for Baseline Covariates, Committee for Proprietary Medicinal Products, London.

EMA (2004) Points to Consider on the Choice of Non-inferiority Margin, Committee for Proprietary Medicinal Products, London.

EMA (2005) Guideline on the Choice of Non-inferiority Margin, Committee for Proprietary Medicinal Products, London.

EMA (2009) Guideline on Missing Data in Confirmatory Trials, Committee for Proprietary Medicinal Products, London.

EMA (2010) Concept Paper on the Need for a Guideline on the Use of Subgroup Analyses in Randomized Controlled Trials, Committee for Proprietary Medicinal Products, London.

FDA (2001) Statistical Approaches to Establishing Bioequivalence, Food and Drug Administration, Silver Spring, MD.

FDA (2003) Exposure-Response Relationships – Study Design, Data Analysis, and Implications for Dosing and Labeling, Food and Drug Administration, Silver Spring, MD.

FDA (2004) Innovation or Stagnation: Challenge and Opportunity on the Critical Path to New Medical Products, Food and Drug Administration, Silver Spring, MD.

FDA (2006) Critical Path Opportunities List, Food and Drug Administration, Silver Spring, MD.

FDA (2008) The Sentinel Initiative: A National Strategy for Monitoring Medical Product Safety, Food and Drug Administration, Silver Spring, MD.

FDA (2010a) Non-Inferiority Clinical Trials, Food and Drug Administration, Silver Spring, MD.

FDA (2010b) Adaptive Design Clinical Trials for Drugs and Biologics, Food and Drug Administration, Silver Spring, MD.

FDA (2011) Process Validation: General Principles and Practices, Food and Drug Administration, Silver Spring, MD.

Fuchs, C. and Kenett, R.S. (1998) Multivariate Quality Control: Theory and Application, Quality and Reliability Series, Vol. 54, Marcel Dekker, New York.

Fuchs, C. and Kenett R.S. (2007) Multivariate process capability indices, in Encyclopaedia of Statistics in Quality and Reliability (eds F. Ruggeri, R.S. Kenett and F. Faltin), John Wiley & Sons, Ltd, Chichester.

Kenett, R.S. (2009) By Design. Six Sigma Forum Magazine (November), pp. 27–29.

Kenett, R.S. and Kenett D.A. (2008) Quality by Design applications in biosimilar pharmaceutical products. ACQUAL, Accreditation and Quality Assurance, 13(12), 681–690.

Kenett, R.S. and Raanan, Y. (2010) Operational Risk Management: A Practical Approach to Intelligent Data Analysis, John Wiley & Sons, Ltd, Chichester.

Kenett, R. and Zacks, S. (1998) Modern Industrial Statistics: Design and Control of Quality and Reliability, 2nd edn, Chinese edition 2004, Duxbury Press, San Francisco.

Kola, I. and Landis, J. (2004). Can the pharmaceutical industry reduce attrition rates. Nature Review Drug Discoveries, 3, 711–716.

Koyama, T., Sampson, A. and Gleser, L. (2005a) A calculus for design of two-stage adaptive procedures. Journal of the American Statistical Association, 100, 197–203.

Koyama, T., Sampson, A. and Gleser, L. (2005b) A framework for two-stage adaptive procedures to simultaneously test noninferiority and superiority. Statistics in Medicine, 24, 2439–2456.

MHLW (2004) Ministerial Ordinance on Standards for Manufacturing Control and Quality Control for Drugs and Quasi-drugs, Ministry of Health, Labour and Welfare, Japan.

Nasr, M. (2007) Quality by Design (QbD) – A Modern System Approach to Pharmaceutical Development and Manufacturing – FDA Perspective, FDA Quality Initiatives Workshop, North Bethesda, MD.

Nasr, M. (2009) Status and Implementation of ICH Q8, Q9, and Q10 Quality Guidelines: Topic Introduction and FDA Perspective, Pharmaceutical Science and Clinical Pharmacology Advisory Committee Meeting, Rockville, MD.

Peterson, J.J. (2004) A posterior predictive approach to multiple response surface optimization. Journal of Quality Technology, 36, 139–153.

Peterson, J. (2008) A Bayesian approach to the ICH Q8 definition of design space. Journal of Biopharmaceutical Statistics, 18, 959–975.

Peterson, J.J., Snee, R.D., McAllister, P.R. *et al.* (2009a) Statistics in pharmaceutical development and manufacturing (with discussion). *The Journal of Quality Technology*, **41**(2), 111–147.

Peterson, J.J., Miro-Quesada, G. and del Castillo, E. (2009b) A Bayesian reliability approach to multiple response optimization with seemingly unrelated regression models. *Quality Technology and Quantitative Management*, **6** (4), 353–369. http://www.cc.nctu.edu.tw/~qtqm/qtqmpapers/2009V6N4/2009V6N4_F1.pdf

PFSB (2007) Guideline for Descriptions on Application Forms for Marketing Approval of Drugs. Pharmaceutical and Food Safety Bureau, Ministry of Health, Labour and Welfare, Japan.

Stockdale, G. and Cheng, A. (2009) Finding design space and a reliable operating region using a multivariate Bayesian approach with experimental design. *Quality Technology and Quality Management*, **6**(4), 391–408.

Tsou, H., Chow, S., Lan, G. *et al.* (2010) Proposals of statistical consideration to evaluation of results for a specific region in multi-regional trials – Asian perspective. *Pharmaceutical Statistics*, **9**, 201–206.

Uvama, Y., Shaibata, T., Nagai, N. *et al.* (2005) Successful bridging strategy based on ICH E5 guideline for drugs approved in Japan. *Clinical Pharmacology & Therapeutics*, **78**(2), 102–113.

Yu, L. (2008). Pharmaceutical quality by design: product and process development, understanding and control. *Pharmaceutical Research*, **25**(4), 781–791.

# 2

# Statistical methods in clinical trials

**Telba Irony[1], Caiyan Li[2] and Phyllis Silverman[1]**
[1]*Center for Devices and Radiological Health, US Food and Drug Administration, Silver Spring, MD, USA*
[2]*Baxter Healthcare Corporation, Round Lake, IL, USA*

## Synopsis

Chapter 1 was an introduction to the regulatory approach for planning, conducting and analyzing outcomes of clinical research. It was focused on statistical aspects in the ICH and FDA guidelines that provide harmonization of regulations among Europe, Japan and the USA. This chapter complements Chapter 1 and provides a comprehensive treatment of statistical methods in drug product and medical device clinical trials. It covers aspects of design and analysis of clinical trials including the definition of endpoints, randomization and study designs, adjustments for covariates, the power of statistical tests, multiplicity, Bayesian inference, handling missing data, propensity scores, adaptive designs and survival analysis.

## 2.1 Introduction

Although Meinert (1986) defines a clinical trial as 'a planned experiment designed to assess the efficacy of a treatment in humans by comparing the outcomes in a group of patients treated with the test treatment with those observed in a comparable group of patients receiving a control treatment', clinical trials in healthcare take on many forms and sizes. Following 'preclinical trials', which may involve animals or laboratory testing, the earliest of clinical

*Statistical Methods in Healthcare*, First Edition. Edited by Frederick W. Faltin, Ron S. Kenett and Fabrizio Ruggeri.
© 2012 John Wiley & Sons, Ltd. Published 2012 by John Wiley & Sons, Ltd.

research involving human subjects may be begun for a new drug or medical device on a small number of subjects. With medical devices, for example, this early clinical research occurs in the form of *feasibility* or *pilot* studies, and serves to obtain some measure of treatment effectiveness and variability. These are followed by one or more '*confirmatory*' or pivotal clinical trials to assess the effectiveness and safety of treatment. Finally, since not all questions can be answered before a treatment comes on the market, there is often a *post-approval study* to look at long-term effectiveness and/or adverse events. With drug trials, the study stages are labeled Phases I to IV, and these phases are discussed in more detail in Section 2.12, Drugs versus devices.

### 2.1.1   Claims

There are three types of claims that can be made for a new drug or medical device treatment relative to a comparison treatment: *superiority, non-inferiority or equivalence*. Each of these claims must be supported by a statistically significant result based on hypothesis testing or confidence intervals. Although a statistically significant result in a superiority trial actually only demonstrates that the treatment difference is not zero (i.e., that there is an effect not due to chance), the study must be sized to detect a clinically meaningful difference as statistically significant. Otherwise, statistically significant differences may be found that are not clinically meaningful, and interpretation is difficult. Similarly, in a non-inferiority study, a *non-inferiority margin*, (commonly called delta ($\delta$)), must be selected that represents the maximum amount by which a new treatment can be numerically inferior to the standard treatment without being considered clinically inferior. In order to accept a lower effectiveness rate, there should be some benefit to the new treatment over the old, such as a better safety profile. More details about superiority and non-inferiority trials are discussed in Section 2.2.1, Hypothesis testing. A claim of equivalence basically says that the new treatment results are clinically indistinguishable from the comparator in either direction. This is most common with trials for diagnostic devices, such as a glucose monitor.

### 2.1.2   Endpoints

The *primary endpoint*, that is, the target outcome of the trial, may be *single, multiple or composite*. With a single primary endpoint, there is one outcome of interest, and overall study success is dictated by that endpoint. For example, the endpoint may be reduction in tumor size, artery patency at a specific time point, or survival of a patient or a hip implant at 10 years. Alternatively, there can be co-primary endpoints, or even three or more primary endpoints. It must be made clear whether all endpoints have to be met for study success, because the overall significance level is affected. This will be discussed more in Section 2.7.1, Multiplicity. Secondary endpoints can serve multiple purposes. They can be used for the purpose of relaying additional information and may not be statistically compared to a control group. These results can be reported descriptively in drug or device labeling. Alternatively, they can be hypothesis driven, with claims against a comparator. The methods discussed in Section 2.7.1 on multiplicity also apply to multiple secondary endpoints. Whether primary or secondary, multiple endpoints require special handling, or spurious significant findings can result.

One way to avoid multiple primary endpoints is to form a *composite endpoint* consisting of an aggregate of the multiple endpoints. Each patient would be classified as a success or failure depending on whether he/she met all of the patient-level success criteria defined for each of the endpoints. For example, the patient success criteria for a hip replacement study might be (1) a Harris Hip score $\geq 80$, (2) no revision or re-operation, (3) radiographic success, and (4) no device-related complications. A patient meeting all four of these criteria would be classified a success, and then the success rates in the two treatment groups could be compared. It is not uncommon, then, to look at each of the individual components of a composite endpoint separately as the secondary endpoints. The selection of appropriate endpoints is a crucial part of a good study design.

## 2.1.3    Types of study designs and controls

Three common types of clinical trial design are the parallel, concurrently controlled design, the paired design and the historically controlled design. The *parallel, concurrently controlled trial* usually has two treatment arms (an investigational arm and a comparator arm), and is prospective, randomized and masked. This type of trial presents the strongest level of scientific evidence. If the randomization is performed correctly, the treatment groups will tend to be balanced for both the known and unknown factors that could instill bias. In this type of study, the control arm could be another active treatment, or a placebo treatment (either a pill or a sham device). Sometimes a three-arm trial is warranted, where there will be an investigational treatment, active control and placebo control.

In a *paired design*, each patient serves as his/her own control. With medical devices, a patient may receive both treatments, such as a different type of wrinkle filler on opposite sides of the face. One strength of this design is that patient-to-patient variability is eliminated. A paired study design can also comprise before-and-after assessments, where follow-up results are compared to baseline. With this design, however, it is difficult to rule out a placebo effect. Matching subjects one-to-one on certain characteristics and then randomly assigning treatments to each pair is another way of conducting a paired study. In general, paired designs are very efficient, requiring a smaller sample size relative to a study with parallel groups due to the reduction in variability. However, they are not without their disadvantages. For example, in the wrinkle filler example given above, it would not be possible to attribute any systemic adverse events to a specific treatment.

*Historically controlled* trial designs seem to be used more in medical device trials than in drug trials. A historically controlled study is essentially a single arm study where the control comes from one or more completed studies. Often the control is an earlier version of the current treatment. Historical controls are problematic in that they are prone to temporal bias. Since the control patients were treated at an earlier point in time, there may have been differences in standard of care, differences in disease stage or prognosis, or differences in patient demographics. Often patient-level data is not available and additional analyses cannot be performed. Sometimes a meta-analysis is performed to derive an 'objective performance criterion (OPC)', which is a number or success rate that must be met by the single investigational arm. There must be agreement in the clinical community on the OPC chosen.

There are many other study designs, such as cross-over designs, which will not be discussed here. Regardless of the study design, it is important that systematic error (bias) be controlled, that random variation be reduced, and that precision of estimates be as high as possible. Clinical trials should be multi-centered, and treatment-by-site interaction should be assessed as part of any data analysis.

## 2.2    Hypothesis testing, significance levels, *p*-values, power and sample size

In clinical trials, we typically ask questions about the effectiveness of a new treatment on an outcome defined by continuous, dichotomous or time-to-event variables. These questions can be formulated into the framework of statistical *hypothesis testing*. In this section, we will introduce the general concepts of hypothesis testing and related topics.

### 2.2.1    Hypothesis testing

Hypothesis testing has played a major role in the design and analysis of clinical trials. It is used to assess the effectiveness and safety of a new treatment by appropriately defining the *null hypothesis $H_0$* and the *alternative hypothesis $H_1$*. A null hypothesis represents the statement that we are trying to reject, and an alternative hypothesis is the claim that we are targeting to prove in clinical trials. A simple example of such hypothesis testing in a controlled clinical trial would be a study of hypertension with active (new treatment) and control (standard treatment) arms. In most studies, the question asked is whether the new treatment is better (superior) than the standard. While *superiority trials* are most common, *non-inferiority trials* are also frequently conducted. For example, in cases where the new treatment may be safer, easier to administer or less expensive than the standard treatment, a non-inferiority trial can be designed to demonstrate that the new treatment is non-inferior to the standard. Using the example above to illustrate the differences between these two types of trials, let's denote the mean reduction in blood pressure in the new and standard treatments as $T$ and $C$, respectively. In a superiority trial, the null and alternative hypotheses could be expressed as: $H_0 : T - C \leq \Delta; H_1 : T - C > \Delta$, where the superiority margin $\Delta \geq 0$. While in most cases $\Delta$ is set as 0 for a superiority test, a $\Delta > 0$ can be used to show that the new treatment is superior by a fixed amount (*super superiority*). If the observed data show enough evidence to reject the null hypothesis, we claim that the new treatment is better than the standard treatment in treating high blood pressure. In a non-inferiority trial, where the objective is to demonstrate that the new treatment is non-inferior to the standard treatment by a clinically insignificant margin $\delta$, the null and alternative hypotheses are defined as: $H_0 : C - T \geq \delta; H_1 : C - T < \delta$. By rejecting the null hypothesis, we claim that the active treatment is less effective than the control treatment by no more than $\delta$, an amount deemed to be clinically insignificant. The margin $\delta$ is one of the key elements in designing a non-inferiority trial. The bigger the margin, the easier it is to reject the null hypothesis. However, from the clinical perspective, we want a margin small enough to be able to ignore the clinical difference. Ideally, the non-inferiority margin should be compensated by the improvement of other aspects (e.g., safety or cost) of the new treatment. The determination of the non-inferiority margin has become a frequently discussed topic in the literature.

### 2.2.2    Statistical errors, significance levels and *p*-values

There are two types of *statistical errors* one can make when conducting a hypothesis test. A *type I error,* also known as a *false positive,* is the error of rejecting the null hypothesis when it is actually true. In the example of a superiority test, above, a type I error occurs if we claim superiority for the active treatment when it is not. A *type II error*, also known as a *false negative,* is the error of failing to reject the null hypothesis when it is not true. An example of this would be failing to claim superiority for the active treatment when it is actually superior to the control treatment. It is, unfortunately, almost impossible to minimize the probabilities of both types of errors with a fixed *sample size.* Therefore, the conventional approach is to restrict the type I error rate to a predetermined level (also known as *significance level*, or $\alpha$ *level*) and, subject to this constraint, try to minimize the type II error rate. The $\alpha$ level is the maximum type I error rate that you are willing to tolerate when rejecting the null hypothesis. It serves as a cut-off point for the type I error rate, below which we agree that an effect is statistically significant. In practice, when we say 'significant at the 0.05 level', we mean that the probability of making a type I error when rejecting a true null hypothesis is less than 0.05. More precisely, one can report a *p-value* for the test, say 0.027, which would mean that the test is significant at the 0.027 level. The *p*-value is the probability of obtaining a result that is at least as extreme as the observed result (towards the alternative hypothesis) assuming that the null hypothesis is true. It quantifies how likely it is that the observed effect is due to chance alone. Thus, the smaller the *p*-value, the less likely it is to observe the effect due to chance alone; that is, the effect is likely real. In practice, a *p*-value which is smaller than or equal to the predetermined significance level $\alpha$ leads to rejection of the null hypothesis and claim of an effect.

### 2.2.3   Confidence intervals

Instead of estimating the parameter of interest by a single value, say the observed difference between treatment arm A and treatment arm B, a more informative approach in clinical trials is to calculate the precision of the estimate by a *confidence interval (CI)*. The idea of a confidence interval was developed by Neyman and Pearson. It is calculated as a range around a population parameter (e.g., mean or proportion) at a given *confidence level* (usually denoted as $100 \times (1 - \alpha)\%$) to convey the precision of the estimate. When one speaks of a '$100 \times (1 - \alpha)\%$ confidence interval', a technical understanding would be that if you repeated your trial many times under exactly the same conditions with identical sample size, $100 \times (1 - \alpha)\%$ of the calculated confidence intervals would contain the true value of the population parameter. Strictly speaking, the confidence level is not a probability that the corresponding confidence interval contains the true parameter value. A confidence interval either does contain the true parameter value or does not. In most cases, confidence intervals are calculated symmetrically around the point estimate of the parameter at a given confidence level. The endpoints of the confidence intervals are called *confidence limits,* which can be used in hypothesis testing. The concept of a $100 \times (1 - \alpha)\%$ confidence level for an interval corresponds to the concept of a significance level $(\alpha)$ for hypothesis testing. For example, if $\alpha = 0.05$, the confidence level would be 95% (i.e., $100 \times (1 - 0.05)\%$). Take the hypertension trial described above as an example. The parameter of interest is the difference in the reduction of blood pressure between the two treatment groups $(C - T)$. Assume that the clinical data gives us a point estimate of $-10$ for this difference, with a 95% confidence interval of $(-18, -2)$. Superiority can then be claimed for the new treatment at a 95% confidence level (or a 5% significance level), because the upper limit of the confidence interval is less than 0. Generally, in superiority testing, if the upper limit of the $100 \times (1 - \alpha)\%$ confidence interval for $(C - T)$ is less than 0 (or in the case of $T - C$, the lower limit would need to be greater than 0), we reject the null hypothesis and claim superiority at $\alpha$ level. Similarly, in non-inferiority testing, if the upper limit of the

$100 \times (1 - \alpha)\%$ confidence interval for $(C - T)$ is less than the non-inferiority margin $\delta$, we reject the null hypothesis and claim non-inferiority at $\alpha$ level. Figure 2.1 shows the results of various 95% confidence intervals for $(C - T)$, and their interpretations. Please note that our discussion here is based on favorable outcomes (e.g., decreased death rate, reduction in blood pressure) for which bigger values are better.

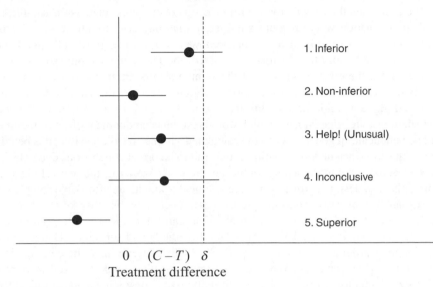

**Figure 2.1**   Results of various 95% confidence intervals for $(C - T)$, and interpretations.

1. Upper limit of the 95% CI for $(C - T)$ is greater than $\delta$, so non-inferiority is not demonstrated; lower limit of the 95% CI for $(C - T)$ is greater than 0, so T is inferior to C.
2. Upper limit of the 95% CI for $(C - T)$ is less than $\delta$, so T is non-inferior to C.
3. Upper limit of the 95% CI for $(C - T)$ is less than $\delta$, so T is non-inferior to C. Lower limit of the 95% CI for $(C - T)$ is greater than 0, so C is superior to T. This outcome would be very unusual and could present interpretive problems.
4. Upper limit of the 95% CI for $(C - T)$ is greater than $\delta$, so non-inferiority is not demonstrated; lower limit of the 95% CI for $(C - T)$ is less than 0, so C is not superior to T. This outcome leads to an inconclusive interpretation about whether T is better, worse or non-inferior to C.
5. Upper limit of the 95% CI for $(C - T)$ is less than 0, so T is superior to C.

## 2.2.4   Statistical power and sample size

*Statistical power* is defined as the probability of rejecting the null hypothesis when it is not true, and is commonly denoted as $1 - \beta$, where $\beta$ is the type II error rate. It quantifies the ability of the trial to detect a true effect when it exists. When planning clinical trials, clinicians often ask statisticians how much power the trial has to detect a treatment effect of a specified size. In general, there are five major factors that affect the power of the trial:

(1) the variability of outcome measurements, (2) the size of the effect one is trying to detect, (3) the probability risk one can tolerate in claiming an effect is present when it is not (significance level $\alpha$), (4) the power to detect a true effect ($1 - \beta$), and (5) the *sample size* of the trial ($n$). These factors are all interrelated in that, if any four of them are fixed, the fifth one can be calculated. If one agrees that the variability of measurements can be appropriately estimated (perhaps from a pilot study or historical data), that the targeted effect size can be estimated, and also that common values for the significance level (e.g., 0.05) and power (e.g., 0.8) are to be used, then the only factor left for investigators to manipulate is the sample size of the trial. In a situation where resources are fixed, one may need to adjust other factors, in particular the effect size to be detected or the power, to meet the 'practical' sample size requirements. Typically, all other factors being fixed, the larger the sample size, the more powerful the trial if the effect is present. If the sample size is dramatically overestimated, the trial may be judged as clinically or economically unfeasible. If the sample size is badly underestimated, there is a good possibility that the trial will fall short of finding statistical evidence to demonstrate effectiveness, which would result in abandonment of a new treatment that could be beneficial. In general, when the calculated sample size is plausible, it is better to overestimate the size since underestimation could lead to incorrect conclusions due to lack of power. It is, therefore, an important duty for biostatisticians to work together with clinicians in the planning phase to design a properly powered clinical trial with an affordable sample size.

Approximate formulas to express sample sizes as a function of the other four basic factors are well developed for different types of trials. One can refer to existing literature (e.g., Friedman, Furberg and Demets, 1996) for detailed methods and formulas. There are also excellent computer programs available (e.g., PASS 2008) that eliminate the computational burden of sample size calculation. While now computationally trivial, it is well recognized that sample size estimation is one of the most difficult tasks in designing a good clinical trial. There are many factors that need to be estimated or assumed when determining sample size. Sometimes one may have to use a best guess based on existing data and experiences, which introduces many uncertainties to sample size estimation.

A sample size estimation formula is an approximation based on statistical models and an assumed probability distribution for the outcome (e.g., normal distribution). In practice, we don't know the distribution of the outcome variable (if there is one) and the corresponding test statistic in hypothesis testing. For larger sample sizes, however, the normal approximation is rather accurate. Also, the sample size formula involves the true sample standard deviation of the measurement. The problem is that we do not know the true variability until after we have carried out the trial. This adds another dimension of uncertainty to the sample size estimation. Although statisticians try to obtain a reasonable estimate of the variability from previous trials, the assumption that the variability of the current trial is the same as that of historical trials is questionable. A more cautious way to incorporate the uncertainty from this source is to study the robustness of the sample size estimation by assuming a range of reasonable sample standard deviations. This would allow for a more conservative sample size choice. A third factor is that the unknown true treatment effect complicates the estimation of sample size. In practice, clinicians often guess the effect size based on their experiences, and weigh this against practical sample size requirements. Lastly, non-compliance of the subjects during the trial must be considered. Typically, an adjustment would be applied to compensate for loss-to-follow-up and dropouts. As a result, the final sample size will be larger than the calculated one. To conclude, the investigators should take into account the different dimensions of sample size calculations, such as statistical power, variability and clinical perspectives, when obtaining a practical sample size for the trial.

## 2.3    Bias, randomization and blinding/masking

Error in clinical trials has two components: a purely random error (also referred to as *variability*) and a systematic error (also referred to as *bias*). Variability describes the precision of a measurement or estimate. Increasing sample size or repeating the experiment can reduce the variability of the mean of the measurements and increase the accuracy of estimates. Bias describes deviations from true treatment effects due to all causes other than random variation. Bias can occur in several places during a clinical trial, from the design and implementation of the trial to data analysis and the interpretation of results. A good understanding of the causes of bias is very helpful in reducing it and obtaining a reasonable estimate of the treatment effect.

### 2.3.1    Bias

Important sources of bias in clinical trials include selection bias, assessment bias and bias caused by selectively missing data.

**Selection bias** arises when individuals in the trial are not representative of the target population. For example, would a sample of NBA basketball players be appropriate to estimate the average height of the American male? Selection bias can happen in the pre-screening of participants, self-selection as to whether or not to participate, selection of historical studies in meta-analysis or even rejection of 'bad' data arbitrarily. A randomized controlled trial (RCT) with well-defined inclusion/exclusion criteria can reduce selection bias. The most important advantage of *randomization* is that it creates balance between study groups with respect to known and unknown characteristics and removes bias in the allocation of treatments. In a properly randomized trial, it is more likely that an observed difference between groups is due to a treatment effect.

**Assessment bias** can occur when participants, investigators or third party evaluators know the actual treatment assignments. This knowledge may cause subjective behavior in assessing the results. The general solution to this problem is *blinding or masking*; that is, keeping the participants, investigators or third-party evaluators unaware of the treatment assignments.

**Selective missing**, also called *informative missing*, of the outcome data is another cause of biased estimates of treatment effect. Inappropriate exclusion of participants from the analysis could break the experimental paradigm and possibly lead to biased estimation of effects. For example, some participants in the treatment group may be too sick to continue the follow-up and may drop out of the study. In this case, exclusion of these sick people from the final data analysis may overestimate the treatment effect. Similarly, exclusion of patients that are missing because they are doing well can have the opposite effect. Proactive follow-up examinations and detailed documentation of case report forms can help to provide a better understanding of the missing mechanism, which may inform the imputation of the missing data using appropriate statistical methods. In addition, there are other sources of bias that are only relevant in some particular circumstances. For example, in a cross-over design, where each subject receives both treatments sequentially, a carry-over effect might introduce additional bias. A *washout* or waiting period between treatments can sometimes be used to counteract this effect.

Bias towards the null hypothesis (i.e., no treatment effect) can happen if the investigational group is slightly worse at the beginning of the trial with respect to baseline characteristics that affect the outcome. This bias is generally considered conservative and not of great concern.

For all potential sources of bias, it is important to consider the relative magnitude and direction of the bias when interpreting the observed effects. For example, if the data indicate that the new treatment is effective, but there is a suspicion of bias towards the direction of effectiveness, careful assessment of the relative magnitude of the bias and effect size should be made before conclusions are drawn.

## 2.3.2  Randomization

Randomization is an effective method to reduce selection bias in a comparative trial. It produces comparable study groups in terms of known and unknown covariates that may be related to outcome. An RCT is considered to be the most reliable and impartial study design used to compare treatments. Some common randomization procedures include simple randomization, blocked randomization, stratified randomization and adaptive randomization.

**Simple randomization:** simple randomization has no restriction; for example, a single sequence of random allocations. Simple randomization is expected to produce balanced study groups for a large sample trial.

**Blocked randomization:** blocked randomization (with a block size of $b$) is a randomization scheme which ensures that for every $b$ participants enrolled in the trial, the number of participants in each treatment group will be equal. It is used to avoid serious imbalance in the number of participants between study groups. However, a known block size $b$ tends to increase the predictability of the assignment. In this case, using a variable block size (a.k.a. permuted random blocks), or determining the size for each block randomly during the randomization process, is recommended.

**Stratified randomization:** stratified randomization is achieved by performing a separate randomization procedure in each stratum determined by stratification variables, such as age group, or prognostic factors. This randomization scheme assures that there is equal representation of prognostic factors in all treatment groups. For example, a study on wound healing might stratify the randomization by initial wound size, below and above a certain threshold.

These three randomization schemes are classified as fixed allocation procedures. They assign each treatment to participants with a pre-specified probability that remains the same throughout the randomization process. In contrast, adaptive randomization procedures change the allocation probabilities during the course of the study. Two types of adaptive randomization procedures are introduced here.

**Baseline adaptive randomization:** adjusts the allocation probabilities according to the imbalances in baseline characteristics between the study groups to prevent severe baseline imbalances in important prognostic factors. Biased coin randomization adjusts the allocation probability so that the probability is higher for the group with fewer participants. Another commonly used baseline adaptive randomization scheme is referred to as an urn design, where we imagine an urn filled with $m$ red and $m$ black balls. When a red ball is drawn, assign the participant to group A, then return the ball to the urn and add a black ball; when a black ball is drawn, assign the participant to group B, then return the ball and add a red ball. Both schemes attempt to keep the number of participants in each group balanced as the randomization proceeds.

**Response-adaptive randomization:** adjusts allocation probabilities according to the responses of participants to assigned treatments. For example, the play-the-winner procedure assigns the next participant to the same treatment if the previous participant turns out to be a success; otherwise, the participant is assigned to the other treatment. Another response-adaptive randomization scheme is called the two-armed bandit method, where allocation probabilities are adjusted in such a way that a higher proportion of future participants would receive the treatment currently deemed 'better'. Both the play-the-winner procedure and the two-armed bandit method tend to maximize the number of participants that receive the best treatment. These randomization techniques, however, would require that the treatment response is quickly observed.

In a two-arm, controlled trial, one-to-one (1 : 1) randomization is most commonly used, because it produces approximately equal-sized treatment groups and is statistically more powerful than other randomization ratios. However, if much is already known about the control treatment, k-to-one ($k : 1$, $k > 1$) randomization can be used to collect more information on the investigational device, particularly for safety.

The actual implementation of the chosen randomization scheme is extremely important in order to maintain the advantages of using randomization to balance known and unknown prognostic factors between groups. Setting up an independent central center to develop the randomization process and allocate the participants to appropriate treatments is recommended.

## 2.3.3    Blinding or masking

An effective way to eliminate assessment bias in clinical trials is to blind or mask the participants and/or the investigators in such a way that they are not aware of the treatment that is assigned to each participant. Blinding (also called masking) becomes especially important to obtain an unbiased estimate of the treatment effect when the outcome endpoints are subjective (patient self-reports, questionnaires, etc.) or when there is an expectation of better performance for a new treatment effect.

**Open-label trial:** also called unblinded trial. In this case the assigned treatments are known to both participants and investigators.

**Single-blind trial:** only the participants are unaware of the assigned treatments.

**Double-blind trial:** both the participants and the investigators are unaware of the treatment assigned to each participant.

**Triple-blind trial:** not only the participants and investigators, but also the third party evaluator, if used, is unaware of the treatment assignment.

Blinding success is a fundamental issue in clinical trials. The validity of a trial may be questioned if blinding is not assured. Assessment of the degree of blinding after the completion of a trial is usually achieved by asking the participants and the investigators to guess the treatment assignments. In an equal-sized, two-arm study with an active control, the guesses would be correct approximately 50% of the time if the trial is well blinded. Substantial deviation from 50% may imply that some participants and/or investigators may be aware of treatment assignments. Ideally, a double-blind trial should be designed to avoid potential assessment bias. In cases when a double-blind trial is impossible, a single-blind trial and the use of other measures to reduce bias are recommended. For example, photographs are often used for assessments of treatment effectiveness for devices with aesthetic outcomes, such as wrinkle fillers. This keeps the evaluator masked as to the treatment timeline.

## 2.4     Covariate adjustment and Simpson's paradox

A *covariate* is defined as a secondary variable or factor that could affect the relationship between the dependent variables (e.g., primary endpoints) and other independent variables (e.g., treatment effect). The terms 'covariates', '*prognostic variables*' and '*independent variables*' are used interchangeably to refer to predictors. There are several reasons why covariate adjustment is useful and important in the analysis of clinical trials. One reason for studying covariates is to explore the relationship between important prognostic variables that can affect the primary outcome measures. If the covariate is strongly associated with the disease outcome (e.g., the stage of cancer is strongly associated with survival), adjustment for the covariate effect could yield stronger and more precise evidence in favor of or against the treatment. In addition, important interaction between the treatment and covariates or between the covariates themselves can be detected through including covariates into statistical models. A second important reason for studying covariates is to improve the comparability between treatment groups and reduce the bias in estimating the treatment effect. In randomized trials, knowledge of prognostic variables can improve the study design. For example, in cancer trials, the stage of cancer is strongly associated with survival, and one might consider a randomization stratified on the baseline severity of cancer patients to improve balance and comparability between treatment groups. In non-randomized clinical trials where treatment groups might be heavily imbalanced in certain important prognostic variables, adjustment for these variables can reduce the bias of the estimated treatment effect. The adjustment for important prognostic variables in the analysis of clinical trials can produce a more credible and precise conclusion. Failure to adjust might lead one to a conclusion in the opposite direction. A classic example is *Simpson's paradox,* which provides an insightful illustration of the importance of covariate adjustment.

### 2.4.1     Simpson's paradox

In an article published in 1952, E. H. Simpson pointed out a simple fact about fractions that has important applications. In clinical studies, *Simpson's paradox* (or the Yule–Simpson effect) arises when a prognostic variable is overlooked at the design phase. In that case, the success rates in the groups determined by different values of the prognostic variable seem to be reversed when the groups are combined. This fact is best illustrated by an example.

Suppose a clinical study is conducted to compare a new intervention with standard of care for a particular disease. One hundred and sixty patients are randomized, with 80 assigned to the new intervention and 80 assigned to standard of care. The results of the study can be displayed as in Table 2.1.

**Table 2.1**   Total population ($n = 160$).

|  | Successful | Not successful | Percentage successful |
| --- | --- | --- | --- |
| New intervention | 40 | 40 | 50% |
| Standard of care | 48 | 32 | 60% |

**Table 2.2** Young patients ($n = 80$).

|  | Successful | Not successful | Percentage successful |
|---|---|---|---|
| New intervention | 16 | 4 | 80% |
| Standard of care | 42 | 18 | 70% |

Based on these results, the new intervention appears inferior to standard of care. However, the clinical investigators know that age is an important prognostic variable and decide to stratify the analysis according to the age of the patients: young patients (less than 40 years old) and senior patients (above 40 years old). Splitting the overall data into two disjoint subgroups of the population is called disaggregation. The results in each subgroup can be displayed as in Tables 2.2 and 2.3.

Note that when the results of Tables 2.2 and 2.3 are combined, we obtain the original aggregated data found in Table 2.1. However, the new intervention appears to be superior to standard of care both for young and for senior patients when analyzed separately. One may be surprised by these results, and here is the source of Simpson's paradox. According to Table 2.1, the new intervention is inferior to standard of care when all subjects are combined. However, after stratifying by patient age (see Tables 2.2 and 2.3), the new intervention is superior to standard of care both for young and senior patients. Clearly, this seeming paradox stems from the fact that young patients have a higher rate of success than senior patients, regardless of whether they receive standard of care or the new intervention. Although the numbers of young and senior patients in the study were the same, the randomization of treatments was not stratified by age, and more young patients than senior patients were randomized to the standard of care arm. As a consequence, the number of young patients that received the new intervention (20) was much smaller than the number of senior patients (60). Since the young patients have a higher rate of success regardless of treatment, it is found in Table 2.1 that the standard of care shows a higher rate of success than the new intervention.

To ensure that this phenomenon does not occur, it is important that the proportion of young and old patients that receive the new intervention be approximately the same. That can be achieved via stratifying the randomization of treatment assignments by the age subgroups (i.e., young and senior patients). In other words, in a well-designed study, the randomization should be stratified by all demographic/prognostic variables that are believed to have a significant association with treatment outcome, or covariate adjustments need to be made at the time of the statistical analysis.

**Table 2.3** Senior patients ($n = 80$).

|  | Successful | Not successful | Percentage successful |
|---|---|---|---|
| New intervention | 24 | 36 | 40% |
| Standard of care | 6 | 14 | 30% |

## 2.4.2    Statistical methods for covariate adjustment

For a single discrete covariate, the covariate adjustment could be simplified to a stratified analysis, which directly compares treatment groups within each subdivided stratum and then averages the results across all strata to get an overall covariate-adjusted estimate. However, in clinical trials, often several prognostic variables are believed to be associated with the outcome variables, and investigators are interested in assessing the effects of all variables together. A *statistical model* is one of the most powerful and flexible tools to assess the effects of multiple covariates on the outcome variable simultaneously. These models combine theoretical knowledge (e.g., hypotheses) with empirical knowledge (observed data) to describe a plausible relationship between the covariates and the outcome variable in terms of one or more parameters which have useful clinical interpretations. To illustrate the use of such models, let's denote $Y$ as the outcome variable, $Z$ as the indicator variable representing the treatment groups ($Z = 1$, treatment group; $Z = 0$, control group), $X = (X_1, \ldots, X_k)$ as the covariate vector, $\alpha$ as the treatment-effect coefficient, and $\beta = (\beta_1, \ldots, \beta_k)$ as the covariate coefficient. The specific adjustment models depend on the type of outcome variables being analyzed. This section will briefly introduce several of the most commonly used models in clinical trials. More complicated models can be found in the statistical literature.

- If the outcome variable is continuous (e.g., blood pressure), a *linear regression model* can be used: $Y = \alpha Z + X_1\beta_1 + \cdots + X_k\beta_k$.

- If the outcome variable is binary (e.g., $Y = 1$ refers to the occurrence of an event), a *logistic regression model* could be built:

$$\log\left(\frac{p}{1-p}\right) = \alpha Z + X_1\beta_1 + \cdots + X_k\beta_k,$$

  where $p$ is the probability of the event; that is, $p = \Pr(Y = 1)$.

- If the outcome variable is time-to-event, then survival analysis models are used. One of the popular models is the *Cox proportional-hazards model*: $h(t) = h_0(t)\exp(\alpha Z + X_1\beta_1 + \cdots + X_k\beta_k)$, where $h(t)$ and $h_0(t)$ are the hazard rate of interest and hazard rate at baseline, respectively. The details of survival model building are described in Section 2.8.

These statistical models can be used not only to study the main effects of a covariate, but also to assess interactions between these covariates and treatment groups by including second-order covariates (e.g., $X_1X_2$) in the models. When estimating interaction effects, it is important to always include the main effects or lower-order terms in the model.

After choosing the mathematical formula to describe the relationship between the outcome variable and covariates, the next step is to build a parsimonious model with the appropriate variables. Although there are software packages (such as SAS) available that have tools for automated model selections, constructing a statistically parsimonious and clinically useful model is, nevertheless, not a simple automated process. Statistical model building techniques as well as clinical judgments are involved. One of the difficulties in model building is that there may be some correlation among variables (i.e., collinearity). Strong collinearity in covariates can cause problems in the statistical estimation process and in interpretation of parameter estimates. For example, with two correlated covariates, including either one of them in the model could significantly improve the model prediction. However, if both variables are included, then both may appear unimportant. Another difficulty arises from the large number of possible covariates and associated higher-order terms. Including all available covariates and interaction terms in the model could cause an identifiability problem in estimation. Also, including all of the measured covariates in the model may make the clinical interpretation difficult. Therefore, selecting appropriate variables is a critical step in model building. It is usually unrealistic to expect one regression model to be clearly superior to all others, and models cannot always be distinguished in terms of statistical evidence. A feasible way of building a good statistical model is for the clinicians who have expert knowledge about the prognostic variables to work closely with the statisticians. Clear clinical interpretation of a prognostic variable should be considered while building the model. Even if a particular variable seems to yield a slight statistical improvement in model prediction over another more clinically important variable, one should choose to include the latter in the model. Clinical expertise, pre-clinical data and observations about the trial data could provide important guidance when choosing which covariates should be adjusted for in the analysis. Generally, variables that are strongly unbalanced between treatment groups, and variables that are believed to be strongly associated with the outcome variable, should be adjusted for in the analysis.

## 2.5    Meta-analysis, pooling and interaction

### 2.5.1    Meta-analysis

*Meta-analysis* is a systematic method that uses statistical analysis to integrate data from a group of independent studies that address a set of related research questions. Often, for a particular clinical research question, several independent studies have been conducted at different times. Some of these studies may be large multi-center trials; while others may be too small to yield a valid conclusion on their own. One of the most important uses of meta-analysis is to synthesize results when individual studies are too small to be conclusive. It can increase the precision of effect estimates and produce more powerful conclusions than any individual study. Frequently, researchers are interested in small treatment effects in common diseases where even modest treatment benefits can have a big impact on public health (e.g., cancers). Through combining large amounts of data from a number of studies, meta-analysis can detect small treatment effects with high statistical power, providing a higher level of evidence that the effect, although modest, exists. Meta-analysis could also be used to construct a historical control rate such as an objective performance criterion (OPC) or performance goal to help design a new clinical trial.

There are generally four steps in a meta-analysis. The first step is a literature search for identifying relevant studies; the second step is the definition of the eligibility criteria for inclusion and exclusion of the studies; the third step is to decide on the summary measurements and data to be abstracted from the studies; and the fourth step is to perform statistical analysis to draw conclusions from the abstracted data.

**Literature search:** the development of a systematic and explicit procedure to identify studies with relevant data is critical in meta-analysis. Usually a large number of published studies can be found by computerized search of literature databases, such as MEDLINE. The reference lists from selected articles are then reviewed as important additional resources for identifying relevant data. In addition, personal knowledge and subject matter experts are important resources from which to gather information about studies that have not yet appeared in the traditional media, such as unpublished studies and institutional research.

**Eligibility criteria for studies:** the purpose of defining eligibility criteria for studies to be included in a meta-analysis is to reduce selection bias (e.g., choosing only the most favorable studies) and to increase the reproducibility of the analysis. Just as not all subjects are eligible to enter a clinical trial, not all studies should be included in a meta-analysis. To select a study for the meta-analysis, researchers must consider the specific treatment in the study and justify that the study is similar in design to other selected studies. The studies selected for the meta-analysis should have similar participants with similar protocols (e.g., similar endpoints).

**Abstraction of data from studies:** this procedure should be pre-planned to ensure reliability. A pretested data abstraction form should be used to organize and collect the information from each study to help control the selection and removal of participants from the analysis, to determine the relevant outcome and to identify information on important prognostic factors.

**Statistical analyses:** after obtaining the abstracted data from all studies, the last step of meta-analysis is to perform the statistical analysis. The main issues in statistical analysis include choosing an effect estimate, such as mean differences (continuous data), risk differences (binary data) and hazard ratios (survival data); deciding on the analysis unit (trial versus individual patient); weighting the quality of each study and selecting statistical models to combine the results from all studies. One frequently used meta-analysis approach in healthcare research is referred to as the 'inverse variance method', which averages the effect estimate using a weighted mean, whereby the weight is the inverse variance of each study's effect estimator. Larger studies with smaller variations are given greater weights than smaller studies with larger variations. Other commonly used methods include the Mantel–Haenszel method and the Peto method. In any case, the overall effect estimate can be adjusted for prognostic factors using statistical models. Generally, three types of statistical models are applied in meta-analysis: simple regression where neither within-study variation nor between-study variations is included; fixed-effects meta-regression where within-study variation is specified, but between-study variation is ignored; and random-effects meta-regression where both within-study variation and between-study variations are taken into consideration. Bayesian hierarchical modeling is a modern statistical technique used in meta-analysis (see Section 2.10). The idea is to 'borrow strength' among the studies to be meta-analyzed with the goal of obtaining overall 'shrunken' estimates. Intuitively, there is more shrinkage if the variability among studies is similar to the variability within studies. The borrowing among studies decreases as the variability among studies increases as compared with the variability within the studies. Like individual studies, meta-analysis also suffers from the missing-data problem and requires pre-planning of subgroup analyses.

The appeal of meta-analysis is to reduce the uncertainty about the effect estimates, to generalize the findings to a group of different studies and to control between-study variations. However, meta-analysis suffers from some theoretical and practical limitations. Not all researchers agree on the theoretical validity of meta-analysis and its practical interpretation. The selection of studies and the methods used to synthesize the results can cause potential bias in the results. Researchers should keep in mind that no meta-analysis can effectively validate evidence from flawed studies. Therefore, clinical investigators are not encouraged to conduct under-powered studies with the hope of combining them later in a meta-analysis.

### 2.5.2 Pooling and interaction

While a meta-analysis combines a large collection of results from the analysis of independent studies for the purpose of integrating the findings, the issue of *poolability* also comes up in all clinical trials which involve more than one investigational site. It is generally assumed that, in a multi-centered clinical trial, all patients are treated under the same protocol with the same endpoints and with the same inclusion/exclusion criteria. Patients are simply pooled together so that statistical power is increased, the trial can be completed in shorter time, and so that it is easier to summarize the results and generalize the findings. This assumes all patients are the same with respect to the prognostic variables. This assumption can be checked by assessing baseline characteristics, particularly those that could be related to outcome. If the patients are not the same, important differences will be missed that could change the study results. Not only could there be differences among the investigational sites, such as differences in standard of care, but there could be differences in other covariates such as gender or age that may affect the results as well. There could be what is known as the presence of an *interaction*. Interaction is a statistical term that means the treatment effect is not the same for all groups defined by some covariate. It is often broken down into two types: *quantitative* and *qualitative*. With a quantitative interaction, the effect has the same direction across all groups, but differs by amount. For example, in a 20-center study, the investigational group may have performed 20% better than the control group at 10 centers and 50% better at the other 10 centers. With a qualitative interaction, the effect differs by direction; for example, the investigational product may have been superior at 12 centers while the control product may have been superior at the other 8 centers. Sometimes the overall result is in favor of one treatment, but there is a significant treatment-by-center interaction that must be further explored. It can be due to differences in physician training, familiarity with the treatment, or differences in baseline characteristics such as geographic region or indication.

Interactions can be detected by a formal statistical test which includes the interaction term in the model. However, this generally has low power since studies are not sized to assess interaction. A non-significant interaction term does not prove there was no interaction. For this reason, it is helpful to also assess outcomes broken down by the relevant groups using descriptive statistics to determine if anything looks odd or unusual. Clinical input should be called upon, as assessing a possible interaction is not solely a statistical decision.

If the data are not deemed poolable, one option is to combine the data but adjust for the variable that might explain the difference. An example would be to include a center effect in the model that should adjust for differences in effects that are due to the centers and not to the treatment. Another option would be a stratified or subgroup analysis, with the strata defined by site or gender, for example. It is important to pre-specify subgroup analyses so that they are not considered exploratory. Otherwise, a confirmatory study or altered indication could be required.

Pooling involves assumptions such as that the same protocol was followed at each site and that the patients are 'exchangeable'. These should be validated by showing comparability of patients and study outcomes across subgroups, whether it is investigational site, gender, age or other relevant covariates. Often foreign data are used to support clinical trials within the USA. Pooling across countries may be justified similarly to pooling across sites within a country. Pooling is best addressed prospectively by limiting the number of centers. It is recommended not to let any one center be too large (preferably <20% of subjects) or too small. If there are a number of centers that have only a few patients, these can be pooled into a 'pseudo-center' for the purpose of statistical analysis. Although the assessment of poolability usually focuses on the investigational sites, other clinically relevant covariates should not be overlooked.

## 2.6    Missing data, intent-to-treat and other analyses cohorts

### 2.6.1    Missing data

Missing data in clinical trial conduct and analysis is, unfortunately, a common problem that is difficult to avoid. Patients drop out, or become lost to follow-up, in which case all subsequent data points are lost. In other cases, a component of a composite clinical success criterion may be missing, such as a radiograph, lab report, or functional score, which makes it difficult, if not impossible, to classify that subject as a success or failure. The analysis can be biased if subjects with missing data are simply excluded. The protocol for any clinical trial should pre-specify how the missing data are to be handled. As a rule of thumb, a study should not have more than 15% loss to follow-up in order to preserve the interpretability of the results. Both the pattern and the balance of missing observations are important. For example, if more controls are missing (i.e., unbalanced missing), and the study was not blinded, the controls may have dropped out because they either were disappointed to receive the control treatment or believed their treatment was not working. This is called non-ignorable missing. If more patients with a particular indication or baseline characteristic (e.g., age) drop out, this would be an example of a missing pattern that requires more evaluation. As a consequence, there are formal definitions of three types of missing data:

> **missing completely at random (MCAR):** missing data are independent of both the observed values and the unobserved (missed) values;
>
> **missing at random (MAR):** missing data are independent of the missed values but depend on observed values (or covariates);
>
> **missing not at random (MNAR):** missing data are not independent of the treatment effect (non-ignorable missing);

There are several methods used to handle missing data in the analysis of clinical trial data. *Simple imputation* imputes a single value for the missing value. It might be obtained from a regression equation, or the mean of two adjacent values. It is not recommended to use the treatment group mean as the imputed value since this reduces the perceived variance and therefore increase chances of spurious significance. A commonly used approach is to impute all missing values as failures (or all missing = success). A '*best case imputation*' would be described as imputing missing outcomes for treated patients as successes and missing outcomes for control patients as failures. Handling missing data this way, however, biases the results in favor of the study intervention. A '*worst case imputation*' is described as imputing the missing treated as failures and the missing controls as successes. This procedure is biased against the study intervention. Often when an intermediate value is missing, *rollback imputation* is used. This would be, for example, rolling back an observed 30-month follow-up to a missing 24-month follow-up. In the case of outcomes such as implant survival, this approach is generally acceptable.

*Multiple imputation* is often the preferred method of imputation. This method imputes a range of values from a selection of probable values weighted by a probability distribution, thus accounting for the variability of missing values. This method requires the assumption that the data are either MAR or MCAR.

*Last observation carried forward* (*LOCF*) is another common method used to impute missing values. It is generally not well received for a number of reasons. It assumes the patient or the treatment effect is stable over time, which is not often the case. It is particularly not advisable when the treatment effect deteriorates over time, such as with a cosmetic wrinkle filler. It underestimates the variance, which gives more chance for a spurious statistically significant result. Only in the case where patients are expected to improve over time would this method be considered conservative.

*Sensitivity analysis* is very helpful in determining the robustness, or tenacity of the study results. This involves performing several sets of analyses under different scenarios for handling missing values, such as those mentioned above. If there is broad agreement in the results obtained using several methods, this provides some assurance that the results are robust to missing-data assumptions. A *tipping point* analysis is a special case of sensitivity analysis. This essentially explores, at a minimum, how many treated successes would need to be switched to failures or control failures switched to successes for the statistical significance to be lost.

Though all these techniques are available to handle missing data, the best approach is to minimize 'missingness' through better trial design and rigorous follow-up methods. For a general introduction to the handling of missing data, see Fuchs and Kenett (2007).

## 2.6.2    Intent-to-treat (ITT) and other analysis cohorts

The *Intent-to-Treat principle* is the method of analysis in clinical trials that groups each participant according to the treatment arm to which they were initially assigned (e.g., experimental therapy, standard therapy, placebo), regardless of whether they actually received that treatment or remained in that arm for the duration of the study. The main advantages are that it preserves the balance of randomization, avoids some biases and optimizes power. The disadvantages include diluting the treatment difference because patients may be analyzed in a group for which they did not receive that treatment, including major protocol violations, and requiring imputation of missing values.

The effect of using an ITT analysis actually varies depending on the type of trial. For a *superiority trial*, where the goal is to show a large treatment difference, performing an ITT analysis where missing values are imputed similarly for both treatment groups (e.g., missing = failure), would render the groups more similar and less likely to show a difference. This type of analysis is considered conservative, but also may result in a false negative (concluding there is no difference when one really exists). On the other hand, in a *non-inferiority trial,* where the goal is to show similarity of treatments, one is more likely to meet that goal when using an ITT analysis because it renders the groups more similar. This is considered 'anti-conservative' and may produce a false positive (i.e., concluding non-inferiority when, in fact, the investigational product is actually inferior). All this depends, however, on how much data are actually missing.

A *per-protocol analysis* is a method of analysis that groups participants according to the treatment they actually received and excludes major protocol violators. The main advantage is that it may reflect the actual performance of the device outside the trial (assuming the numbers of exclusions and mis-randomizations are small). The disadvantages are that the exclusion of patients can render the treatment groups unbalanced with respect to important characteristics (i.e., covariates); that this analysis may be biased if the investigator changes treatment assignment after randomization; and that there can be a loss of power due to exclusion of patients. For patients who have no major protocol violations but have missing data points, one can consider imputation. For a valid per-protocol analysis, one would need a reason to assume the missing data were ignorable, especially if missing data are imputed. Performing both an ITT and per-protocol analysis is one way to check the robustness of the study results.

A *completed cases analysis* groups each participant according to the treatment actually received and only includes the completed cases, disregarding the 'drop outs'. This is one of the riskiest types of analyses. It is biased when missing is not completely at random; that is, the 'missingness' is related to outcome, perhaps due to an adverse event or failed treatment benefit. It disregards information by exclusion of subjects, which sometimes is a considerable proportion of the study sample, and it includes the major protocol violators. Similarly to the per protocol analysis, the completed cases analysis also can compromise the balance of the randomization by analyzing subjects in treatment groups to which they were not randomized.

Another type of analysis cohort falls under the term *modified ITT analysis*. Examples of this would be to exclude patients who were not treated, even if they were randomized; to analyze patients according to treatment received even if there were major protocol violations (i.e., as treated); or to analyze patients according to treatment received provided there was at least one, or some other specified number of follow-up visits (i.e., all 'evaluable' patients). Regardless, it is very important that the analysis cohort be pre-specified in the investigational plan so that the analyses are not considered exploratory.

# 2.7    Multiplicity, subgroup and interim analyses

## 2.7.1    Multiplicity

> Just as the Sphinx winks if you look at it too long, so, if you perform enough significance tests you are sure to find significance even when none exists. *Jerome Cornfield (1976)*

Multiplicity considerations arise in experimental research when it is desired to make inferences about several aspects of a problem from a single study. In clinical studies, these aspects could be: multiple endpoints (primary or secondary), multiple testing of the same endpoint at different time points, multiple treatment comparisons (e.g., three arm study), multiple analyses on the same data, or multiple subgroup testing. Attempting to interpret the results of numerous tests becomes problematic because 5% of the tests (or 1 in 20) will reject the null hypothesis by chance alone if all tests are performed at the 5% significance level; thus resulting in 'spurious significances' (false positives). In other words, one would expect that, on average, if there are 20 null hypotheses rejected, 1 rejection will be a mistake. As a consequence, steps must be taken to adjust the individual significance levels ($\alpha$), or employ other testing procedures to preserve the overall *type I error rate*. These will be discussed further below.

One simple method of significance level adjustment is to divide the desired '*experiment-wise' error rate* (e.g., 5%) by the number of significance tests performed and use the quotient as the adjusted significance level. This is called the *Bonferroni* method. For example, if five tests were being performed on the same data and the desired experiment-wise error rate is 5%, one would perform each test at the 1% level. This method can be considered overly conservative because it does not take into account the dependence among the tests. If the number of tests is large, the significance threshold can become quite small and difficult to attain. The Bonferroni method, as well as the following methods, is most often used to assess a set of secondary endpoints, as the primary endpoint is usually singularly defined. Another method would be a hierarchical testing procedure, which orders the endpoints in order of clinical importance and tests each one at the 5% level. The testing stops when the first non-significant endpoint is found. Two other popular methods are the *Holm's Step Down* procedure and the *Hochberg Step Up* procedure. Rather than adjusting the significance levels, the Holm's method orders the $p$-values from smallest to largest, and then only those $p$-values smaller than the pre-specified overall significance level (e.g., 5%) are considered significant. With the Hochberg procedure, the $p$-values are ordered from largest to smallest. If the largest $p$-value is significant at the pre-specified overall $\alpha$ level (e.g., 5%), all subsequent (smaller) $p$-values would also be significant. If it fails, then the next largest $p$-value is compared to $\alpha/2$. If significant, all subsequent (smaller) $p$-values would also be significant. If not, the next largest $p$-value is compared to $\alpha/3$ and so forth. If the last, let's say '$m$th', $p$-value fails at the level $\alpha/m$, then all comparisons are declared not statistically significant.

Adjustment of the significance level for multiplicity is not always necessary. If there is more than one primary endpoint (e.g., co-primary endpoints) and both have to be met for study success, then each one can be tested at the desired overall significance level (e.g., 5%). If the purpose of an interim analysis is to stop the study early for futility, but not effectiveness, or to re-evaluate the sample size, then adjustment may not be necessary. Adjustment is also not necessary for tests of nested hypotheses (i.e., following a *Gatekeeper* strategy), such as first testing for non-inferiority, and, if met, then testing for superiority. Multiplicity adjustment is not typically done when testing safety endpoints because the adjustment would make it more difficult to detect significances, and would thus be considered anti-conservative.

Analysis of multiple endpoints requires careful planning in terms of the number of endpoints, the study success criteria, the experiment-wise error rate, and the testing procedure for determining statistical significance. Some statistical methods, such as longitudinal data analysis techniques or generalized estimating equations (GEE), can be used for data with repeated measurements over time, or with correlated data. However, it is prudent to design a study so as to avoid multiplicity whenever possible.

## 2.7.2   Subgroup analyses

Subgroup analysis, in the context of the design and analysis of experiments, refers to testing for a statistically significant association or treatment effect in a subset of patients who share a common characteristic. This generally is a baseline characteristic, for example age, gender, disease severity or indication. The researcher might want to know if the treatment effect varies among the different levels of the baseline factor. For example, does the treatment work differently in males versus females, old versus young, NYHA (New York Heart Association) categories, or perhaps rheumatoid arthritis versus osteoarthritis? Labeling for a drug or medical device can be specific to a subgroup, and the claims have to be validated by proper subgroup analyses.

There are several problems associated with subgroup analyses. Multiplicity or multiple testing naturally occurs in subgroup analyses since the analyses usually involve factors with many levels, such as age group or race. This increases the overall probability of a type I error. For example, if four independent subgroups are tested each at the 5% level, there is a 20% chance of falsely finding a significant subgroup. Another problem with subgroup analyses is the phenomenon of regression to the mean. If a subgroup of only patients with extreme values prior to treatment is selected, the mean of their measurements after treatment will be closer to the mean of the whole population due to natural clustering around the mean in the normal distribution. This change should not be interpreted as showing a treatment effect. Statistical power is a third issue with subgroup analysis, as most studies enroll just enough patients to test the primary hypothesis. Therefore, statistical tests on subgroups will only have sufficient power to detect larger effects. By the same token, genuine differences in treatment effect across subgroups may go undetected due to insufficient power.

In order to mitigate the problems inherent in subgroup analyses, it is important to pre-specify the subgroups at the design phase. Otherwise, the subgroup analyses can be considered exploratory and should be validated with a confirmatory study. Sometimes trials are sized for the subgroup analysis. If several subgroups will be tested, the adjustment for multiplicity should also be pre-planned, as should tests for treatment-by-subgroup interactions.

*Post-hoc* subgroup analyses refer to choosing subgroups after looking at the data. This relates back to the 'seek and ye shall find' problem of multiplicity, and they are often done when there is no evidence of an overall effect, in an attempt to salvage a failed study. Some subgroups picked among many will be significant by chance alone. Post-hoc subgroup analysis can be akin to data dredging or data mining. If there is no overall treatment effect, subgroup analyses are risky and should be avoided.

### 2.7.3   Interim analyses

An *interim analysis* is the evaluation of the data prior to the end of the study for the purpose of assessing the treatment effect, site-to-site variability, quality of the data collected, or even for the purpose of sample size re-estimation. It can be done during the enrollment or follow-up phases of the study. The purpose can vary, from wanting to stop the trial early for efficacy, stop for futility, or just to re-assess the assumptions that went into the sample size calculation, such as the expected size of the treatment effect or variability. If the initial assumptions were inaccurate, there is a possibility for sample size re-estimation. To ensure the integrity of trial results, the blind should not be broken and results of the interim analysis should not be disseminated to investigators or patients. A well-designed trial will often have a Data Safety Monitoring Board (DSMB) independent of the study investigators. The DSMB will monitor the occurrence of adverse events.

Because interim analyses involve two or more looks at the data during the course of the study, the problem of multiplicity applies. The experiment-wise type I error rate could be inflated with multiple looks for efficacy, because there will be multiple chances of stopping the trial for success. Taken to the extreme, if one theoretically looked at the data after every patient, there is a very high chance that at some point, due to random variation, there will be a statistically significant effect in favor of the new treatment. That is why any interim analyses must be pre-specified and the type I error rate should be controlled. An interim analysis may be planned for when a pre-specified *proportion* of the study population reaches the final follow-up, such as when 100 of 200 enrolled patients reach the final follow-up evaluation (end of study). Or, it may be planned when the *entire* study cohort reaches an *intermediate time point*, such as when all 200 patients complete one year of follow-up in a two-year study. If the object of the interim analysis is to stop the study early and declare success, then the significance level must be adjusted for multiplicity. If an investigator has no intention of stopping a study early, but just wants an interim analysis to see if the sample size assumptions were on track, then it is not necessary to adjust the significance level. However, if the study was planned as an adaptive design with a possible increase in sample size after the interim analysis, then adjustment may be necessary.

In summary, subgroup and interim analyses are both subject to the problems of multiplicity because they entail multiple looks at the data. Pre-specifying the subgroups and the timing of interim analyses at the design phase along with the pre-planned multiplicity adjustment is necessary for most commonly used study designs.

## 2.8   Survival analyses

In clinical trials assessing therapeutic effectiveness, the ultimate measure of success is patient survival over the study period, or recurrence of morbid events like the relapse of cancer or the rejection of a hip transplant. Often in these trials, the primary endpoints are selected as the event rates of mortality or morbidity, with each patient being recorded as 'success or failure' using a dichotomous variable. The comparison of such event rates of the new treatment to a control treatment could involve statistical methods for two proportions; for example, the two-sample exact binomial test. However, such a simple comparison of whether or not the events happen over the study period ignores the time effect in the treatment process, since the length of observation and the follow-up experience for each subject often differ. For example, in a five-year study for cancer, the primary interest is whether subjects in the new treatment group have higher survival rates than subjects in the control group. A subject who died after one month of receiving the treatment had a much shorter survival time than a subject who died at the five-year endpoint. However, the simple five-year survival proportion comparison will treat both of them exactly the same; that is, as a 'failure'. Furthermore, even though the five-year survival rates of two treatments are the same, the survival experiences for two groups of subjects during the five-year follow-up period can be very different. Figure 2.2 illustrates the survival experiences for the treatment group and control group. Although the survival rates at five years are the same, the treatment group showed a steady decline in survival over the follow-up period, while the control group's survival rate only decreased between years two and three. Therefore, a simple comparison of proportions for the event rates at five years cannot show that the two treatments are comparable. *Survival analysis* is an effective way to assess the entire 'survival' experience during the follow-up period and can be applied to any time-to-event variable, such as time to death or time to failure of a transplanted organ.

*Time to event* (usually denoted as $T$) is defined as the length of time from entry into the study to the occurrence of an event. In a trial where subjects are entered over a period of time and have varying lengths of observation windows, the time-to-event variable is a more informative way to record the whole follow-up throughout the study than a simple dichotomous variable at one specific time point. In clinical trials with time-to-event endpoints, the situation

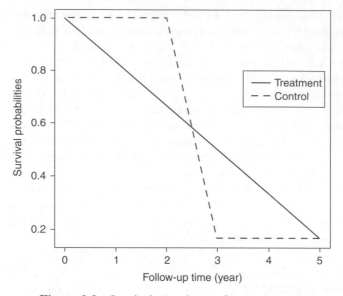

**Figure 2.2**   Survival experiences for two groups.

where a substantial fraction of subjects remain free of events at the end the study could introduce various degrees of incomplete data and make the analysis even more complicated. This type of incomplete information is referred to as *censoring* (or *right censoring* since the true time-to-event exceeds the observed time), and the measured endpoint for those subjects is defined as *time to censoring*. Another type of incomplete data is called *truncation*, when the subject's event time exceeds a known time (left truncation) or less than a known time (right truncation). Time to event, time to censoring and time to truncation are treated differently in survival analysis. The primary interest is the survival function, $S(t)$, defined as the probability that the time to event exceeds a specified time, $t$.

The research on survival analysis emerged in the twentieth century and there have been some enormous achievements over the past century. The developments of the non-parametric *Kaplan–Meier estimator* for estimating a survival curve, the parametric *Cox proportional-hazards model* to account for the effects of covariates in the survival analysis, and the *log-rank test statistic* for comparing two survival experiences have had a most profound impact on clinical trials. A complete and technical review of survival analysis can be found in the recommended Further reading listed at the end of the chapter. This section will briefly introduce some of the most commonly used methods to estimate the survival functions and tests to compare two survival distributions in clinical trials.

## 2.8.1   Estimating survival functions

With the tremendous growth in the field of survival analysis, many complicated methods for estimating survival functions were developed in order to account for different factors, such as continuous covariates, time-dependent variables, multiple events (i.e., competing risks) and random effects. In this section, we will only discuss the two most frequently used methods in clinical trials: the Kaplan–Meier estimator and Cox proportional-hazards model.

**Kaplan–Meier estimator:** also known as the product-limit estimator. In this method, the follow-up time period is divided into small intervals using, for example, the ordered event times as the interval endpoints. For each interval, the probability of surviving through that interval, given that the subject has survived the previous interval, is calculated based on the number of subjects 'at risk' (i.e., alive) at the beginning of the interval and the number of subjects having the event in the interval. Censored subjects in the interval are considered 'at risk', but are excluded from the 'at risk' set in the following intervals. The overall survival is the product of the interval survival probabilities. A major advantage of the Kaplan–Meier estimator is that it takes into account certain types of survival data (e.g., left-truncated and right-censored data) in the calculation of the survival-function estimate. A graphical presentation of the Kaplan–Meier estimator is a series of horizontal steps of declining magnitude which, when a large number of subjects are sampled, approaches the true survival function.

**Cox proportional-hazards model:** if some baseline characteristics such as gender or age differ between groups, investigators may be concerned that the survival functions in each group could be affected by those differences. One way to adjust for these covariate differences is to conduct a stratified survival analysis. For example, for simple stratification with an appropriate number of strata, one could use Kaplan–Meier methods to incorporate the effect of the covariates. However, in cases when there are many covariates, each with several levels, or if the covariates are continuous, a stratified analysis may not be appropriate. There will be too many strata and too few subjects in each stratum. For such cases, Cox proposed a regression model to analyze censored survival data that adjusts for both continuous and discrete covariates in estimating the survival function. Define the hazard rate $h(t)$ as the instantaneous rate of failure (e.g., death or some event) at time $t$. In the Cox model, the hazard rate $h(t)$ is expressed through regression: $h(t) = h_0(t) \exp(\alpha Z + X_1\beta_1 + \cdots + X_k\beta_k)$, where $Z$ is the indicator variable representing treatment groups; $X_1, \ldots, X_k$ are covariates that may affect the survival (e.g., gender, age); and $\beta_1, \ldots, \beta_k$ are the corresponding regression coefficients. The survival function can then be expressed as

$$S(t) = \exp\left(-\int_0^t h(t)\,dt\right).$$

The Cox model is also called the Cox proportional-hazards model since the key assumption for this model is that the hazard rate $h(t)$ is proportional to a baseline hazard rate $h_0(t)$ by a constant factor (i.e., a factor independent of time $t$). This means that deaths or events are assumed not to be clustered, so that failures would not be more prevalent in the early years, for example. This assumption needs to be checked and sometimes may not be valid when some of the covariates (e.g., age) change over time. There are more complicated models that account for time-dependent covariates, which will not be discussed here (see the Further reading section).

## 2.8.2    Comparison of survival functions

We have discussed above how to estimate the survival function for each group. The other central question to ask is whether the two survival functions for a new treatment and a control are statistically different. This question can be assessed by comparing the two estimated survival functions. There are many ways to compare the results depending on different interests. For example, one could conduct a point-by-point comparison if there are some important time points that are clinically meaningful (e.g., five-year survival in cancer trials). Test statistics are developed for point survival comparison, such as a $z$-test. The problems with point-by-point comparisons lie in the multiplicity introduced by multiple looks and interpretation. Take Figure 2.2 as an example. What conclusion should one draw about the new treatment?

Due to the limitations of point comparisons, global comparison methods to test differences between two survival functions were originally proposed by Gehan and Mantel, and have been widely used in clinical trials since. Both the Wilcoxon and log-rank statistics test the hypothesis of whether one survival function is consistently better or worse than the other throughout the follow-up time period. These tests have the most power when the two survival functions are monotonic (i.e., one is greater than the other at all times). Caution should be taken in the interpretation of these tests if the two survival functions cross. Both test statistics can be viewed as a weighted sum of the differences between the observed and expected number of events at all unique event times. There are other test statistics developed to compare two survival functions and they can be found in some text books in the Further reading section at the end of the chapter.

## 2.9    Propensity score

Investigators often aim to make inferences about the causal effects of a new treatment exposure from clinical studies. In randomized studies, it is expected that all observed and unobserved covariates are balanced between treatment groups by the randomization, and that the differences between groups are only due to the treatment effects. However, in observational studies, investigators have no control over the treatment assignments. As a result, treatment groups may be imbalanced with respect to some observed covariates (e.g., age, gender) which may be associated with the treatment assignment and, therefore, may not be directly comparable. A direct comparison between imbalanced groups may result in biased estimation of treatment effects. For example, in an observational study comparing the mortality rate between cigarette smokers and cigar/pipe smokers, a naïve direct comparison between the two groups showed that the mean mortality rate for cigarette smokers is lower than for cigar/pipe smokers (13.5 vs. 17.4 per 1000 person-year). Investigators found that age is associated with both smoking behavior and mortality rate. The mean age in the cigar/pipe group is higher than that in the cigarette group (59.7 vs. 53.2) and the data analysis needs to be adjusted for the confounding of covariate 'age' with mortality. One frequently used method of controlling for covariates is subclassification; that is, grouping subjects into subclasses based on observed covariates, and then directly comparing the treatment groups within each subclass. However, the number of subclasses increases exponentially as the number of covariates increases. Thus, if there are $k$ variables, even if they are all binary there would be a total of $2^k$ subclasses. When $k$ is large, some subclasses would contain few or no subjects, and some may only contain subjects from one treatment group, making it unfeasible to compare treatment effects within certain subclasses.

In 1983, Rosenbaum and Rubin introduced the propensity score as a function of the covariates which aims to balance the distribution of all observed covariates between groups with a single scalar score. For subject $i$ with a vector of covariates ($x_i$), the conditional probability of assigning the subject to a treatment ($Z_i = 1$) versus a control ($Z_i = 0$) is given by the propensity score $e(x_i) = \Pr(Z_i = 1 \mid x_i)$. A logistic regression model is usually used to estimate the propensity score. Intuitively, the propensity score is a measure of the likelihood that a subject would have been assigned to the investigational treatment group based solely on the subject covariates. In a controlled study with a randomization ratio of 1 : 1, the likelihood of a subject being treated is 50%. In an observational study, if a treatment-group subject and a control-group subject have the same propensity score, we could imagine that these two subjects are 'randomly' assigned to each group and have the same distribution of covariates.

A treatment assignment is 'strongly ignorable' if the treatment assignment and the response variable are conditionally independent given the covariates; that is, the relationship between the treatment assignment and the response variable does not depend on the covariates. Rosenbaum and Rubin showed that under a 'strongly ignorable' treatment assignment, if the treatment group and control group have the same propensity score, the difference in means between the two groups is an unbiased estimate of the average treatment effect at that particular propensity score. Because of this property, propensity scores can be used to balance covariates between groups and reduce bias in the estimate of the treatment effect in observational studies.

The rest of this section assumes that the treatment assignment is 'strongly ignorable'. The three most commonly used techniques with propensity scores are matching, subclassification and regression adjustment.

**Matching:** in studies where there are a limited number of treated subjects and a much larger number of potential control subjects, matching is a commonly used sampling technique to produce a control group to 'match' the treated group via similar distributions of covariates. Ideally, matched treated and control pairs would have exactly the same covariates so that their distributions of covariates are identical. When there are many covariates, it is almost impossible to obtain an exact match for each set of covariates. Fortunately, propensity score matching allows the investigator to simultaneously control for all observed covariates through matching subjects on a single scalar balancing score. Rosenbaum and Rubin proved that exact matching on the propensity score guarantees the same probability distribution of covariates for treated and control subjects in matched samples and leads to an unbiased estimate of the average treatment effect. However, even for one scalar score, exact matching is usually not feasible, so an approximate matching, such as 'nearest available matching on the estimated propensity score' must be used.

**Subclassification (also referred to as stratification):** this is another commonly used method to control for differences in covariates between control and treated groups in observational studies. All subjects are grouped into several strata defined by observed covariates. After the strata are formed, treated and control subjects who are in the same stratum are compared directly and an average treatment effect across strata is summarized. Traditional subclassification defines strata using all covariates that are believed relevant, which may result in too many strata when the number of stratifying covariates is large. Again, the propensity score is a very useful tool in such cases. Rosenbaum and Rubin showed that subclassification on the propensity score alone can produce strata where the distribution of all observed covariates in the treated and control groups within strata are balanced and lead to unbiased average treatment effects within strata. Based on Cochran's observation, stratifying on five subclasses can remove at least 90% of the bias. Rosenbaum and Rubin state that Cochran's result applies to propensity score subclassification; that is, creating five subclasses determined by the quintiles of the estimated propensity score can remove at least 90% of the bias in each covariate used to estimate the propensity score.

**Regression adjustment:** this is a third adjustment for confounding covariates in observational studies. The propensity score is a useful variable and can be incorporated into a regression adjustment in simple or multivariate regression models. In the simple regression model, one only needs to adjust the propensity score for the final estimate of the treatment effect. In the multivariate regression model, one first uses all covariates to estimate the propensity score, but then includes only a subset of these covariates and the propensity score in the regression model. One advantage of using the propensity score as a variable in the regression model is that one can use as many covariates as desired to estimate the propensity score without worrying about model over-fitting, instead of building a large model with too many covariates. This smaller model allows the investigator to perform model fit checks more reliably. Under some conditions when the covariance matrices in the treated and control groups are unequal, Rubin showed that regression adjustment may, in fact, increase the expected squared bias. Therefore, one may consider using propensity scores for matching and subclassification, while using regression adjustment with caution.

The propensity score has gained more use in the research of applied medicine, since more investigators turn to observational studies due to increased costs of randomized clinical trials. Propensity score methods work well when there are large numbers of subjects, especially in the control group, and many important covariates are measured. However, propensity score methods can only adjust for observed confounding covariates and have no control over unobserved confounding covariates. Consequently, results can be seriously degraded when important covariates influencing treatment assignment are not included in estimating the propensity score. Propensity score methods lack the discipline and rigor of randomized trials, and do not provide results as reliable as the ones provided by randomized trials. Therefore, randomized trials are still considered as the highest level of evidence for treatment comparison and should be encouraged whenever possible. Propensity score methods should only be thought of as an additional tool to estimate the treatment effects when randomized trials are not available.

# 2.10    Bayesian versus frequentist approaches to clinical trials

Bayesian statistics is a rigorous mathematical approach for learning from evidence as it accumulates. The traditional statistical approach to clinical trials, also called frequentist, may use information from previous studies only at the design stage. Then, at the data analysis stage, the information from previous studies is not part of the formal statistical analysis, although it may be used informally. In contrast, the Bayesian approach uses Bayes' theorem to mathematically combine prior information, possibly from other trials, with current information on the parameter of interest (i.e., effect of a medical treatment). The Bayesian idea is to continuously update prior information with information obtained from the current trial as part of a continual data stream, in which inferences are being updated each time new data become available.

There are several differences between the Bayesian and frequentist approaches:

1. **Interpretations of probability**

   **Bayesians** interpret probability as the measure of one's uncertainty about an unknown state of nature (i.e., parameter). An example of an unknown state of nature (parameter) is the difference in effectiveness between A and B. Consequently, it is natural that probabilities for the same unknown state of nature vary from person to person. For Bayesians, the probability of a parameter changes as information accrues via Bayes' theorem.

   **Frequentists** interpret the probability of an event as the long-run number of times the event happens relative to the total number of observations. In the case of a clinical trial comparing treatments A and B, the probability of A being more effective than B would be interpreted based on numerous repetitions of identical clinical trials comparing A to B. The probability that A is more effective than B is construed as the long-run relative frequency of times in which A performed better than B.

2. **Exchangeability in clinical trials**

   Exchangeability is a fundamental concept in Bayesian inference. In the case of clinical trials, one may have exchangeability of patients or exchangeability of trials.

   **Exchangeability of patients:** in a clinical trial, patients within the trial are usually assumed to be exchangeable or, in lay words, very similar. Under exchangeability, patient outcomes are not expected to depend on the order in which the patients were enrolled or the order in which the outcomes are observed. If patients in the trial are exchangeable with patients in the population from which they were sampled (e.g., the intended-use population), then inferences can be made about the population on the basis of data observed on the trial patients. Thus, the concept of a *representative sample* can be expressed in terms of exchangeability.

   **Exchangeability of trials:** a Bayesian clinical trial can be assumed to be exchangeable with other trials when the other trials are *similar enough* in design and execution to the current trial. The assumption of trial exchangeability enables the current trial to 'borrow strength' from the previous trials, while acknowledging that the trials are not identical in all respects. Exchangeable trials can be thought of as a representative sample of some *super-population* of clinical trials.

3. **Use of prior information**

   **Bayesians** use available prior information and update it with new information using Bayes' theorem. In other words, Bayesians may 'borrow strength' from other clinical studies. A control group may use information from a historical control, a new treatment may use information from similar treatments or, in the case of multi-center trials, information may be borrowed across different centers. When there is *exchangeability* of patients across different trials, prior information may be used completely through a straightforward use of Bayes' theorem. Whenever patients across trials are not exchangeable, but the trials are exchangeable, prior information is used partially via Bayesian hierarchical models.

   **Frequentists** start everything *de novo* and do not use prior information at the analysis stage.

4. **Inferences**

   **Bayesian** inferences are based on the posterior distribution of the parameter of interest. The posterior distribution is obtained from the prior distribution and the data from the clinical trial, via Bayes' theorem. From the posterior distribution one can obtain the posterior mean, mode, median and a credible interval. A 95% credible interval is an interval that contains the unknown state of nature (i.e., parameter) with 95% probability.

   **Frequentist inferences** are based on $p$-values, and confidence intervals. A $p$-value is a product of hypothesis testing. It gives the probability of obtaining the results at least as extreme as those obtained in the clinical trial, assuming that the null hypothesis is true (e.g., treatment is not effective). A small $p$-value indicates that the probability of obtaining the results that were actually obtained, if the treatment were not effective, is small. When the $p$-value is small, one may conclude that the hypothesis that the treatment is not effective should be rejected (see Section 2.2). The interpretation of the 95% confidence interval is different from the interpretation of the 95% credible interval. If the clinical trial is repeated numerous times, the resulting confidence intervals will contain the value of the true parameter 95% of the time and will miss it 5% of the time.

5. **Sample size determination**

   **Bayesians** usually use adaptive designs and the sample size is determined as information accrues (see Section 2.11). Data are collected until the investigator knows enough in order to make a decision (i.e., until the width of the credible interval is small enough). If the variability is small, the sample size will be smaller. If the effect size is large, the sample size will be smaller.

   **Frequentists** guess the variability and the effect size at the design stage, usually based on pilot studies. The sample size is pre-determined based on the guessed variability, effect size, significance level and desired power. It is more difficult, yet possible (see Section 2.11), to modify the sample size in the midcourse of a trial.

6. **Modifications of trials in midcourse (adaptive designs – see Section 2.11)**

   **Bayesians** follow the likelihood principle (Berger and Wolpert, 1988), and modifications of trials in midcourse are natural. If there is a need to control type I error rate for regulatory purposes, or to assess the *operating characteristics* (type I error rate and power) of the experimental design, this is done through simulations. Bayesians will use posterior distributions or *predictive distributions* to make decisions about modifications of trials in midcourse.

   **Frequentists** use statistical techniques to penalize interim looks and use modifications such as O'Brian–Fleming boundaries or $\alpha$-spending functions in order to control type I error rates.

7. **Decision analysis**

   Bayesian posterior and predictive distributions are tailored to perform decision analysis, which does not happen with the frequentist $p$-values.

## 2.11   Adaptive designs

In practice, there is a great deal of uncertainty at the design phase of a clinical trial. The effect size is a conjecture, the variability is unknown and the compliance with the therapy is uncertain. In the case of a long-term study, medical practice may change and such changes may affect the relevant parameters that were used for the study design. As a consequence, investigators may opt for an adaptive or flexible design that allows for learning as the study goes along. An adaptive trial design is a multistage study design that uses accumulating data to decide how to modify aspects of the study without undermining its validity or integrity. Such adaptations should be pre-planned; that is, an adaptive design should be adaptive 'by design' since ad-hoc changes to the trial conduct or analysis could challenge the validity of the results. This section provides an introduction to adaptive design; whereas Chapter 5 is a comprehensive treatment of the subject by Shelley Zacks, who was one of it pioneers. See also Zacks (2009).

## 2.11.1    Sequential designs

The most common type of adaptive design, the sequential design, is a method which consists of several interim analyses. At each interim analysis, the following modifications may occur.

**Sample size re-estimation:** investigators could decide to re-estimate the sample size (increase or decrease) or to increase the length of follow-up of the trial in response to interim estimates of either the variability or the effect size. Designs that allow for such changes are called *internal pilot designs*. During the design phase, one should identify the parameters with greatest uncertainty and select midcourse changes specifically to address those uncertainties.

**Stopping early:** a trial may stop early either for futility or for success. The benefits of stopping early are both ethical and economical. In order to stop early, the probability that the new intervention will or will not show benefit must be computed at an interim look. This probability may be computed through a *Bayesian predictive probability* or through *stochastic curtailment*. The Bayesian predictive probability is the probability of trial success (or failure) given the interim data. Stochastic curtailment will provide the probability of trial success (or failure) conditional on the interim data and on the null or alternative hypothesis.

1. **Stopping early for futility:** this happens when the probability that the new intervention will show benefit at the end of the trial is low.

2. **Stopping early for success:** this happens when the probability that the new intervention will show benefit at the end of the trial is so high that it becomes unethical to continue the trial due to lack of equipoise. Both the patients in the trial and in the public should be able to benefit from the best treatment as soon as possible. Stopping a trial early may allow declaration of success for the primary endpoints, but information on the secondary endpoints may be compromised. This may be problematic particularly when the secondary endpoints are safety endpoints. In that case, stopping the trial early for success may not be possible.

*Group sequential methods* are frequentist methods that deal with the dilemma of repeated interim analyses of the accumulating data by addressing the issue of inflation of the type I error rate due to the multiple looks. These methods consist of several interim analyses with the possibility of stopping for either success or futility. However, each interim analysis will have a nominal significance level for successful stopping that is less than 5% (or other chosen overall significance level), such that the overall nominal significance level will add up to no more than 5%. Bayesians handle the inflation of type I error rate by performing simulations of the trial at the design stage. Based on the simulations, adjustments are made to the stopping criteria for success at each interim look in such a way that the overall type I error rate does not exceed 5%. In other words, for regulatory purposes, the *operating characteristics* (i.e., type I error rate and power) of the adaptive design should be assessed when either frequentist or Bayesian approaches are adopted.

Sequential designs may be perceived as less efficient than the standard fixed-sample design because penalties are paid for multiple looks. However, such small losses in efficiency could be more than compensated for by the benefit of adapting the trial to obtain the maximum amount of information without having to re-start a brand new trial. Such trials may provide a hedge against having poor estimates of effect size or variability at the design stage.

The monitoring of a sequential clinical trial is best viewed as part of the design phase. It provides a flexible sample size calculation that avoids unnecessary sampling while guaranteeing the desired power. Sequential methods are currently widely used in practice, especially in large-scale studies for serious and life-threatening diseases, for which finding the best treatment as soon as possible is of foremost importance.

Several other types of adaptations are also possible:

- changing the allocation or randomization rate (e.g., play-the-winner or drop-the-loser): this aims to increase the probability of assigning the best treatment to most participants of the trial;

- adaptation to incorporate both dose-finding and confirmatory phases in the same study;

- dropping an arm during the course of the study;

- changing or redefining endpoints (primary or secondary) during the course of a study;

- modifying the inclusion/exclusion criteria (i.e., changing the study population);

- switching from a superiority study to a non-inferiority study;

- changing multiplicity adjustment methods for primary or secondary endpoints.

All adaptive studies must be carefully designed and conducted in order to mitigate operational bias. The operating procedures should be well documented, and the details that may reveal evolving treatment differences should be kept unknown to investigators and participants. The interim analyses may generate operational biases that could affect trial integrity and the validity of the results. Such interim looks may introduce:

- **selection bias:** the investigator may decide to assign the current best treatment to his patient independently of the randomization;

- **investigator bias:** the investigator may record the patient as a success if he knows the patient is receiving the treatment that, at the time, is performing better;

- **patient bias:** the patient may believe he is doing better just because he is receiving the treatment that is currently performing better (placebo effect).

In order to avoid operational biases, the clinical study should have third-party investigators perform interim analyses and make sure that firewalls are implemented.

# 2.12   Drugs versus devices

Medical device and drug trials have their differences, despite sharing many common elements that go along with good clinical trial design and analysis practices. *Drug trials* have four formal phases that follow preclinical research: *Phase I* – a small group (~10–50) of (usually) healthy human subjects to determine dose range, tolerability and safety of the drug; *Phase II* – a medium-sized (>50) study on diseased subjects to determine optimal dosing schedule and evidence of safety and effectiveness; *Phase III* – pivotal trials (two or more), usually controlled, randomized and blinded, involving a large number (>1000) of diseased subjects to confirm the efficacy observed in Phase II and compare it to standard treatment; and *Phase IV* – to determine how the drug works in the general population and to observe long-term side effects, safety, efficacy and benefits of the drug outside of the restrictive sample of the clinical trials.

*Medical device trials* also have multiple phases, although not so formally labeled. For therapeutic devices, following preclinical bench or animal testing, there will sometimes be a *feasibility* or *pilot* study on a small number (<30) of diseased subjects to gain information on device safety, size of effect and variability, so that a pivotal study can be better designed and powered. Medical device pilot studies are usually uncontrolled. Following a successful pilot study, a sponsor will usually perform only one *pivotal study*. Sample sizes are often in the range of 100–500 subjects. As a condition of FDA approval, there may be a *post-approval study* required for generally the same reasons as drug licensing requires a Phase IV study. A post-approval study may last for 10 years or more, as they have with breast implants, for example.

Medical device trials have unique challenges that are not found with drug trials. For some devices, such as breast implants for augmentation or reconstruction, randomization is not possible. Sometimes blinding is not possible, for example if one treatment arm is surgical and the other is medical therapy. Further, doctors can see devices on x-rays, and patients can sometimes feel stimulation or pain that would alert them to their treatment group assignment. For this reason, third-party evaluators are often used. Sometimes there is no suitable control, as a sham (or placebo) surgery is not likely to be approved by an *Investigational Review Board (IRB)* due to ethical reasons. In the case of a drug trial, a placebo pill can always be used. Historical controls are used in medical device trials, but this is not without bias. There can be differences in the patient populations with respect to demographics, diagnostic or prognostic factors. There can be a temporal bias in that the standard of care has changed over time. Historical controls often lack *patient-level data*, which limits the capabilities for statistical analysis. The preference is for a randomized, concurrently controlled and blinded study, but this is not always possible with medical device trials.

When medical device trials involve a surgical procedure, there can be a *physician learning curve*, from the administration of a wrinkle filler to a complicated neurosurgical technique. It is not uncommon to have one or two training cases at each site. Physician skill can also differ across investigational sites. *Investigational site effect* must be dealt with in the analysis of the data. *Patient compliance* to treatment regimen is also an issue, and this can result in a lot of missing data. Some medical device trials require frequent trips to the doctor or hospital for administration of the treatment. Even when a device treatment can be administered at home, it is much easier just to take a pill. When dealing with medical device trials, one must balance what is statistically ideal with what is feasible in real life. Fortunately, statistical techniques often allow for controlling or adjusting factors that cannot be controlled in the clinical setting.

# References

Berger, J. and Wolpert, R. (1988) *The Likelihood Principle*, IMS Lecture Notes – Monograph Series, Vol. 6, The Institute of Mathematical Statistics, Haywood, CA.

Cornfield, J. (1976) Recent methodological contributions to clinical trials. *American Journal of Epidemiology*, **104**, 408–421.

Friedman, L.M., Furberg, C.D. and Demets, D.L. (1996) *Fundamentals of Clinical Trials*, Mosby.

Fuchs, C. and Kenett, R.S. (2007) Missing data and imputation, in *Encyclopedia of Statistics in Quality and Reliability* (eds F. Ruggeri, R.S. Kenett and F. Faltin), John Wiley & Sons, Ltd, pp. 1090–1099.

Meinert, C.L. (1986) *Clinical Trails, Design Conduct and Analysis*, Oxford University Press.

Rosenbaum, P.R. and Rubin, D.B. (1983) The central role of the propensity score in observational studies for causal effects. *Biometrika*, **70**(1), 41–55.

Zacks, S. (2009) *Stage-Wise Adaptive Designs*, John Wiley & Sons, Inc.

# Further reading

Armitage, P. and Berry, G. (1994) *Statistical Methods in Medical Research*, Blackwell Science Ltd.

Armitage, P. and Colton, T. (2005) Bayesian methods in clinical trials, in *Encyclopedia of Biostatistics*, Vol. **1** (eds P. Armitage and T. Colton), 2nd edn, John Wiley & Sons, Ltd, p. 338.

Bernardo, J.M. and Smith, A.F.M. (1993) *Bayesian Theory*, John Wiley & Sons, Ltd.

Berry, D.A. (1985) Interim analysis in clinical trials: classical vs. Bayesian approaches. *Statistics in Medicine*, **4**, 497–508.

Berry, D.A. (1996) *Statistics, A Bayesian Perspective*, Duxbury Press.

Berry, D.A. and Stangl, D.K. (eds) (1996) *Bayesian Biostatistics*, Marcel Dekker, New York.

Bland, J.M. and Altman, D.G. (1998) Bayesians and frequentists. *BMJ*, **317**(24), 1151.

Brophy, J.M. and Joseph, L. (1995) Placing trials in context using Bayesian analysis: GUSTO, revisited by Reverend Bayes. *JAMA*, **273**, 871–875.

Carlin, B.P. and Louis, T. (2008) *Bayesian Methods for Data Analysis*, 3rd edn, Chapman and Hall.

Cochran, W.G. (1965) The planning of observational studies of human populations. *Journal of the Royal Statistical Society, Series A*, **128**, 234–255.

Cox, D.R. (1972) Regression models and life-tables. *Journal of the Royal Statistical Society. Series B (Methodological)*, **34**(2), 187–220.

D'Agostino, R.B. (1998) Tutorial in biostatistics: propensity score methods for bias reduction in the comparison of a treatment to a non-randomized control group. *Statistics in Medicine*, **17**, 2265–2281.

DerSimonian, R. and Laird, N.M. (1986) Meta-analysis in clinical trials. *Controlled Clinical Trials*, **7**, 177–188.

FDA (2010) *Guidance for the Use of Bayesian Statistics in Medical Device Clinical Trials*, Department of Health and Human Services, Food and Drug Administration, Rockville, MD.

Gelman, A., Carlin, J.B., Stern, H.S. and Rubin, D.B. (2004) *Bayesian Data Analysis*, 2nd edn, Chapman and Hall, London.

Goodman, S. (1999a) Toward evidence-based medical statistics, 1: the p value fallacy. *Annals of Internal Medicine*, **130**, 995–1004.

Goodman, S. (1999b) Toward evidence-based medical statistics, 2: the Bayes factor. *Annals of Internal Medicine*, **130**, 1005–1013.

Hochberg, Y. and Tamhane, A. (1987) *Multiple Comparison Procedures*, John Wiley & Sons, Inc.

Hosmer, D.W. and Lemeshow, S. (1999) *Applied Survival Analysis: Regression of Modeling of Time to Event Data*, Wiley Series in Probability and Statistics, John Wiley & Sons, Inc.

Irony, T.Z. and Simon, R. (2006) Application of Bayesian methods to medical device trials, in *Clinical Evaluation of Medical Devices, Principles and Case Studies*, 2nd edn (eds K. Becker and J. Whyte), Humana, p. 99.

Kadane, J.B. (1996) *Bayesian Methods and Ethics in A Clinical Trial Design*, John Wiley & Sons, Inc.

Kaplan, E.L. and Meier, P. (1958) Nonparametric estimation from incomplete observations. *Journal of the American Statistical Association*, **53**, 457–481.

Klein, J.P. and Moeschberger, M.L. (1997) *Survival Analysis: Techniques for Censored and Truncated Data*, Springer-Verlag, New York.

Lee, P.M. (1997) *Bayesian Statistics: An Introduction*, John Wiley & Sons, Inc., New York.

Malakoff, D. (1999) Bayes offers a 'new' way to make sense of numbers. *Science*, **286**, 1460–1464.

Mantel, N. (1966) Evaluation of survival data and two new rank order statistics arising in consideration. *Cancer Chemotherapy Reports*, **50**, 163–170.

Molenberghs, G. and Kenward, M. (2007) *Missing Data in Clinical Studies*, John Wiley & Sons, Ltd .

Normand, S.-L.T. (1999) Tutorial in biostatistics: meta-analysis: formulating, evaluating, combining, and reporting. *Statistics in Medicine*, **18**, 321–359.

Piantadosi, S. (2005) *Clinical Trials: A Methodologic Perspective*, 2nd edn, John Wiley & Sons, Inc.

Proschan, M. and Hunsberger, S. (2002) Practical midcourse sample size modification in clinical trials. *Controlled Clinical Trials*, **24**, 4–15.

Rubin, D.B. (1979) Using multivariate matched sampling and regression adjustment to control bias in observational studies. *Journal of the American Statistical Association*, **74**, 318–324.

Senn, S. (2007) *Statistical Issues in Drug Development*, 2nd edn, John Wiley & Sons, Ltd.

Simpson, E.H. (1951) The interpretation of interaction in contingency tables. *Journal of the Royal Statistical Society (Series B)*, **13**, 238–241.

Spiegelhalter, D.J., Abrams, K.R. and Myles, J.P. (2004) *Bayesian Approaches to Clinical Trials and Health-Care Evaluation*, John Wiley & Sons, Inc., New York.

Spiegelhalter, D.J., Myles, J.P., Jones, D.R. and Abrams, K.R. (2000) Bayesian method in health technology assessment: a review. *Health Technology Assessment*, **4**, 38.

Whitehead, J. (1983) *The Design and Analysis of Sequential Clinical Trials*, Ellis Horwood, Chichester.

Whitehead, J. (2005) Sequential methods for clinical trials, in *Encyclopedia of Biostatistics* (eds P. Armitage and T. Colton), 2nd edn, vol. **7**, John Wiley & Sons, Ltd, pp. 4896–4905.

Wittes, J. (2005) Adaptive designs for clinical trials, in *Encyclopedia of Biostatistics* (eds P. Armitage and T. Colton), 2nd edn, vol. **1**, John Wiley & Sons, Ltd, pp. 51–55.

Wittes, J. and Brittain, E. (1990) The role of internal pilot studies in increasing the efficiency of clinical trials, *Statistics in Medicine*, **9**, 65–72.

Yule, G.H. (1903) Notes on the theory of association of attributes in Statistics. *Biometrika*, **2**, 121–134.

# 3

# Pharmacometrics in drug development

**Serge Guzy[1] and Robert Bauer[2]**
[1] *POPPHARM, Albany, CA, USA*
[2] *ICON Development Solutions, Ellicot City, MD, USA*

## Synopsis

In this review, we focus on both theoretical and practical aspects of pharmacometrics. We emphasize the thinking process behind the pharmacometric analysis. After defining the main components of pharmacometrics, we formalize mathematically the engineering-based dynamic processes that characterize most biological systems. The mathematical model includes model parameters that can be estimated once data are observed. This leads us to the introduction of the nonlinear mixed-effect modeling as the statistical modeling approach, which, coupled with optimization procedures like the Monte Carlo expectation maximization algorithm, enables the estimation of the distribution of these model parameters. Finally a case study is presented that shows how pharmacometric analysis was pivotal in deciding the optimal design condition of a Phase 2b study in multiple sclerosis patients.

## 3.1  Introduction

### 3.1.1  Pharmacometrics definition

Pharmacometrics uses models based on pharmacology, physiology and disease for quantitative analysis of interactions between drugs and patients. This involves  pharmacokinetics

---

*Statistical Methods in Healthcare*, First Edition. Edited by Frederick W. Faltin, Ron S. Kenett and Fabrizio Ruggeri.
© 2012 John Wiley & Sons, Ltd. Published 2012 by John Wiley & Sons, Ltd.

(PK), pharmacodynamics (PD) and disease progression with a focus on populations and variability.

Pharmacometrics is emerging as a science that quantifies drug, disease and trial information to aid efficient drug development and/or regulatory decisions. Drug models describe the relationship between exposure (PK), response (PD) for both desired and undesired effects, and individual patient characteristics.

Disease models describe the relationship between biomarkers and clinical outcomes, time course of disease and placebo effects. The trial models describe the inclusion/exclusion criteria, patient discontinuation and adherence. Typically the focus of pharmacometrics has been on drug models, also referred to by terms such as: concentration-effect, dose-response or PK/PD relationships.

## 3.1.2    Dose-response relationship

The PK/PD and/or dose-response relationship describes the change in effect (response) on individuals caused by differing levels of exposure (or doses) after a certain exposure time. Studying dose response, and developing dose-response models, is central to determining 'safe' and 'hazardous' levels and dosages for drugs. This information can help identify an appropriate starting dose, the best way to adjust dosage to the needs of a particular patient, and a dose beyond which increases would be unlikely to provide added benefit or would produce unacceptable side effects. Dose-concentration, concentration- and/or dose-response information is used to prepare dosage and administration instructions in product labeling. In general, useful dose-response information is best obtained from trials specifically designed to compare several doses. Conducting dose-response studies at an early stage of clinical development may reduce the number of failed Phase 3 trials, speeding the drug development process and conserving development resources. It is important to choose as wide a range of doses as is compatible with practicality and patient safety to discern clinically. A widely used, successful and acceptable design, but not the only study design for obtaining population average dose-response data, is the randomized parallel, dose-response study with three or more dosage levels, one of which may be zero (placebo). From such a trial, if dose levels are well chosen, the relationship of drug dosage, or drug concentration, to clinical beneficial or undesirable effects can be defined. Note that a single dose level of drug versus placebo allows a test of the null hypothesis of no difference between drug and placebo, but cannot define accurately the dose-response relationship.

## 3.1.3    FDA perspective of pharmacometrics

The pharmacometric division at the FDA reviews a variety of pharmacometric analysis types including population PK, exposure-response (or PK/PD), biomarker-clinical outcome modeling and simulations, to determine optimal dosing based on benefit–risk assessment, and therefore the need for early interaction between the FDA and sponsors has been emphasized, to plan the development more efficiently. An FDA review was performed in 2006. The authors surveyed fiscal years 1995 and 1996 and found that 23% of NDA submissions contained population pharmacokinetics and/or pharmacodynamic reports [1]. The use of the population approach (population pharmacokinetics/pharmacodynamics) provided useful information for the drug label in 83% of the 47 submissions on safety, efficacy and dosage optimization. However, in 17% of the 47 applications, the use of the approach did not yield any positive impact because the population approach was not integrated into the original plan of the drug development program.

Another review was performed by V. A. Bhattaram [2], where he assessed the role of pharmacometrics in making drug approval and labeling decisions. Cardio-renal, oncology and neuropharmacology drug products divisions were surveyed from 2000 to 2004. About 20% of the studies included a pharmacometric component and, of these, about 50% had pharmacometric analyses which were considered pivotal in regulatory decision making.

The overall conclusion was that population pharmacokinetics should, therefore, be integrated into drug development.

### 3.1.4    When should we perform pharmacometric analysis?

Pharmacometric analyses are designed, conducted and presented in the context of drug development, therapeutic and regulatory decisions. The single-most important strength of such an analysis is its ability to integrate knowledge across the entire development program and compounds, and biology. In drug development, the population approach can help increase knowledge of the quantitative relationships between drug input patterns, patient characteristics, drug disposition and responses. The population approach may be used to estimate population parameters of a response-surface model in Phases 1 and 2b of clinical drug development, where information is gathered on how the drug will be used in subsequent stages of drug development and after release (through the use of estimated population dose-response relationships). The population approach may increase the efficiency and specificity of drug development by suggesting more informative designs and analyses of experiments. The population approach can also be applied to Phases 2A and 3 of drug development to gain information on drug safety (efficacy) and to gather additional information on drug pharmacokinetics (and pharmacodynamics) in special populations, such as the elderly. It is also useful in postmarketing surveillance (Phase 4) studies.

### 3.1.5    Pharmacometric software tools

Five important software packages have been developed to facilitate pharmacometric analysis. These are NONMEM, S-ADAPT, PDx-MC-PEM, MONOLIX and WinBUGS [3,4]. A special section of this review focuses on the characteristics of each of these programs.

### 3.1.6    Organization of the chapter

The chapter is organized as follows: we first define the main components of pharmacometrics. We then review in detail the thinking process behind the pharmacometric analysis. This includes construction of the engineering-based dynamic processes that characterize the system considered, which are obtained by translating the biological processes into a mathematical framework; the nonlinear mixed-effect modeling as the statistical modeling approach to define the distribution of the model parameters (PK/PD); the model formulation; and the optimization procedures, like the Monte Carlo expectation maximization algorithm, used to estimate the distribution of these model parameters. Finally a case study is presented that shows how pharmacometric analysis was pivotal in deciding the optimal design condition of a Phase 2b study in multiple sclerosis patients.

## 3.2    Pharmacometric components

The components of pharmacometrics are pharmacokinetics, pharmacodynamics, disease progressions and trial simulation.

### 3.2.1    Pharmacokinetics (PK)

Pharmacokinetics (PK) includes the study of the mechanisms of absorption and distribution of an administered drug, the rate at which a drug action begins and the duration of the effect, the chemical changes of the substance in the body (e.g., by enzymes) and the effects and routes of excretion of the metabolites of the drug [5].

### 3.2.2    Pharmacodynamics (PD)

Pharmacodynamics (PD) is the study of the physiological effects of drugs on the body, or on microorganisms or parasites within or on the body, and the mechanisms of drug action and the relationship between drug concentration and effect [6].

Pharmacokinetics is often studied in conjunction with pharmacodynamics. Pharmacodynamics explores what a drug does to the body, whereas pharmacokinetics explores what the body does to the drug.

Population pharmacokinetics [7] is the study of the sources and correlates of variability in drug concentrations among individuals who are the target patient population receiving clinically relevant doses of a drug of interest. Certain patient demographic, pathophysiologic and therapeutic features, such as body weight, excretory and metabolic functions, and the presence of other therapies, can regularly alter dose-concentration relationships. For example, steady-state concentrations of drugs eliminated mostly by the kidney are usually greater in patients suffering from renal failure than they are in patients with normal renal function receiving the same drug dosage. Population pharmacokinetics seeks to identify the measurable pathophysiologic factors that cause changes in the dose-concentration relationship, and the extent of these changes, so that, if such changes are associated with clinically significant shifts in the therapeutic index, dosage can be appropriately modified.

### 3.2.3    Disease progression

A disease state is an impairment of the normal state or functioning of the body as a whole or of any of its parts. Some diseases are acute, producing severe symptoms that terminate after a short time, for example pneumonia; others are chronic disorders, for example arthritis, that last a long time; and still others return periodically and are termed recurrent, for example malaria.

The time course of the disease refers to disease progression, which reflects how the disease state changes with time, due to either the natural progression of the disease or to drug intervention (e.g., disease-modifying agents) [8].

### 3.2.4    Simulation of clinical trials

Simulation of a clinical trial can provide a dataset that will resemble the results of an actual trial. Multiple replications of a clinical trial simulation can then be used to make statistical inferences, like estimating the power of the upcoming trial, predicting the expected percentage of the population that should fall within a predefined therapeutic range, and finally proposing optimal trial design conditions based on predefined criteria [9].

## 3.3    Pharmacokinetic/pharmacodynamic analysis

Pharmacokinetic analysis can be performed by either noncompartmental or compartmental methods. Noncompartmental methods [10] estimate the exposure to a drug by estimating the area under the curve of a concentration-time graph. Some important PK parameters are often estimated when performing a noncompartmental analysis and are the following.

1. **Half-life:** the half-life is the time taken for the plasma concentration to fall to half its original value. The symbol is $T_{1/2}$ and the units are time units.

2. **AUC:** the AUC is the area under the plasma concentration-time curve and has the units of concentration by time units.

3. **Clearance:** clearance can be defined as the volume of plasma which is completely cleared of drug per unit time. The symbol is CL and the units are volume units/time units.

4. **Blood volume of distribution:** the blood volume of distribution is the ratio of the total amount of drug in the body and the concentration of drug in blood. The symbol is $V_d$ and it has volume units.

### 3.3.1    Compartmental methods

Compartmental methods [5] estimate the concentration-time graph using kinetic models. The simplest PK compartmental model is the one-compartmental PK model with intravenous (IV) bolus administration and first-order elimination. The concentration-time profile following a single IV dose can be described by equation (3.1):

$$C = \frac{D}{V} \exp\left(-\left(\frac{Cl}{V}t\right)\right), \qquad (3.1)$$

where:

$C$ is the concentration of drug at time $t$. It is defined as the dependent variable.

$t$ is the time and defines the independent variable.

$D$ is the dose and is assumed to be known.

$Cl, V$ are called the model parameters and are usually estimated based on the observed concentrations in a trial.

The most complex PK models (called physiologically-based pharmacokinetic or PBPK models) rely on the use of physiological information to ease development and validation. These so-called 'true' models describe all the dynamic processes that lead to a change in the responses with time (concentration, effect, toxicity etc.) [11]. The PBPK modeling is a mathematical modeling technique for predicting the absorption, distribution, metabolism and excretion (ADME) of a compound in humans and other animal species. PBPK modeling is used often in pharmaceutical research and development. PBPK models are intended to be mechanistic by mathematically transcribing anatomical, physiological, physical and chemical descriptions of the phenomena involved in the complex ADME processes. PBPK models try to rely *a priori* on the anatomical and physiological structure of the body. These are usually also multi-compartment models, but the compartments correspond to predefined organs/tissues, or their components for which the interconnections correspond to blood or lymph flows, transfer across endothelium or across cell membrane. A system of differential equations can still be written, but its parameters represent blood flows, pulmonary ventilation rate, organ volumes and so on, for which information is available in scientific publications.

However, in general not enough data are available to estimate accurately the population variability in the model parameters that characterize these complex systems. In addition, these models are usually fitted to the observed data with most of the model parameters fixed. Interestingly enough, most of the drugs can have their PK described and estimated accurately using fitting procedures with the use of only one, two or three compartments, although the real biological system is comprised of a large number of compartments (organs).

Compartment-free methods are useful to describe the data in that they do not assume any specific compartmental model, but do not have the prediction power of the compartmental approach. In this review, we will concentrate only on the compartmental approach applied to a population of individuals, from which the 'population PK/PD modeling' term has been derived.

## 3.4 Translating dynamic processes into a mathematical framework

The compartmental analysis [12] approach allows one to easily write a mass balance for the drug amount (or concentration) at any time. The main processes that lead to a change in the amount(concentration) of drug in blood with time are absorption of the drug into the blood stream (applies to any extravascular drug input), distribution of drug into tissue and return from tissue to blood, binding to receptors sites, and elimination of drug through either excretion or by metabolism (Figure 3.1) [6]. As an example, let us assume that the drug is given through an IV infusion (accesses blood stream instantly) and that the drug is immediately mixed into the blood stream and then eliminated by a first-order process (excretion by first-order kinetics). First-order kinetics means that the rate of change of drug concentration by any process is directly proportional to the drug concentration remaining to

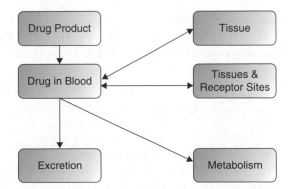

**Figure 3.1** Schematic representation of main drug disposition processes.

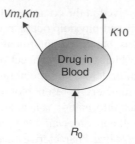

**Figure 3.2**  The one-compartment model with IV infusion input ($R_0$) and first-order elimination (rate $K10$), and Michaelis–Menten elimination ($Vm$, $Km$).

undertake that process. Figure 3.1 can therefore be simplified into Figure 3.2, where the only processes involved are the IV infusion dosing and first-order elimination of the drug.

These processes occur simultaneously and lead to a change in the drug concentration ($C$) in blood with time ($t$). The idea of mass balance resides in looking at the change in drug concentration with time ($dC/dt$) within a very small time window ($\Delta t$). We want to predict how these processes will result in a new concentration at the end of that time window: $C_{new} = C_{old} + dC/dt$. We know $C_{old}$ (initial concentration which is 0), and therefore computing $dC/dt$ will allow determination of $C_{new}$, with $C_{new} = C_{old} + dC/dt$.

This equation, $dC/dt$, is a differential equation. We now go from the processes identification to the mathematical formulation using the differential equation setting (3.2).

$$\frac{dC}{dt} = +R_0 \qquad - K10 \cdot C, \tag{3.2}$$

Infusion (drug in)    first-order linear elimination (drug out)

where $C = 0$ ($C_{old}$) at $t = 0$.

Because the $\Delta t$ is small, we can hold $C$ constant for the calculation in (3.2), and the new $C$ can now be determined at the new $t$.

$$C_{new} = C_{old} + \frac{dC}{dt}.$$

For most of the systems where linear kinetics apply, it is possible to integrate the differential equation and get an analytical solution for the concentration-time profile. For example, the integrated form of the one-compartment model with constant IV infusion and first-order elimination is given by equation (3.3):

$$C = \frac{R_0}{VK10}[1 - \exp(-K10 \cdot t)],$$

with:

$R_0$ = rate of infusion in mass units per unit of time

$V$ = volume of distribution in volume unit (for example ml)       (3.3)

$K10$ = elimination rate constant in per-units of time (e.g., 1/hour)

$t$ = time.

Although very simple, the above example helps translate more complex biological processes into a mathematical framework by defining the appropriate differential equation settings that can be integrated to give the predicted response(s) at any time.

## 3.5   Nonlinear mixed-effect modeling

This approach considers the population study sample, rather than the individual, as a unit of analysis for the estimation of the distribution of parameters and their relationships with covariates within the population. Analysis according to the nonlinear mixed-effects model provides estimates of population characteristics that define the population distribution of the PK and/or PD parameters. The collection of population characteristics is composed of population mean values (derived from fixed-effects parameters) and their variability within the population (generally the variance-covariance values derived from between-subject random-effects parameters). The fixed component is what is common among the individuals and can be associated with the population mean. The between-subjects random components are terms specific to each individual and therefore allow differentiation between one individual and another. Another type of random effect often estimated during a population analysis accounts for changes of a model parameter within an individual. We refer to it as the 'inter-occasion random effect'. Finally, observed concentrations are also subject to error and define random effects occurring at the observation level.

Nonlinear mixed-effect modeling [13,14] is indeed the most common statistical model used in population analysis. It uses one-stage analysis that simultaneously estimates all parameters (e.g., fixed effect parameters, inter-individual variability, inter-occasion variability and measurement errors).

## 3.6   Model formulation and derivation of the log-likelihood

So far, we have learned about how to translate the biological processes into a mathematical framework which lead us to the generation of a PK/PD model which includes the response(s) as dependent variables, the time as independent variable and the model parameters. The observed response also has two components: the predicted model-based response and the measurement noise. The PK/PD model parameters have both fixed (that can be covariate-controlled) and random components, but are usually unknown while the responses are observed at different times and for different dosing conditions. The question now is how to estimate the fixed effects (population means), the random effects (population variances and covariance) and also the measurement noise (usually assumed to be normally distributed around each predicted response with its standard deviation modeled as a function of the predicted responses) [15]. In order to provide the population characteristics given the response data, we need to define a criterion that when increasing or decreasing reflects better or worse fit. This criterion is called the 'objective function'. An objective function value measures the statistical distance between the model predictions and the observations. Examples of objective functions are sums of squares, and likelihood functions. Given the data, you will try to find the best set of population means, variances and error-variance-based model parameters that best explain the data. This search is called an optimization procedure. The optimization procedure is a process of finding that estimate of the sets of parameters that maximizes/minimizes the objective function. If the objective function reflects a probability, you will try to maximize it, while reflection of a distance will lead to a minimization. We often use the $-\log(\text{likelihood})$ with the likelihood linked to a probability, and, since we are using the negative of it, we will have to minimize that objective function. The use of the logarithmic function is only for numerical convenience as it does not change the final estimate of the model parameters.

We will concentrate in this review mainly on the maximum likelihood methods. In order to do so, we must first formulate our model, the objective function to be optimized and then the different methods of optimization.

Data from a subject consists of measured responses at selected times after administration of a drug, such as drug concentration in plasma, and/or some measure of pharmacodynamic response. A PK/PD model $f(t, \theta)$ is proposed to describe the changes in response with time $t$, where $\theta$ is a vector of individual parameters, such as volume of distribution, clearance and so on. A specific function is proposed for each response type, one for drug levels, another for PD response, another for efficacy and so on. Typically, the subject's data is modeled to include intra-subject error as follows:

$$y_i = f(t_i, \theta) + G^{1/2}(t_i, \theta)\varepsilon \qquad (3.4)$$

where $y_i$ is an $m_i \times 1$ vector of the $m_i$ total data collected at times $t_i$ for subject $i$; $f(t_i, \theta)$ is an $m_i \times 1$ vector of predicted values based on the family of essential PK and PD functions $f(t, \theta)$ specific for each data point; $G(t_i, \theta)$ is an $m_i \times m_i$ matrix of modeled (based on predicted values $f(t_i, \theta)$) residual variances and covariances to the data $y_i$; and $\varepsilon$ is an $m_i \times 1$ vector of random values, normally and independently distributed with mean 0 and variance 1. The negative logarithm of the joint probability density for all of the $m_i$ data points for subject $i$, not including a constant term, is then (suppressing notation showing dependence on $t_i$ and $\theta$):

$$-\log(l(y_i|\theta)) = \frac{1}{2}(y_i - f_i)'G_i^{-1}(y_i - f_i) + \frac{1}{2}\log|G_i|. \qquad (3.5)$$

where we shall designate $l(y_i|\theta)$ as the likelihood or data density for data vector $y_i$ of subject $i$, given model parameters $\theta$.

In turn, the variability of the vector of parameters $\theta$ among the population is also assumed to be normally distributed, or perhaps some simple transformation of the parameters is normally distributed (such as via logarithmic transformation), with population mean vector $\mu$, and population variance matrix $\Omega$. The negative logarithm of the probability density of a given $\theta$ is therefore, not including a constant term,

$$-\log(h(\theta|\mu, \Omega)) = \frac{1}{2}\log|\Omega| + \frac{1}{2}(\theta - \mu)'\Omega^{-1}(\theta - \mu) \qquad (3.6)$$

where we shall designate $h(\theta|\mu, \Omega)$ as the parameter population density for $\theta$, given $\mu$ and $\Omega$. Then, the joint probability density for some vector $\theta$ and a set of data $y_i$ is

$$p(y_i, \theta|\mu, \Omega) = l(y_i|\theta)h(\theta|\mu, \Omega). \qquad (3.7)$$

For a particular subject, the data $y_i$ are observed and therefore fixed throughout the analysis; whereas the parameter vector $\theta$ describing the pattern in the data is unknown (and therefore considered 'missing' in some discussions of the expectation-maximization algorithm) but imputable, based on the model and the observed data. It is therefore best to consider all possible values of $\theta$, taking into consideration the probability of occurrence of each $\theta$ for the particular population in question. To do so, we integrate the density over all possible $\theta$, producing the following contribution of the objective function by subject $i$:

$$L_i = -\log(p(y_i|\mu, \Omega)) = -\log\left(\int_{-\infty}^{+\infty} l(y_i|\theta)h(\theta|\mu, \Omega)d\theta\right), \qquad (3.8)$$

which is the negative logarithm of the marginal density of the data $y_i$ for subject $i$, up to a constant. The negative logarithm of the joint marginal density for all $m$ subjects is then

$$L = -\log(p(y|\mu, \Omega)) = \sum_{i=1}^{m} L_i = -\sum_{i=1}^{m} \log\left(\int_{-\infty}^{+\infty} l(y_i|\theta)h(\theta|\mu, \Omega)d\theta\right), \qquad (3.9)$$

where $L$ is the total objective function.

## 3.7  Review of the most important pharmacometric software characteristics

The latest versions of the three programs NONMEM (NONMEM7), PDx-MC-PEM and S-ADAPT currently use a newly implemented method called the 'Monte Carlo parametric expectation maximization' algorithm or MCPEM. Therefore, we will review the MCPEM algorithm in detail, while referring to other papers for the other algorithms such as SAEM or Bayesian methodologies [4].

### 3.7.1  NONMEM

The gold standard, NONMEM, is distributed by ICON/Globomax [16]. Users may select from predefined models, or write their own by inserting Fortran-type code in the control stream file. The code may describe analytical model functions, or differential equations, which NONMEM then presents to its numerical integration routine. Furthermore, the population parameters may be modeled as a function of covariates such as gender, age, creatinine clearance and so forth, using a syntax that represents the statistical basis of the model. The latest version of NONMEM includes both deterministic (FO (first-order), FOCE (first-order conditional estimation) and Laplacian) and stochastic (MCPEM, SAEM and Bayesian) methods for population analysis, making it currently the most versatile software.

### 3.7.2  PDx-MC-PEM

PDx-MC-PEM is a program written by Serge Guzy and distributed by ICON/Globomax (Ellicott, MD) that provides population analysis using direct and importance sampling Monte Carlo expectation maximization methods. A user-friendly interface is provided from which the user may select predefined PK and PD models. The user may also create his own PK/PD models. While a Fortran compiler is not needed for the predefined models, the user-defined Fortran model file must be compiled by Intel Fortran, Compaq Fortran, or gfortran, a freeware compiler supplied with PDx-MC-PEM. With the user-defined feature, the versatility of the types of PK and PD models one can build in PDx-MC-PEM is extended considerably, including models defined by differential equations. Diagnostic goodness-of-fit plots may easily be obtained, and the progress of the analysis can be monitored by a running plot of the objective function versus iteration number. The intersubject variance may be defined as a normal or log-normal distribution.

### 3.7.3    MONOLIX

MONOLIX implements an algorithm that combined the stochastic approximation expectation maximization (SAEM) with a Markov chain Monte Carlo procedure for maximum likelihood estimation of the PK/PD parameters in nonlinear mixed-effect models without any linearization techniques. At each iteration, only one to five random samples per subject are simulated (expectation step). Markov chains are used to generate these samples, and the likelihood ratio between two subsequent samples is used to accept or reject the new sample that was generated. This is performed for about 200 iterations and is called the burn-in period. There is no integration at each iteration as in MCPEM, where we simulated many random vectors and estimated the full individual posterior distributions. Thereafter, at each subsequent iteration, the maximization step is then used to update the population mean and variance, but the program accumulates random sample results among the next 300 iterations, to obtain a more precise estimate of the population means and intersubject variances. The advantage of the SAEM is the speed compared to MCPEM. On the other hand, the main disadvantage is that it does not have the same driving force toward the maximum as MCPEM. MCPEM works better for complex PK/PD models.

### 3.7.4    WinBUGS

WinBUGS has implemented a full Bayesian technique employing three-stage hierarchical analysis. To each population parameter (population means and population variance-covariance matrix) is also associated a distribution from which the sampling occurs (these are called hyper priors). Therefore the programs simulate many population means and many variance covariance matrices and then use the data to estimate the relative likelihood that these distributions explain the data. The advantage is that it provides in one step not only a single estimate of the population mean and variances but a full distribution for all these relevant population parameters. The disadvantage is again the lack of driving force for complex PK/PD models. Therefore, in the WinBUGS program, not just a single best-fit population parameter set is provided, but rather a collection of several thousand population parameter sets is reported, clustered in proportion to their likelihood of representing the data. Descriptive statistics of the collection of representative parameters may then easily be obtained, such as mean, variance, covariance between any two parameters, and quantile ranges (such as 2.5%, median, 97.5% levels). There is no maximization procedure but only a big expectation step.

### 3.7.5    S-ADAPT

S-ADAPT is a Fortran 95 open-source, free program distributed by the University of Southern California, Biomedical Simulations Resource department (USC, BMSR). The S-ADAPT program was developed by R. Bauer as an extension of the ADAPT II PK/PD modeling software provided by USC, BMSR, and has been successfully used to analyze clinical data for Raptiva (efalizumab), consisting of 6 differential equations and 16 model parameters.The S-ADAPT program is designed for the advanced PK/PD modeler who likes to have an interface with complete access to all variables and actions at run-time. It also has extensive simulation tools. It is the most flexible and interactive program based on the current available software. It provides population analysis using direct sampling, importance sampling, stochastic expectation maximization and full Bayesian approaches. In addition, it has a built-in scripting capability that allows the user to perform different tasks one after the other. Finally it has parallel processing capabilities, as it allows the dataset to split across multiple computers or CPUs during the expectation step. Once the expectation step is completed, the information from each computer (or CPU) comes back to the central computer which performs the maximization step. Then the split is performed at the next iteration again during the expectation step. If, for example, six computers are available, S-ADAPT will run the same problem almost six times faster than it would be analyzed with only one computer (or CPU).

## 3.8    Maximum likelihood method of population analysis

A detailed description of the different maximum likelihood methods of population analysis can be found elsewhere [4, 15]. We focus here on one of the most powerful maximum likelihood method, the Monte Carlo parametric expectation maximization (MCPEM) method. The MCPEM algorithm is based on the expectation maximization (EM) algorithm [17]. The EM algorithm is used for finding maximum likelihood estimates of parameters in probabilistic models, where the model depends on unobserved latent variables (the population means and variances). The idea of the MCPEM method is very intuitive. As a first step, we choose a prior set of population means and variances for each of the model parameters (for example, mean and variance for clearance and volume). We start the algorithm implementation with the data coming from the first individual, and sample one set of model parameters (e.g., one clearance and volume value) from the above prior distributions. The likelihood (proportional to the probability) that this set of model parameters explains the observed data for that first individual is calculated. The same process is then repeated ($n_r$ times), each time with a different set of sampled model parameters. At the end of this first step, we have stored $n_r$ likelihood values for that individual. We then divide each of the stored likelihoods by the sum of all the $n_r$ likelihoods, leading to a weighting function (bounded between 0 and 1) associated with each of the sampled model parameters. The same steps are then performed on all the remaining individuals. This is called the expectation step. At the end of the expectation step, the knowledge of the $n_r$ weighting values for each individual allows one to estimate a distribution for each individual. These distributions are called the individual posterior distributions. The set of means and variances (more exactly variance-covariance) associated with the individual $i$ posterior distribution are denoted $\bar{\theta}_i$ and $\bar{B}_i$, respectively. The next step is called the maximization step and allows the updating of the prior distributions to new values that are probabilistically better than our initial guesses.

It can be shown that, if the parameter population density is of the form of a multivariate normal distribution with respect to $\theta$, (or some transformation of $\theta$), then the updated population means ($\mu$) can easily be calculated by just averaging the individual distribution means ($\bar{\theta}_i$)

$$\mu = \frac{1}{m} \sum_{i=1}^{m} \bar{\theta}_i, \qquad (3.10)$$

and the population variance-covariance matrix is updated using the following equation (3.11):

$$\Omega = \frac{1}{m} \sum_{i=1}^{m} \bar{\Omega}_i,$$

(3.11)

with:

$$\bar{\Omega}_i = (\bar{\theta}_i - \mu)(\bar{\theta}_i - \mu)' + \bar{B}_i$$

(3.12)

The only difference between the standard EM algorithm and the MCPEM algorithm is in the way the individual posterior distributions are estimated. The MCPEM method relies on stochastic simulation of model parameters, while the standard EM algorithm estimates these distributions using a pure deterministic algorithm [17].

# 3.9   Case study: Population PK/PD analysis in multiple sclerosis patients

The sponsor is working on the development of a drug believed to inhibit some protein expression, which would result in a therapeutic benefit in treating human diseases characterized by aberrant cell trafficking and local tissue damage, such as multiple sclerosis (MS) [18].

MS patients show areas of demyelination (lesions or plaques) that can be detected using magnetic resonance imaging (MRI) of the brain and spine. Gadolinium can be administered intravenously as a contrast, to highlight active plaques called T1 lesions. These plaques are generated and then disappear after some time. The disease is defined as progressing when the average number of T1 lesions increases over time. Therefore the drug is intended to decrease T1 lesion progression. The cumulative number of T1 lesions, which is the clinical response of interest, is defined as the sum of T1 lesions from the first to the last selected observation times. Since the cumulative number of T1 lesions depends heavily on the choice of observation times, we first modeled the time course of T1 lesions and then calculated the corresponding cumulative number for any desired sampling-time schedule.

Clinical data were obtained from a subcutaneous (SC)/IV Phase 2a human data study. Based on that study, both the time course of T1 lesions and side effect as reflected by drug-related platelet count reduction were modeled and linked to the pharmacokinetics of the drug.

## 3.9.1   Study design

The patient population was divided into two cohorts, with the first including 40 patients that were dosed subcutaneously with three 'induction' doses of 200 mg of the drug each on days 1, 4 and 7 of the study and then a 'maintenance' dose regimen of 200 mg twice a week (days 4 and 7 of the week) for seven weeks. The second cohort had 40 patients with SC placebo injections according to the schedule of Cohort 1. The duration of the study was 16 weeks: 8-week treatment period (first week induction phase followed by 7 weeks maintenance period) followed by 8 weeks without treatment. There were four visits (Day 1, 28, 56 and 112) where PK measurements were taken. On these days, six samples were collected as follows: one

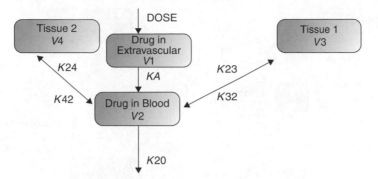

**Figure 3.3** Schematic representation of the PK processes, assuming a three-compartment model. *Kij* is the transfer rate of drug from compartment *i* to compartment *j*. *K*10 is the elimination rate constant from the plasma compartment. *Vk* is the volume of distribution corresponding to compartment *k*. *KA* is the absorption rate.

sample before administration of medication and after 1, 2, 3, 4 and 6 hours post-dose. MRI measurements were on Day 28, 56, 84 and 112.

### 3.9.2 Model building

A population PK/PD (platelet)/efficacy (T1 as clinical response for multiple sclerosis) model was developed in order to link between the PK dynamics and the associated platelet level suppression as well as the corresponding calculated reduction in the cumulative number of T1 lesions over the study period.

### 3.9.3 The PK model

The PK model was characterized by a three-compartment model with linear kinetics and SC route of administration (Figure 3.3).

### 3.9.4 Platelet modeling

The Platelet suppression was quantified using an indirect response model with the production of platelets assumed to be inhibited by the drug (Figure 3.4).

### 3.9.5 T1 lesions model

A Poisson regression model was linked to the PK model in order to quantify the correlation between the number of T1 lesions and PK time profiles. The T1 analysis used a population mixture model to separate the active from inactive patients with respect to T1. The cumulative number of T1 lesions was then derived directly from the T1 predictive model (Figure 3.5).

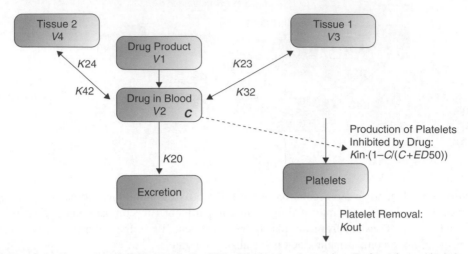

**Figure 3.4** Processes defining both the PK and platelet dynamics. Before drug administration, platelets are produced at a constant rate ($K$in) and removed at a rate ($K$out) proportional to the platelet concentration. Once the drug is given, the production of platelets is inhibited, leading to a temporal suppression of the platelet concentration. $ED50$ is the drug concentration at which the platelet inhibition is half *Emax*, where *Emax* is the maximum inhibition in the production of platelets.

## 3.10    Mathematical description of the dynamic processes characterizing the PK/safety/efficacy system

Equations (3.13) to (3.20) comprise all the processes that lead to a dynamic time change of the drug concentration and responses with time. This includes: the first-order transfer of the drug from the extravascular compartment to the plasma compartment; the absorption of a

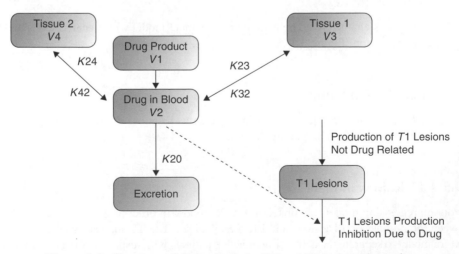

**Figure 3.5**    Processes defining both the PK and T1 lesions dynamics.

fraction of the drug $(F. A(1))$ from the extravascular to the plasma compartment; the first-order transfer rate of the drug from plasma to both tissue compartments and from both tissues back to plasma; the mass balance in both tissue compartments which is characterized by first-order transfer of the drug from plasma to tissues and back from tissue to plasma; finally the two mass balances for the responses, T1 lesions and platelets. The T1 lesion time profile is assumed to follow a linear relationship with time (constant slope $\alpha$), but with that slope being reduced by the drug through an $Emax_{T1}$ model ($Emax_{T1}$ is the maximum change in slope). The initial condition is $t = t_0$, $A(5) = \alpha \cdot t_0 +$ intercept, and is derived for each patient by plugging the first recorded time $(t_0)$ into that equation for a given slope and intercept value. Finally the platelet mass balance includes the natural production of platelets that is assumed to occur at a constant rate, the inhibition of this production rate by the drug through an $Emax$-type model, and the natural removal of the platelets by a first-order process. The initial conditions assume steady state before drug administration, which lead to the initial platelet counts being equal to the ratio of the placebo production rate $(Kin)$ to the elimination rate $(Kout)$.

SC compartment:

$$\frac{dA(1)}{dt} = -K01 \cdot A(1). \tag{3.13}$$

Plasma compartment:

$$\frac{dA(2)}{dt} = K01 \cdot A(1) \cdot F - K20 \cdot A(2) - K23 \cdot A(2)$$
$$+ K33 \cdot A(3) - K24 \cdot A(2) + K42 \cdot A(4). \tag{3.14}$$

The concentration of drug in plasma is then given by $C = A(2)/V2$, $V2$ being the volume of distribution of the plasma compartment.

Peripheral tissue 1:

$$\frac{dA(3)}{dt} = K23 \cdot A(2) - K32 \cdot A(3). \tag{3.15}$$

Peripheral tissue 2:

$$\frac{dA(4)}{dt} = K24 \cdot A(2) - K42 \cdot A(4). \tag{3.16}$$

Mass balance for the number of T1 lesions: $A(5)$ is the logarithm of the Poisson mean. The rate of change of $A(5)$ is assumed to be a constant $(\alpha)$ for placebo (constant slope), while the slope is affected by the drug through a Michaelis–Menten equation type.

$$\frac{dA(5)}{dt} = \alpha \cdot \left( 1 - Emax_{T1} \cdot \frac{C}{C + ED50_{T1}} \right), \tag{3.17}$$

where $Emax_{T1}$ is the maximum inhibition in the production of platelets, $ED50_{T1}$ is the drug concentration at which the platelet inhibition is half $Emax_{T1}$, and with the corresponding initial conditions:

$$t = t_0, \quad A(5) = \alpha \cdot t_0 + \text{intercept}, \tag{3.18}$$

with $t_0$ being the first recorded time for each patient, and intercept being the value of $A(5)$ at $t = 0$.

Mass balance for platelets: $A(6)$ is the platelet counts.

$$\frac{dA(6)}{dt} = Kin \cdot \left(1 - Emax \cdot \frac{C}{C + ED50}\right) - Kout \cdot A(6), \tag{3.19}$$

where *Emax* is the maximum inhibition in the production of platelets, *ED50* is the drug concentration at which the platelet inhibition is half *Emax*, and with the corresponding initial conditions:

$$t = 0, \quad A(6) = \frac{Kin}{Kout}. \tag{3.20}$$

(For more on Michaelis-Menten kinetics see Kenett, 1978, Kenett, 1979 and Karlin and Kenett, 1980)

### 3.10.1   Optimization procedure and Phase 2b simulation procedures

The parameters of the model were estimated using a powerful optimization methodology (MCPEM) implemented in the PDx-MC-PEM [4] program, and were used to simulate the expected PK/PD/efficacy time profiles for different potential dosage regimen scenarios. The simulation strategy served as guidance for optimally designing the next Phase 2b study with respect to both safety and efficacy, as well as to justify the selection of the dosing groups for the next trial.

### 3.10.2   Clinical simulation results and discussion

The Phase 2b tentative design is a six-month treatment period, with two to three dose groups and placebo. MRI would be observed once a month, with the primary endpoint being the percentage reduction in the average cumulative number of T1 lesions (starting on Month 4 and cumulated every month until Month 7), relative to placebo. The optimal regimen would have preferably the following characteristics:

at least 60% reduction of cumulative T1 lesions compared to placebo;

platelets: not more than 10% of subjects $<150$ ($\times 10^9$/l) at any time, 5% of subjects $<100$ ($\times 10^9$/l) at any time, and no subject $<50$ ($\times 10^9$/l) at any time.

The doses to be explored are 100 mg, 200 mg and 400 mg, with dosage intervals varying from weekly to every four weeks. The goal of the simulation exercise was to have insight into the following issues.

What dosing regimens can provide the required outcome based on the boundaries of MRI detection and acceptable platelet counts?

What is the outcome simulating the predefined regimens?

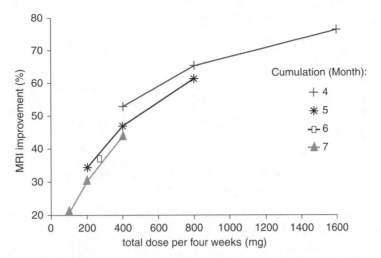

**Figure 3.6** Percentage MRI improvement vs. total dosing per four weeks, for dosage intervals between 1 and 4 weeks: MRI cumulated on Month 4, 5, 6 and 7.

### 3.10.3   Calculation of the cumulative number of T1 lesions and the percentage MRI improvement

The PK/PD model was used to predict, on Month 4–7, the expected average number of T1 lesions. Therefore, the cumulative number of T1 lesions for the treated group is simply calculated by just summing up the number of T1 lesions starting on Month 4, until Month 7. We call it cum_T1_drug. The same calculation proceeds for the placebo group (same model with a zero dose). We call it cum_T1_placebo.

The percentage MRI improvement (%MRI) is directly computed using the following formula:

$$\%\mathrm{MRI} = (\mathrm{cum\_T1\_placebo} - \mathrm{cum\_T1\_drug})/\mathrm{cum\_T1\_placebo} \times 100.$$

(See Figure 3.6.)

### 3.10.4   Estimation of the percentage of patients to reach platelet counts below a certain threshold value

The PK/PD model characteristics include the PK/PD average parameters as well as the parameters quantifying the variability across the population. The average and variability information can be used to simulate hypothetical patients that would behave similarly to the actual population for any specific dosage regimen. We simulated a large number of patients and recorded the platelet counts for each of them at the expected measurements times (usually predose). Each patient that had at least one recorded platelet count less than X (X being either 150, 100 or 50) was considered as passing the threshold value. The percentage of patients

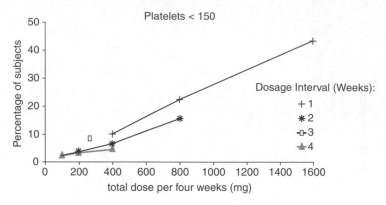

**Figure 3.7**   Percentage of subjects with platelets <150 versus total dose per four weeks, and dosage interval (1, 2, 3 and 4 weeks).

passing the specific threshold value at least once was then plotted versus the total dosing per four weeks for different dosage intervals (see Figures 3.7, 3.8, 3.9).

### 3.10.5   Tentative proposal for the Phase 2b trial design

The above graphs lead us to the following conclusions. PK and platelet time profiles are highly correlated. The only safety concerns are with the percentage of patients expected to have platelet counts <150, which is larger than 10% for a total dose per 4 weeks exceeding 400 mg. However, 200 mg every week (800 mg per 4 weeks) should not lead to more than 5% of the population with platelet counts <100. Therefore, for the tentative Phase 2b trial design, we have one arm with 200 mg every week with safety concerns only for platelet counts <150 (about 20% of the population), but less than 5% of the population will have platelet counts <100 for that regimen. MRI reduction is expected to be about 60%.

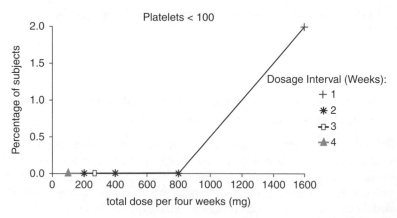

**Figure 3.8**   Percentage of subjects with platelets <100 versus total dose per four weeks, and dosage interval (1, 2, 3 and 4 weeks).

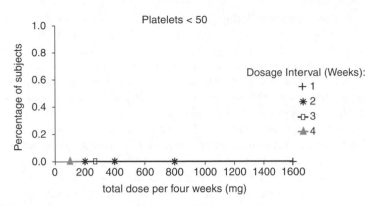

**Figure 3.9**   Percent subjects with platelets <50 versus total dose per four weeks, and dosage interval (1, 2, 3 and 4 weeks).

The second group could be 200 mg every two weeks (no safety concerns), and MRI reduction is expected to be about 45%. Finally the third arm could be 200 mg every three weeks (no safety concerns), and MRI reduction is expected to be about 35%. The proposed design of 200 mg every week, two and three weeks should lead to enough separation in the MRI response (60, 45 and 35% MRI reduction) to model a dose-response relationship. The characterization of a dose-response relationship will lead to an optimal design of Phase 3. The safety concern for a 200 mg dose every week has been addressed and quantified. The results of simulations suggest you cannot meet all the original criteria, and a tradeoff is necessary to generate the adequate dose-response relationship.

## 3.11   Summary

Pharmacometric modeling is an increasingly used method for analyzing the outcome from clinical trials in drug development. The model building process is complex and involves testing, evaluating and diagnosing a range of plausible models, aiming to make an adequate inference from the observed data and predictions for future studies and therapy. We attempted in this review to emphasize the thinking processes that lead to that model selection. We then focused on the model development, where the basic concepts of the nonlinear mixed-effect approach, the most common statistical model used in population analysis, were reviewed. After defining the model structure as well as the statistical distribution of the parameters, we then reviewed the different optimization procedures and the associated software that are currently available.

We emphasized the Monte Carlo EM methodology and other similar optimization procedures. Robustness, unbiased population estimates and stability make these new techniques attractive and the reason for their implementation in most of the software for population analysis (S-ADAPT, PDx-MC-PEM, NONMEM, SAEM).

Pharmacometrics is a quantitative pharmaco-statistical analysis to answer clinical drug development and regulatory questions, and influence decisions. A strong background in clinical pharmacology and biostatistics, with good judgment in therapeutics, drug development and regulatory decisions, is essential for this field.

The case study on patients suffering from multiple sclerosis was a good example where pharmacometric tools could be used to optimize the design of a Phase 2b clinical trial. Pharmacokinetic, safety and efficacy dynamic processes were defined and a mathematical framework was generated which contained model parameters that were estimated using the MCPEM approach. Criteria defined by the team as well as upper management were given to the pharmacometric team, who then proposed the Phase 2b dosing conditions that best satisfied the defined efficacy and safety criteria.

Pharmacometrics is an evolving science. Different aspects of pharmacometrics are today, and will continue to be, subject to intensive research, such as in the development and evaluation of methods for efficient and robust model building, development of estimation algorithms, methods for model diagnosis and sequential procedures for model building, and model development for the time-course of a system biomarker or a set of such biomarkers during normal, diseased or provoked situations. Pharmacometrics is useful from preclinical studies to Phase 3 clinical trials, and helps in the designing of studies, deciding upon dosing strategies and other developmental decisions and analyses of dose-concentration-response data from trials to understand therapies with existing drugs, with the aim of allowing improved therapy.

# References

1. Williams, P.J. and Ette, E.I. (2007) Pharmacometrics: impacting drug development and pharmacotherapy, in *Pharmacometrics: the Science of Quantitative Pharmacology* (eds E.I. Ette and P.J. Williams), John Wiley & Sons, Inc., Hoboken, NJ, pp. 1–21.

2. Bhattaram, V.A., Bonapace C., Chilukuri D.M. *et al.* (2007) Impact of pharmacometric reviews on new drug approval and labeling decisions—a survey of 31 new drug applications submitted between 2005 and 2006. *Clinical Pharmacology and Therapeutics*, **81**, 213–221.

3. Racine-Poon, A. (1998) Statistical methods for population pharmacokinetic modeling. *Statistical Methods in Medical Research*, **7**, 63–84.

4. Bauer, R.J., Guzy, S. and Ng, C. (2007) A survey of population analysis methods and software for complex pharmacokinetic and pharmacodynamic models with examples. 1. *AAPS Journal*, **9**, 60–83.

5. Wagner, J. (1971) *Biopharmaceutics and Relevant Pharmacokinetics*, Drug Intelligence Publications, Hamilton, IL.

6. Bonate, P.L. (2009) *Pharmacokinetic-Pharmacodynamic Modeling and Simulation*, Springer.

7. Ette, E.I. and Williams, P.J. (2004) Population pharmacokinetics I: background, concepts, and models. *The Annals of Pharmacotherapy*, **38**(10), 1702–1706.

8. Mould, D.R., Denman, N.G. and Duffull, S. (2007) Using disease progression models as a tool to detect drug effect. *Clinical Pharmacology and Therapeutics*, **82**, 81–86.

9. Holford, N.H.G., Kimko, H.C., Monteleone, J.P.R. and Peck, C.C. (2000) Simulation of clinical trials. *Annual Review of Pharmacology and Toxicology*, **40**, 209–234.

10. Nüesch, E.A. (1984) Noncompartmental approach in pharmacokinetics using moments. *Drug Metabolism Reviews*, **15**(1–2), 103–131.

11. Reddy, M., Yang R.S., Andersen, M.E. and Clewell H.J. III (2005) *Physiologically Based Pharmacokinetic Modeling: Science and Applications*. John Wiley & Sons, Inc., Hoboken, NJ.

12. Anderson, D.H. (1983) *Compartmental Modeling and Tracer Kinetics*, Springer-Verlag, Berlin.

13. Davidian, M. and Giltinan, D.M. (2003) Nonlinear models for repeated measurement data: an overview and update. *Journal of Agricultural Biological and Environmental Statistics*, **8**, 387–419.

14. Karlsson, M.O. and Sheiner, L.B. (1993) The importance of modeling interoccasion variability in population pharmacokinetic analyses. *Journal of Pharmacokinetics and Pharmacodynamics*, **21**, 735–750.

15. Bauer, R.J. and Guzy, S. (2007) Monte Carlo parametric expectation maximization (MC-PEM) method for analyzing population pharmacokinetic/pharmacodynamic data, in *Advanced Methods of Pharmacokinetic and Pharmacodynamic Systems Analysis* (ed. D.Z. D'Argenio), Springer, p. 135.

16. Beal, S.L., Sheiner, L.B. and Boeckmann, A.J. (2006) *NONMEM Users Guides*, Icon Development Solutions, Ellicott City, MD.

17. Aarons, L. (1993) The estimation of population pharmacokinetic parameters using an EM algorithm. *Computer Methods and Programs in Biomedicine*, **41**, 9–16

18. Compston, A. and Coles, A. (2002) Multiple sclerosis. *Lancet*, **359**(9313), 1221–1231.

19. Kenett, R.S. (1978) Studies in Enzyme Kinetics, PhD Thesis, Theoretical Mathematics Dept., Weizmann Institute, Rehovot, Israel.

20. Kenett, R.S. (1979) Statistical Analysis of Enzyme Kinetic Data, Tech. Report 580, Dept. of Statistics, University of Wisconsin, Madison, WI.

21. Karlin S. and Kenett, R.S. (1980) Shapes of Velocity Curves in Multiunit Enzyme Systems, Mathematical Biosciences, 52: 97–115.

# 4

# Interactive clinical trial design

## Zvia Agur

*Optimata Ltd., Ramat Gan, Israel and Institute for Medical Biomathematics (IMBM), Bene Ataroth, Israel*

## Synopsis

Clinical trials have traditionally been carried out in a 'trial and error' fashion, which is highly inefficient in measures of human and animal suffering, cost and time to market of the newly discovered compounds. Currently, pharmaceutical companies investigate various methods for increasing their productivity in drug development, in order to compensate for increasing costs and to avoid regulatory fiascos.

The major drawback of the traditional system lies in the lack of *a priori* guidance about the potentially successful treatments. The need for a change in paradigm of clinical trial design has been reiterated, and it has been suggested that the new paradigm should be based on formal methods for predicting disease progression under specific treatment regimens of given drugs or drug combinations.

A complex set of mathematical models, denoted the Virtual Patient Model, retrieving the dynamics of key biological, pathological and pharmacological processes in the body of a patient undergoing anti-cancer drug treatment, has been developed. The Virtual Patient Model has been employed for studying improved regimens for cytotoxic and cytostatic mono- and combination drug regimens and for selecting optimal personalized treatments. By simulating using the Virtual Patient Model in a population of patients, one can conduct virtual clinical trials recreating and improving drug development. To this end a collection of Virtual Patient Models is created (denoted the Synthetic Human Population). Each Virtual Patient in the population is represented by a set of parameters for the Virtual Patient Model. The inclusive set of parameters represents the distributions of disease, physiological and PK/PD parameters in the population. The virtual clinical trials can be employed in drug development in conjunction

*Statistical Methods in Healthcare*, First Edition. Edited by Frederick W. Faltin, Ron S. Kenett and Fabrizio Ruggeri.
© 2012 John Wiley & Sons, Ltd. Published 2012 by John Wiley & Sons, Ltd.

with an elaborate algorithm, Interactive Clinical Trial Design (ICTD), which provides a method for a step-by-step process of model prediction and *in vivo* verification. The user can employ the ICTD for fine-tuning and testing the drug/disease/population models interactively with the 'real' clinical trials, so that relatively early during development the Virtual Patient Model can be employed for checking the most appropriate treatment schedules for the drug, or for making an early 'No Go' decision. The ICTD algorithm is expected to replace the current drug trial-and-error policy with a new policy of clinical trials, which will be based upon a gradual improvement and zeroing-in on the best prediction-directed treatment schedules.

## 4.1  Introduction

The number of new drugs brought into the market has dropped significantly in the last few years, despite the substantial effort of pharmaceutical companies in medical research and development and in capital investments. In addition, the regulatory agencies have become more cautious about approving new molecular entities, in the wake of several fiascos of new. The resulting depleted pipelines may have serious consequences for industry, society and government, and a big crisis is foreseen if drug development becomes too risky and unprofitable. If the pharmaceutical industry is to remain at the forefront of medical research and continue helping patients, it must become more innovative in reducing the development time and costs of new therapies ('Pharma 2020 – Which path will you take?' (PriceWaterhouseCoopers, 2008)).

Currently, the physical and toxicological properties of drug candidates are mostly studied *in vitro*, by screens to find molecules that 'hit' a designated target. The most promising candidates are then selected to be tested in animals, and, subsequently, in large-scale clinical trials, essentially conducted by 'trial and error'. Pharmacometric research develops models for the response-time profiles observed in a clinical trial. These models may then be used for designing further clinical studies, for deciding upon dosing strategies and for other developmental decisions. Pharmacometrics also analyzes dose-concentration-response data from trials to understand therapies with existing drugs, with the aim of allowing improved therapy. However, pharmacometrics analyses are mostly retrospective, relying on large data bases obtained during the clinical trials. The pharmaceutical industry needs a faster, cheaper and more predictive way of testing molecules before they go into the clinic.

One strategy is to use 'virtual R&D', that is, research and development aided by computer simulations of the human body, to dramatically shorten the period of development of new drugs, and substantially reduce the chance of clinical failure, for substantially reducing costs across clinical development.

Research shows that drug effects may crucially depend on the internal dynamics of cancer growth processes, as well as on the relevant patient's physiology. These aspects might often be too complex to be estimated by the naked eye, and slight changes in the treatment schedule may be critical for the effect [1–4]. In theory, if all potential treatment schedules could be tested, considering all the available information on the involved biological processes, pathological processes and the momentary effect of the drug on every element of these processes, one could, *a priori*, suggest a theoretical set of the most promising treatment schedules for a given indication, or, even, for a given patient. Subsequently, these promising schedules would be clinically tested, thus saving human resources and time, and helping to achieve maximal possible therapeutic effects of the tested drug.

Moreover, such a method would enable one to take off the shelf drugs with valid properties, which failed during the development process, due to insufficient efficacy, or limitations of toxicity, which could possibly be overcome by modifying the treatment schedule. In addition, it would enable a Go–No Go decision to be made early during the clinical trial process.

In this chapter we will discuss the development of the Virtual Patient Model, and its use for identifying improved drug schedules. The Virtual Patient Model of a solid cancer disease includes a mathematical model of tumor progression, and we will explain how such a model is constructed and simulated. We will briefly describe retrospective clinical validation of the basic Virtual Patient Model. Subsequently, we will discuss how Synthetic Human Populations (SHPs) are created that transfer the real-life distribution of parameters into the Virtual Patient Model. *Interactive Clinical Trial Design*™ (ICTD; [5]), for use of the SHP-implemented Virtual Patient Model in virtual clinical trials, will be discussed and compared to adaptive clinical trials. The ICTD involves massive simulations of a population of the Virtual Patient Models, reflecting the patient population (to be denoted *Synthetic Human Population*). The ICTD enables the drug developer to generate, fine-tune and validate a reliable drug/disease/host model for forecasting improved treatments during an ongoing 'real' clinical trial. Thus, relatively early during development, that is, by the end of Phase I, and no later than in mid-Phase II, the model already contains the PK/PD drug parameters, to be embedded in the Virtual Patient Model. At this stage numerous drug schedules, termed 'infinite regimen space', are simulated for any desired indication, and optimization methods are employed for selecting, among the vast number of simulation scenarios, those yielding best results according to the list of specifications set by the drug developer. This method carries little risk of yielding false predictions, since the algorithm has been designed so as to be continuously validated and improved by information derived in parallel from clinical trials.

In this way one can identify the most appropriate patient-population/schedule for the drug, or alternatively, make a 'No Go' decision. The method is expected to replace the current drug trial policy, essentially one of 'shots in the dark', by a new policy of rationally designed clinical trials, which will be based upon a gradual improvement and zeroing-in on the best prediction-directed treatment schedules.

## 4.2    Development of the Virtual Patient concept

The Virtual Patient Model (Figure 4.1) is a set of multi-scale mathematical models that describe disease progression and the progression of relevant physiological toxicity processes. These models are simulated in conjunction with pharmacological models, fully accounting for the pharmacokinetics/pharmacodynamics (PK/PD) and dosing regimens of specific drugs or drug combinations. Simulation results are used for predicting the efficacy and toxicity of the drug under multitudes of putative treatment regimens. In addition, the platform of the Virtual Patient Model includes powerful optimization algorithms, which select the best treatment for a specific patient population, out of a large number of potential treatments.

### 4.2.1    The basic Virtual Patient Model

In the 1980s, a mathematical model was suggested that takes account of tumor and host cell-cycle dynamics. The model suggested that intermittent delivery of cell-cycle-phase-specific drugs, at intervals equivalent to the mean cell-cycle time, might minimize harmful toxicity

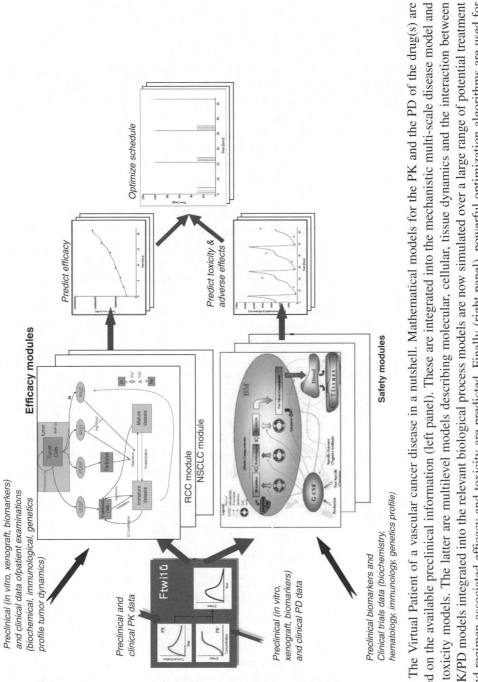

**Figure 4.1** The Virtual Patient of a vascular cancer disease in a nutshell. Mathematical models for the PK and the PD of the drug(s) are derived based on the available preclinical information (left panel). These are integrated into the mechanistic multi-scale disease model and the relevant toxicity models. The latter are multilevel models describing molecular, cellular, tissue dynamics and the interaction between them. The PK/PD models integrated into the relevant biological process models are now simulated over a large range of potential treatment regimens, and regimen-associated efficacy and toxicity are predicted. Finally (right panel), powerful optimization algorithms are used for identifying the most appropriate drug regimen for particular endpoints set by the drug developer.

without compromising therapeutic effects on target cells (*Z-Method* [6, 7]). Subsequently, explicit general formulae have been derived for the growth or decay of cell populations that are subjected to repeated pulse delivery of cell-cycle-phase-specific drugs [2], and an algorithm has been developed for calculating the required length of treatment for this regimen [8].

On the basis of the above theory, a heuristic optimization method has been developed [9], which uses operational research techniques for identifying improved drug schedules in any group of patients. The work focuses on developing the general concept of the optimization method, rather than on the particular implementation and, hence, the much simplified, but already validated, cell-cycle model, briefly mentioned above and described below, was selected for describing disease progression. The heuristic optimization method resulting from this simplified approach admits dynamic mathematical models of any desired level of complexity and is employed by the ICTD method, also described below.

The cell-cycle model considers two types of target cells in the human body. The host cells, denoted h-cells, and the malignant cells, denoted m-cells, which are, in fact, the tumor. Both types of cells may be damaged when exposed to drug treatment. Our aim is to reduce the number of m-cells, while maintaining a certain level of h-cells in the body. We assume that the lengths of the cell-cycle phases are deterministic and known, both for host and malignant cells. Both host and malignant cells are susceptible to the drug during some of the cell-cycle phases, denoted here the critical cell cycle phases. If a cell is exposed to drug treatment, typically chemotherapy, during part of its critical phase there is a chance that it will be eliminated. Specifically, we assume that during each unit of time in which treatment is applied, a fraction of the cells which are in their critical phase will be eliminated. Our aim is to reduce the number of m-cells to a certain fraction of their initial level. However, in order not to cause irreversible damage to the patient, we must schedule treatments so that the number of h-cells will always remain above a fraction of its initial level. Cells of both types multiply, but not necessarily at the same rate. If the number of m-cells is reduced below the desired level, we assume that the remaining m-cells will not multiply anymore.

We assume that treatments can be of variable length and can be given at any time. A solution, that is, a treatment schedule, determines those time intervals in which treatment is to be applied. This model is computationally intractable, as it is proved to be NP-complete, even in extremely simplified special cases. Consequently, an approach was put forward, aimed at obtaining good solutions that are not necessarily optimal. The approach solves the model by applying local search heuristics [9].

### 4.2.1.1   A simple cancer progression model

Let us denote by $\tau_i$ and $s_i$ the length of the cell cycle and the critical phase, respectively, of $i$-cells, $i \in \{m, h\}$. At the end of the cell cycle the cell may produce daughter cells. The average number of daughter cells produced by a single $i$-cell that reaches age $\tau_i$ is the growth rate in the $i$-cells' population, and we denote it by $r_i$.

If the proportion of m-cells is reduced to a fraction $\beta_m$ of its initial level, then the patient is considered cured and the treatment may be stopped. In practice, the proportion of h-cells must remain above a fraction $\beta_h$ of its initial level during the entire treatment. If the proportion of h-cells falls below this level, the patient is considered dead. However, we will allow solutions that do not satisfy this condition to be tested, with the aim of achieving good solutions at a later stage of the process. In our model, the patient can only die as a result of the treatments' toxicity – death is not caused by the tumor. This model assumption would not result in solutions that leave a patient without treatment, since growing cancer cells will quickly reduce the fitness to $-\infty$. Hence, solutions that result in a patients' death due to treatment have higher fitness values than solutions that do not treat the patient at all.

For each $t \in [0, T]$, the state of the system is characterized by two 'density' functions, $n_i(w, t)$, $i \in \{m, h\}$, that are defined for $w \in [0, \tau_i)$. For $0 \leq p \leq q \leq \tau_i$, the number of $i$-cells whose age is in the interval $[p, q]$ at time $t$ is $\int_{w=p}^{q} n_i(w, t)dw$. In particular, the total number of $i$-cells at $t$ is $x_i(t) = \int_{w=0}^{\tau_i} n_i(w, t)dw$. The units by which cells are counted are normalized so that the initial quantity is $x_i(0) = 1$.

Initially, before treatments begins, it is assumed that the cell ages distribute uniformly along the life cycle; that is, $n_i(w, 0) = \frac{1}{\tau_i}$, $w \in [0, \tau_i]$. When chemotherapy is applied, the cell age distribution obtains some non-uniform shape, depending on the treatment schedule.

With no treatment, the number of $m$-cells is assumed to double during each cell cycle; that is, $r_m = 2$. In reality we may find that the actual growth rate is lower. However, a growth rate of 2 defines the worst-case scenario, and the solutions found for this case still hold when the rate is lower. The host cells' growth rate depends on their number. The growth rate at time $t$ is $r(x_h(t))$, where $r(x)$ is a (non-linear) decreasing function that tends to 1 as $x$ goes to 1. Therefore, the growth of the host cells slows as they multiply. Note that our model assumes that, although influenced by the total number of host cells, their growth rate is independent of the age distribution.

We denote by $\alpha_i$ the proportion of all $i$-cells that that are destroyed during one time unit of treatment (host or malignant). Note that different rates for h- and m-cells may be eliminated by newly developed drugs that are more aggressive to m-cells than to h-cells. A treatment policy (schedule) consists of the times at which specific doses are applied.

Any policy that cures the patient without damaging more h-cells than is clinically affordable is a good policy, and can be accepted as a solution of high quality to our problem. However, defining a most desirable policy is not an easy task, since both the time of cure, and the number of h-cells at time determine the quality of a treatment: the relative importance of each one of these factors has to be defined in order to refine the performance of the algorithm. The fitness function constructed to meet these criteria is:

$$
\begin{aligned}
fitness(s) = & (x_h(T) - \beta_h)(2 + \beta_h - x_h(T)) - x_m(T) \\
& + c_1 I_{alive} + c_2 I_{cured} + c_3 I_{alive} I_{cured} \\
& + \frac{time\_of\_death}{K}(1 - I_{alive}) - \frac{time\_of\_cure}{K} I_{cured}.
\end{aligned}
$$

where $I_{alive}$ and $I_{cured}$ are indicator functions stating the patients condition at the end of the treatment period. Detailed analysis of this fitness function follows in Section 4.2.1.2.2.

Our approach is to compute a regimen through numerical computations, since theoretical analysis is possible only for very simplified models [8]. To make the process computationally tractable, we measure time and age by discrete units of a given length. To make computations reasonably quick, we divide the cells' cycle into discrete time units, and assume that the number of cells is constant over this unit. Thus, treatment policy consists of the times, $t_1, \ldots, t_m \in [0, T]$, at which treatments are given.

The distribution of the cells' age is generated using the following simulation rule: when no treatment is given, all cells mature by one time unit, and the cells that have reached the end of their cell cycle multiply. When chemotherapy is applied, all cells mature by one time unit, cells that are in the critical phase are reduced by a given fraction, and the cells that have reached the end of their cycle multiply.

The growth rates are calculated using the following rules: the m-cells double their number at each cycle; therefore the m-cell growth rate always equals 2. In contrast, the population of h-cells can never exceed its initial level – there is no uncontrolled growth in the h-cells. Their growth rate is assumed to be the highest number not greater than 2 that will keep the total number of host cells at most 1. This growth rate becomes smaller as the host cells replicate.

### 4.2.1.2    Optimization

The generality of the above model renders it computationally intractable. Therefore, good, but not necessarily optimal, solutions have been computed by different local search heuristics.

#### 4.2.1.2.1    Search algorithms    Simulated annealing (SA) is one of the three search heuristics used in the study [9].

It is a well-known heuristic (for details see [10, 11]). Here, we briefly describe the two other heuristics used in the aforementioned study.

Threshold acceptance (TA) is a deterministic version of SA. The difference between the two heuristics lies in the criterion for making a downhill descent – accepting a solution $s$ for which $fitness(s) < fitness(s_0)$, $s_0$ being the current best solution. In SA, downhill descent is made with a certain probability that depends on $fitness(s) - fitness(s_0)$ and on the temperature that is gradually reduced as the simulated annealing process continues. In TA, the temperature is replaced by a series of descending thresholds $t_0, \ldots, t_n$. A solution $s$ such that $fitness(s) < fitness(s_0)$ will replace $s_0$ as current solution at stage $i$ of the process if $fitness(s) > fitness(s_0) - t_i$. We refer the reader to [12] for further details.

The TA parameters were tested in the aforementioned work by running a series of different instances of the problem, and comparing the performances of the algorithm under different parameter values. The series of thresholds that was taken was geometrically descending, and several values of a descent rate, noted as the reduction factor, were tried. The threshold was reduced after two complete searches of the entire neighborhood, which is similar to the rule used for reducing the temperature in SA. The algorithm terminates when two consecutive thresholds end with the same fitness value, which is also similar to the SA termination rule.

Old bachelor acceptance (OBA) is a modification of TA, where the threshold doesn't always decrease. In this method, the threshold depends on the acceptance or rejection of the several most recently tried solutions. The heuristic is described in [13], and was slightly changed to suit the specific problem at hand. Thus, the original algorithm used $T_0 = 0$ as the initial threshold, but here $T_0 > 0$ was used. The reason for this modification is that the first solutions tested always cause an increase in the fitness, and, therefore, lower the threshold rapidly. When these consecutive improvements stop, many solutions are rejected until the threshold enables another acceptance.

#### 4.2.1.2.2    Fitness function    In the generic algorithms each treatment schedule is represented by a binary string of length $T$. Each bit in this string is equivalent to one time unit, say one hour, where a 0 means that no treatment is applied during this hour, and 1 means that treatment is applied. For example, the string 110001 shows that treatment is applied for two hours, following which there is no detectable drug in the system during three hours, and again treatment is applied over a period of one hour. The length of this string can be determined by

the user. Such a string is equivalent to a series of treatments, not necessarily of equal length, with drug-free system at variable intervals.

The fitness of a solution includes several factors: $x_h(t)$ and $x_m(t)$ denote the relative numbers of h- and m-cells, respectively, at time $t$. We measure these numbers as proportions which are taken with respect to the initial level, so that by definition $x_m(0) = x_h(0) = 1$. When all m-cells are eliminated we assume that the patient is cured. Our discrete representation of the cell age distribution implies that:

$$x_h(t) = \sum_{w=0}^{\tau_h-1} n_h(w, t)$$

and

$$x_m(t) = \begin{cases} \sum_{w=0}^{\tau_m-1} n_m(w, t) & \sum_{w=0}^{\tau_m-1} n_m(w, t) \geq \beta_m \\ 0 & \sum_{w=0}^{\tau_m-1} n_m(w, t) < \beta_m. \end{cases}$$

In addition, let us define two indicators (using obvious notation): $I_{cured}$ and $I_{alive}$, that indicate the patient's status during the treatment series. $I_{cured}$ indicates that, at some moment during the treatment, the number of m-cells decreased under the required threshold, and from this point on we considered the patient cured. As mentioned earlier, we assume that once a patient is cured the m-cells do not replicate any longer, so that we consider the tumor totally eliminated. The indicator $I_{alive}$ shows that the patient was alive during the entire treatment period, and that at no time did the number of h-cells decrease below the permitted limit. If the patient is cured, time_of_cure is the time elapsing until cure happens, and if the patient dies time_of_death is the period until the patient's death.

Our aim is to cure the patient as quickly as possible, when a certain level of h-cells must be maintained throughout the entire treatment period in order not to threaten the patient's life. Until the patient is cured, we attempt to preserve as many h-cells as possible. No more treatments need to be given after the patient is cured, and it is assumed that, given sufficient time, the h-cells will recover.

As stated, if the patient is cured, we prefer that cure will occur as early as possible. Similarly, in case of the patient's death, we prefer to delay the death as much as we can. These preferences are made under the assumption that solutions that prolong a patient's life can be more easily modified into solutions that keep the patient alive.

All these considerations having been taken into account, the following fitness function was constructed:

$$fitness(s) = (x_h(T) - \beta_h)(2 + \beta_h - x_h(T)) - x_m(T)$$

$$+ c_1 I_{alive} + c_2 I_{cured} + c_3 I_{alive} I_{cured}$$

$$+ \frac{time\_of\_death}{K}(1 - I_{alive}) - \frac{time\_of\_cure}{K} I_{cured}.$$

Let us now examine how this fitness function depends on each one of the required variables.

The fitness increases as $x_h(T)$ increases. However, this increase is not linear. The quadratic argument which includes $x_h(T)$ in the function is equal to 0 when $x_h(T) = \beta_h$, and is maximized when $x_h(T) = 1$. Thus, the function changes more rapidly around the critical value of $\beta_h$, where h-cells are very valuable, than around the maximal value of 1, where h-cells can easily be spared. Its derivative changes from 2 when $x_h(T) = \beta_h$ to $2\beta_h$ when $x_h(T) = 1$. Comparing this to the derivative of the argument representing $x_m(T)$ in the fitness function, which always equals 1, we see that many h-cells can be sacrificed in order to eliminate one m-cell when $x_h(T)$ is around 1. When $x_h(T)$ is close to $\beta_h$, we will sacrifice an h-cell only if many target cells will be eliminated at the same time. This way, h-cells affect the fitness more when they are most needed.

A 'bonus' of $c_1$ is given if the patient survives the treatment, and $c_2$ if the patient is cured. In addition, if both goals are achieved, an additional bonus of $c_3$ is given. Note that *cured* doesn't necessarily mean *alive*. Two thresholds exist, one for the h-cells and one for m-cells, that determine the patient's status: if the h-cells are reduced below their threshold then the patient is considered dead. If the m-cells are reduced below their threshold, the patient is cured.

Since the effect of the *time_of_death* variable should never exceed the effect of any of the indicators that were mentioned earlier, its contribution to the fitness is normalized such that it will never be greater than 1. This is achieved by dividing the *time_of_death* by a constant $K > T$.

Following the same logic, if a patient is cured we would like the cure to occur as early as possible. In this case this demand is not just a means of comparing 'good' solutions in order to modify them, but an actual benefit to the patient. The contribution of the *time_of_cure* variable is also normalized as mentioned before, for the same reasons.

Possible solutions to the above-defined optimization problem are scheduling plans represented by strings of '0's (no treatment) and '1's (treatment). The possible schedules have been tested by three local search-based heuristics, to find a solution that will locally optimize the fitness function. The comparison between the three approximation methods mentioned above shows that they are competitive, but the computational effort is much higher in SA than in the other two methods. All three methods produced solutions of similar quality, and therefore the choice among them should be made according to their computational efficiency.

**4.2.1.2.3 Discussion**    The general approach for selecting desired chemotherapy schedules, described in the above section, can satisfy a realistically complex medical optimization problem. In order to enable its implementation in the clinic, elaborate mathematical models of pathology and physiology have been developed, yielding precise quantitative predictions of cancer progression and the drug-susceptible physiological processes, notably hematopoiesis. One of these models describing vascular tumor growth will be described briefly below.

# 4.3    Use of the Virtual Patient concept to predict improved drug schedules

## 4.3.1    Modeling vascular tumor growth

The progress in understanding the biology of tumor neovascularization (angiogenesis) enables formalization of the known properties of this process. A detailed model is required to reflect the role of growth factors (cytokines) in the signaling cascade of tumor vascularization, so as to depict the non-monotonic and unstable angiogenic behavior, observed even under no anti-cancer treatment [14–16].

The first simple model that incorporates the mediating role of angiogenic signaling by tumor cells is explored in Agur *et al.* [17, 18]. It consists of three ordinary differential equations (ODEs) describing the dynamics of three variables: the tumor size, $N$, the concentration of the protein involved in angiogenic signaling, $P$, and the volume of blood vessels, $V$.

The tumor growth rate is assumed to depend on nutrient supply, which is proportional to vessel density, defined by $E = V/N$, as follows.

$$\dot{N} = f_1(E)N. \tag{4.1}$$

Here, the function $f_1$ is increasing, $f_1(0) < 0$, $\lim_{E \to \infty} f_1(E) > 0$; that is, the tumor will regress for zero vessel density and will grow with bounded rate for high vessel density.

The signaling protein is assumed to be secreted by the tumor as a result of nutrient deficiency:

$$\dot{P} = f_2(E)N - \delta P. \tag{4.2}$$

Here, the function $f_2$ is decreasing, $f_2(0) > 0$, $\lim_{E \to \infty} f_2(E) = 0$; that is, when vessel density is large, the secretion of the pro-angiogenic protein drops, while at small vessel density each tumor cell secretes more protein. The second term accounts for first-order decay of the protein.

The size of the vessels is determined by the protein, as follows:

$$\dot{V} = f_3(P)V. \tag{4.3}$$

Here, the function $f_3$ is increasing, $f_3(0) < 0$, $\lim_{E \to \infty} f_3(E) > 0$; that is, a small amount of protein causes vessel regression, while large amounts induce growth of vasculature.

The model given by equations (4.1–4.3) is studied in [17, 18] in numerical computations using sigmoid-like functions. It turns out that, in contrast to previously published models, here no positive stable biologically relevant steady state exists. Note that the steady state $N = P = E = 0$ is of no interest, since the model describes the dynamics of existing vascular tumors. It was analytically proven in this model that both the tumor and the vessel volume always grow monotonically showing no oscillations. The vessel density can either increase unlimitedly or stabilize at some level, so that the tumor and the vessels grow proportionally. Since these modeled tumor and vascular dynamics fail to capture the full range of the observed real-life cancer growth behavior, such as oscillations, one has to consider the introduction of additional assumptions that may enrich the model behavior. In [17, 18] the above model is extended by introducing time delays into the equations. Specifically, it is assumed that the current tumor growth rate and vessel formation rate depend on the prior vessel density and protein concentration some time before. Mathematically, this leads to the following system of delayed differential equations (DDEs).

$$\dot{N} = f_1(E(t - \tau_1))N \tag{4.4}$$

$$\dot{P} = f_2(E)N - \delta P \tag{4.5}$$

$$\dot{V} = f_3(P(t - \tau_2))V. \tag{4.6}$$

Here all the functions are the same as in the system of equations (4.1–4.3); $\tau_1$ and $\tau_2$ are time delays, so, for example, tumor growth rate depends on vessel density some $\tau_1$ time units ago, rather than depending on the current vessel density. In Agur et al. [17] it is shown that this model exhibits a specific behavior, termed Hopf bifurcation: namely periodic oscillations of tumor size and vessel volume under some specific conditions. Since such behavior is observed in laboratory experiments in untreated animals [19], it can thus be concluded that the system of equations (4.4–4.6) is a minimal model able to reproduce the experimentally observed non-monotonic behavior of the angiogenic tumor.

In Bodnar and Foryś [20], the models expressed in equations (4.1–4.3) and (4.4–4.6) are modified by introducing the logistic term into the equation for tumor growth. The addition of this term is justified by the observed deceleration in tumor growth and the existence of natural limits for the tumor size, even if no limitations are imposed by the vascular system. Thus, for the system of equations (4.1–4.3), the first equation now becomes

$$\dot{N} = \alpha N \left( 1 - \frac{N}{1 + f_1\,(E)} \right),$$

(4.7)

and for the system of equations with delay (4.4–4.6), the first equation becomes

$$\dot{N} = \alpha N \left( 1 - \frac{N}{1 + f_1\,(E\,(t - \tau_1))} \right).$$

(4.8)

where $f_1$ is the same as in equation (4.1) and $\alpha$ is the maximal tumor growth rate. The analysis in [20] shows that these two models always exhibit at least one stable steady state with $N > 0$, thus representing a realistic saturation in tumor growth. The model with delays also exhibits oscillatory behavior, similar to the model given by equations (4.4–4.6).

It should be noted that the simple concept of carrying capacity as used in [21] was replaced in the models presented above by the more elaborate notion of vessel density, reflecting the relationship between the vessel volume and tumor size. In fact, the crucial factor governing tumor growth is the efficiency of the vascular support. To account for this, in [22, 23] the notion of effective vessel density (EVD) was introduced. It differs from the previously used vessel density in that it takes into consideration that different types of vasculature can contribute differently to nutrient supply. Following this notion, the blood vessels involved in tumor angiogenesis are divided into two groups – the immature vessels and the mature vessels. The more detailed description of the angiogenic process takes this distinction into account. The new vessels are formed by endothelial cells, which proliferate and migrate upon angiogenic signals. These newly formed vessels are unstable and inefficient in nutrient supply. They are termed immature vessels. However, these vessels can stabilize by undergoing a maturation process, essentially coating the endothelial cells by smooth muscle cells, named pericytes. This process is governed by a different type of molecular signal – the maturation signal. Mature vessels can also destabilize, as a result of decaying maturation signals or the appearance of anti-maturation signals. Experimental observations [14–16] suggest that the dynamics of maturation and destabilization may be responsible for the non-monotonicity in tumor and vasculature growth. Following this suggestion an additional model of five DDEs was proposed in Agur et al. [17]. This model describes the growth of immature and mature vessels, $V_1$ and $V_2$, respectively, as two inter-related processes. Two types of signaling proteins are considered. The first, $P_1$ is secreted by tumor cells and assumed to stimulate immature vessels' growth. Its role is equivalent to that of $P$ in the previous models. The second protein, $P_2$, stimulates maturation. It is also assumed to be secreted by tumor cells. This model takes the following form:

$$\dot{N} = f_1 \left( E \left( t - \tau_1 \right) \right) N \tag{4.9}$$

$$\dot{P}_1 = f_2 \left( E \right) N - \delta_1 P_1 \tag{4.10}$$

$$\dot{P}_2 = \alpha N - \delta_2 P_2 \tag{4.11}$$

$$\dot{V}_1 = f_3 \left( P_1 \left( t - \tau_2 \right) \right) V_1 - f_4 \left( P_2 \right) V_1 + f_5 \left( P_2 \left( t - \tau_3 \right) \right) V_2 \tag{4.12}$$

$$\dot{V}_2 = f_4 \left( P_2 \right) V_1 + f_5 \left( P_2 \left( t - \tau_3 \right) \right) V_2. \tag{4.13}$$

Here equations (4.9, 4.10, 4.12) are similar to equations (4.4–4.6), except for the indices of $P_1$ and $V_1$ added here. The function $f_4$, accounting for the maturation rate, is positive and increasing. The function $f_5$ computes mature vessels' destabilization; it is positive and decreases to zero. In addition, the computation of $E$ is changed. Now it depends on both types of vessels, $E = (\alpha_1 V_1 + \alpha_2 V_2)/N$; $\alpha_1$ and $\alpha_2$ being the relative contribution of immature and mature vessels to the EVD. In this work, both were taken to be 1. This model also exhibits oscillatory behavior, suggesting the possible role of blood vessels' maturation and destabilization in tumor growth.

Finally, a more comprehensive model of the processes discussed above has been developed in order to better represent experiments where human ovary carcinoma spheroid were implanted in mice and tumor growth as well as immature and mature vascular dynamics were monitored *in vivo* [22, 23]. This model is formulated in terms of difference equations discrete in time and, also, by ODE formalism. The model captures the dynamics of the angiogenic tumor, calculating the following variables over time: tumor size, immature vessels' density, mature vessels' density, number of endothelial cells, number of pericytes, concentration of vascular endothelial growth factor (VEGF), concentration of platelet-derived growth factor (PDGF), concentration of pro-maturation factor Angiopoietin1 (Ang1), and concentration of its competitor, anti-maturation factor Angiopoietin 2 (Ang2). The equations for these variables reflect the biological understanding of the role of the system components, similar to the models described above. We refer the reader to Arakelyan *et al.* [23] for more detailed description.

In Arakelyan *et al.* [23] it is shown that, consistent with the simpler models, if the maturation process is neglected, tumor and vasculature growth become monotonic. In contrast, the introduction of vessel maturation and their destabilization dynamics into the model reduces tumor growth and leads to highly non-monotonic behavior, including irregular oscillations of tumor and vasculature size. Further, by simulating anti-VEGF and anti-PDGF treatments, it was demonstrated that anti-angiogenic treatment alone will not suffice to eliminate the tumor and has to be combined with anti-maturation treatment. As will be described below, this prediction has been corroborated in the preclinical setting by showing, in pancreatic cancer mouse models, that the combination of a VEGF receptor inhibitor with another distinctive kinase inhibitor targeting PDGF receptor activity (Gleevec (imatinib)) was able to regress late-stage tumors [24].

In summary, an accurate and detailed description of system dynamics can be obtained using complex models, which account for known relevant components and processes. Even more importantly, mathematical modeling allows one to determine the minimal necessary components required to produce the observed phenomena and to understand how the complex behavior emerges from basic system properties. Once experimentally validated, the model can be used to assist researchers to improve and accelerate drug development and help identify the most promising treatment regimens for different drugs that may vary subtly in drug action mechanism. See [25] for a more comprehensive review of the development of angiogenesis models.

### 4.3.1.1    A multi-scale vascular tumor growth model retrieves the clinical scenario and suggests efficacious regimens

Mathematical analysis and numerical simulations of Arakelyan *et al.*'s 2002 model shed important light on vascular tumor dynamics. Thus, it was suggested that there are circumstances in which small tumors oscillate in size instead of growing steadily. If such circumstances can be medically replicated then this may be a powerful way of controlling cancer growth [23, 26]. Notably, it was suggested that monotherapy by anti-angiogenic drugs alone can slow tumor growth, but cannot altogether eliminate it, and that anti-angiogenic drugs combined with drugs that target mature vessels may be superior to anti-angiogenic monotherapy [19, 27, 28]. As was mentioned above, these conclusions were later corroborated experimentally [24].

In order to check whether or not the model is a high-fidelity portrayal of vascular tumor growth, its predictions are to be experimentally validated. This is essential if one is to use the model in the context of the Virtual Patient, where new drugs are examined for their efficacy. In [28], the vascular tumor model was verified in xenograft experiments. Thus tumor growth, vascular maturation and functionality were studied noninvasively by magnetic resonance imaging (MRI) in human epithelial ovarian carcinoma spheroids, xenografted in mice. Individual tumor growth curves were input into the model for evaluating the tumor-specific parameters, and predictions of vascular dynamics were compared with the MRI readings. The revealed accuracy and critical importance of model predictions is demonstrated by the following example. The model predicts complete maturation of all neovasculatures in a tumor, within about one month. Indeed, the experimental results support model predictions quite remarkably and further explain the model-predicted and clinically observed short-term effects of the anti-VEGF drug bevacizumab [29, 30].

The accuracy of the mathematical model of vascular tumor dynamics was further validated clinically, by comparing its predictions to the clinical response of metastatic breast cancer (MBC) patients to docetaxel; this drug is among the few monotherapy options available for patients that are resistant to other alkylating agents. Predicting individual response to docetaxel may improve the efficacy of treating MBC patients. The mathematical model of solid tumor dynamics, previously validated in preclinical studies, was employed in a retrospective study of MBC patients.

Clinical and histopathological data were collected from 25 MBC patients treated with tri-weekly docetaxel. The patients were randomly divided into a training set (18 patients), for adjusting population-specific PD, and a validation set (7 patients), for predicting disease progression under individually assigned docetaxel regimens. Once-weekly docetaxel regimens were also simulated for the patients and compared with their actual clinical performance.

The model accurately predicted the observed tumor sizes over the entire observation period ($R^2 = 0.7$; $p < 0.001$) and the objective tumor response, assessed according to the internationally accepted Response Evaluation Criteria In Solid Tumors, RECIST (85.7% of match between the observed and predicted, Kappa $= 0.72$, $p < 0.05$; Figure 4.2).

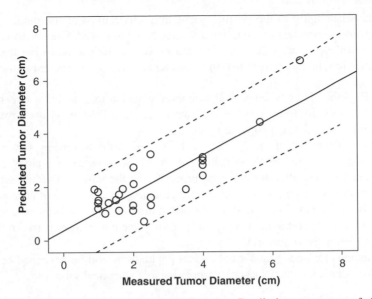

**Figure 4.2** Predicted vs. measured tumor diameter. Prediction accuracy of the vascular tumor model. Tumor size at the end of treatment, $R^2 = 0.7$ ($p < 0.001$); objective tumor response assessed according to RECIST; 85.7% (Kappa $= 0.72$, $p < 0.05$). Regression model line (solid line); 95% confidence interval (dashed line).

Significantly improved efficacy was predicted for the once-weekly schedule in 48% of the patients. Model analysis revealed that angiogenesis-intensive tumors can be controlled by more frequent docetaxel dosing, whereas angiogenesis-poor tumors may be treated by less-dense regimens [29].

## 4.3.2    Synthetic Human Population (SHP)

In the preceding sections, we described the concept of the Virtual Patient Model using simple models of tumor growth and patient toxicity, as well as optimization problem formalism in order to identify treatment regimens which will maximize drug efficacy while minimizing its toxicity. We noted that the Virtual Patient can admit more complex biological progression models, and went on to describe the methodology underlying the development of a multi-scale mathematical model for vascular tumor growth. We then pointed out that the use of the Virtual Patient Model in drug development requires preclinical and clinical validation, and showed examples of such validation experiments. In the same way as described for the efficacy model, namely for drug effects on tumor progression, one embeds toxicity models in the Virtual Patient 'platform'. That is to say that models describing physiological processes that are known to be a target of the drug under study are simulated in parallel to the pathology models, and specific optimization problems are then solved, as described above.

To use the Virtual Patient platform in order to predict the effect of a drug treatment on the entire patient population (or sub-population), a Virtual Patient *population* needs to be generated. To this end one must replace the parameters evaluated for a single patient model by a distribution representing the population distribution of each of the parameters. In practice, the individuals belonging to the 'virtual population' share most of the model parameters. However, several parameters are individually selected from a predefined distribution. These parameters and their actual values are selected based on studies indicating that they may have a prognostic value, and given that most of them are readily measured in the laboratory [31–33].

The SHP method is to be employed whenever we wish to generate a larger sample of patients that probes different areas in the parameter space and may also provide higher accuracy in predicting the real population response.

The general definition of the problem to be solved is the following. Given a set of $p$ parameters that is assigned to $N$ individual patients: how to generate a larger set, $M > N$, of the $p$ parameters such that the statistical properties of the initial set are preserved. Three restrictions should be made. The first determines that the average value of each parameter is the same in the real set and in the SHP set. Secondly, the standard deviation of each parameter in the SHP should reflect that in the real world. Lastly, the covariance matrix in the SHP set should reflect that in the real world.

Three methods for obtaining Virtual Patient populations will be described below. These are parameter inflation, convex biased interpolation and statistical sampling.

### 4.3.2.1    Parameter inflation ('cherries and flies')

Initially, we define each input 'individual' as a point, $\vec{P} \equiv |p_1, p_2, \ldots, p_n|$, in the parameter hyperspace, according to the parameter values $(p_i)$ obtained in the parameter evaluation process. Subsequently, multiple, normally distributed, random points $\vec{R}$ are generated around each of the input 'individuals', such that $r_i \sim N\left(p_i, \sigma_i^2\right)$, where $p_i$ and $r_i$ are the values of the $i$th input and output parameters, respectively, and $\sigma_i$, the standard deviation, determines the degree of variability. Empirically, we have selected $\sigma_i$ to be between 1 and 5% of the estimated value $p_i$. This parameter inflation approach is relatively fast and little error-prone (see Figure 4.3).

### 4.3.2.2    Convex biased interpolation

In this method we generate additional experiments by taking a linear combination of the initial set of $\chi$ experiments, as follows:

$$E_i = \left\{ P_{\{j\}}^i = \sum_{k=1}^{\chi} r_{i,k} P_{\{j\}}^i : 1 \leq j \leq N \right\} : i > \chi.$$

The requirement that the coefficients, $r_{i,k} : 1 \leq k \leq \chi$, sum up to 1, provides new experiments which fall inside the convex hull, defined by the $\chi$ points in the $N$-dimensional space that represents the initial experiments. In other words the parameter range restriction is met.

When the values of $r_{i,k}$ are randomly chosen within the range [0, 1], the parameter values of the resulting new experiments would not meet the standard deviation restriction mentioned above. The standard deviation of the new experiments would be smaller than that of the original experiments.

To handle the $\sigma$ restriction, as well as the correlation restriction, the linear combination coefficients $r_{i,k}$, have to be taken from the 'tails' of the range [0,1]. This is accomplished

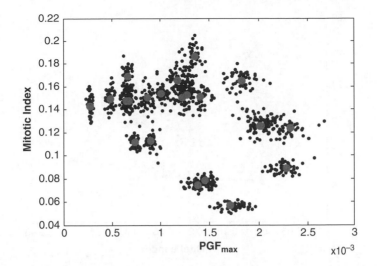

**Figure 4.3** Demonstration of parameter inflation in two dimensions (two parameters). Thick gray points represent values obtained during the parameter evaluation process. Thin black dots represent the generated values. The term 'cherries and flies' method was inspired by the shape of this plot.

by raising $r_{i,k}$ to the power of $q_0$, $R_{i,k} = (r_{i,k})^{q_0}$, for some constant $q_0$, where the $R_{i,k}$ are normalized.

The generated additional experiments are points in the $N$-dimensional space, located 'close' to the $\chi$ points (which stand for the initial 'real' experiments) inside their convex hull (see Figure 4.4).

### 4.3.2.3 Statistical sampling

This method generates a multivariate normal random series. First, we define the distributions of each parameter, $p_1, \ldots, p_n$, by calculating the mean, $\mu$, and variance $\sigma^2$ of the estimated values of the observations for each parameter. Then a new set of values for the parameters, $p_1, \ldots, p_n$, can be randomly sampled based on the mean and the covariance matrix of the parameters.

### 4.3.2.4 Application considerations

The SHP should not be used when the size of the original real-life population is too small. Specifically, there is no point in trying to generate SHPs when the size of the original population is smaller than 10 patients. Moreover, the estimation of the parameter covariance should not be considered reliable when the number of measurements is less than 10-fold the number of independent parameters (e.g., for 3 parameters we have 3 non-diagonal covariances, for 5 we have 10 non-diagonal covariances, and for 7 individual parameters we have 21 independent parameters). Thus the non-diagonal covariances should not be considered reliable unless we have at least 30 patients for 3 individual variables, 50 patients for 5 individual variables and 210 for 7 individual variables. In the last case, and in general, if the original

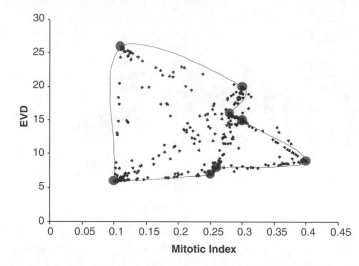

**Figure 4.4** Demonstration of the convex biased interpolation method in two dimensions (two parameters). Thick gray points represent values obtained in the parameter evaluation process. Thin black dots represent the generated values.

population is large enough (>100), no SHP is necessary for evaluating the distribution of patients' parameters to be implemented in the Virtual Patient Models which will be simulated.

# 4.4    The Interactive Clinical Trial Design (ICTD) algorithm

Above, we have sketched the basic concept of the Virtual Patient using a very simple model. Subsequently we described the development of more complex and more accurate models for vascular tumor growth, which need to be implemented in the Virtual Patient platform in order to retrieve quantitative predictions of disease progression under drug treatment. We have described methods for expanding the Virtual Patient to a Virtual Patient population, SHP, in order to represent a specific population of patients, and below we go one step further and briefly describe the Interactive Clinical Trial Design (ICTD) algorithm by which an SHP is used for carrying out virtual clinical trials that predict the response in the various stages of the clinical trials.

## 4.4.1    Preclinical phase: Constructing the PK/PD module

The preclinical phase of drug development concerns the retrieval of the drug's PD and PK in animals, and the initialization of human PD research. In this phase a virtual population of the experimental animal, usually that of human cancer xenografted mice, is created, and adjusted to the drug under development, as is detailed below.

Based on the *in vitro* studies, the drug PD module of the virtual animal is constructed. Thus, putative mechanisms of drug action are simulated, retrieving the most appropriate action mechanisms. The mechanism showing best fit to the experimental results is selected as most probable. From the results of the *in vitro* studies, the parameters of the drug's effect on the different target tissues are empirically estimated and input into the module. These include the data from experiments using different tumor types, also in combination with another drug. Conversely, the model here can simulate and comparatively estimate the efficacy of treatment in combination with other known drugs, as well as the effect of the drug on different tumor types. By evaluating parameters to be implemented in the model of the average animal bearing a given cancer disease, and by evaluating the distribution of this parameters in the experimental population, one can create a virtual experimental population, which can direct the preclinical research to the most effective avenues. The model is continuously fine-tuned, by 'online' implementation in the Virtual Animal Population of the preclinical research results. In this way, the model can interactively guide the preclinical research.

Using animal studies, the PK module of the virtual animal is adjusted to describe the PK of the given drug, as evaluated in animal studies. The PD module, which up to this point was based solely on the *in vitro* data, is adjusted to represent the *in vivo* animal results, and is supplemented by animal parameters for the functions of drug-effect time series. This, again, includes data on different tumor types and on the effects of combinations with other drugs. From animals treated with multiple doses, some data on cumulative effect can be obtained and implemented in the model.

The toxicity module is designed on the basis of the qualitative and quantitative data on side effects observed during the animal studies. For example, the Virtual Patient's module describing hematopoietic processes is provided with evaluated values of the parameters of the drug effect on hematopoiesis, if observed in animals. From animals treated by multiple drug doses, some data on cumulative toxicity may be obtained and implemented in the model as well.

At this stage the model already has the capacity to simulate the administration of the drug to humans. Known inter-species differences in the target tissue characteristics are taken into account when simulating the human PK model, in order to consider a reasonable dose range for Phase I human studies. This procedure is expected to offer an improvement on the traditional LD10 initial dose for Phase I trials (i.e., the dose lethal for 10% of mice administered the drug), which is often too low to show effect on the disease. That is to say that, already in this stage, based on *in vitro* and *in vivo* data the model can be used for predicting the minimal dose within therapeutic range; that is, the lowest dose which has a rationale to be tested. It is possible at this point to use the model for predicting failure for the drugs with therapeutic doses too toxic to be tolerated.

### 4.4.2    Phase I: Finalizing and validating the PK/PD module

During dose escalation testing in the Phase I clinical trials, the PK/PD module in the Virtual Patient Model is interactively fine-tuned and validated according to the results of the dose escalation experiments. This could, possibly, save steps during the dose escalation process, necessary for obtaining the toxicity profile and an initial efficacy profile. During Phase I trials, while using intra-patient dose escalation methods, the model is to be provided with data on cumulative effect and cumulative toxicity, if observed.

In this way, by the end of Phase I, a fully *in vivo*-verified human model is available, integrating all the existing data on PK and PD of the drug. The general algorithm for conducting interactive clinical trials during Phase I is shown in Figure 4.5. In the last stage of the Phase I ICTD work, one uses the SHP formalism to yield a population distribution model for the PK/PD model.

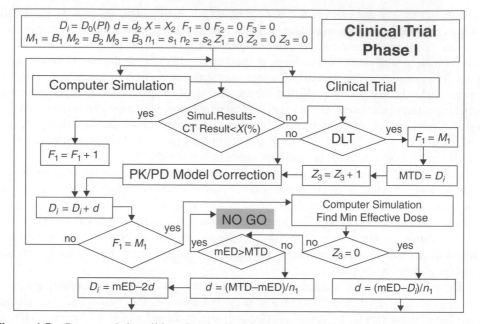

**Figure 4.5**  One panel describing the detailed interactive trial design (out of a total of 12 panels for the whole trial period); $X$ – a difference between simulated results and clinical trial (CT) results; $F_i$ – a counter; $D_i$ – a dose 'step' in dose elevation; $d$ – dose elevation per 'step'; $D_0(PI)$ – initial dose, predetermined for Phase I; $M_1$ – a criterion for model validity; $B_i$ – integer; DLT – dose-limiting toxicity; $Z_i$ – a counter; Min Effective Dose (mED) – a dose at which the effect was first observed; MTD – maximal tolerated dose (after which the DLT is observed); $n_i$ – number of steps to be defined for going from mED to MTD; $s_i$ – integer; NO GO – no rationale to continue developing the drug.

### 4.4.3   Interim stage between Phase I and Phase II: Intensive simulations of short-term treatments

Following Phase I, the model can yield reasonable, short-term predictions for the population effects of specific drug administration schedules on disease progression for specific indications. This allows one to perform an exhaustive search in the regimen space (i.e., within all the treatment schedule possibilities), for those mono- and combination therapy schedules expected to yield the highest response and lowest toxicity for any potential cancer type to be treated. This may help the drug developer to predict the most effective treatment schedule and the most promising indication, thus saving patient health, time and cost.

### 4.4.4   Phase II and Phase III: Focusing the clinical trials

At the onset of Phase II trials and following the interim stage outlined above, a few potential treatment schedules for the selected indication(s) are applied in short pilot trials testing a relatively small number of patients. After the first results are obtained (lasting six months, on the average), the SHP model is further adjusted by implementing the new data on the observed effects.

Subsequently, a new set of intensive simulations are carried out, predicting population response to the drug during an extended period of up to two years, and predicting which of the schedules, tested in short-term trials, are expected to yield the best results in the long-run. At this stage the predicted effect for each selected schedule is compared with that of the 'Gold Standard' therapy for the same indications.

Already at this time, the SHP model can predict failure, that is, recommend a No Go decision, for the drugs that are incapable of showing benefit over the 'Gold Standard' therapy. The schedule(s) predicted to carry the most significant benefit over the 'Gold Standard' are selected for further testing in Phase III. After the efficacy and safety profile of the selected schedule(s) is confirmed in further Phase II trials (for another six months), the selected schedules should be further tested in a larger patient population in Phase III trials.

The general algorithm of ICTD was compared to a classical clinical trial design of anti-cancer drugs (denoted 'original'). Figure 4.6 illustrates the average differences in the number of patients expected to be recruited for the clinical trials designed according to each of the two methods.

One can notice in Figure 4.6. a significant potential saving in time and in the number of patients recruited for ICTD. Figures 4.7a and b schematically present the results of our theoretical comparison between the classical design in the development of a recently approved drug, to be nicknamed 'O', which was in development in a big pharmaceutical company, and

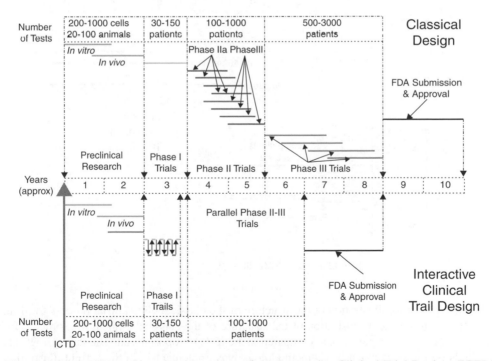

**Figure 4.6** An illustration of the structure of the Interactive Clinical Trial Design (ICTD) as compared to the classical design for the duration and number of patients (averages).

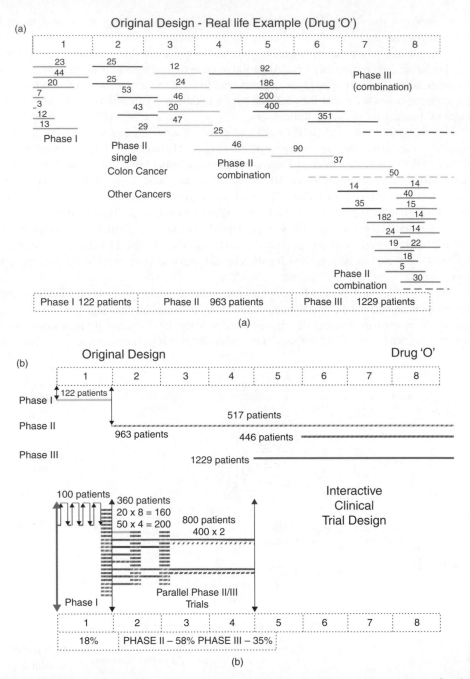

**Figure 4.7** (a) An illustration of the structure of the classical clinical trial process for drug 'O'. (b) A summarized illustration of the structure of the classical clinical trial process for drug 'O' (see detail in part (a)), as compared to the ICTD-proposed trial. The saving by ICTD depends on the stage when ICTD methodology was implemented; in the current illustration ICTD is implemented in Phase I. Numbers specify the number of patients in the specific arm (averages).

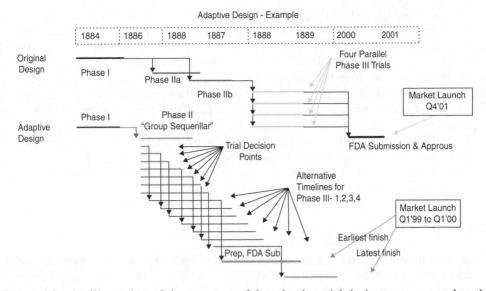

**Figure 4.8**  An illustration of the structure of the adaptive trial design, as compared to the classical design.

the putative design of the same drug under the ICTD method; the differences (in percentage) in the number of patients and the total duration of drug development are noted at the bottom of the figure.

## 4.4.5   Interactive Clinical Trial Design method as compared to Adaptive Clinical Trial Design methods

The use of adaptive clinical trial design (ACTD; Figure 4.8) methods in clinical research and development has become popular in recent years, due to their flexibility and efficiency. ACTD allows modifications to be made to trial and/or statistical procedures of ongoing clinical trials. ACTD suggests an improvement to the classical design, as it offers the ability to stop trials relatively early, to drop or add treatment groups, to change group proportions or shift seamlessly into a later phase, and so on. These models aid in planning trials by predicting the probability distribution of trial outcomes conditional on current knowledge and assumptions, and thus evaluating the ability of the trial to support a certain decision. These models rely upon prior knowledge of population probability distribution [34–36].

However, since ACTD is based on the assumptions of Bayesian statistics, it is a concern that major adaptations of trial and/or statistical procedures of ongoing trials may result in a totally different trial that is unable to address the scientific/medical questions the trial is intended to answer. We believe that this difficulty is much reduced in the ICTD, which is based on mechanistic models of disease and physiology progression and on the drug mechanism of action and PK/PD, and is therefore significantly less dependent on the trial data than is ACTD.

Another significant difference between the ACTD and the ICTD method suggested here lies in the effort required for each suggested clinical trial design method. The trials according to ICTD are started as early as the preclinical stage, or Phase I; whereas those according to the ACTD begin in Phase II. Moreover, while the first and potentially most important decision-making impact of the ICTD already takes effect at the end of Phase I, the ACTD's impact can be effectuated almost only towards the end of Phase III. The reason for these differences lies in the significant distinction between the tools employed by each of the designs. The major asset offered by the Virtual Patient technology is the predictive power associated with simulation of disease progression in large patient populations that are subjected to many hypothetical treatment schedules. In contrast, the major asset of ACDT is flexibility in trial design, relying on statistical analyses of accruing clinical data. In other words, our design is primarily prospective, integrating all the available biological, medical and pharmacological, theoretical and clinical information. In contrast, ACTD is primarily retrospective, integrating statistical methods with the information from the clinical trials.

## 4.5   Summary

Drug development is a challenging, costly and time-consuming process. Drugs that fail in clinical trials, often due to low efficacy and/or high toxicity levels, are shelved or altogether discontinued. Together with the recent stringency of the regulatory authorities, the high attrition in drug development increasingly exhausts the new product pipelines. Therefore, it becomes mandatory for pharmaceutical companies to revisit their decision-making process at all stages of drug development.

In this chapter we have introduced the concept of the Virtual Patient, and further illustrated its construction by briefly describing mathematical models for tumor progression at different levels of biological detail and at different levels of system complexity. We have described the consideration by which a Synthetic Human Population (SHP) is constructed; that is, a population of Virtual Patients that embodies a specific patient population, and is used to test the potential cost-efficiency of mono- or combination drug therapy. We then described the Interactive Clinical Trial Design (ICTD) method for conducting virtual clinical trials intertwined with and directing the real-life clinical trials. This method does not replace the adaptive clinical trial design (ACTD). Rather, we firmly believe that the two methods should be integrated in order to provide drug developers with a comprehensive and powerful tool to navigate drug development towards improved success and improved aid to the well-being of our society.

## Acknowledgements

I wish to thank L. Arakelyan, R. Ben-Av, R. Hassin, Y. Kogan, Zmira Silman and S. Levy for developing the work described in this chapter.

## References

1. Agur, Z., Arnon, R. and Schechter, B. (1992) Effect of the dosing interval on myelotoxicity and survival in mice treated by cytarabine. *European Journal of Cancer*, **28A**, 1085–1090.
2. Cojocaru, L. and Agur, Z. (1992) A theoretical analysis of interval drug dosing for cell-cycle-phase-specific drugs. *Mathematical Biosciences*, **109**, 85–97.

3. Ubezio, P., Tagliabue, G., Schechter, B. and Agur, Z. (1994) Increasing 1-beta-D-arabinofuranosylcytosine efficacy by scheduled dosing intervals based on direct measurements of bone marrow cell kinetics. *Cancer Research*, **54**, 6446–6451.

4. Agur, Z. (1998) Resonance and anti-resonance in the design of chemotherapeutic protocols. *Journal of Theoretical Medicine*, **1**, 237–245.

5. Arakelyan, L., Selitser, V. and Agur, Z. Inventors; interactive technique for optimizing drug development from the pre-clinical phases through phase-IV. *Pending*.

6. Agur, Z. (1986) The effect of drug schedule on responsiveness to chemotherapy. *Annals of the New York Academy of Sciences*, **504**, 274–277.

7. Agur, Z., Arnon, R. and Schechter, B. (1988) Reduction of cytotoxicity to normal tissues by new regimens of cell-cycle phase-specific drugs. *Mathematical Biosciences*, **92**, 1–15.

8. Agur, Z. and Dvir, Y. (1994) Use of knowledge on $\{\varphi n\}$ series for predicting optimal chemotherapy treatment. *Random & Computational Dynamics*, **2**, 279–286.

9. Agur, Z., Hassin, R. and Levy, S. (2006) Optimizing chemotherapy scheduling using local search heuristics. *Operations Research*, **54**, 829–846.

10. Aarts, E.H.L. and Lenstra, J.K. (1997) *Local Search in Combinatorial Optimization*, John Wiley & Sons, Ltd, Chichester.

11. Johnson, D.S., Aragon, C.R., McGeoch, L.A. and Schevon, C. (1989) Optimization by simulated annealing: an experimental evaluation; Part I, graph partitioning. *Operations Research*, **37**, 865–892.

12. Dueck, G. and Scheuer, T. (1990) Threshold accepting: a general purpose optimization algorithm appearing superior to simulated annealing. *Journal of Computational Physics*, **90**, 161–175.

13. Hu, T.C., Kahng, A.B. and Tsao, C.-W.A. (1995) Old Bachelor acceptance: a new class of non-monotone threshold accepting methods. *INFORMS Journal on Computing*, **7**, 417–425.

14. Gilead, A., Meir, G. and Neeman, M. (2004) The role of angiogenesis, vascular maturation, regression and stroma infiltration in dormancy and growth of implanted MLS ovarian carcinoma spheroids. *International Journal of Cancer*, **108**, 524–531.

15. Gilead, A. and Neeman, M. (1999) Dynamic remodeling of the vascular bed precedes tumor growth: MLS ovarian carcinoma spheroids implanted in nude mice. *Neoplasia*, **1**, 226–230.

16. Holash, J., Wiegand, S.J. and Yancopoulos, G.D. (1999) New model of tumor angiogenesis: dynamic balance between vessel regression and growth mediated by angiopoietins and VEGF. *Oncogene*, **18**, 5356–5362.

17. Agur, Z., Arakelyan, L., Daugulis, P. and Ginosar, Y. (2004) Hopf point analysis for angiogenesis models. *Discrete and Continuous Dynamical Systems. Series B*, **4**, 29–38.

18. Forys, U., Kheifetz, Y. and Kogan, Y. (2005) Critical-point analysis for three-variable cancer angiogenesis modeling. *Mathematical Biosciences and Engineering: MBE*, **2**, 511–525.

19. Arakelyan, L., Merbl, Y., Daugulis, P. *et al.* (2003) *Multi-Scale Analysis of Angiogenic Dynamics and Therapy*, CRC Press.

20. Bodnar, M. and Foryś, U. (2009) Angiogenesis model with carrying capacity depending on vessel density. *Journal of Biological Systems (JBS)*, **17**, 1–25.

21. Hahnfeldt, P., Panigrahy, D., Folkman, J. and Hlatky, L. (1999) Tumor development under angiogenic signaling: a dynamical theory of tumor growth, treatment response, and postvascular dormancy. *Cancer Research*, **59**, 4770–4775.

22. Arakelyan, L., Merbl, Y. and Agur, Z. (2005) Vessel maturation effects on tumour growth: validation of a computer model in implanted human ovarian carcinoma spheroids. *European Journal of Cancer*, **41**, 159–167.

23. Arakelyan, L., Vainstein, V. and Agur, Z. (2002) A computer algorithm describing angiogenesis and vessel maturation and its use for studying the effects of anti-angiogenic and anti-maturation therapy on vascular tumor growth. *Angiogenesis*, **5**, 203–214.

24. Bergers, G., Song, S., Meyer-Morse, N. *et al.* (2003) Benefits of targeting both pericytes and endothelial cells in the tumor vasculature with kinase inhibitors. *The Journal of Clinical Investigation*, **111**, 1287–1295.

25. Agur, Z., Bloch, N., Gorelik, B. *et al.* (2011) Developing oncology drugs using virtual patients of vascular tumor diseases, in *Systems Biology in Drug Discovery and Development* (eds D. Young and S. Michelson), John Wiley & Sons, Inc., New York, pp. 203–231.

26. Arakelyan, L., Daugulis, P., Ginosar, Y. *et al.* (2003) Multi-scale analysis of angiogenic dynamics and therapy, in *Cancer Modelling and Simulation* (ed. L. Preziosi), CRC Press, pp. 185–219.

27. Arakelyan, L., Vainstain, V. and Agur, Z. (2002) Optimizing anti-angiogenic therapy using mathematical tools. *Proceedings of the American Society of Clinical Oncology (ASCO)*, **21**, 440a.

28. Vainstein, V., Ginosar, Y., Shoham, M. *et al.* (2005) The complex effect of granulocyte colony-stimulating factor on human granulopoiesis analyzed by a new physiologically-based mathematical model. *Journal of Theoretical Biology*, **234**, 311–327.

29. Agur, Z. (2010) From the evolution of toxin resistance to virtual clinical trials: the role of mathematical models in oncology. *Future Oncology*, **6**, 917–927.

30. Walker, E.P. (2010) FDA Panel Nixes Bevacizumab for Breast Cancer, www.breastcancer.org/treatment/targeted_therapies/new_research/20100720b.jsp (accessed March 27, 2012)

31. Assikis, V.J., Do, K.A., Wen, S. *et al.* (2004) Clinical and biomarker correlates of androgen-independent, locally aggressive prostate cancer with limited metastatic potential. *Clinical Cancer Research*, **10**, 6770–6678.

32. Caine, G.J., Ryan, P., Lip, G.Y. and Blann, A.D. (2007) Significant decrease in angiopoietin-1 and angiopoietin-2 after radical prostatectomy in prostate cancer patients. *Cancer Letters*, **251**, 296–301.

33. Maruyama, Y., Ono, M., Kawahara, A. *et al.* (2006) Tumor growth suppression in pancreatic cancer by a putative metastasis suppressor gene Cap43/NDRG1/Drg-1 through modulation of angiogenesis. *Cancer Research*, **66**, 6233–6242.

34. Simon, R. (1994) Some practical aspects of the interim monitoring of clinical trials. *Statistics in Medicine*, **13**, 1401–1409.

35. Simon, R. (1999) Bayesian design and analysis of active control clinical trials. *Biometrics*, **55**, 484–487.

36. Simon, R. and Norton, L. (2006) The Norton-Simon hypothesis: designing more effective and less toxic chemotherapeutic regimens. *Nature Clinical Practice. Oncology*, **3**, 406–407.

# 5

# Stage-wise clinical trial experiments in Phases I, II and III

**Shelemyahu Zacks**
*Department of Mathematical Sciences, Binghamton University, Binghamton, NY, USA*

## Synopsis

This chapter reviews various important methods in Phase I, II and III of clinical trials. In Phase I the main objective is to find the maximum tolerated dose (MTD) of a new agent (drug). We discuss and evaluate the up-and-down methods, the continuous reassessment method and the EWOC (escalation with overdose control) method. For Phase II designs we discuss the individual dosing approach, which depends on individual covariates (markers). We discuss also the problem of the time of termination of the Phase II trials. In Phase III trials we have problems of adaptive randomization procedures. We discuss in this chapter six different adaptive designs and conclude with a short review of group sequential methods.

## 5.1   Introduction

Clinical trials are designed to test a new drug or therapy on human subjects. There are several important aspects to test: the toxicity of the drug and what dosage could be tolerated by the subjects without endangering their life. In cancer chemotherapy it is generally desired to administer a high dosage in order to kill as many cancer cells as possible. The first thing to investigate is the value of the maximal safety dose. After that one would like to investigate the efficacy of the new drug at the dosage that was determined as safe for applications.

*Statistical Methods in Healthcare*, First Edition. Edited by Frederick W. Faltin, Ron S. Kenett and Fabrizio Ruggeri.
© 2012 John Wiley & Sons, Ltd. Published 2012 by John Wiley & Sons, Ltd.

A third problem is to establish whether the new drug is better or worse than those which are already in use. Also side effects should be explored, and so on.

Clinical trials proceed in phases which have different objectives and are conducted differently. Phase I trials are designed to explore the toxicity and the side effects of a new drug. Typically, the sample consists of 20–80 cancer patients in progressive stages of the disease. The aim is to find the *maximum tolerated dose* (MTD) of the new drug to avoid life-threatening toxicity and other unacceptable side effects. Phase II of clinical trials are generally pilot studies of moderate size concerned with evaluating efficacy and safety of the new drug. The MTD established in Phase I is usually the applied dose in Phase II. Phase III trials are of longer duration. The objective is to compare the new therapeutic to an established standard or to several other treatments, and the presence of long-term side effects is monitored. In this phase, patients are allocated to different treatments by adaptive randomization procedures. Phase IV is that of additional testing of a treatment that has been approved for general use.

In the present chapter we discuss the theoretical aspects connected with each one of the phases, and indicate some new trends and developments. We show also some results from the theory of sequential allocation of resources (the bandits problem) which are relevant to clinical trials. For additional technical details the reader is referred to Chapters 6–8 of the recent book (Zacks, 2009), entitled *Stage-Wise Adaptive Designs*.

## 5.2    Phase I clinical trials

As mentioned in the introduction, we concentrate on Phase I clinical trials which involve new drugs for cancer chemotherapy. Different individuals have, typically, different tolerance levels to drugs. These tolerance levels for a new agent are unknown. It is desired that no more than one-third of the population will reveal a life-threatening toxicity. The maximal dose assuring this is called an MTD. In the search for the MTD we will discuss methods which avoid, with high probability, overdosing. This is, however, not a concern in many studies, since the patients participating in cancer Phase I clinical trials are already in life-threatening situations due to the advanced stages of their disease.

There are two approaches to dose escalation in cancer Phase I clinical trials. One is a nonparametric approach, like the up-and-down procedure and isotonic regression estimates. The other one is the modeling approach. The modeling approach connects the dosage to the probability of dose-limiting toxicity (DLT) via a tolerance distribution. Examples will be given later. A dose escalation scheme determines the dose for the $n$th patient as a function of the previous $(n-1)$ dosages and the observed level of toxicity manifested by the first $(n-1)$ subjects. Generally the trials start at a low dose which is considered 'safe'. It is desired that the doses assigned to the following patients will be as close as possible to the MTD, but below it. This is a challenging problem. Babb, Rogatko and Zacks (1998) developed a Bayesian procedure, called escalation with overdose control (EWOC), which is designed to fulfill these objectives. For a review of Bayesian methods in cancer Phase I clinical trials, see the article of Babb and Rogatko (2003). We start with a discussion of the up-and-down procedure, since it is the oldest one, and proceed to isotonic regression procedures. We then discuss Bayesian escalation schemes. The Bayesian approach is called for since the number of patients participating in Phase I studies is small, and procedures based on asymptotic results may not be appropriate. The literature on Phase I clinical trials contains hundreds of papers, most of which employ the up-and-down procedure. We list a few of these at the end of the chapter.

## 5.2.1   Up-and-down adaptive designs in search of the MTD

Up-and-down (UD) designs were first suggested by Anderson, McCarthy and Tukey (1946), Dixon and Mood (1948), Dixon (1965), Tsutakawa (1967) and more. The common feature to these designs is the following. The response of each subject to a given dose, $x$, is binary: either a DLT response or not. Starting with a low 'safe' dose, rules are given for escalating or de-escalating the dosage for the next trial. The dose at which the trial ends is estimated as the MTD. The following are some UD procedures.

1. **UD1:** the patients are treated in groups of size $n = 3$ (cohort groups). All patients in the same cohort receive the same dose. If no DLT is observed in a given dose, $x_1$, the next cohort receives the next higher dose, $x_2$. Otherwise, if only one patient exhibits a DLT, the next cohort remains at the same dose, $x_1$. If the next cohort does not exhibit any DLT, the dose is then escalated to $x_2$. If there are one or more DLTs among the next cohort, the trial is terminated, and the estimate of the MTD is $x_1$. In UD1 there is an immediate escalation, one repeat of the same dose, or termination.

2. **UD2:** treat patients in cohorts of size $n = 3$. If no DLT is observed, escalate the dose. If more than one patient manifests DLT, de-escalate the dose. Otherwise, remain at the same dose. Terminate the trial when a specified number of patients, $N$, have been observed.

3. **UD3:** treat the patients one at a time. If DLT is manifested, de-escalate the dose. Otherwise, if at two consecutive trials no DLT is shown, escalate the dose. Terminate after a specified number of patients, $N$, have been treated.

4. **UD4:** escalate continuously until the first DLT. Then, implement UD3.

Durham and Flournoy (1995) considered UD designs with randomization. They called these biased coin designs (BCDs). Two such designs were considered:

5. **BCD1:** patients are treated one at a time. At a dose $x$, let $0 < b(x) < 1$ be a randomization probability. If there is *no* DLT at $x$, escalate with probability $b(x)$ and stay at $x$ with probability $1 - b(x)$. If there is a DLT at $x$, de-escalate the dose.

6. **BCD2:** patients are treated one at a time. If there is *no* DLT at dose $x$, escalate. If there is DLT, stay at $x$ with probability $b(x)$ and de-escalate with probability $1 - b(x)$.

Let

$$Q(x) = P\{\text{DLT} \mid \text{dose} = x\}. \tag{5.1}$$

To evaluate the characteristics of the various UD procedures, we should assign the dosages values of $Q(x)$. We adopt here the logistic model employed by Durham and Flournoy (1995); namely,

$$Q(x) = \frac{\exp(-3.569 + 0.549x)}{1 + \exp(-3.569 + 0.549x)}. \tag{5.2}$$

We consider a set of six dosages with the associated values of $Q(x)$:

| $x$ | 2.5 | 4.5 | 5.24 | 5.76 | 6.5 | 7.25 |
|------|------|------|------|------|------|------|
| $Q(x)$ | 0.1 | 0.25 | 0.33 | 0.4 | 0.5 | 0.6 |

For a target of $Q(x) \leq \gamma = \frac{1}{3}$, the MTD is 5.24. Suppose that in all procedures other than UD1 there are $N = 24$ patients in the trial. We estimate by simulation the bias of the estimators of the MTD, the MSE (mean square error) of these estimators, and the proportion of cases where $x >$ MTD. This is denoted by proportion of overdose cases POD. We repeat it for each one of the four UD designs and for the BCD1 design. In the BCD designs, $b(x) = Q(x)/(1 - Q(x))$. All procedures start at the lowest dose of $x = 2.5$. We employed $M = 5000$ simulation runs in each case. In Table 5.1 we present the results of these simulations.

One can develop formulae for exact computations of the Bias, MSE and POD of these up-and-down procedures. For such formulae, see Zacks (2009, Ch. 6).

Several important studies have been published recently concerning UD designs for Phase I clinical studies, in particular on the estimation of the MTD. The reader is referred to Stylianou, Proschan and Flournoy (2003); Ivanova et al. (2003); and in particular the article of Ng, Mohanty and Balakrishnan (2007). In this paper, the authors study, in addition to the BCD rule mentioned before, also a $k$-in-a-row (KROW) rule, the Naroyana rule (NAR), and the CRM rule, which is discussed in the next section. The KROW is appropriate only if $\gamma = 1 - (\frac{1}{2})^k$, $k \geq 1$, which is at least 0.5. This is generally too large. The NAR rule was introduced for $\gamma = 0.5$.

In our previous discussion we applied as an estimator of the MTD the last dosage used in the design. This is obviously a nonparametric estimator. Stylianou and Flournoy (2002) introduced an empirical mean estimator (EME), which is the average of the last $(N - r)$ dosages used. Another type of nonparametric estimator is the *isotonic regression* estimator suggested by Stylianou and Flournoy (2002). Suppose that $h$ out of the $K$ dosages were used in a trial. Let $Q_j = X_n/n_j$, $j = 1, \ldots, h$, where $X_j$ is the number of patients exhibiting DLT and $n_j$ is the number of patients subjected to dosage $d_j$. For $i = 1, \ldots, h$, define $\hat{Q}_j^* = \hat{Q}_{j-1}I\{\hat{Q}_j \leq \hat{Q}_{j-1}\} + \hat{Q}_jI\{\hat{Q}_j > \hat{Q}_{j-1}\}$. Notice that $\hat{Q}_0 \equiv 0$ and $\hat{Q}_1^* \leq \hat{Q}_2^* \leq \cdots \leq \hat{Q}_h^*$.

Let $m$ be such that $\hat{Q}_m^* \leq \gamma \leq \hat{Q}_{m+1}^*$. The isotonic linear estimator of the MTD is

$$\widehat{MTD}_{LI} = d_m + \frac{\gamma - \hat{Q}_m^*}{\hat{Q}_{m+1}^* - \hat{Q}_m^*}(d_{m+1} - d_m) \tag{5.3}$$

**Table 5.1** Bias, MSE and proportion of overdose cases (POD). MTD $= 5.24$, $\gamma = {}^1/_3$, $N = 24$.

| Procedure | Bias | MSE | POD |
|-----------|--------|--------|-------|
| UD1 | −0.316 | 1.0869 | 0.241 |
| UD2 | −0.233 | 0.8732 | 0.267 |
| UD3 | −0.190 | 1.6134 | 0.367 |
| UD4 | −0.217 | 1.7169 | 0.362 |
| BCD1 | 0.078 | 2.2837 | 0.456 |

if $\hat{Q}^*_{m+1} > \hat{Q}^*_m$, and $\widehat{MTD}_{\text{LI}} = d_m$ if $\hat{Q}^*_m = \hat{Q}^*_{m+1}$. Another type of isotonic estimator is given by a *logistic-type* interpolation. Recall that, for $0 < p < 1$, $\text{logit}(p) = \log[p(1-p)]$. Accordingly,

$$\widehat{MTD}_{\log I} = d_m + \frac{\text{logit}(\gamma) - \text{logit}(\hat{Q}^*_m)}{\text{logit}(\hat{Q}^*_{m+1}) - \text{logit}(\hat{Q}^*_m)} \cdot (d_{m+1} - d_m). \tag{5.4}$$

In the case $\gamma > \hat{Q}^*_h$, the estimator is $d_h$, and if $\gamma < \hat{Q}^*_1$ the estimator is $d_1$. The maximum likelihood estimators (MLEs) were also studied in the above-mentioned papers, with likelihood based on the logistic distribution. According to the numerical results of Ng, Mohanty and Balakrishnan (2007), the isotonic and the maximum likelihood estimators of the MTD have smaller MSE than the estimators based on the last dosage.

## 5.2.2   The continuous reassessment method

The continuous reassessment method (CRM) has been applied by many researchers. This method is based on modeling a tolerance distribution in order to have a likelihood function. After observing $k$ patients, an estimator of the MTD is obtained as a function of the previous results. The treatment is applied one by one and the dosage for the next patient is the last estimator of the MTD or a function of it. In the present section we focus attention on Bayesian procedures. CRM methods were investigated by O'Quigley, Pepe and Fisher (1990); Storer (1989); Eichhorn and Zacks (1973); Tsutakawa (1980); Gastonis and Greenhouse (1992); Babb, Rogatko and Zacks (1998); and Zacks, Rogatko and Babb (1998). In particular see the article of Babb and Rogatko (2003) on Bayesian methods in cancer Phase I clinical trials (CPICTs).

There are different formulations of the tolerance distributions in the literature. Let $F(z)$ be a cumulative distribution function (cdf) in standard form. The relationship between a dose $x$ (or log-dose) and the response which is a binary variable $Y(x)$, is given by

$$P\{Y(x) = 1 \mid x\} = F(\beta_0 + \beta_1 x), \tag{5.5}$$

where $\beta_1 > 0$. Recall that $Y(x) = 1$ if the response is DLT, and $Y(x) = 0$ otherwise. The MTD is the dosage for which the probability of DLT is $\gamma$. Thus, the MTD is a function of $F(\cdot)$, $\beta_0$, $\beta_1$, and is given by

$$x_\gamma = \frac{F^{-1}(\gamma) - \beta_0}{\beta_1}. \tag{5.6}$$

In Zacks (2009, Ch. 6) we developed the CRM with the logistic distribution (5.2). Here we do it with the standard normal distribution, $\Phi(z)$; that is,

$$Q(x) = \Phi(\beta_0 + \beta_1 x). \tag{5.7}$$

The dosages considered are 2.5, 4.5, 5.24, 5.76, 6.5 and 7.25. As before we assume that $Q(2.5) = 0.1$ and $Q(4.5) = 0.25$. With these values we get $\beta_0 = 2.0404$ and $\beta_1 = 0.3035$.

Thus, our tolerance distribution is

$$Q(x) = \Phi(-2.0404 + 0.3035x).$$

The MTD is $x_\gamma = Q^{-1}(\frac{1}{3}) = 5.303$. As shown in Zacks (2009, p. 178) the MTD for the logistic tolerance distribution is $x_\gamma = 5.24$. The $Q(x)$ values for all six dosages are

| $x$ | 2.5 | 4.5 | 5.24 | 5.76 | 6.5 | 7.25 |
|------|-----|------|-------|-------|-------|-------|
| $Q(x)$ | 0.1 | 0.25 | 0.326 | 0.385 | 0.473 | 0.564 |

If only $p_1 = Q(2.5)$ is known, and $x^* = 2.5$, the model becomes

$$\tilde{Q}(x) = \Phi(-1.2816 + \beta(x - 2.5)), \tag{5.8}$$

where $0 < \beta < \infty$. According to the $\tilde{Q}(x)$ model, the MTD is

$$x_\gamma = 2.5 + \frac{\Phi^{-1}(\gamma) + 1.2816}{\beta}. \tag{5.9}$$

The CRM method determines a Bayesian estimator of $1/\beta$ after each trial, and substitutes it in (5.9) to obtain the next recommended dose. More specifically, let $D_k = \{(x_j, Y_j), \ j = 1, \ldots, k\}$ be the data after the first $k$ trials, where $x_j$ is the dose administered to the $j$th patient, and $Y_j = 1$ if DLT is observed and $Y_j = 0$ otherwise. The likelihood function of $\beta$, after $k$ trials is

$$L_k(\beta; \ D_k) = \prod_{j=1}^{k} \tilde{Q}(x_j)^{Y_j}(1 - \tilde{Q}(x_j))^{1-Y_j}. \tag{5.10}$$

If $h(\beta)$ is a prior density for $\beta$, then the Bayesian estimator of $(1/\beta)$ after $k$ trials is

$$E_H\{\beta^{-1} \mid D_k\} = \frac{\int_0^\infty \frac{1}{\beta} L_k(\beta; \ D_k) h(\beta) d\beta}{\int_0^\infty L_k(\beta; \ D_k) h(\beta) d\beta}. \tag{5.11}$$

Thus, the dose assigned to the $(k + 1)$st patient, according to the CRM method is the closest one to

$$\hat{x}^{(k+1)} = 2.5 + (1.2816 - 0.4307)E_H\{\beta^{-1} \mid D_k\}. \tag{5.12}$$

In Table 5.2 we present a sequence of 30 simulated values of $\hat{x}_\gamma^{(k)}$. The prior distribution of $\beta$ is the gamma distribution, with scale parameter 0.15175 and shape parameter 2. The integrals in (5.11) were computed by simulation from the $0.15175G(2,1)$ distribution. The values of $Y_j$, for a given $x_j$, were simulated from a Binom$(1, Q(x))$.

Interestingly, only one dose is extreme, and 80% of the dosages are in the range (MTD $\pm$ 0.1 MTD) or (4.773–5.833).

**Table 5.2**  Simulated values of $\hat{x}_\gamma^{(k)}$, $\gamma = {}^1/_3$.

| k | 1 | 2 | 3 | 4 | 5 | 6 | 7 | 8 | 9 | 10 |
|---|---|---|---|---|---|---|---|---|---|----|
| $\hat{x}_\gamma^{(k)}$ | 2.5 | 3.29 | 8.23 | 5.94 | 4.84 | 4.30 | 4.56 | 4.79 | 5.04 | 5.34 |
| k | 11 | 12 | 13 | 14 | 15 | 16 | 17 | 18 | 19 | 20 |
| $\hat{x}_\gamma^{(k)}$ | 4.89 | 5.10 | 5.28 | 5.64 | 5.11 | 5.31 | 4.91 | 5.09 | 5.23 | 4.98 |
| k | 21 | 22 | 23 | 24 | 25 | 26 | 27 | 28 | 29 | 30 |
| $\hat{x}_\gamma^{(k)}$ | 5.14 | 4.85 | 4.96 | 5.05 | 5.12 | 5.24 | 5.08 | 5.18 | 5.31 | 5.26 |

### 5.2.3   Efficient dose escalation scheme with overdose control (EWOC)

Eichhorn and Zacks (1973) introduced the notion of a $1 - \alpha$ feasible sequence of dosages. This was later extended to Bayesian feasibility.

A sequence $\{x_n^{(\alpha)}, \ n \geq 1\}$ is called *Bayesian feasible* at level $1 - \alpha$ if

$$P_H\{x_n^{(\alpha)} \leq x_\gamma \mid \mathsf{D}_{n-1}\} \geq 1 - \alpha \text{ for all } n \geq 1. \tag{5.13}$$

where $P_H\{\cdot \mid \mathsf{D}_{n-1}\}$ denotes the posterior probability for a prior $H$. Zacks, Rogatko and Babb (1998) proved that the $\alpha$-quantile of the posterior distribution of $x_\gamma$ given $\mathsf{D}_{n-1}$ is the optimal Bayesian-feasible dose for stage $n$.

Let $\beta_{1-\alpha}$ denote the $1 - \alpha$ quantile of the posterior distribution of $\beta$ given $\mathsf{D}_{n-1}$. Then the $\alpha$-quantile of the posterior distribution of $x_\gamma$ given $\mathsf{D}_{n-1}$ is

$$x_n^{(\alpha)} = x^* + (\Phi^{-1}(\gamma) + 1.2815)/\beta_{1-\alpha, n}. \tag{5.14}$$

We approximate $\beta_{1-\alpha, n}$ by

$$\beta_{1-\alpha, n} \cong E_H\{\beta \mid \mathsf{D}_{n-1}\} + \lambda(V_h(\beta \mid \mathsf{D}_{n-1}))^{1/2}. \tag{5.15}$$

Since $1/\beta$ is a convex function of $\beta$, by Jensen's inequality

$$E_H\left(\frac{1}{\beta} \mid \mathsf{D}_n\right) \geq \frac{1}{E_H\{\beta \mid \mathsf{D}_n\}} \geq \frac{1}{\beta_{1-\alpha, n}}. \tag{5.16}$$

Hence, the CRM procedure always yields estimates of the MTD *greater* than those of the EWOC procedure. The EWOC was designed to protect against assigning dosages greater than the MTD. Babb, Rogatko and Zacks (1998) conducted extensive simulations to compare the properties of the EWOC procedure with those of the CRM and the up-and-down procedures UD1–UD4. The results show that the proportion of patients treated at dosages close to the MTD, but below it, is greater under EWOC than any other procedure. Moreover, there was clear indication that EWOC protected against overdosing relative to the CRM.

## 5.3    Adaptive methods for Phase II trials

Phase II is generally a one-armed trial, the main objective of which is to test or estimate the efficacy of a new drug. Generally it is difficult to measure the efficacy of a drug after a short time of treatment. One could phrase the objective as 'the agent (new drug) will be of interest if *at least* 50% of the patients are cured after one year'. The term 'cured' is used here in the broad sense, to mean 'significant improvement'. A patient might be declared 'uncured' at any time before a year of treatment if death occurs, or if it is clear that the treatment has not made any significant improvement. Thus, stopping rules should be developed so that, as soon as it is evident that the cure rate is smaller than $p_0 = 0.5$, the trial is terminated.

In many trials, the MTD determined in Phase I is applied on all individuals throughout the treatments. This may however be too low for many patients, who could tolerate higher doses, and thus may be ineffective. The first part of Phase II treatments should be devoted to finding individual dosing, and applying for each patient his individual MTD, so that the treatments would be more effective.

### 5.3.1    Individual dosing

Babb and Rogatko (2001) extended the EWOC to allow the inclusion of individual covariates. The model applied is the logistic regression

$$P\{Y = 1 \mid \text{Dose} = x, \text{ Covariate} = w\} = \frac{\exp(\beta_0 + \beta_1 x + \beta_2 w)}{1 + \exp(\beta_0 + \beta_1 x + \beta_2 w)}. \tag{5.17}$$

The individual MTD is then

$$x_\gamma(w) = \frac{\log \dfrac{\gamma}{1 - \gamma} - \beta_0 - \beta_2 w}{\beta_1}. \tag{5.18}$$

The data associated with the first $k$ patient is

$$D_k = \{(x_1, Y_1, w_1), \ldots, (x_k, Y_k, w_k)\}.$$

where the dose given to the first (or first few) patient(s) is the MTD found in Phase I. Given $D_k$, the value of $x_{k+1}$ is determined, similarly to the EWOC Bayesian procedure, by computing the $\alpha$-quantile of the posterior distribution of $x_\gamma(w_{k+1})$. Here $w_{k+1}$ is the covariate of the $(k + 1)$st patient. The $\alpha$-quantile of $x_\gamma(w_{k+1})$ is found in three steps.

***Step I:*** Determine the joint posterior distribution of $(\beta_0, \beta_1, \beta_2)$; namely

$$\pi(\beta_0, \beta_1, \beta_2 \mid D_k) = \frac{L(\beta_0, \beta_1, \beta_2 \mid D_k)h(\beta_0, \beta_1, \beta_2)}{\int \int \int_\Theta L(\beta_0, \beta_1, \beta_2 \mid D_k)h(\beta_0, \beta_1, \beta_2)\mathrm{d}\beta_0 \mathrm{d}\beta_1 \mathrm{d}\beta_2} \tag{5.19}$$

where $h(\beta_0, \beta_1, \beta_2)$ is the prior probability distribution function (pdf), and $\Theta = \{(\beta_0, \beta_1, \beta_2) : \beta_1 > 0, \beta_2 < 0\}$.

**Step II:** Make the transformation

$$
\begin{aligned}
\beta_0 &= \beta_0 \\
\beta_1 &= \beta_1 \\
\beta_2 &= \frac{\beta_1 x_\gamma + \beta_0 - \log \frac{\gamma}{1 - \gamma}}{w_{k+1}}.
\end{aligned}
\tag{5.20}
$$

The Jacobian of this transformation is

$$
J = \frac{\beta_1}{w_{k+1}}.
\tag{5.21}
$$

The posterior joint density of $\beta_0$, $\beta_1$, $x_\gamma (w_{k+1})$ is

$$
\left| \frac{\beta_1}{w_{k+1}} \right| \pi \left( \beta_0, \beta_1, \frac{\beta_1 x_\gamma (w_{k+1}) + \beta_0 - \log \frac{\gamma}{1-\gamma}}{w_{k+1}} \Big| D_k \right).
$$

**Step III:** Compute the marginal posterior density of $x_\gamma (w_{k+1})$; namely

$$
\pi^*(x|D_k) = \int_{\beta_0=\infty}^{\infty} \int_{\beta_1=0}^{\infty} \pi \left( \beta_0, \beta_1, \xi(\beta_0, \beta_1, w_{k+1}) \right) \cdot \left| \frac{\beta_1}{w_{k+1}} \right| \cdot d\beta_0 d\beta_1,
\tag{5.22}
$$

where

$$
\xi(\beta_0, \beta_1, w_{k+1}, x) = \frac{1}{w_{k+1}} \left( \beta_1 x + \beta_0 - \log \frac{\gamma}{1 - \gamma} \right).
\tag{5.23}
$$

Finally find the $\alpha$-quantile of (5.22); namely

$$
x_{\gamma,\alpha}(w_{k+1}) = \inf \left\{ \xi > 0 : \int_0^\xi \pi^*(x \,|\, D_k) dx = \alpha \right\}.
\tag{5.24}
$$

An algorithm for numerical determination of $x_{\gamma,\alpha}(w_{k+1})$ can be easily determined. The difficulty is to determine, for a new agent, the significant covariates. Babb and Rogatko (2001) described a PNU trial in which the covariate was an anti-SEA/E120. Ubezio *et al.* (1994) considered direct measurement of bone marrow cell kinetics.

## 5.3.2   Termination of Phase II

Another important problem is when to terminate a Phase II study, when there is evidence that the new drug is not effective. We describe here a possible approach for the efficacy objective stated at the beginning of the section.

A patient may be declared uncured at any time before a year of treatment if death occurs, or if it is clear that the treatment will not cure the patient. As soon as this happens, the patient is removed from the trial. In addition, any patient who is uncured after a year of treatment is removed from the trial and labeled 'uncured'.

Patients enter the study at random times, following a Poisson process, $\{N(t), t \geq 0\}$, with intensity $\lambda$, $0 < \lambda < \infty$. $\lambda$ is the expected number of patients entering the trial in a unit time (a month). Let $q$, $0 < q < 1$, denote the probability that a patient will be dropped from the trial uncured, and let $\{X(t), t \geq 0\}$ be the number of patients dropped uncured during the time interval $(0, t]$. $\{X(t), t \geq 0\}$ is a Poisson process, with intensity $\lambda q$. If $q > 0.5$ we should reject the new agent. We construct a one-sided Wald SPRT (sequential probability ratio test), for testing the hypotheses

$$H_0 : q \leq q_0 = 0.45$$

against

$$H_1 : q \geq q_1 = 0.55$$

with error probabilities $\alpha$ and $\beta$. The likelihood ratio at time $t$ is

$$L_t = \left( \frac{q_1}{q_0} \right)^{X(t)} \exp\left( -\lambda(q_1 - q_0)t \right), \, t \geq 0. \tag{5.25}$$

Consider the stopping time $T_x = \min\{T_1, T^*\}$, where

$$T_1 = \inf \left\{ t > 0 : L_t \geq \frac{1 - \beta}{\alpha} \right\}, \tag{5.26}$$

and $T^*$ is the end of the trial period. Notice that $T_1 = \inf\{t > 0 : X(t) \geq B_u(T)\}$, where

$$B_u(t) = \frac{\log\left( \frac{1 - \beta}{\alpha} \right)}{\log\left( \frac{q_1}{q_0} \right)} + \lambda \frac{q_1 - q_0}{\log\left( \frac{q_1}{q_0} \right)} t. \tag{5.27}$$

$T_1$ is a stopping time (early stopping) due to *rejection* of the hypothesis that the cure probability $p$ is at least 0.5.

## 5.4   Adaptive methods for Phase III

### 5.4.1   Randomization in clinical trials

Randomization in Phase III clinical trials is a very important feature of allocating the patients to the various treatments under comparison. Randomization means that patients entering the study are randomly assigned to the treatments. This is done in order to avoid biasing the results by some uncontrollable factors. There is a principle that should be followed in designing an experiment: block over factors under control and randomize what cannot be controlled. If controllable patient characteristics like age, gender and stage of the disease are relevant to the study, the patients should be grouped first into strata defined by such factors.

Within each stratum the patients should be assigned to the different treatments at random, trying to avoid the creeping of unforeseen bias into the results. Various methods of randomly assigning patients to treatments have developed during the last 50 years. The reader is referred especially to the books of Rosenberger and Lachin (2002) and Hu and Rosenberger (2006). In the present chapter we present just the essentials.

Suppose there are only two treatments on test, a standard one and a new one. If there is a pool of $N$ patients, and it is decided that $M$ patients will be treated with the standard and $N - M$ with the new, one could choose a random sample of $M$ patients out of $N$ without replacement. In this case there are exactly $M$ patients in one group (the control group) and $N - M$ in the second one (the test group). This should be executed also under double masking so that both the patients and the doctors will not know which treatment is given to whom. This is often impractical. Many Phase III clinical studies extend over several years. Patients arrive as candidates for treatments at random times, and the total number of patients entering the study is a random variable. Thus, in most studies an entering patient is assigned to a given treatment with certain probability vector $\psi$. This probability vector might be the same for all patients or might change from one patient to another. For example, suppose that there are only two treatments, $A$ and $B$. Let $\psi$ be the probability of assigning a new patient to treatment $A$. In a 'completely randomized' study $\psi = \frac{1}{2}$ for all patients. But then, the number of patients assigned to treatment $A$, among the first $n$ patients, is a random variable $J_n^{(A)}$ having a binomial distribution $B(n, \frac{1}{2})$. With probability close to 1,

$$\frac{n}{2} - \frac{3}{2}\sqrt{n} < J_n^{(A)} < \frac{n}{2} + \frac{3}{2}\sqrt{n}.$$

Thus, if $n = 100$, $35 < J_{100}^{(A)} < 65$. This may result in a strongly imbalanced trial. We will list below several methods which have been devised in order to alleviate this problem. These methods change the probabilities $\psi_n$ as a function of the observed values of $J_{n-1}^{(A)}$; that is, $\psi_n = \psi(J_{n-1}^{(A)})$, $n \geq 2$, where $\psi_1 = \frac{1}{2}$. Another source of imbalance is *covariates imbalance*. We may find at the stage of analysis that more women were assigned at random to treatment $A$ then men, or some other type of imbalance (more older patients than young, etc.).

## 5.4.2   Adaptive randomization procedures

In the present section we discuss designs listed in Rosenberger and Lachin (2002, Ch. 2). We start with adaptive randomization designs, which attempt to keep the balance.

### 5.4.2.1   Random allocation rule

The following procedure was suggested by Lachin (1988). This procedure can be applied only if the total number of trials, $N$, is fixed and known from the beginning. In this case, the randomization probabilities are given by

$$\psi_n\left(J_{n-1}^{(A)}\right) = \frac{\frac{N}{2} - J_{n-1}^{(A)}}{N - (n-1)}, \quad n \geq 1, \tag{5.28}$$

where $J_0^{(A)} \equiv 0$. Recall that $J_n^{(A)}$ denotes the random number of patients assigned to treatment $A$ among the first $n$ assignments. The problem with this rule is that if $J_m^{(A)} = N/2$ then $\psi_n = 0$

for all $n > m$. This creates a source of possible selection bias. We examine below whether this bias is serious. Notice that this random allocation rule (5.28) is equivalent to the sampling at random without replacement which was mentioned in the previous section. Accordingly, the distribution of $J_n^{(A)}$ following (5.28) is hypergeometric with pdf

$$p_n^{(A)}(j) = \frac{\binom{N/2}{j}\binom{N/2}{n-j}}{\binom{N}{n}}, \quad j = 0, \ldots, n. \tag{5.29}$$

It is interesting to study the distribution of the first time one of the treatments gets the allotment of $N/2$ patients under the rule (5.28). This is the stopping variable

$$T_N = \min\left\{ n \geq \frac{N}{2} : \max\left(J_n^{(A)}, n < J_n^{(A)}\right) = \frac{N}{2} \right\}. \tag{5.30}$$

It is proven in Zacks (2009, p. 188) that the probability distribution of $T_N$ is

$$P\left\{ T_N = \frac{N}{2} + j \right\} = \frac{2\binom{N/2 + j - 1}{j}}{\binom{N}{N/2}}, \quad j \geq 1, \tag{5.31}$$

and

$$P\left\{ T_N = \frac{N}{2} \right\} = \frac{2}{\binom{N}{N/2}}. \tag{5.32}$$

(See Table 5.3.)

### 5.4.2.2 Truncated binomial design

This procedure was suggested by Blackwell and Hodges (1957):

$$\psi_n\left(J_{n-1}^{(A)}\right) = \begin{cases} \frac{1}{2} & \text{if } \max\left\{J_{n-1}^{(A)}, n - 1 - J_{n-1}^{(A)}\right\} < \frac{1}{2}N, \\ 0 & \text{if } J_{n-1}^{(A)} = \frac{1}{2}N, \\ 1 & \text{if } n - 1 - J_{n-1}^{(A)} = \frac{1}{2}N, \end{cases} \tag{5.33}$$

**Table 5.3** Distribution of $T_N$, $N = 20$.

| n | 10 | 11 | 12 | 13 | 14 |
|---|---|---|---|---|---|
| $P\{T_N = n\}$ | 0.00001 | 0.00011 | 0.00059 | 0.00238 | 0.00774 |
| n | 15 | 16 | 17 | 18 | 19 |
| $P\{T_N = n\}$ | 0.02167 | 0.05418 | 0.12384 | 0.23616 | 0.52632 |

**Table 5.4**  Distribution of $T_N^*$, $N = 20$.

| n | $P\{T_N^* = n\}$ | n | $P\{T_N^* = n\}$ |
|---|---|---|---|
| 10 | 0.00195 | 15 | 0.12219 |
| 11 | 0.00977 | 16 | 0.15274 |
| 12 | 0.02686 | 17 | 0.17456 |
| 13 | 0.05371 | 18 | 0.18547 |
| 14 | 0.08728 | 19 | 0.18547 |

with $\psi_1 = \frac{1}{2}$. Since the smallest value of $n$ for which $\max\{J_n^{(A)}, n - J_n^{(A)}\} = \frac{1}{2}N$ is $\frac{1}{2}N$, according to (5.33), $\psi_n(J_{n-1}^{(A)}) = \frac{1}{2}$ for all $n = 1, 2, \ldots, T_N^*$, where

$$T_N^* = \min\left\{ n \geq \frac{1}{2}N : \max\{J_n^{(A)}, n - J_n^{(A)}\} = \frac{1}{2}N \right\}. \tag{5.34}$$

The distribution of $T_N^*$ is

$$P\left\{ T_N^* = \frac{1}{2}N + j \right\} = \binom{\frac{1}{2}N + j - 1}{j} \left(\frac{1}{2}\right)^{\frac{N}{2}+j-1}, \tag{5.35}$$

for $j = 0, 1, \ldots, \frac{1}{2}N - 1$. (See Table 5.4.)

The expected value of $T_N^*$ is

$$E\{T_N^*\} = \frac{N}{2}\left( 1 + \sum_{j=0}^{\frac{N}{2}-2} \binom{\frac{N}{2}+j}{j} \left(\frac{1}{2}\right)^{\frac{N}{2}+j} \right). \tag{5.36}$$

For example, for $N = 200$, $E\{T_{200}^*\} = 188.73$. Thus, under randomization rule (5.33), the danger of bias due to the fact that the last few assignments are all to one treatment is not negligible.

### 5.4.2.3  Efron's biased coin design

Efron (1971) suggested a randomization procedure which is based on the difference $D_n = J_n^{(N)} - (n - J_n^{(A)}) = 2J_n^{(A)} - n$. This procedure is called the *biased coin design* and is given by

$$\psi_n(D_{n-1}) = \begin{cases} \frac{1}{2} & \text{if } D_{n-1} = 0, \\ p & \text{if } D_{n-1} < 0, \\ 1 - p & \text{if } D_{n-1} > 0, \end{cases} \tag{5.37}$$

where $\frac{1}{2} < p < 1$, and $D_0 \equiv 0$.

The process $\{D_n, n \geq 1\}$ is a birth-and-death process symmetric about $D_n = 0$ in the sense that, for $n$ odd, $P\{D_n > 0\} = P\{D_n < 0\} = \frac{1}{2}$. One can show then that $E\{\psi_n(D_{n-1})\} = \frac{1}{2}$ for all $n \geq 1$. For further properties see Zacks (2009, p. 190).

#### 5.4.2.4   Wei's urn design

Wei (1977, 1978) developed a procedure with probabilities $\psi_n$ which change from one patient to another. Starting with a pair of nonnegative integers $(\alpha, \beta)$, the conditional probability $\psi_n(J_{n-1}^{(A)})$ is

$$\psi_n\left(J_{n-1}^{(A)}\right) = \frac{\alpha + \beta\left(n - 1 - J_{n-1}^{(A)}\right)}{2\alpha + \beta(n - 1)}, \quad n \geq 1, \tag{5.38}$$

where $J_0^{(A)} \equiv 0$. Thus, if $J_n^{(A)} > J_{n-1}^{(A)}$, then $\psi_{n+1}(J_n^{(A)}) < \psi_n(J_{n-1}^{(A)})$, but if $J_n^{(A)} = J_{n-1}^{(A)}$, then $\psi_{n+1}(J_n^{(A)}) \geq \psi_n(J_{n-1}^{(A)})$. Such a design is designated as UD$(\alpha, \beta)$. If $\alpha = 0$ we define $\psi_1 = \frac{1}{2}$. The UD$(\alpha, 0)$ is equivalent to complete randomization. Since $E\{J_1^{(A)}\} = \frac{1}{2}$, we immediately obtain that $E\{\psi_2(J_1^{(A)})\} = \frac{1}{2}$. Thus, we can prove by induction on $n$ that $E\{\psi_n(J_{n-1}^{(A)})\} = \frac{1}{2}$ for all $n \geq 1$; or $E\{J_n^{(A)}\} = n/2$ for all $n \geq 1$. One can show that this procedure is asymptotically (as $n \to \infty$) equivalent to complete randomization.

#### 5.4.2.5   Response adaptive designs

Generally, Phase III trials are conducted in order to compare the probabilities of success (positive response) of different treatments. In particular, if a new treatment is compared to a standard one, ethics require one to assign more patients to the treatment having a higher probability of success.

Let $p_A$ denote the probability of success of the new treatment and $p_B$ that of the standard. Given that $J_n^{(A)}$ patients have been assigned to the new treatment, let $X(J_n^{(A)})$ denote the number of successes among them and $X(n - J_n^{(A)})$ the number of successes among the patients assigned to treatment $B$. We assume that the conditional distribution of $X(J_n^{(A)})$ given $J_n^{(A)}$ is binomial $B(J_n^{(A)}, p_A)$; similarly with the distribution of the number of successes in treatment $B$.

$$\text{Let } \hat{p}_n^{(A)} = \frac{X\left(J_n^{(A)}\right)}{J_n^{(A)}} \text{ and } \hat{p}_n^{(B)} = \frac{X\left(n - J_n^{(A)}\right)}{\left(n - J_n^{(A)}\right)}.$$

For the randomization methods we discussed before, $J_n$ is either equal to $n/2$ or its distribution is concentrated near $n/2$. Thus, the asymptotic distribution of $Z_n$ is the standard normal. To minimize the conditional variance $V\{\hat{p}_n^{(A)} - \hat{p}_n^{(B)} \mid J_n^{(A)}\}$, $J_n^{(A)}$ should be equal to

$$n_A^0 = n\frac{\sqrt{p_A(1 - p_A)}}{\sqrt{p_A(1 - p_A)} + \sqrt{\hat{p}_B(1 - \hat{p}_B)}}. \tag{5.39}$$

Thus, as long as we cannot reject the null hypothesis $H_0 : p_A = p_B$, the optimal allocation is $n_A = n/2$ and we should randomize the assignment to treatments with $\psi_n(J_{n-1}^{(A)})$ such that

$E\{\psi_n(J_{n-1}^{(A)})\} = \frac{1}{2}$. As soon as $H_0$ is rejected, one could switch to a randomization with

$$\psi_{n+1}\left(J_n^{(A)}, X_n^{(A)}, X_n^{(B)}\right) = \frac{\sqrt{\hat{p}_n^{(A)}\left(1 - \hat{p}_n^{(A)}\right)}}{\sqrt{p_n^{(A)}\left(1 - \hat{p}_n^{(A)}\right)} + \sqrt{\hat{p}_n^{(B)}\left(1 - \hat{p}_n^{(B)}\right)}}. \qquad (5.40)$$

Notice that $\hat{p}_n^{(A)}(1 - \hat{p}_n^{(A)})$ is greater than $\hat{p}_n^{(B)}(1 - \hat{p}_n^{(B)})$; therefore $\psi_{n+1}(J_n^{(A)}, X_n^A, X_n^B) > \frac{1}{2}$. This is satisfied only if $|\hat{p}_n^{(A)} - \frac{1}{2}| < |\hat{p}_n^{(B)} - \frac{1}{2}|$. Thus (5.40) does not meet the ethical requirement to allocate more patients to the treatment with the larger success probability. The randomization

$$\psi_{n+1}\left(J_n^{(A)}, X_n^{(A)}, X_n^{(B)}\right) = \frac{\sqrt{\hat{p}_n^{(A)}}}{\sqrt{\hat{p}_n^{(A)}} + \sqrt{\hat{p}_n^{(B)}}} \qquad (5.41)$$

satisfies the ethical requirement but does not minimize the variance. Notice also that these kinds of randomization rules are only asymptotically stable.

### 5.4.2.6  Sequential allocations in clinical trials

Sequential allocation of patients to two or more treatments is a very important feature in clinical trials. We emphasized allocation problems associated with randomization procedures to maintain balance and valid inference. Due to ethical considerations it is desired to maximize the expected number of patients receiving the better treatment. The question is whether optimal procedures for bandit problems, see Zacks (2009, Ch. 8), can be applied to clinical trials. In bandit models the result of each trial should be available before the next trial can be allocated. This is often not the case in clinical trials, where the success or failure of treatments takes a long time to be established. Also, when one arm (treatment) is being applied, other arms are generally not frozen, as it is in the multiarmed bandit procedures. One could develop, however, stopping rules according to which trials on a certain arm terminate as soon as it is realized that the treatments on that arm yield inferior results relative to the other arms. Many papers (see Wang, 1991; Bather, 1981; Hardwick, 1995; Jones, Lewis and Hartley, 1995; and others) formulate additional criteria for clinical trials, like probability of correct selection, expected number of patients receiving an inferior treatment, and more; Jones, Lewis and Hartley (1995) considered the following stopping rule: after $n_1$ trials on $A_1$ and $n_2$ trials on $A_2$, they compute the predictive probabilities $\hat{p}_i = (X_i + 1)/(n_i + 2)$ $(i = 1, 2)$. As soon as $|\hat{p}_1 - \hat{p}_2| > \Delta$, they switch all the remaining observations to the arm having the larger value of $\hat{p}_i$. Suppose that $N$ is the total number of trials allowed. If $(a_1, b_1, a_2, b_2)$ is the state of the system, the posterior probability that $\theta_1 < \theta_2$ for the independent beta priors is

$$\psi(a_1, b_1, a_2, b_2) = P_H\{\theta_1 < \theta_2 \mid (a_1, b_1, a_2, b_2)\}$$
$$= \sum_{j=a_1}^{a_1+b_1-1} \binom{a_1 + b_1 - 1}{j} \frac{B(a_2 + j, a_1 + b_1 + b_2 - j - 1)}{B(a_2, b_2)}. \qquad (5.42)$$

where $a_1 = X_i + 1$ and $b_i = n_i - X_i + 1$ ($i = 1, 2$). Indeed,

$$P\{\theta_1 < \theta_2 \mid a_1, b_1, a_2, b_2\}$$
$$= \frac{1}{B(a_2, b_2)} \int_0^1 v^{a_2-1}(1-v)^{b_2-1} I_v(a_1, b_1) dv. \tag{5.43}$$

Furthermore,

$$I_v(a_1, b_1) = \sum_{j=a_1}^{n_1+1} \binom{n_1 + 1}{j} v^j \left(1 - v^{n_1+1-j}\right). \tag{5.44}$$

Define the stopping variables

$$M_1 = \min\{n \geq k \ : \ \psi(a_1, b_1, a_2, b_2) \geq 1 - a_1\} \tag{5.45}$$

and

$$M_2 = \min\{n \geq k \ : \ \psi(a_1, b_1, a_2, b_2) \leq a_2\}. \tag{5.46}$$

Notice that $n = n_1 + n_2$. Here $\alpha_1$ and $\alpha_2$ are small values; for example, $\alpha_1 = \alpha_2 = 0.01$. We stop at $M = \min(M_1, M_2)$. Suppose also that, for $n \leq M$, $n_1 = n_2 = n/2$.

If $M = M_1$, then all the additional $N - M$ trials are allocated to $A_2$. On the other hand, if $M = M_2$, all the additional $N - M$ trials are on $A_1$. Let $N_1$ denote the number of trials on $A_1$. This is given by

$$N_1 = I\{M = M_1\}\frac{M_1}{2} + I\{M = M_2\} \left(N - \frac{M_2}{2}\right). \tag{5.47}$$

For example, in a simulation of $N = 100$ trials, with $k = 40$, when $\theta_1 = 0.5$ and $\theta_2 = 0.8$, we obtained $M = M_1 = 50$. In this case $N_1 = 25$. In Table 5.5 we present simulation estimates of $E\{N_1\}$ under different values of $p_1$ and $p_2$ with $k = 20, 40$. Each estimate is based on 100 runs.

In the above simulations we estimated also the *probability of correct selection* (PCS) of the superior arm. Let $\widehat{PCS}(p_1, p_2)$ denote the estimator of this probability. Thus, for the case of

**Table 5.5**   Simulation estimates of $E\{N_1\}$, $N = 100$, $\alpha_1 = \alpha_2 = 0.05$, $k = 20, 40$.

| $p_1$ | $p_2$ | $k = 20$ | $k = 40$ |
|-------|-------|----------|----------|
|       |       | $E\{N_1\}$ | $E\{N_1\}$ |
| 0.5   | 0.6   | 39.1     | 40.8     |
| 0.5   | 0.7   | 25.8     | 33.6     |
| 0.5   | 0.8   | 17.7     | 24.4     |

**Table 5.6**  Simulation and estimates of $E\{N_1\}$ and PCS, $N = 100, p < 0.5$.

| $p_2$ | $E\{N_1\}$ | PCS |
|-------|-----------|-----|
| 0.60 | 27.6 | 0.74 |
| 0.65 | 22.6 | 0.79 |
| 0.70 | 18.3 | 0.84 |
| 0.75 | 16.3 | 0.86 |
| 0.80 | 11.8 | 0.91 |

$\alpha_1 = \alpha_2 = 0.05, N = 100$ and $k = 40$, we obtained $\widehat{PCS}(0.5, 0.6) = 0.55, \widehat{PCS}(0.5, 0.7) = 0.92$ and $\widehat{PCS}(0.5, 0.8) = 1.00$. In order to minimize $E\{N_1\}$ and maximize PCS, one should use an optimal allocation determined by dynamic programming with uniform discounting truncated at $N$. This, however, is impractical. Bather and Simons (1985) showed that if we start with $M_1 = M_2 \cong 0.3\sqrt{N}$ and then use, for the rest of the trials, the arm with the maximal value of $\hat{p}_i$, then the risk is minimax. Notice that if $N = 100, 0.3\sqrt{N} = 3$. In Table 5.6 we present simulation estimates of $E\{N_1\}$ and of PCS $(p_1, p_2)$ following the Bather and Simon procedure. These are also based on 100 simulation runs.

### 5.4.3   Group sequential methods: Testing hypotheses

The so-called group sequential method is actually a multistage testing procedure. Instead of evaluating the results after each observation, we wait until a whole group of $m$ patients are tested on the two treatments. Afterwards, the hypothesis $H_0 : p_A = p_B$ is tested. If $H_0$ is rejected, then the trial is stopped: otherwise, another group of $m$ patients is treated on each one of the treatments, and so on. In other words, the total number of $N$ patients is tested in $K$ stages. In each stage $m$ patients are assigned at random to treatment $A$ and $m$ patients to treatment $B$. If in *all* $K$ stages the hypothesis $H_0$ is not rejected, the trial terminates after $K$ stages, with a total of $N = 2mK$ patients treated. On the other hand, if $H_0$ is rejected after the $k$th stage, $1 \leq k < K$, the trial is terminated with $N_k = 2mk$ patients treated. The problem is to devise the repetitive tests so that the level of significance will not exceed a prescribed value $\alpha$. There are many papers on the subject. The reader is referred to the book of Jennison and Turnbull (2000) for details and tables. For further theory of group sequential testing, see Zacks (2009, pp. 198–205).

## 5.5   Summary

In this chapter we reviewed and examined various procedures associated with Phases I–III of clinical trials. In Phase I the main objective is to find the MTD of a new agent (drug or combination of drugs). We evaluated six up-and-down (UD) procedures, and discussed some recent estimators of the MTD under UD designs. We then discussed the CRM procedures, which are essentially Bayesian. These were compared to the EWOC procedure, which was designed to control overdosing. For Phase II we reviewed the new approach of individual dosing to increase efficacy. We also discussed termination rules based on one-sided SPRT.

In Phase III we generally compare several treatments. One of the important facets is the randomized allocation of patients to treatments. Six different allocation procedures were presented: five randomization procedures, and one based on optimal sequential allocation. Group sequential methods for possible early termination were reviewed.

# References

Anderson, T.W., McCarthy, P.J. and Tukey, J.W. (1946) 'Staircase' method of sensitivity testing, in *Naval Ordinance Report*, Princeton Statistical Group, Princeton, NJ, pp. 46–65.

Babb, J. and Rogatko, A. (2001) Patient specific dosing in cancer Phase I clinical trials. *Stat. Med.*, **20**, 2079–2090.

Babb, J. and Rogatko, A. (2003) Bayesian methods for cancer Phase I clinical trials, in *Advances in Clinical Trial Biostatistics* (ed. N.L. Geller), Marcel Dekker, New York, pp. 1–39.

Babb, J., Rogatko, A. and Zacks, S. (1998) Cancer phase I clinical trials: efficient dose escalation with overdose control. *Stat. Med.*, **17**, 1103–1120.

Bather, J.A. (1981) Randomized allocation of treatments in sequential experiments (with discussion). *J. Roy. Stat. Soc. B*, **43**, 265–292.

Bather, J.A. and Simons, G. (1985) The minimax risk for clinical trials. *J. Roy. Stat. Soc. B*, **47**, 466–475.

Blackwell, D. and Hodges, J.L. (1957) Design for the control of selection bias. *Ann. Math. Stat.*, **28**, 449–460.

Dixon, W.J. (1965) The up-and-down method for small samples. *J. Am. Stat. Assoc*, **60**, 967–978.

Dixon, W.J. and Mood, A.M. (1948) A method of obtaining and analyzing sensitivity data. *J. Am. Stat. Assoc.*, **43**, 109–126.

Durham, S.D. and Flournoy, N. (1995) Up-and-down designs I: stationary treatment distributions. *Adapt. Des. IMS Lect. Notes Monogr. Ser.*, **25**, 139–157.

Efron, B. (1971) Forcing a sequential experiment to be balanced. *Biometrika*, **58**, 403–417.

Eichhorn, B.H. and Zacks, S. (1973) Sequential search of an optimal dosage I. *Am. Stat. Assoc.*, **68**, 594–598.

Gastonis, C. and Greenhouse, J.B. (1992) Bayesian methods for Phase I clinical trials. *Stat. Med.*, **11**, 1377–1389.

Hardwick, J.P. (1995) A modified bandit as an approach to ethical allocation in clinical trials. *Adaptive Des. IMS Lect. Notes Monogr. Ser.*, **25**, 65–87.

Hu, F. and Rosenberger, W.F. (2006) *The Theory of Response-Adaptive Randomization in Clinical Trials*, John Wiley & Sons, Inc., New York.

Ivanova, A., Montazar-Haghighi, A., Mohanty, S.G. and Durham, S.D. (2003) Improved up-and-down designs for Phase I trials. *Stat. Med.*, **22**, 69–82.

Jennison, C. and Turnbull, B.W. (2000) *Group Sequential Methods with Applications in Clinical Trials*. Chapman & Hall/CRC, Boca Raton, FL.

Jones, P.W., Lewis, A.M. and Hartley, R. (1995) Some designs for multi-criteria bandits. *Adapt. Des. IMS Lect. Notes Monogr. Ser.*, **25**, 88–94.

Lachin, J.M. (1988) Properties of simple randomization in clinical trials. *Control. Clin. Trials*, **9**, 312–326.

Ng, H.K.T., Mohanty, S.G. and Balakrishnan, N. (2007) An assessment of the up-and-down designs and associated estimators in Phase I trials, in *Advanced Statistical Methods in Health Sciences* (eds J.L. Auget, N. Balakrishman and G. Molenberghs), Burkhäuser, Boston.

O'Quigley, J., Pepe, M. and Fisher, L. (1990) Continual reassessment method: a practical design for Phase I clinical trials in cancer. *Biometrics*, **46**, 33–48.

Rosenberger, W.F. and Lachin, J.M. (2002) *Randomization in Clinical Trials, Theory and Practice*, John Wiley & Sons, Inc., New York.

Storer, B. (1989) Design and analysis of Phase I clinical trials. *Biometrics*, **45**, 925–937.

Stylianou, M. and Flournoy, N. (2002) Dose finding using the biased coin up-and-down design and isotonic regression. *Biometrics*, **58**, 171–177.

Stylianou, M., Proschan, M. and Flournoy, N. (2003) Estimating the probability of toxicity at the target dose following an up-and-down design. *Stat. Med.*, **22**, 535–543.

Tsutakawa, R.K. (1967) Random walk design in bio-assay. *J. Am. Stat. Assoc.*, **62**, 842–856.

Tsutakawa, R.K. (1980) Selection of dose levels for estimating a percentage point of a logistic response curve. *J. Roy. Stat. Soc. Ser. C Appl. Stat.*, **29**, 25–33.

Ubezio, P., Tagliabue, G., Schechter, B. and Agur, Z. (1994) Increasing 1-b-D-Arabinofuranosylcytosine efficacy by scheduled dosing intervals based on direct measurement of bone marrow cell kinetics. *Cancer Res*, **54**, 6446–6451.

Wang, Y.-G. (1991) Gittins indices and constrained allocation in clinical trials. *Biometrika*, **78**, 101–111.

Wei, L.J. (1977) A class of designs for sequential clinical trials. *J. Am. Stat. Assoc.*, **72**, 382–386.

Wei, L.J. (1978) The adaptive biased coin design for sequential experiments. *Ann. Stat.*, **6**, 92–100.

Zacks, S. (2009) *Stage-Wise Adaptive Designs*, John Wiley & Sons, Inc., New York.

Zacks, S., Rogatko, A. and Babb, J. (1998) Optimal Bayesian-feasible dose escalation for cancer Phase I clinical trials. *Stat. Prob. Lett.*, **38**, 215–220.

# 6

# Risk management in drug manufacturing and healthcare

**Ron S. Kenett**
*KPA Ltd, Raanana, Israel*

## Synopsis

Healthcare quality clearly affects everyone, at one point or another. Risks in healthcare have been abundantly documented and many efforts are invested in order to identify, assess and mitigate such risks. In this chapter we cover several areas related to risk management in drug manufacturing and healthcare delivery. These include reporting and tracking of adverse events, healthcare decision systems with an example in the area of hemodialysis, and risk-based quality audits. We begin with a discussion on the quality of data on adverse events; that is, risks that have materialized. We then provide an example of how risks assessment can be integrated in healthcare management of diabetic patients, and conclude with a section on facility audits that are conducted to ensure the efficacy and safety of pharmaceutical products delivered to the market. These three sections provide an extensive overview of risk management in drug manufacturing and healthcare. We conclude with a discussion and summary section.

## 6.1 Introduction to risks in healthcare and trends in reporting systems

The quality of healthcare processes is a key determinant of the quality of care and related risks. Delays in test results, mistakes in administering medicine, lack of information about a patient's health history and radiology retakes are only a few such examples.

*Statistical Methods in Healthcare*, First Edition. Edited by Frederick W. Faltin, Ron S. Kenett and Fabrizio Ruggeri.
© 2012 John Wiley & Sons, Ltd. Published 2012 by John Wiley & Sons, Ltd.

Healthcare represents 17.6% of the US economy and grows 8 to 10% annually. The Institute of Medicine (IOM) published two high-impact reports that shed light on the phenomenon of medical errors in the USA – 'To Err is Human: Building a Safer Health System' Kohn, Corrigan and Donaldson, 1999) and 'Crossing the Quality Chasm: A New Health System for the 21st Century' (Corrigan, Donaldson and Kohn, 2001). These reports show that at least two million hospital patients acquired dangerous infections and diseases during their hospital stays. Moreover, surgical errors, including improper surgical instruments or techniques, wrong-site surgery, improper anesthesia and improper monitoring contribute to an estimated 98 000 deaths each year at US hospitals. About 5% (150 million) prescriptions are filled incorrectly. This alone results in about 7000 deaths a year in the USA.

In order to address risks in healthcare one needs data. In the remaining of this section we will focus on the reporting and collection of healthcare-related adverse events. Studies conducted in the USA have shown that immediate reporting of adverse events by clinicians can serve as a forewarning in the identification of future claims regarding medical negligence and generate knowledge for improving the quality of medical care (Lindgren, Christensen and Mills, 1991).

These empirical studies aimed to test the hypothesis that immediate reporting of adverse events can improve claim management and its results. Research confirmed the hypothesis that indeed, immediate reporting reduces the time needed for handling claims and their costs. According to Lindgren, Christensen and Mills (1991). There are three alternatives for the establishment of reporting structure for adverse events in the healthcare systems:

1. **Systematic survey of medical records in order to screen out adverse events in advance.** According to this approach, instead of waiting for physicians' reports on their own error, one should actively review patients' files and manage them professionally. This method is, however, difficult to implement.

2. **Active risk surveys of the medical environment designed to screen risks before they are expressed in an adverse event.** This alternative is a typical quality control activity, but it is usually not sufficient for minimizing damages or proactive risk management.

3. **A reporting system in which physicians and other professionals report adverse events and near misses, immediately after they occur.**

A blame-free approach is an essential condition for the establishment of physician error-reporting systems. Frankel (2001) remarked in a symposium dedicated to patient safety that the golden rules of the reporting system in aviation, ASRS (Aviation Safety Reporting System), should be adopted by the medical field. These are:

1. limited immunity

2. time limitation for disciplinary action

3. analysis of reports: two analysts read each report

4. involves everyone

5. ensures protection: prohibits the use of any reports submitted (on any disciplinary action, except for information concerning criminal offenses)

6. de-identification.

Coles, Pryce and Shaw (2001) conducted a study in the UK regarding clinicians' attitudes toward reporting adverse events, by interviewing clinicians and risk management experts. A quote from one of those interviews shows the complexity of the problem:

> I think you have to address the fears and say why people don't do these things. I am sure some people don't do it for fear that they might lose their jobs, or being pilloried in the press. There could be a chief executive who says anyone in my Trust who instead of employee of the month is risk taker of the month and his or her names will be put around the Trust. They wouldn't lose their jobs, but they would lose the respect of their colleagues. I think you have to address those issues and give someone security – say we all make errors, no one is perfect.

The code of ethics (E-8.12) of the American Medical Association (2000) states that:

> ... Situations occasionally occur in which a patient suffers significant medical complications that may have resulted from the physician's mistake or judgment. In these situations, the physician is ethically required to inform the patient of all the facts necessary to ensure understanding of what has occurred.

Understanding what might motivate and what might prevent a physician from reporting an error is a major issue in risk management. A system with physicians reporting errors is fundamental to risk management, since it is the basis for every reactive and proactive activity of risk management, both in the short and long term.

The motivation to report adverse events can be intrinsic or extrinsic. Issues regarding nursing activity are usually addressed first (Mills and von Bolschwing, 1995), while adverse events related to a physician are taken care of at later stages. Risk managers in hospitals are often focused on events due to nursing services and not on clinical events due to doctor treatment. A study of the causes for this bias might help elucidate the forces motivating reporting of events by physicians.

The physician's main role is perceived as decision-making. The doctor–patient encounter, conducted in the form of SOAP (Subjective, Objective, and Assessment Plan), is a classical example of a decision-making process. The doctor listens to the patient's complaints (subjective), checks the patient and his medical record (objective), analyses the data and makes an assessment, according to which he makes decisions regarding the care management plan. Since it is a decision-making process, the alternatives are numerous and, in most cases, there isn't a clear-cut solution.

## 6.2   Reporting adverse events

Decisions are usually classified as reasonable or unreasonable. Thus, in cases where errors were made, the physician is not necessarily aware of the quality of his decisions. Even in cases of clear harm with consequences to the patient's health, a causative relationship between the available information the physician had at the time of making the decision, the decision made and the negative consequences of the decision is very difficult to establish.

The implication of this discussion is that, in a large portion of the cases where an error is made by a physician, he/she is not aware of it, whether because the error didn't result in significant or obvious harm, or because of the difficulty in establishing an association between the physician's decisions and the patients' deteriorating health.

Unlike physicians, the nurses' duty is to carry out doctors' orders, and implement the 'plan'. They are also expected to provide doctors with feedback regarding the treatment outcomes and the patient's condition. Therefore, in the nurses' work, there is a reference point to which it is possible to compare the nurse's actions. For example, if the doctors order was to inject the patient with a certain drug, at a certain dosage, it is relatively easy to find out if the nurse performed the order accurately and according to certain standards, or not.

Still, a very high proportion of doctors refrain from reporting adverse events. Estimates of reporting rates, prior to claims, range from 5 to 30% in the USA and 0 to 2% in the UK. The data refer to reporting events that end up with legal claims. Reporting rates of events that do not result in claims are probably lower.

Studies of physicians reporting clinical errors indicate many barriers to reporting, including fear, shame, lack of trust in the system, lack of time, arrogance and individualism (Anderson and Starzynski, 2001; Coles, Pryce and Shaw, 2001).

The main reasons for physicians not reporting adverse events are the following.

- Fear of damage to their medical reputation – the medical community is a relatively small and intimate community in which intense professional relationships exist. The doctor's reputation is a significant asset for him or her, both with regard to patients and with regard to colleagues. Doctors fear that reporting events might damage their reputation. The organizational culture of most health organizations doesn't distinguish between blaming and learning from errors.

- Fear of legal claims – the issue of legal immunity for doctors reporting errors still remains unresolved, and doctors fear being sued after reporting an adverse event. Some solutions to this problem include reporting to an insurer, whose relationships with the doctor can be formulated as confidential.

- Fear of being 'the village fool' – physicians are expected to perform with no errors, and the tolerance of senior physicians towards interns or younger doctors is low. The first report of the Institute of Medicine (Kohn, Corrigan and Donaldson, 1999) indicated a need to break the cultural paradigm according to which doctors do not err and those who make errors are not considered 'good doctors'. Breaking this paradigm is a necessary condition for creating a proper foundation for improving the quality of care and patient safety. A doctor who volunteers to report his errors should not be considered the 'village fool'.

Leape (2002), in an article regarding reporting adverse events at the USA national level, notes that despite the advantages of developing the system, it can also confront a serious problem of lack of resources for handling the increasing number of reports. According to some estimates, the number of severe adverse events in the USA reaches about a million a year, and, adding near misses, the number may reach up to five million a year. If only 10% of the events were reported and handled, it would be 15 times more than the number of events handled by the ASRS in the USA. According to ASRS estimates, the average cost of handling an event is $70, so, assuming similar costs and a reporting rate of 10%, the cost of a national healthcare reporting system in the USA could reach 35 million dollars a year. This is in addition to the need to recruit and train a very large number of experts in the field. Leape argues that a more practical approach is to encourage local reporting systems to focus on specific areas such as labor and delivery, neonatal units and adult intensive care units.

The comprehensive handling of adverse events necessitates an appropriate infrastructure and involves significant investments and resources that require economic considerations. Achieving immediate reporting of adverse events shortens the time needed to handle claims and reduces the payment for claims (Lindgren, Christensen and Mills, 1991). These findings are based on the implementation of reporting systems in 30 healthcare institutions during a period of 14 years. In a striking example, Leape (2002) states that rates of nosocomial infections in hospitals with a fully implemented reporting program were 32% lower than in hospitals that did not implement the program.

Western healthcare systems have gone through radical changes in the last decades of the twentieth century. McKinlay and Marceau (2002) analyzed those changes extensively. One of the prominent changes is the bureaucratization of medicine. Between 1983 and 1997, the proportion of physicians employed as salaried in the USA increased from 24 to 43%. Among young physicians (up to five years of experience), this tendency is even more noticeable – from 37 to 66%. More physicians are employed today by large organizations that are motivated mainly by financial interests, as opposed to the past, when the physician's loyalty was given first of all to the patient.

Following this background on adverse event reporting systems, we proceed by describing methods for analyzing such data, with examples.

# 6.3    Risk management and optimizing decisions with data

## 6.3.1    Introduction to risk management

The two previous sections provide a context for risk management in healthcare. This section is focused on statistical decision theory with healthcare applications. It formalizes the intuitive decision-making process of healthcare providers. We begin with a review of basic elements of risk management and optimal decisions.

Buying insurance is a typical passive form of risk management. Loss prevention and technological innovations are active means of managing risks. Loss prevention is a means of altering the probabilities of undesirable, damaging states. For example, maintaining one's own car properly is a form of loss prevention seeking to alter the chances of having an accident due to equipment failure such as a tire blowout at high speed on a freeway. Similarly, driving carefully, locking one's own home effectively, installing fire alarms, and so on, are all forms of loss prevention. Of course, both insurance and loss prevention are types of risk protection. Taking up an insurance policy implies that the risk is being accepted and cash provisions are being made to handle the risk if it materializes. Car insurance rates tend to be linked to a driver's past driving record. Certain drivers are classified as 'high-risk drivers', and required to pay higher insurance fees. Inequities in insurance rates occur because of uncertainty in the probabilities of damage, and imperfect distribution of information between the insured and insurers. Thus, situations may occur where persons might be 'over-insured' and have no motivation to engage in loss prevention. Passive risk management is often practiced in business and industry, especially when proactive prevention initiatives are difficult to justify on the basis of return on investment.

In the passive mode of risk management, one tries to measure the risk of an adverse event. If the cost of the event occurring is $c$ and the probability of the event occurring is $p$, then the risk of the event is its expected loss: $R = cp$.

Lets us call the event $A$, and the loss function $L$. To model the situation we consider a binary random variable $X \in \{0, 1\}$, which is 1 if event $A$ happens and 0 if it does not happen. Think of $L$ as attached to $X$, with $L(0) = 0$ and $L(1) = 1$: $R = E\{L(X)\} = cp$, where $E\{\cdot\}$ stands for the mathematical expectation, or average loss. Indeed, we typically think of risk as expected loss. Even if $A$ does not happen, we may have loss and then we may have $L(0) = c_0$, $L(1) = c_1$, and the method is the same:

$$R = E(L(X)) = c_0(1 - p) + c_1 p.$$

Now let us think actively. We observe some data $X$ and we make a decision $d(X)$. That is to say, we do not just sit back and accept our loss, we take some positive action. The loss $L$ (or reward) then depends on the value of the action, and we can attach the loss to $d(X)$. The risk becomes:

$$R = E(L(d(X))).$$

A somewhat more precise version says that a decision maps the data $X$ into a set of possible actions called the action space $A$: $d(X)$ which is in $A$. We can also think of $d$ as being a decision *rule*, which means that it specifies what we do if we see $X$ (i.e., a rule is just a mathematical function). So our problem is to *find the rule (i.e., make the decision) which has smallest risk.*

However we need to know the probability distribution generating the data. In the above example we need to know $p$.

One approach is to describe uncertainty about the value of $p$ by a probability distribution function. To describe this model of randomness, we introduce yet another parameter, $\theta$. This generates a family of distribution functions, and now the risk becomes: $R(\theta) = E(L(d(X)), \theta)$.

So, if we know what $\theta$ is, we can compute the risk. What we can do is conduct a thought experiment: if $\theta$ is the true value representing the uncertainty about $p$, what is the best decision rule? Is there a rule which has smallest risk for all values of $\theta$? Is there a decision rule whose worst risk, over all values of $\theta$, is better (no worse than) other rules about worst risk? Such a rule is called a minimax rule.

With minimax, management considers risks in various decision scenarios and picks the one which minimizes the maximum possible risk. Another approach is to consider Bayesian statistics. The choice of the loss function used to make the decision rule depends on what we want to achieve. There are three basic possibilities depending on our objectives.

**Option 1:** a loss function which helps us learn about $\theta$. This is the bedrock of statistics. We change notation and say, for example, $d(X) = \theta_{est}$, an estimator for $\theta$. The loss penalizes us according to how distant, in some sense, $\theta_{est}$ is from the true $\theta$.

**Option 2:** a loss which has to do not so much with $\theta$ itself but more to do with some special characteristic of the distribution of $X$. For example if $X$ is the response time of a Web System in which we plan to submit a request, then if we think that $X = 2\ seconds$ is a good maximum response time, we may decide to aim for it. We have a loss if we fill in the request forms in the system and it is too slow to respond.

**Option 3:** in this category we let the decision-making extend to data collection. We let the distribution of $X$ (the parameter $\theta$), depend on the data collection procedure. In its simplest form, this refers to the sample size $n$. In general, it depends on the whole *experimental design* including where, what and how we measure. Clearly, a proper measuring method can improve our decision-making.

## 6.3.2    Bayesian methods in risk management

Bayesian methods are used for getting around the issue of not knowing $\theta$ (for more details on Bayesian methods, see Kenett and Zacks, 1998). With Bayesian statistics, our intuitive or data-based knowledge can be represented by a *prior distribution* for $\theta$ and a mathematical expression for the Bayesian risk defined as:

$$E(L(d(X); \theta)) = E_X E_{\theta|X}(L(d(X); \theta|X)).$$

The internal expectation in the expression on the right is the *posterior risk*. If we choose a decision rule that always minimizes the posterior risk, then we minimize the overall Bayesian risk. Such a rule is called a Bayes rule. This simple statement is the basis of Bayesian risk theory. It can be shown (under some conditions) that using a Bayes rule is equivalent to behaving rationally. In other words, any decision rule whose risk is not dominated by some other rule for all $\theta$ is equivalent to a Bayes rule for some prior distribution.

If we do not have enough data to estimate parameters, we may be forced to become 'Bayesian'. However, we should distinguish between unknown parameters in observable systems and an open system for which we will never have enough data. Bayesian methods can address the practical issue of eliciting probabilities when no data are available. Prior elicitation is a difficult task in practice, as thoroughly discussed in O'Hagan et al. (2006). Indeed, there is a formal mathematical statistics method, called *decision analysis*, which concentrates on eliciting utilities by presenting alternative *gambling options* to subjects.

The statistical methods outlined above are thought to fail when there is the perception of a very large risk. This applies when the loss $L$ is extremely large but the probability $p$ is very small so that the risk $R = Lp$ is virtually undetermined. This is the case in catastrophes such as global warming, nuclear war, pandemic events, environmental disasters and threats to critical systems. These events have been referred to as 'Black Swans' (Taleb, 2007).

The growing interest in risk management is driven partly by regulations related to corporate governance in the private and public sector. However, much of risk management is still based on informal scoring using subjective judgment.

Modern risk management systems incorporate several activities such as the following.

1. **System mapping.** Organizational charts and process maps are standard practice. A more comprehensive approach is the application of enterprise knowledge development (EKD) to map actors, roles, activities and goals (Kenett and Baker, 2010).

2. **Risk identification.** A list of main risk events classified by area and sub-area. Risk identification does not stop at the first stage; it should be a continuous process. It is best to reduce dimensionality by grouping similar items.

3. **Risk measurement and risk scoring.** Ideally we want to assess the loss or impact of a risk event and its probability. Note that a score is the value of a *metric*.

4. **Risk prioritization.** Prioritization is done on the basis of the risk scores. A one-dimensional score may be too general; consequently, here one often considers several dimensions and multiple objectives. Technically this process allows us to identify the main *risk drivers* (Kenett and Raphaeli, 2008).

5. **Decision.** Any risk management system is basically a *decision support system*. Usually, decisions are not made automatically (there are possible exceptions like automatic trading in finance). One needs to take decisions and try to keep a record of the decisions taken.

6. **Action.** This is not the same as decision. Actions take place after a decision. It is critical to record the actual action.

7. **Risk control.** Risk control is the ongoing process of monitoring the effect of the actions, including re-scoring the risks, introducing new risks (more prioritization), removing old risks from the list, and taking new or repeat decisions and actions. This is a process of feedback and iteration. It should be a continuous process.

Additional general risk management components include the following.

1. **Risk champions:** facilitators who have ownership of the process or individual areas of risk.

2. **Stakeholders:** these can be employees, customers, experts, partners, shareholders, patients, students, the general public, special subgroups of the public (e.g., old, young, handicapped), the government, regulatory agencies, and so on. It is very important to draw all the stakeholders into the risk management process.

3. **Experts:** these are key personnel in risk management. However, one should not solely rely on the experts. Public perceptions of risks are often profound, somewhat erratic and sensitive to media sensation.

4. **Senior management commitment:** very similar to what is said about quality. One needs champions at the board-of-director's level, not just a back-office risk function. Ideally risk is a regular item at board meetings.

5. **Risk communication:** to all stakeholders.

6. **Practical control:** there may be no legal rights or it might be physically impossible to take some of the actions. For example, one cannot prevent a hurricane.

### 6.3.3  Basics of financial engineering and risk management

Mathematical economics and financial engineering provide complementary aspects to risk management. They consist of discussions on complete/incomplete markets and rational expectation models and include *equilibrium theory*, *optimization theory*, *game theory* and several other disciplines. The concept of a complete market has various technical definitions. In general, it means that every player in the market has the same information, and that new information reaches every player at the same time and is instantaneously incorporated into prices. Roughly, no player can get an advantage from an information point of view (as in insider trading). If the market is not in equilibrium, then there is opportunity to make an *arbitrage*, a something-for-nothing profit just by taking a buy or sell action.

Rational expectations assume that an efficient market should be in equilibrium. The proof is that if it is not efficient, some players would have an advantage and drive the market in a particular direction. Under rational expectation one behaves according to the best prediction of the future market equilibrium point. Note that this is quite close to the Bayes rule which states that the conditional expectation $\theta_{est} = E(\theta \mid X)$ is the best rule for estimation of $\theta$ under quadratic loss:

$$L = (\theta_{est} - \theta)^2.$$

Rational expectation implies that the conditional expectation under all available (past) information should be the basis for (rational) decisions. These economic principles lie behind the desire to minimize some risk metrics. Very roughly, if we like a particular risk metric and we fail to minimize it, there is a better rule than the one we are using. Even worse, someone else may be able to take advantage of us. Some modern economic theories are about operating with *partial information*. Mathematical economics is an extension of the decision theory we discussed above, with specific decisions taken at certain times. Typical actions are: buy, sell, swap and price (the act of setting a price). For more on these topics see Tapiero (2004).

The freedom to make a decision is called an *option*. Note the connection with risk management in which we may or may not have this freedom (we do not have the freedom to stop a hurricane but we may have some prevention or mitigation options for the effect of the hurricane). The key point is that the option will have a time element for example, to buy or sell at or before a certain date, and perhaps at a certain price. A *real option* is where the option is investment in a 'real' object like a factory or technology. When time elapses, certain things happen: the value of assets may change, or we may have to pay interest. The things that happen are usually random (stochastic), and we typically have no control over their occurrence. We do have control over the choice of what to buy or sell and the time at which to do it. Once we buy or receive an option we are in the grip of the market until we sell. A whole body of work in economics and portfolio theory is connected to mean-risk or mean-variance theory (see Tapiero, 2004).

When dealing with operational issues, aspects of operational risks are evaluated using similar techniques, including Value at Risk and related scoring methods. These techniques are beyond the scope of this introductory section. For more on operational risks see Panjer (2006) and Kenett and Raanan (2010).

The next section is at the interface between financial engineering, economics, statistics and operational risk management. We present it here because of its importance to modern risk management methodology and because it has many implications for systems and software development. It relates to the work of Nassim Taleb, a hedge fund manager who dared to question the system, before the dramatic events of September 15, 2008 when Lehman Brothers announced that it was filing for Chapter 11 bankruptcy protection, with significant ripple effects: Iceland declared bankruptcy as a country on October 8, 2008, and CitiBank laid off 51 000 people.

### 6.3.4  Black Swans and the Taleb quadrants

In 2007, Taleb published a book that predicted the 2008 economic meltdown (Taleb, 2007). Taleb labeled the meltdown and similar major impact events, such as the 9/11 terrorist attack, the Katrina hurricane, or the rise of Google, as 'Black Swans'. A Black Swan is a highly improbable event with three principal characteristics: (1) it is unpredictable; (2) it carries a massive impact; and (3) after the fact, we concoct an explanation that makes it appear less random, and more predictable, than it was. The Western world did not know about Black Swans before 1697, when they were first spotted in Australia. Up to then, all swans where white. Why do we not acknowledge the phenomenon of Black Swans until after they occur? Part of the answer, according to Taleb, is that humans are hardwired to learn specifics when they should be focused on generalities. We concentrate on things we already know, and time and time again fail to take into consideration what we don't know. We are, therefore, unable to truly estimate opportunities, too vulnerable to the impulse to simplify, narrate, and categorize, and not open enough to rewarding those who can imagine the 'impossible'. Taleb has studied how we fool ourselves into thinking we know more than we actually do. He claims that we focus our thinking on the irrelevant and inconsequential, while large events continue to surprise us and shape our world.

Taleb proposed a mapping of randomness and decision-making into a quadrant with two classes of randomness and two types of decisions. Decisions referred to as 'simple' or 'binary' lead to data-driven answers such as 'very true' or 'very false' or that 'a product is fit for use or defective'. In these cases, statements of the type 'true' or 'false' can be stated with confidence intervals and $p$-values. A second type of decision is more complex, emphasizing both its likelihood of occurrence and its consequences. The other dimensions of the Taleb quadrant characterize randomness. A first layer is based on 'forecastable events', implied by uncertainty described with finite variance (and thus from thin-tail probability distributions). A second dimension relates to 'unforecastable events', defined by probability distributions with fat tails. In the first layer, exceptions occur without significant consequences since they are predictable. The traditional random walk, converging to Gaussian-Poisson processes, provides such an example. In the second domain, large consequential events are experienced but are also more difficult to predict. 'Fractals' and infinite variance models provide such examples (see Kenett and Tapiero, 2010). These are conditions with large vulnerability to Black Swans. The reader is referred to Taleb (2007) for more insights on Black Swans.

## 6.4   Decision support systems for managing patient healthcare risks

Healthcare organizations understand the importance of risk management as a key element to improve service deliveries and patient outcomes. This, however, requires that clinical and operational risks are quantified and managed. A risk assessment involves two elements, which are a probability or frequency with which an event might take place and an assessment of impact severity or consequences from such events.

Physicians usually want to evaluate and to forecast adverse events that may provoke morbidity, mortality or a longer hospital stay for a patient; moreover, they want to quantify a patient's risk profile. The latter is the assessment of the patient's medical parameters by using probability distributions, given the patient's status and prior domain knowledge. Physicians typically summarize risk probability distributions through a percentile and decide acceptability of risks. Detection of unacceptable risks and the resulting risk mitigation analysis completes the risk management process. Healthcare organization evaluate economic losses and costs due to adverse events are in order to choose convenient forms of insurance;

furthermore, for better governance it is useful to understand risk levels and how each risk contributes to economic losses.

When data are scarce, the experience of physicians often offers a good source of information. The use of prior information is actually recommended by the Food and Drug Administration (FDA, 2006) for achieving more accurate estimation of risks.

Bayesian methodology can be used for the estimation of operational and clinical risk profiles. The approach is described in the next section with an example involving healthcare of end stage renal disease (ESRD). This application is an example explicitly designed to manage operational and clinical risks in healthcare environments. The main goal is to support the nephrologist and risk managers who have to manage operational and clinical risk in healthcare (ESRD Group, 2006). Many statistical models applied to risk management estimate only risks, without consideration for decision-making. Decisions models have to be considered in order to realize a fully integrated risk management process. The integration between risk estimations and decision-making can be achieved with Bayesian Networks, which will be now introduced.

Making inferences about uncertain conditions is complex when limited information is available; moreover, clinical and operational risks have high-dimensional distributions, and decision problems are difficult to formalize in a convenient way.

Given medical parameters $X_1, \ldots, X_n$, physicians want to estimate both mortality and hospitalization risk of a patient, and the failure risks of a device. For examples of similar problems see Chapter 10 and Chapter 16. In the ESRD case presented in Section 6.5, more than one target variable is analyzed under the hypothesis that $X_1, \ldots, X_j$ $(j \leq n)$ are positive dependent, with targets, and the combinations $(X_i, X_k)$, where $X_1, \ldots, X_q$ $q \leq j \leq n$, $i \neq k$, are either positive dependent or independent. Dependencies and independence between variables is typically determined in medicine through scientific studies and clinical research. In general, unknown dependency can be extracted from data using data-mining techniques and statistical models (Hand, Mannila and Smyth, 2001). Different sources of knowledge such as subjective information (e.g., expert opinions of nephrologists, knowledge from literature) and data can be integrated with Bayesian Networks (BNs). In our case, BNs offer several advantages: (1) the method allows one to easily combine prior probability distributions; (2) the complexity of the ESRD domain and the relationships among medical parameters can be intuitively represented with graphs; and (3) utility or loss functions can be included in the model.

Bayesian Networks belong to the family of probabilistic *graphical models* used to represent knowledge about an uncertainty domain. Specifically, each node in the graph represents a random variable, and the edges between the nodes represent probabilistic dependencies among the corresponding random variables. These conditional dependencies in the graph are often estimated by using known statistical and computational methods. Hence, BNs combine principles from graph theory, probability theory, Computer Science and Statistics. They implement a graphical model structure known as a *directed acyclic graph* (DAG) that is popular in Statistics, Machine Learning and Artificial Intelligence. Bayesian Networks are both mathematically rigorous and intuitively understandable. They enable an effective representation and computation of the joint probability distribution over a set of random variables (Pearl, 2009).

The structure of a DAG is defined by two sets: the set of nodes and the set of directed edges. The nodes represent random variables and are drawn as circles labeled by the variable names. The edges represent direct dependence among the variables and are represented by arrows between nodes. In particular, an edge from node $X_i$ to node $X_j$ represents a statistical dependence between the corresponding variables. Thus, the arrow indicates that a value taken by variable $X_j$ depends on the value taken by variable $X_i$, or roughly speaking that variable $X_i$ 'influences' $X_j$. Node $X_i$ is then referred to as a 'parent' of $X_j$ and, similarly, $X_j$ is referred to as the 'child' of $X_i$. An extension of these genealogical terms is often used to define the set of 'descendents' – the set of nodes that can be reached on a direct path from the node, or 'ancestor' nodes – the set of nodes from which the node can be reached on a direct path. The structure of the acyclic graph guarantees that there is no node that can be its own ancestor or its own descendent. Such a condition is of vital importance to the factorization of the joint probability of a collection of nodes, as seen below. Note that although the arrows represent direct causal connection between the variables, the *reasoning process* can operate on a BN by propagating information in any direction. A BN reflects a simple conditional independence statement; namely that each variable is independent of its non-descendents in the graph, given the state of its parents. This property is used to reduce, sometimes significantly, the number of parameters that are required to characterize the joint probability distribution of the variables. This reduction provides an efficient way to compute the posterior probabilities given the evidence (Lauritzen and Spiegelhalter, 1988; Pearl, 2009; Jensen, 2001).

In addition to the DAG structure, which is often considered as the 'qualitative' part of the model, one needs to specify the 'quantitative' parameters of the model. The parameters are described by applying the Markovian property, where the conditional probability distribution at each node depends only on its parents. For discrete random variables, this conditional probability is often represented by a table, listing the local probability that a child node takes on each of the feasible values – for each combination of values of its parents. The joint distribution of a collection of variables can be determined uniquely by these local conditional probability tables.

Formally, a Bayesian Network $B$ is an annotated acyclic graph that represents a joint probability distribution over a set of random variables $\mathbf{V}$. The network is defined by a pair $B = \langle G, \Theta \rangle$, where $G$ is the directed acyclic graph whose nodes $X_1, X_2, \ldots, X_n$ represents random variables, and whose edges represent the direct dependencies between these variables. The graph $G$ encodes independence assumptions, by which each variable $X_i$ is independent of its non-descendents given its parents in $G$, denoted generically as $\pi_i$. The second component $\Theta$ denotes the set of parameters of the network. This set contains the parameter $\theta_{x_i|\pi_i} = P_B(x_i|\pi_i)$ for each realization $x_i$ of $X_i$ conditioned on $\pi_i$, the set of parents of $X_i$ in $G$. Accordingly, $B$ defines a unique joint probability distribution over $\mathbf{V}$, namely:

$$P_B(X_1, X_2, \ldots, X_n) = \prod_{i=1}^{n} P_B(X_i|\pi_i) = \prod_{i=1}^{n} \theta_{X_i|\pi_i}.$$

For simplicity of representation we omit the subscript $B$. If $X_i$ has no parents, its local probability distribution is said to be *unconditional*; otherwise it is *conditional*. If the variable represented by a node is *observed*, then the node is said to be an evidence node, otherwise the node is said to be hidden or latent.

The complexity of a domain may be reduced by models and algorithms that describe an approximated reality. When variable interactions are too intricate for application of an analytic model, we may represent current knowledge about the problem, such as a cause generating at least one effect (Pearl, 2009), where the final effect is the target of the analysis. For example, consider a person that might suffer from a back injury, an event represented

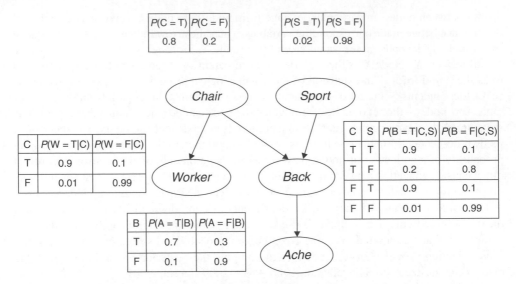

**Figure 6.1**   The Backache problem.

by the variable *Back* (B). Such an injury can cause a backache, an event represented by the variable *Ache* (A). The back injury might result from some sport activity, represented by the variable *Sport* (S) or from an uncomfortable office chair represented by the variable *Chair* (C). In the latter case, it is reasonable to assume that a co-worker will suffer and report a similar backache syndrome, an event represented by the variable *Worker* (W). All variables are binary, thus, are either true (denoted by 'T') or false (denoted by 'F'). The conditional probability table of each node is listed beside the node in Figure 6.1. The probability of a backache following a back injury is 0.7. The probability of a co-worker reporting a backache due to the office chair is 0.9. The probability of a back injury due to both the office chair and the sport activity is 0.9. For more on this example and BNs see Ben Gal (2007).

The domain knowledge allows experts to draw an arc to a variable from each of its direct causes. Given a BN that specifies the joint probability distribution in a factored form, one can evaluate all possible inference queries by marginalization; that is, summing out over 'irrelevant' variables. Two types of inference support are often considered: *predictive support* for node $X_i$, based on evidence nodes connected to $X_i$ through its parent nodes (called also *top-down reasoning*), and *diagnostic support* for node $X_i$, based on evidence nodes connected to $X_i$ through its children nodes (called also *bottom-up reasoning*). In general, the full summation (or integration) over discrete (continuous) variables is called *exact inference* and known to be an NP-hard problem. Some efficient algorithms exist to solve the exact inference problem in restricted classes of networks. In many practical settings the BN is unknown and one needs to learn it from the data. This problem is known as the *BN learning problem*, which can be stated informally as follows: given training data and prior information (e.g., expert knowledge, causal relationships), estimate the graph topology (network structure) and the parameters of the joint probability distribution in the BN.

Learning the BN structure is considered a harder problem than learning the BN parameters. Moreover, another obstacle arises in situations of *partial observability* when nodes are hidden or when data are missing. In the simplest case of known BN structure and full observability, the goal of learning is to find the values of the BN parameters (in each conditional probability distribution) that maximize the (log)likelihood of the training dataset. This dataset contains $m$ cases that are often assumed to be independent. Given training dataset $\Sigma = \{x, \ldots, x_m\}$, where $x_l = (x_{l1}, \ldots, x_{ln})^T$, and the parameter set $\Theta = (\theta_1, \ldots, \theta_n)$, where $\theta_i$ is the vector of parameters for the conditional distribution of variable $X_i$ (represented by one node in the graph), the log-likelihood of the training dataset is a sum of terms, one for each node:

$$\log L\,(\Theta \mid \Sigma) = \sum_m \sum_n \log P\,(x_{li} \mid \pi_i, \theta_i)$$

The log-likelihood scoring function is decomposed according to the graph structure; hence, one can maximize the contribution to the log-likelihood of each node independently. Another alternative is to assign a prior probability density function to each parameter vector and use the training data to compute the posterior parameter distribution and the Bayes estimates.

Bayesian Networks are gaining popularity in a wide range of application areas such as risk management (Cornalba, Kenett and Giudici, 2007), Web data analysis (Harel, Kenett and Ruggeri, 2008) and management science (Ruggeri, Kenett and Faltin, 2007; Kenett *et al.*, 2008). Availability of software for analyzing BNs is further expanding their role in decision analysis and decision support systems (Jensen, 2001). Some popular software implementations of BNs include GeNie (http://genie.sis.pitt.edu, Decision Systems Laboratory, University of Pittsburgh); Hugin Decision Engine (www.hugin.com, Hugin Expert, Denmark); SPSS Clementine (www-01.ibm.com/software/analytics/spss/, IBM, New York); and the R package *bnlearn* (http://cran.r-project.org/web/packages/bnlearn/index.html, The R Project for Statistical Computing).

During quantitative learning of BNs, conditional and unconditional prior probability distributions represent the belief on $\theta$ before the experiment (i.e., dialysis session). The distribution functions are expressed for each node (i.e., medical parameter) of the DAG $G$. By updating priors with likelihood functions (i.e., data collection), the corresponding posterior distributions are generated. Available data update prior belief and prior distributions so that posterior distributions converge to a likelihood shape with more and more dialysis sessions.

The choice of prior distributions (Bernardo and Smith, 1994) gives a mathematical shape to *a priori* belief on $\theta$. This can be achieved by different methods such as exponential power distribution, vague priors, and empirical Bayes distributions. In particular, priors are set for public policies, and distortions resulting from personal biases of analysts have to be removed. Typically only one method is employed for prior selection, which limits the subjective contribution of a model developer.

Among these approaches is the *maximum entropy method*, proposed by Jaynes (2003). With this method, the shape distribution is derived from available information and no assumptions are made. Alternatively one can apply *conjugate priors* where prior and posterior distributions belong to the same family of distributions. The ease of tractability of the distributions is highly recommended in a complex domain like ESRD.

The *maximum entropy prior* function is what maximizes the Shannon–Jaynes information entropy, defined as:

$$S = -\sum_{i=1}^{n} p_i \ln p_i, \quad \sum_{i=1}^{n} p_i = 1,$$

where $S$ is the knowledge over the distribution and $S$ is equal to 0 for a degenerate distribution, that is, full knowledge over the value of interest; the larger $S$, the greater is the ignorance about the uncertain value of interest.

In the case of no constraints other than normalization, $S$ is maximized by the uniform distribution, $p_i = 1/n$; see Jaynes (2003), Fomby and Hill (1997) and Grandy and Schick (1999) for the proof with Lagrange multipliers.

For continuous variables, and when the only information about the distribution is either the expected value or both the expected value and the variance, two maximum-entropy priors are applied; these are based on the moments of the distribution, $M_r$. For $r = 1$, $M_r$ is equal to the expected value; furthermore, the first and the second moment together provide the variance. The knowledge about the expected value is the extension to continuous variables of the discrete case.

The *conjugate prior family* is chosen on the basis of mathematical convenience. The posterior distribution belongs to the same family of the prior distribution; the family is a closed class under transformation from prior to posterior (Raiffa, 1997).

Once the posterior probability distribution of risks is estimated on the given BN's topology, the goal is the identification of a decision which is expected to best satisfy the stated objectives, for both the $j$th patient and the department. Let $\Theta$ denote the discrete space of all possible parameters $\theta$ representing the uncertainty in ESRD, $D$ denote the space of all possible decisions $d$ to the problem and $A$ denote the corresponding set of available actions $a$, given $d$. For each decision $d \in D$, let $p(\theta|d)$ denote the probability that $\theta$ will take its various values given the decision $d$, that is, the probability mass function on $\theta \in \Theta$ with $p(\theta|d) \geq 0$ for all $\theta \in \Theta$ and $\sum_{\theta \in \Theta} p(\theta|d) = 1$.

A consequence $c$ of the set $C$ corresponds to each decision $d \in D$ and parameter $\theta \in \Theta$. The consequence is quantified, usually in monetary terms, by loss function $L(d, \theta)$. The decision $d^* \in D$, also called the *Bayes decision*, is what minimizes the expected loss $L(d)$ defined as follows:

$$L(d) = \sum_{\theta \in \Theta} L(d, \theta) p(\theta|d).$$

A preference order ($\leq$) has to be set in $D$ and it takes the form of a binary relation between some elements of $D$. If the objectives of the analysis are correctly determined and a loss function of the nephrologist is given, $d^*$ is an optimal decision under loss $l$; that is, $l(d^*) < l(d)$.

Each nephrologist has a different shape for the loss function, and $d^*$ depends on this choice. In general, a risk-prone decision-maker has a concave-shaped loss function in the region of $\theta$, taking big risk to avoid a little possible loss; analogously, a conservative (or risk-averse) decision-maker has a convex-shaped loss function.

Finally, a neutral decision-maker has a loss function that is linearly shaped.

For technical mathematical theorems see Grunwald and Dawid (2004), and Jaynes (2003).

Many loss functions have been suggested in the literature. These include quadratic, linear and piecewise linear and asymmetric loss functions (Bernardo and Smith, 1994). In general, the decision $d^* \in D$ involves the choice of the estimator that minimizes the expected loss $L(d)$. In estimation problems, the action to be taken is to choose an estimator, $\hat{\theta}$, so that, for the action $a = \hat{\theta}$, the loss function is $L(\theta, \hat{\theta})$.

Usually, symmetric functions like *quadratic loss functions* are preferred so that underestimates of $\theta$ have equal consequences to overestimates. Such loss functions are defined as:

$L(\theta, \hat{\theta}) = c(\theta - \hat{\theta})^2$ , where $c$ denotes a constant. If $\theta$ and $\hat{\theta}$ are multidimensional, the equivalent loss function may be written as a positive semidefinite quadratic form: $L(\theta, \hat{\theta}) = (\theta - \hat{\theta})'A(\theta - \hat{\theta})$.

The use of symmetric loss functions is not always appropriate, especially when the risk increases; among the asymmetric loss functions, the *linear loss function* is useful under the hypothesis of a neutral-risk decision-maker. Let $a_i$ and $a_j$ be the $i$th and $j$th possible actions in a decision problem. The linear loss function is assumed to be given, for $b_i > b_j$, by $L(a_i, \theta) = a_i + b_i\theta, L(a_j, \theta) = a_j + b_j\theta$.

The expected losses for taking the two actions are: $\rho(a_i) = a_i + b_iE(\theta)$, $\rho(a_j) = a_j + b_jE(\theta)$.

If relevant data is available, the expectations are taken over the appropriate posterior distribution; otherwise they are taken over the prior distribution. The Bayesian decision $d^*$ is to take action $a_i$ if $\rho(a_i) < \rho(a_j)$; if the reverse is true, take action $a_j$. Otherwise, flip a fair coin if $\rho(a_i) = \rho(a_j)$.

The break-even point, $\theta_0$, is

$$\theta_0 = \frac{(a_i - a_j)}{(b_i - b_j)},$$

so that the decision rule becomes: choose $a_i$ if $E(\theta) > \theta_0$, and choose action $a_j$ if $E(\theta) < \theta_0$. Otherwise, flip a fair coin.

The decision problem may be represented by an influence diagram (ID), which is a directed graph with decisional and value nodes. The former represent the decision space and the latter represent the expected loss on the values of their direct predecessor nodes. The ID has the following properties:

- it contains no directed cycles;

- the only node to have no direct successor is the value node;

- if any chance node $X$ (i.e., the node of the Bayesian Network) is not a predecessor of any decision node $D$, then there is no directed path from $X$ to $D$;

- there is an ordering of the decision nodes $(D_1, \ldots, D_m)$ such that $D_s$ is a directed successor of $D_r$ where $r < s$ and $1 \leq s \leq m$.

The next section presents a case study where the above concepts and tools are implemented.

## 6.5   The hemodialysis case study

A risk management process consists of various steps including risk identification, risk estimation and decision-making. In our case study a general definition of risk was carried out by analyzing the non-adherence of patients and healthcare providers to the treatment plan of nephrologists for end stage renal disease (Cornalba, 2009). An appropriate set of risks was identified as follows.

- Clinical risks that are limited to hospitalization and mortality risks which are caused by bone disease, renal diet and causes related to cardiovascular problems.

- Operational risks that involve both the process and the device. Three clusters are distinguished: *Execution, Delivery and Process Management* (i.e., fistula closure, time failure), *System Failures* (i.e., pulmonary venous resistance (PVR) or pulmonary arterial resistance (PAR) resistance), and *External Event* (i.e., skipped hemodialysis session).

The complex domain of ESRD was represented by the DAG $G$ presented in Figure 6.2, where the size of the set $V$ is equal to 34. The number of vertices results from a trade-off between a deeper description of dialysis and exponential growth of possible DAGs. Each variable is classified into one group of causes, such as *Dialysis Quality Indexes* = {*Dialysis adequacy* (Kt/V), *PTH* pg/ml, *Serum albumin* g/dl} and *HD Department Performances* = {*Serum phosphorus P* mg/dl, *Potassium* mEq/l, *Serum calcium* mg/dl}.

Some dependence relations among variables, which form the set $E$ of edges of $G$, are defined on the basis of medical literature, such as DOPPS (Kim *et al.*, 2003), and guidelines of the DOQI Group (2003). The *Dialysis Outcome Practice and Pattern Study* (DOPPS) is one of the most important sources of experimental results. These are international, observational studies of hemodialysis practices and outcomes that have been realized in countries with large populations of dialysis patients, such as France, Germany, Italy, Spain, Japan, the UK and the USA.

Under the condition of existence of a directed path $X_1 \rightarrow X_2$, the latest posterior distribution is identified for every pair of variables $(X_1, X_2)$. The set of all paths $X_1 \rightarrow \cdots \rightarrow X_n$ is selected under the acyclic condition. As already mentioned, learning a BN is known to be NP-hard. The number of DAGs on $N$ variables is super-exponential in $N$. For instance, there are 543 possible DAGs on four variables and 1018 on ten variables. As all possible subsets cannot be explored, several approaches have been proposed to efficiently learn BNs from data (Cooper and Herskovits, 1992). We rely here on an *a priori* constrained network; that is, an exhaustive exploration of a small subset of possible competitive substructures. An *acceptance measure* (Jensen, 2001) is applied to establish the credibility of the possible structures ($S^h$, $h = 1, \ldots, n$) and, then, to select one of them. In our case, the measure takes into account the trade-off between the size of a model and the distance between the 'true' posterior distribution and the one approximated by the model. The measure assesses a score of acceptability which gives a complete order among the hypotheses $S^h$.

Let $M$ be a Bayesian Network with variables $X$. For each variable $X_j$ with parents $pa(X_j)$, we define $Sp(X_j)$ to be the number of entries in $P(X_j|pa(X_j))$, and the size is $Size(M) = \sum_{X_j \in X} Sp(X_j)$.

Let $P$ denote the distribution over $X$ taken from the sample of the database of cases. Let $M_i$ be the $i$th candidate Bayesian Network for $P$, and let $P_i$ be the joint probability distribution determined by $M_i$.

To compare the two distributions we apply the *Euclidean distance*:

$$Dist_E(P, P_i) = \sum_{x \in X} (P(x) - P_i(x))^2.$$

The best BN minimizes the following acceptance measure: $Acc(P, M_i) = Size(M_i) + kDist(P, P_i)$, where $k$ is a positive real number.

Given $V = \{X_1, \ldots, X_{34}\}$ and the set of directed edges $E$, four variables (serum calcium – Ca, parathyroid hormone – PTH, hemoglobin – Hgb, and serum ferritin – Fe) are left without

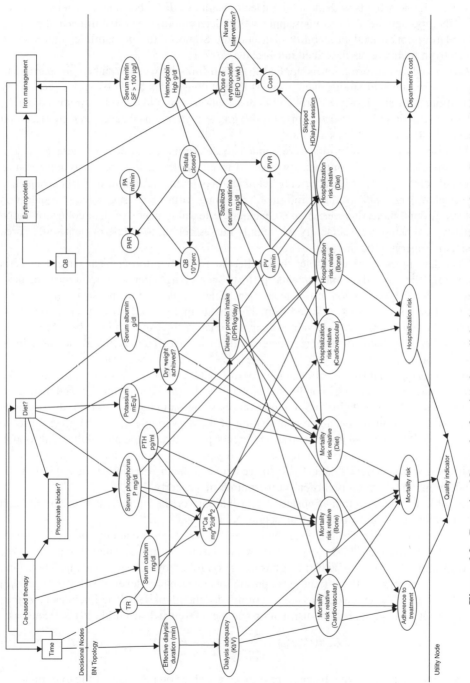
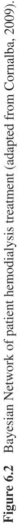

**Figure 6.2**  Bayesian Network of patient hemodialysis treatment (adapted from Cornalba, 2009).

fixing their causal links, since the available prior knowledge is compatible with different BN representations. For this reason, this part of the network was learned from the data derived from all available patients with the model selection strategy described above. After the choice of the BN topology, *batch learning* is applied, thus determining the probabilities of the model and updating conditional probability distributions. Some of the probabilities can also be derived from literature, as described in Cornalba (2009).

*Expert opinion* information is applied to set up links between variables; in particular, results of experimental studies were used as known constraints to choose prior probability distributions. The shape of prior probability distributions was subjectively introduced during model construction. The distribution with the greatest Shannon–Weaver entropy (Lee and Wright, 1994) was selected as a prior.

Mixtures of conjugate priors were applied to determine some priors. These provide a sufficiently rich range of prior density 'shapes' to enable the risk manager to approximate reasonably closely any particular prior belief function of interest. A mixture of *m* beta densities was selected, when *soft* available information coming from belief suggested that data was clustered around more than one mode. Quantitative learning needs of data collection came from a typical hemodialysis facility where only nurses belong to the permanent staff. Three physicians supervise the dialysis sessions.

Two data types were available: data collected from monitoring each patient dialysis session, and personal data and patients' history, such as age, gender and number of days from the first dialysis session in the department. The sample size of the data is $n = 10\,095$ monitored dialysis sessions collected from 47 patients in a period of five years (from 2001 to 2006). Follow-up data were obtained at approximately three-month intervals. Among the large number of available medical parameters, only those that affected clinical and operational risks have been selected.

In summary, given the set of dependences and data, it is possible to assess risk profiles for the *j*th patient $(pr_j)$ both by conditional probability distribution $p(X|pa(X))$ and by unconditional probability distribution $p(X)$; moreover, working on marginal posterior distributions it is possible to evaluate the single contribution of the *i*th variable $X_i$ for the *j*th risk profile $pr_j$. Each prior distribution is assumed as a reference prior; that is, the probability distribution for a mean patient. The latest is compared with the posterior probability distribution, which is learned from the patient's data. The distance between the distributions is quantified by the Euclidean measure, which is chosen for its symmetric property.

In Table 6.1 some marginal posterior distributions for the *j*th patient's risk profile and related effects, given a decision and an action, are reported.

For example, during the first year the patient has a risk profile about *time failure* better than the reference one (99.41 vs. 95.68%); while during the first update (15 months) there is a worsening (94.13 vs. 95.68%) that has to be controlled by decision-making. The action *add 30 minutes* restores the patient's risk profile to an acceptable level of risk (98.59%). Let $X_i$ be the *i*th variable which defines the risk profile for the *j*th patient. The Euclidean distance measured between the *j*th patient distribution and the reference distribution $(R)$ is defined as:

$$Dist(P_j, P_R) = \sum_{x \in X_i} (P_j(x) - P_R(x))^2$$

The score, defined by the distance, prioritizes variables on the basis of the importance to determining the risk profile. In this way nephrologists can cluster key medical variables for causes in a given horizon period. In this example, the most important adverse event is due to

**Table 6.1**  Marginal posterior distributions for the $j$th patient's risk profile and related effects, given a decision and an action (adapted from Cornalba, 2009).

| Variable state | Marginal posterior distribution in % | | | Decision |
| | Reference profile | First year | First update | |
| --- | --- | --- | --- | --- |
| | | Time failure? | | Plus 30 min |
| False | 95.68 | 99.41 | 94.13 | 98.59 |
| True | 4.32 | 0.59 | 5.87 | 1.41 |
| | | | | Plus one dose of |
| | | Hemoglobin, Hgb | | erythropoietin |
| 0–9 | 22.55 | 8.56 | 21.66 | 20.11 |
| 9–10 | 31.22 | 50.61 | 24.09 | 31.71 |
| 10–11 | 19.08 | 31.17 | 51.82 | 20.03 |
| 11–12 | 13.01 | 4.58 | 1.15 | 13.56 |
| 12–13 | 8.67 | 3.2 | 0.82 | 8.77 |
| 13–14 | 3.3 | 1.13 | 0.28 | 3.49 |
| ... | ... | ... | ... | ... |
| | | | | Plus one dose of |
| | | Erythropoietin dose | | erythropoietin |
| 0–1000 | 12.64 | 2.97 | 1.54 | 12.9 |
| 0–6000 | 44.93 | 10.57 | 5.48 | 45.01 |
| 6000–11 000 | 29.12 | 83.32 | 91.36 | 29.89 |
| 11 000–16 000 | 8.26 | 2.18 | 1.13 | 8.39 |
| ... | ... | ... | ... | ... |

an incorrect dose of erythropoietin administered to the $j$th patient, so that resources have to be allocated better in follow-up dialysis.

Moreover, it is possible to explore also marginal posterior probability distributions of the target variables. For example, during the first update both of therapeutic protocol and data collection, the mortality risk of the $j$th patients increases (the probability distribution shifts to the right). To restore the correct risk profile, the nephrologist can *add a dose of erythropoietin*.

To complete the risk management process, physicians have to make a decision either on the patient's treatment or device's substitution. This decision problem has been represented by an influence diagram (ID). The set of decisions $D$ and the corresponding set of actions $A$ for each decision are the following.

- $d_1$ – 'Time': keep or add 30 minutes to dialysis session.

- $d_2$ – 'Ca-based therapy':

  - treat hypercalcemia;

  - continue current therapy;

  - decrease vitamin D dose to achieve ideal Ca; decrease Ca-based phosphate binders;

    – decrease or discontinue vitamin D dose/Ca-based phosphate binders; decrease Ca
    dialysate if still needed; assess trend in serum PTH as there may be low turnover.

- $d_3$ – 'Phosphate binder':

    – assess nutrition, discontinue phosphate binder if being used;

    – begin dietary counseling and restrict dietary phosphate; start or increase phosphate
    binder therapy;

    – begin short-term Al-based phosphate binder use, then increase non-Al-based phos-
    phate binder; begin dietary counseling and restrict dietary phosphate; increase dial-
    ysis frequency.

- $d_4$ – 'Diet?': apply a 'hypo' diet or keep his/her diet.

- $d_5$ – 'QB': increase, keep or decrease QB.

- $d_6$ – 'Erythropoietin': keep, decrease or increase (1 EPO) the current dose.

- $d_7$ – 'Iron management': keep the treatment; iron prescription.

Nephrologists provided an ordering of the decision nodes $(d_1, \ldots, d_7)$. The shape of the loss function, $L(d, \theta)$, depends on individual views of risk; the risk attitude of nephrologists (or clinical governance) can be assumed as neutral, and a linear loss function is chosen. The *Quality indicator* node summarizes $L(d, \theta)$ within the influence diagram.

    *Mortality ratio*, *Hospitalization ratio* and *Adherence to treatment* represent the weighted contribution to the loss function, defined on $D$ and $\theta$. Analyzing the most important causes and the consequence of each action, it is possible to assess each scenario and prioritize actions that should be taken for the *j*th patient. With the approach presented in this section the risk manager can recommend the best treatment.

    We began this chapter by discussing the reporting of adverse events and how such data is used in healthcare risk management. We then proceeded to discuss risk management of individual treatments and provided an in-depth example of dialysis of patients with ESRD. The next section is focused on the manufacturer of drug products and how quality audits can be used to mitigate risks in the quality of the delivered drug product.

## 6.6    Risk-based quality audits of drug manufacturing facilities

### 6.6.1    Background on Facility Quality Audits

Risk events can have significant impact on business activities. After the Food and Drug Administration (FDA) recommended withdrawal of the Avandia (rosiglitazone) diabetes treatment, its maker, GlaxcoSmithKline PLC announced on July 10, 2010, that it would charge $2.4 billion to offset the estimated $6 billion liability exposure, and the abrupt end left many physicians and patients worried. Assessing, tracking and managing risks in the pharmaceutical industry is a complex and multifaceted activity. The scope of this ranges from patient safety to business risks and includes risks in the supply chain, the research and development process, the manufacturing sites' operations and post-marketing monitoring.

In this section we focus on drug manufacturing plants and risk events relative to quality compliance with current good manufacturing practices (cGMP) mandated by the FDA and other regulatory agencies. We show how a risk-based Facility Quality Audit of such plants can provide important information for effective and efficient quality and cGMP compliance risk management. The methodology we present has been developed for a global pharmaceutical company in its continuous improvement effort to generate coherent and precise information of quality and cGMP compliance risks associated with its plants all over the world (Yu *et al.*, 2011).

We begin with a discussion of the various risk dimensions in pharmaceutical plants with respect to quality and cGMP compliance. The following sections describe the risk assessment and the scoring methodology we developed. Using examples, we demonstrate how it accounts for both contextual information and risk-related data from the performance of each audited manufacturing site. As shown later, we determine contextual information with a Quality Function Deployment (QFD)-like matrix. QFD is a collaborative tool used to transform objectives (the 'what') to requirements (the 'how'), and represent their relationship with a two dimensional matrix (El-Haik, 2007). In addition, the impact of key process indicators (KPIs) is ascertained with a desirability function. Some generic examples are provided, including a description of the supporting tools developed by the project team.

## 6.6.2    Risk dimensions of facilities manufacturing drug products

A drug manufacturer is exposed to quality and cGMP compliance risks determined by variables such as the type and mix of products manufactured, the operational process, the age and sophistication of the equipment, the regulatory compliance history, or its organizational infrastructure and culture. One approach to assess exposure to risks, for a specific plant, is to conduct a Facility Quality Audit.

Such audits are conducted both internally, usually by a corporate entity, and externally by regulators and/or customers. Similar models can be applied to nutritional supplements, excipients and various drug product components.

In September 2004, as part of the FDA initiative on 'Pharmaceutical cGMPs for the 21st Century', the FDA launched a pilot for 'Risk-Based Method for Prioritizing cGMP Inspections of Pharmaceutical Manufacturing Sites – A Pilot Risk Ranking Model' (FDA, 2004).

Risk exposure of a drug product manufacturing site consists of three high-level components:

**product:** type and mixture of products, dosage form

**process:** age and sophistication of systems, contamination potential

**facility:** location, age of equipment, audit results.

In our model we have added three additional components; namely:

**regulatory compliance history:** compliance rating, customer complaints;

**quality metrics:** deviations, Cost of Quality;

**organization:** organizational culture indicators, employee turnover.

Some of these components create a context for interpreting risk-related data, while others determine an impact factor that should be considered when interpreting Facility Quality

Audit results. The approach presented here builds on various risk-management initiatives of the FDA and other regulatory agencies aimed at improving the quality of production and delivery of drug products. The overall objective is ensuring delivery of safe and cost-efficient products to the market. The FDA's goal of ensuring safety and efficacy rests on five product attributes defined as SISPQ: Strength, Identity, Safety, Purity and Quality. Facility Quality Audits are conducted to objectively determine quality and compliance risks in order to trigger remedial actions in specific areas of vulnerability.

The FDA pilot study calls for the derivation of a *Site Risk Potential* (SRP) of facilities manufacturing drug products. The audit process used to derive such an SRP is based on a Facility Quality Audit that assesses six quality systems representing various sources of risks in a manufacturing operation.

The methodology we developed weighs the risk contributions of these six quality systems by contextual information derived from the type of products and processes of the facility. The SRP is then determined by weighting the Facility Quality Audit findings and considering impact generation components such as regulatory compliance history, quality metrics or organizational characteristics.

We next present this risk-based Facility Quality Audit methodology and discuss the experience gained in its implementation. The methodology can be applied in a broad context, for example in auditing suppliers and subcontractors of drug manufacturing plants.

### 6.6.3   The site risk assessment structure

As mentioned, there are six top-level risk components affecting the quality and cGMP compliance risk of a specific site. Some of these components determine a context for interpreting the site audit results; while others determine an impact factor affecting the overall findings. These components are:

1. Product

2. Process

3. Facility

4. Regulatory Compliance History

5. Quality Metrics

6. Organization.

The *Product*, *Process*, and some of the elements in the *Facility* component, set the contextual parameters that influence weights of Facility Quality Audit findings. The *Regulatory Compliance History*, *Quality Metrics* and *Organization* components set up an impact factor affecting overall risk levels.

The facility risk elements, in each of the six quality systems, are assessed by Facility Quality Audits for impact level and risk likelihood. The former is determined by the severity of a given observation, while the latter determines the likelihood of such an occurrence by assessing whether or not a robust system exists. Risk exposure of elements of the audit categories are classified as high, medium or low.

The acronyms we use for the indicators we developed are: SRP for *Site Risk Potential*, SRS for *Site Risk Score*, and CRS for *Category Risk Score*. In the following sections we show, with examples, how these scores are determined.

The Site Risk Score (SRS) is a weighted combination of findings in a Facility Quality Audit that produces six Category Risk Scores (CRSs). The weights of the risk categories are determined by the site contextual weights.

In setting such a context, we consider various *Product*, *Process* and *Facility* characteristics. Specifically these are the following.

**Product:** number of products, dosage form, sector, antibiotics, hormones, toxicity, allergens, ANDA/NDA (Abbreviated New Drug Application/New Drug Application) or monograph, route of administration and product stability profiles.

**Process:** complexity, velocity, volume, contamination potential and process capability.

**Facility:** country, recognized certifications, type of facility, age of facility, age of equipment, recognized name in industry, use of recognized industry software and capacity/utilization.

The contextualized weights of the Facility Quality Audit categories are determined by a QFD matrix linking context elements with audit categories. As mentioned above, a QFD is an L-shape matrix representing links between two dimensions. In our case the link mapped in the QFD matrix connects the impact-creating elements with the six risk categories used to audit a site (Hoerl, 2007). Figure 6.3 presents part of this matrix indicating ratings of a specific plant in terms of number and type of products it manufactures.

| Product | Score | Risk Categories | | | | | |
|---|---|---|---|---|---|---|---|
| | | C-1 Quality System/Quality Management | C-2 Production Control | C-3 Materials System | C-4 Facilities/ Equipment System | C-5 Laboratory System | C-6 Packaging & Labeling System |
| # of Products | 10 | 5 | 10 | 10 | 10 | 5 | 10 |
| DOSAGE FORM | | | | | | | |
| Group A | 10 | 10 | 10 | 5 | 10 | 5 | 5 |
| Sterile (Injectable, Opthalmic) | | | | | | | |
| Gas | | | | | | | |
| Group B | 5 | 10 | 5 | 5 | 5 | 5 | 5 |
| Liquid | | | | | | | |
| Suspension | | | | | | | |
| Semisolids | | | | | | | |
| Soft Gel | | | | | | | |
| Solid (Tablet/ Capsule) | | | | | | | |
| Powder | | | | | | | |
| Group C | | 5 | 5 | 5 | 5 | 1 | 1 |
| Plastic Component | | | | | | | |
| Glass Component | | | | | | | |
| Group D | 0 | 10 | 5 | 5 | 5 | 5 | 5 |
| Medical Device | | | | | | | |
| Group E | 0 | 10 | 10 | 5 | 5 | 5 | 5 |
| Transdermal | | | | | | | |
| Nasal Spray | | | | | | | |
| | | | | | | | |
| | | Strong = 10 | | | | | |
| | | Medium = 5 | | | | | |
| | | Weak = 1 | | | | | |
| | | | | | | | |

**Figure 6.3**   A QFD matrix matching context variables with risk categories.

Figure 6.4 presents the calculation of contextualized weights, which are than applied to the calculation of CRSs to produce a contextualized SRS. In this example the weights of categories C-1 to C-6 are, respectively (in %), 15, 19, 19, 19, 11 and 19.

A Facility Quality Audit classifies elements of risk categories as critical, major, minor or not audited.

- **Critical findings** are conditions or practices which may result in rejection of products or regulatory action against products considered non-compliant with good manufacturing practice.

- **Major findings** are conditions or practices with potential adverse effect and that would be most likely cited by regulatory inspections.

- **No findings/minor findings** are conditions with no expected adverse effect, albeit being departures from accepted guidelines and thus may be cited by regulatory inspections, and should be addressed by appropriate corrective action.

- **Not audited,** either by planning or execution, are suggestions for improvements, preventive measures, or proactive control of potential deviations.

Risk elements are scored by auditors on a 1–5 scale for probability of occurrence, and for impact severity. Critical findings are scored as 5, major findings as 3, minor findings as 1, and non-audited items are marked as (n/a).

Findings are classified by the risk-assessment methodology as high risk, medium risk or low risk, depending on their position on a risk map generated by the combined probability and severity scores.

Figure 6.5 presents a sample risk map for the Production Control System category. Category elements are positioned within red (mid gray), yellow (light gray) and green (dark gray) zones, representing high, medium or low risk, respectively. Category element names are listed on the side legend of the map. The risk maps were generated using the TRIMS software (Technical Risk Identification and Mitigation; www.bmpcoe.org/pmws/trims.html)).

The outcome of a Facility Quality Audit is therefore a classification of risk elements. From the risk elements score we compute the Category Risk Scores (CRSs). A CRS represents, as a percentage, the seriousness of the findings. If all findings are of high risk (in the red zone), the CRS is 100%. If all findings are minor (in the green zone), the CRS = 0%. For mixed cases, the CRS reflects the level of risk exposure of the risk categories. We showed earlier how weights of the risk categories are determined by the context of the manufacturing facility. These weights are used to compute an SRC. Figure 6.6 presents sample calculations based on weighted scores of facility risk elements, where contextualized weights of the C-1 to C-6 categories produced an SRS of 39%.

We proceed by showing how impact components are accounted for, and conclude with a description of the final Site Risk Potential (SRP) calculator.

Impact components are determined by *Regulatory Compliance History*, *Quality Metrics* and *Organizational Characteristics*. Regulatory Compliance History is determined by regulatory compliance standing, third party audit standing and customer audit standing. Quality History consists for example of Cost of Quality, number of deviations out of specification (OOS), complaints trends, adverse events trends, frequency of rework, overdue corrective and preventive action (CAPA) and open deviations. Finally, Organizational Characteristics are determined by measures of competency levels, resource availability, organizational integrity,

| Product | Score | Risk Categories | | | | | | Importance QFD Scores | | | | | |
| | | C-1 Quality System/Quality Management | C-2 Production Control | C-3 Materials System | C-4 Facilities/ Equipment System | C-5 Laboratory System | C-6 Packaging & Labeling System | C-1 | C-2 | C-3 | C-4 | C-5 | C-6 |
|---|---|---|---|---|---|---|---|---|---|---|---|---|---|
| # of Products | 10 | 5 | 10 | 10 | 10 | 5 | 10 | 50 | 100 | 100 | 100 | 50 | 100 |
| DOSAGE FORM | | | | | | | | | | | | | |
| Group A | 0 | 10 | 10 | 5 | 10 | 5 | 5 | | | | | | |
| Sterile (Injectable, Opthalmic) | | | | | | | | | | | | | |
| Gas | | | | | | | | | | | | | |
| Group B | 5 | 10 | 5 | 5 | 5 | 5 | 5 | 50 | 25 | 25 | 25 | 25 | 25 |
| Liquid | | | | | | | | | | | | | |
| Suspension | | | | | | | | | | | | | |
| Semisolids | | | | | | | | | | | | | |
| Soft Gel | | | | | | | | | | | | | |
| Solid (Tablet/ Capsule) | | | | | | | | | | | | | |
| Powder | | | | | | | | | | | | | |
| Group C | 0 | 5 | 5 | 5 | 5 | 1 | 1 | | | | | | |
| Plastic Component | | | | | | | | | | | | | |
| Glass Component | | | | | | | | | | | | | |
| Group D | 0 | 10 | 5 | 5 | 5 | 5 | 5 | | | | | | |
| Medical Device | | | | | | | | | | | | | |
| Group E | 0 | 10 | 10 | 5 | 5 | 5 | 5 | | | | | | |
| Transdermal | | | | | | | | | | | | | |
| Nasal Spray | | | | | | | | | | | | | |
| QFD Total | | | | | | | | 100 | 125 | 125 | 125 | 75 | 125 |
| QFD% | | | | | | | | 15% | 19% | 19% | 19% | 11% | 19% |

**Figure 6.4**   Calculating contextualized weights of risk categories.

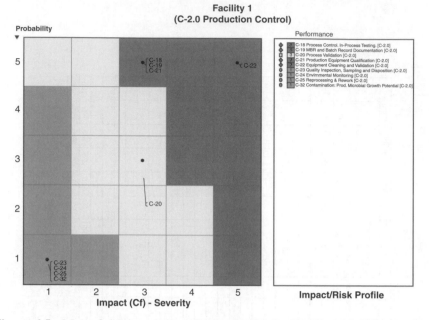

**Figure 6.5**    Map of risk impact/severity for the Production Control audit category.

management engagement and quality culture. Some of these can be assessed by employee surveys.

For each of these measures we compute a desirability function, which reflects how well we are doing with respect to each measure. A value of zero reflects unacceptable performance level, while a value of one indicates that the measurement meets our goal. In mathematical terms, for each measure, $Y_i$, we defined a univariate desirability function, $d_i(Y_i)$, which assigns numbers between 0 and 1 to the possible values of $Y_i$; so that $d_i(Y_i) = 0$ represents a completely undesirable value of $Y_i$ and $d_i(Y_i) = 1$ represents a completely desirable or ideal response value.

The shape of the function $d_i(Y_i)$ can be tailored. Figure 6.7 presents examples of desirability functions by goal. To obtain an individual desirability ($d$) for each response (risk component), we select one of three goals and set up the desirability boundaries:

- minimize the response (smaller is better)

- target the response (target is best)

- maximize the response (larger is better).

For measures one wants to maximize, the function goes from a value of zero up to a lower value threshold to a value of one, beyond a target value. The increase can be linear or abrupt (Figure 6.7 on the right). In this study we apply a linear increase or decrease depending on whether we want to maximize, minimize or set the response value on target.

As an example, the desirability function of the Cost of Quality reflects a goal of minimization, the resource availability indicator should be on a pre-set target, and we would like to see management engagement maximized (see Figure 6.7).

**Golbal Risk Parameters**

| Category | QFD Weighted | Scores | |
|---|---|---|---|
| C-1 Quality System/Quality Managem | 15 | High | 5 |
| C-2 Production Control | 19 | Medium | 3 |
| C-3 Materials System | 19 | Low | 1 |
| C-4 Facilities/Equipment System | 19 | | |
| C-5 Laboratory System | 11 | | |
| C-6 Packaging & Labeling System | 19 | | |

**Contextualized Audit**

| Category | Number of Elements | | | | | Actual Score | | | | Audit Scores |
|---|---|---|---|---|---|---|---|---|---|---|
| | H | M | L | Not Audited | Total Audited | H | M | L | Sum | Risk |
| C-1 Quality System/Quality Managem | 0 | 1 | 10 | 6 | 11 | 0 | 24 | 80 | 104 | 5% |
| C-2 Production Control | 4 | 1 | 4 | 6 | 9 | 160 | 24 | 32 | 216 | 50% |
| C-3 Materials System | 1 | 3 | 4 | 3 | 8 | 20 | 36 | 16 | 72 | 31% |
| C-4 Facilities/Equipment System | 0 | 0 | 11 | 0 | 11 | 0 | 0 | 88 | 88 | 0% |
| C-5 Laboratory System | 10 | 2 | 0 | 2 | 12 | 400 | 48 | 0 | 448 | 92% |
| C-6 Packaging & Labeling System | 2 | 4 | 0 | 3 | 6 | 40 | 48 | 0 | 88 | 67% |
| Overall | 17 | 11 | 29 | 20 | 57 | | | | 1016 | 39% |

**Figure 6.6**  Applying contextualized weights to the SRS calculator.

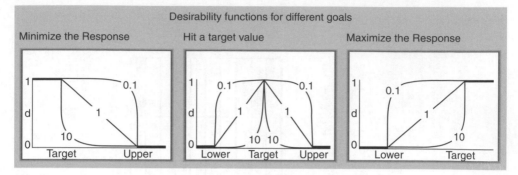

**Figure 6.7**  Desirability functions by goal (adapted from MINITAB™ documentation).

The desirabilities for all measures are then combined to an overall composite desirability using the geometric mean of the individual desirabilities:

$$\text{Composite Desirability}, D = [(d_1(Y_1) \times d_2(Y_2)) \times \cdots \times d_k(Y_k))]^{1/k},$$

with $k$ denoting the number of measures. For more on such functions see Harrington (1965) and Figini, Kenett and Salini (2010).

The outcome of the above analysis is a composite desirability index, which is the basis for computing the impact of various components in the facility risk profile. The composite desirability is used to compute the SRP with the following formula:

$$\text{Site Risk Potential}, \text{SRP (in\%)} = 100(1 - (1 - \text{SRS}) \times D).$$

SRS denotes Site Risk Score, and D is the composite desirability risk factor. Figure 6.8 presents sample calculations of the final SRP for a computed composite desirability of 0.87.

Figure 6.9 represents the impact of the composite desirability on an SRS and the final SRP. In this example, a composite desirability of 0.87 increased the calculated SRS of 39% by 13%, resulting in the final SRP of 46.50%.

| Risk Component | Goal | Lower | Target | Upper | Upper | Importance | Value | Desirability |
|---|---|---|---|---|---|---|---|---|
| Regulatory Compliance Standing | Maximize | 0.3 | 0.7 | | 1 | 1 | 0.65 | 0.88 |
| Third Party Audit Standing | Minimize | | 0.1 | 0.25 | 1 | 1 | 0.11 | 0.93 |
| Customer Audit Standing | Target | 0.1 | 0.15 | 0.2 | 1 | 1 | 0.145 | 0.90 |
| Cost of Quality - Failure Cost | Minimize | | 10 | 15 | 1 | 1 | 8.5 | 1.00 |
| Deviations/Volume | Minimize | | 2 | 4 | 1 | 1 | 2.1 | 0.95 |
| OOS | Minimize | | 5 | 8 | 1 | 1 | 6 | 0.67 |
| Complaints Trend | Minimize | | 5 | 12 | 1 | 1 | 6 | 0.86 |
| Adverse Events Trend | Target | 4 | 5 | 6 | 1 | 1 | 5 | 1.00 |
| Near Misses (Quality Events) | Minimize | | 17 | 23 | 1 | 1 | 18 | 0.83 |
| Frequency of Rework/Reprocess due to Quality Events | Minimize | | 7 | 12 | 1 | 1 | 7 | 1.00 |
| Overdue CAPA | Minimize | | 17 | 23 | 1 | 1 | 18 | 0.83 |
| Open Deviations | Minimize | | 7 | 12 | 1 | 1 | 7 | 1.00 |
| Competency | Target | 65 | 80 | 95 | 1 | 1 | 83 | 0.80 |
| Resources | Target | 85 | 100 | 115 | 1 | 1 | 99 | 0.93 |
| Integrity/Ethics | Maximize | 50 | 80 | | 1 | 1 | 75 | 0.83 |
| Management Engagement | Maximize | 10 | 20 | | 1 | 1 | 17 | 0.70 |
| Quality Culture | Maximize | 35 | 65 | | 1 | 1 | 59 | 0.80 |
| Composite Desirability Score | | | | | | | | 0.87 |

**Figure 6.8**  Composite desirability risk factor calculator.

**Golbal Risk Parameters**

| Category | QFD Weighted | Scores | |
|---|---|---|---|
| C-1 Quality System/Quality Manag | 15 | High | 5 |
| C-2 Production Control | 19 | Medium | 3 |
| C-3 Materials System | 19 | Low | 1 |
| C-4 Facilities / Equipment System | 19 | | |
| C-5 Laboratory System | 11 | | |
| C-6 Packaging & Labeling System | 19 | | |

**Contextualized Audit**

| Category | Number of Elements | | | | | Actual Score | | | | Audit Scores |
|---|---|---|---|---|---|---|---|---|---|---|
| | H | M | L | Not Audited | Total Audited | H | M | L | Sum | Risk |
| C-1 Quality System/Quality Manag | 0 | 1 | 10 | 6 | 11 | 0 | 24 | 80 | 104 | 5% |
| C-2 Production Control | 4 | 1 | 4 | 6 | 9 | 160 | 24 | 32 | 216 | 50% |
| C-3 Materials System | 1 | 3 | 4 | 3 | 8 | 20 | 36 | 16 | 72 | 31% |
| C-4 Facilities / Equipment System | 0 | 0 | 11 | 0 | 11 | 0 | 0 | 88 | 88 | 0% |
| C-5 Laboratory System | 10 | 2 | 0 | 2 | 12 | 400 | 48 | 0 | 448 | 92% |
| C-6 Packaging & Labeling System | 2 | 4 | 0 | 3 | 6 | 40 | 48 | 0 | 88 | 67% |
| Overall | 17 | 11 | 29 | 20 | 57 | | | | 1016 | 39% |
| | | | | | | Composite Desirability | | 0.87 | | 46.50% |

**Figure 6.9**  Calculating Site Risk Potential by applying the composite desirability factor.

As mentioned, a Facility Quality Audit is based on a subset from a comprehensive set of audit elements that are actually audited. This de facto sample of elements can be used to determine overall readiness of the site in terms of risk exposure using statistical inference methods. Moreover, a Bayesian approach can be implemented by considering the Dirichlet conjugate family for multinomial distributions. These topics are, however, beyond the scope of this chapter.

## 6.7   Summary

Risk management is a key activity in many areas such as the finance industry, in chemical plants, transportation systems, telecommunications and Web-based services. In healthcare it is more than critical, since human life and significant budgets are at stake. This chapter on risk management in drug manufacturing and healthcare was designed to trigger the interest and draw attention of readers to this important area. The first two sections discussed risk management of healthcare systems and dwelled on the reporting of adverse events. Without such reports any attempt to conduct effective risk management is obviously severely handicapped. The third section was focused on risk management of a specific healthcare treatment and provides a comprehensive example where risk assessment, decision analysis and utility theory are combined to optimize the treatment of patients with end stage renal disease (ESRD). These two parts of the chapter dealt with the healthcare system in general and a specific treatment protocol. The third part of the chapter was focused on facilities manufacturing drug products. In that part we described a comprehensive methodology for conducting facility audits and analyzing their findings in order to establish a site risk potential (SRP). Deriving risk scores of a manufacturing site is a trigger for remedial action and, thereby, containment of risks.

Overall we have covered parts of a basic supply chain for healthcare services. Risks can be due to the drug product being used, the healthcare establishment, including errors due to doctors and nurses, or to the specific treatment protocol such as hemodialysis. Any exposure to risks in these three parts can have severe detrimental consequences.

Further research needs to be conducted in order to better understand the integration of such components. Eventually, the challenge is to identify effective risk mitigation initiatives that will make healthcare a safe and cost-effective service.

## References

American Medical Association (2000) E-8.12 *Patient Information. Code of Medical Ethics. Current Opinions of the Council of Ethical and Judicial Affairs*, American Medical Association, Chicago, IL.

Anderson, D.O. and Starzynski, B. (2001) Successful strategies for cultural transformation are the essential first steps to increase medical error reporting and identify performance improvement strategies. Partnership symposium 2001, Patient Safety – Stories of Success. Fairmont, Dallas.

Ben Gal, I. (2007) Bayesian networks, in *Encyclopaedia of Statistics in Quality and Reliability* (eds F. Ruggeri, R.S. Kenett and F. Faltin), John Wiley & Sons, Ltd, Chichester.

Bernardo, J.M. and Smith, A.F.M. (1994) *Bayesian Theory*, John Wiley and Sons, Inc., New York.

Coles, J., Pryce, D. and Shaw, C. (2001, October) The reporting of adverse clinical incidents – achieving high quality reporting, CASPE Research, London.

Cooper, G.F. and Herskovits, E. (1992) A Bayesian method for the induction of probabilistic networks from data. *Machine Learning*, **9**(4), 309–347.

Cornalba, C. (2009) Clinical and operational risk: a Bayesian approach. *Methodology and Computing in Applied Probability*, **11**, 47–63.

Cornalba, C., Kenett, R.S. and Giudici, P. (2007) Sensitivity analysis of Bayesian networks with stochastic emulators. ENBIS-DEINDE proceedings, University of Torino, Turin, Italy.

Corrigan, J.M., Donaldson, M.S. and Kohn, L.T. (eds ) (2001) *Crossing the Quality Chasm: A New Health System for the 21st Century*, Institute of Medicine, National Academy Press, Washington, DC.

DOQI Group (2003) K/DOQI clinical practice guidelines for bone metabolism and disease in chronic kidney disease. *American Journal of Kidney Disease*, **42**(3), 1–201.

El-Haik, B. (2007) Quality function deployment, in *Encyclopedia of Statistics in Quality and Reliability* (eds F. Ruggeri, R.S. Kenett and F. Faltin), John Wiley & Sons Ltd, Chichester.

ESRD Group (2006) *End Stage Renal Disease Glossary*, Medicare ESRD Network Organizations.

FDA (2004) *Risk-Based Method for Prioritizing cGMP Inspections of Pharmaceutical Manufacturing Sites – A Pilot Risk Ranking Model*. Department of Health and Human Services, US Food and Drug Administration.

FDA (2006) *Guidance for the Use of Bayesian Statistics in Medical Device Clinical Trials*. Technical Report, Food and Drug Administration, Center for Devices and Radiological Health, Division of Biostatistics.

Figini, S., Kenett, R.S. and Salini, S. (2010) Integrating operational and financial risk assessments. *Quality and Reliability Engineering International*, **26**(8), 887–897.

Fomby, T.B. and Hill, R. (1997) *Applying Maximum Entropy to Econometric Problems*, JAI Press.

Frankel, A. (2001) Reporting system new approaches. Partnership symposium 2001, Patient Safety – Stories of Success. Fairmont, Dallas.

Grandy, W.T. and Schick, L.H. (1999) *Maximum Entropy and Bayesian Methods*. Kluwer Academic Publishers, Dordrecht.

Grunwald, P.D. and Dawid, A.P. (2004) Game theory, maximum entropy, minimum discrepancy, and robust Bayesian decision theory. *Annals of Statistics*, **32**, 1367–1433.

Hand, D., Mannila, H. and Smyth, P. (2001) *Principles of Data Mining (Adaptive Computation and Machine Learning)*, The MIT Press.

Harel, A. Kenett, R. and Ruggeri, F. (2008) Modeling Web usability diagnostics on the basis of usage statistics, in *Statistical Methods in eCommerce Research* (eds W. Jank and G. Shmueli), John Wiley & Sons, Inc., Hoboken, NJ.

Harrington, E.C. (1965) The desirability function. *Industrial Quality Control*, **21**, 494–498.

Hoerl, R. (2007) Critical-to-quality matrices, in *Encyclopedia of Statistics in Quality and Reliability* (eds F. Ruggeri, R.S. Kenett and F. Faltin), John Wiley & Sons, Ltd, Chichester.

Jaynes, E.T. (edited by L. Bretthorst) (2003) *Probability Theory: The Logic of Science*, Cambridge University Press.

Jensen, F.V. (2001) *Bayesian Networks and Decision Graphs*, Springer.

Kenett, R.S. and Baker, E. (2010) *Process Improvement and CMMI for Systems and Software: Planning, Implementation, and Management*, Auerbach Publications.

Kenett, R.S. and Raanan, Y. (2010) *Operational Risk Management. A Practical Approach to Intelligent Data Analysis*, John Wiley & Sons, Ltd, Chichester.

Kenett, R.S. and Raphaeli, O. (2008) Multivariate methods in enterprise system implementation, risk management and change management. *International Journal of Risk Assessment and Management*, **9**(3), 258–276.

Kenett, R.S. and Tapiero, C. (2010) Quality, risk and the Taleb quadrants. *Risk and Decision Analysis*, **1**(4), 231–246. http://ssrn.com/abstract=1433490.

Kenett, R.S. and Zacks, S. (1998) *Modern Industrial Statistics: Design and Control of Quality and Reliability*, Duxbury Press, San Francisco, Spanish edition 2000, 2nd paperback edition 2002, Chinese edition 2004.

Kenett, R.S., de Frenne, A., Tort-Martorell, X. and McCollin, C. (2008) The statistical efficiency conjecture, in *Statistical Practice in Business and Industry* (eds S. Coleman, T. Greenfield, D. Stewardson and D. Montgomery), John Wiley & Sons, Ltd, Chichester, pp. 61–95.

Kim, J.R.L., Pisoni, M., Danese, S. *et al.* (2003) Achievement of proposed NKF-K/DOQI bone metabolism and disease guidelines: results from the dialysis outcomes and practice patterns study (DOPPS). *Journal of the American Society of Nephrology*, **14**(25), 269–270.

Kohn, L.T., Corrigan, J.M. and Donaldson, M.S. (eds ) (1999) *To Err is Human. Building a Safer Health System*, Institute of Medicine, National Academy Press, Washington, DC.

Lauritzen, S.L. and Spiegelhalter, D.J. (1988) Local computations with probabilities on graphical structures and their application to expert systems. *Journal of the Royal Statistical Society, Series B (Methodological)*, **50**(2), 157–224.

Leape, L.L. (2002) Reporting of adverse events. *The New England Journal of Medicine*, **347**(20), 1633–1638.

Lee, R.C. and Wright, W.E. (1994) Development of human exposure-factor distributions using maximum entropy inference. *Journal of Exposure Analysis and Environmental Epidemiology*, **4**, 329–341.

Lindgren, O.H, Christensen, R. and Mills, D.H. (1991) Medical malpractice risk management early warning systems. *Law and Contemporary Problems*, **54**, 22–41.

McKinlay, J.B. and Marceau, L.D. (2002) The end of the golden age of doctoring. *International Journal of Health Services*, **32**, 379–416.

Mills, D.H. and von Bolschwing, G.E. (1995) Clinical risk management: experiences from the United States, in *Clinical Risk Management* (ed. C. Vincent), BMJ Publishing Group.

O'Hagan, A., Buck, C.E., Daneshkhah, A. *et al.* (2006) *Uncertain Judgements Eliciting Experts' Probabilities*, John Wiley & Sons, Inc., New York.

Panjer, H. (2006) *Operational Risk: Modeling Analytics*, John Wiley & Sons, Inc., Hoboken, NJ.

Pearl, J. (2009) *Causality: Models, Reasoning, and Inference*, 2nd edn, Cambridge University Press.

Raiffa, H. (1997) *Decision Analysis: Introductory Readings on Choices Under Uncertainty*, McGraw Hill.

Ruggeri, F., Kenett, R.S. and Faltin F. (2007) *The Encyclopaedia of Statistics in Quality and Reliability*, John Wiley & Sons, Ltd, Chichester.

Taleb, N. (2007) *The Black Swan: The Impact of the Highly Improbable*, Random House, New York.

Tapiero, C. (2004) *Risk and Financial Management: Mathematical and Computational Methods*, John Wiley & Sons, Ltd, Chichester.

Yu, L., Urkin, E., Lum, S. *et al.* (2011, September) Site seeing, *Quality Progress*, 16–25.

# 7

# The twenty-first century challenges in drug development*

**Yafit Stark**

*TEVA Pharmaceutical Industries, Ltd., Netanya, Israel*

## Synopsis

Globalization, rapidly evolving technologies and emerging areas of science are having a major impact on medical products regulated by the Food and Drug Administration (FDA) and the European Medicines Agency (EMA). Evolving technologies in scientific, medical, clinical and statistical areas are making it possible to implement cutting-edge information systems critical to supporting medical innovation and public health safety. This chapter will review the current conditions and outcomes of drug development processes and focus on some challenges that need to be addressed by statistical methodologies and statisticians working in the pharmaceutical industry.

## 7.1    The FDA's Critical Path Initiative

The Critical Path Initiative (CPI) is the FDA's national strategy to drive innovation in the scientific process through which medical products are developed, evaluated and manufactured.

The initiative was launched in March 2004, with the release of the FDA's landmark report: *Innovation or Stagnation: Challenge and Opportunity on the Critical Path to New Medical Products* (FDA, 2004).

---

*This chapter is based on a talk given at the 2nd QbD conference at the Hebrew University of Jerusalem, May 5–6, 2010, Jerusalem, Israel.

---

*Statistical Methods in Healthcare*, First Edition. Edited by Frederick W. Faltin, Ron S. Kenett and Fabrizio Ruggeri.
© 2012 John Wiley & Sons, Ltd. Published 2012 by John Wiley & Sons, Ltd.

The publication diagnosed the reasons for the widening gap between scientific discoveries that have unlocked the potential to prevent and cure some of today's biggest killers, such as diabetes, cancer and Alzheimer's and their translation into innovative medical treatments.

Sounding the alarm on the increasing difficulty and unpredictability of medical product development, the report concluded that collective action was needed to modernize scientific and technical tools, as well as harness information technology to evaluate and predict the safety, effectiveness and manufacturability of medical products.

The report called for a national effort to identify specific activities along the critical path of medicinal product development and use, which, if undertaken, would help transform the critical-path sciences.

In March 2006, the FDA Commissioner announced the release of the FDA's *Critical Path Opportunities* (FDA, 2006). Created with the broad contribution of the public, academia and industry, the list describes specific areas where the sciences of product development have the greatest need for improvement. It lists 76 tangible examples where new scientific discoveries in fields like genomics, imaging, informatics and the analysis of biological information using statistical techniques could be applied during development to improve accuracy of tests that better predict the safety and efficacy of potential medical products.

These two documents summarize a deep introspective process on the state of the art in the pharmaceutical industry. The next section presents some details on the level of innovation in this industry.

## 7.2    Lessons from 60 years of pharmaceutical innovation

- From 1956 to 2008, the FDA has approved 1222 products: 1103 new molecular entities (NMEs) and 119 new biological entities (NBEs).

- The number of new drugs approved in 2010 is not greater now than 50 years ago.

- In 2008 only 21 new drugs were approved by the FDA.

### 7.2.1    New-drug performance statistics

Figure 7.1 (adapted from the FDA Center for Drug Evaluation and Research, CDER) presents the number of new drug products filed and approved by the FDA. For more on this data see www.fda.gov/downloads/Drugs/DevelopmentApprovalProcess/HowDrugsareDevelopedand Approved/DrugandBiologicApprovalReports/UCM242695.pdf. The stagnation in the number of new drugs being developed in order to reach the market is apparent.

### 7.2.2    Currently there are many players, but few winners

At present, there are 4300 companies engaged in drug innovation. Only 261 organizations (6%) have registered at least one product since 1956. Only 32 out of 261 organizations (12%) have been in existence for at least 59 years. The cost of new-product development has soared to $1 billion (0.8 to 1.7 billion) or more, and the average time to market for a new drug/biologic is going up (see Figure 7.2, adapted from Gilbert, Hauske and Singh, 2001).

Another dimension affecting the balance between innovation and stagnation is the time to file new drug products. Some data on this are presented next.

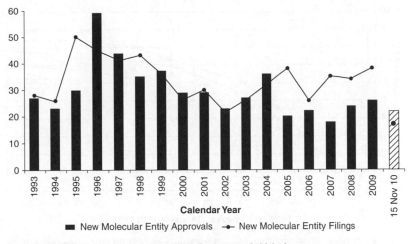

*beginning in 2004 these figures include BLAs for therapeutic biologics

**Figure 7.1**   New molecular entity filings and approvals, CDER.

## 7.2.3   Time to approval – standard new molecular entities

Figure 7.3 (again, adapted from the FDA Center for Drug Evaluation and Research) presents the statistics on time to file (in months) under various time windows of the Prescription Drug User Fee Act (PDUFA). The figure presents cumulative time to approval for five time periods. The median time to file corresponds to the time at 50%.

- Pre-PDUFA (Filing Year (FY) 1968 through FY 1992) – median: 34 months
- PDUFA I (FY 1993 through FY 1997) – median: 18 months

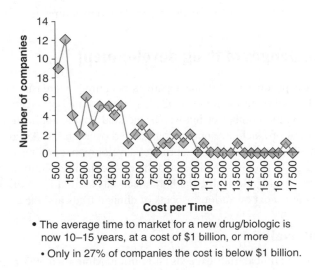

- The average time to market for a new drug/biologic is now 10–15 years, at a cost of $1 billion, or more
- Only in 27% of companies the cost is below $1 billion.

**Figure 7.2**   Cost of new molecular entities' development.

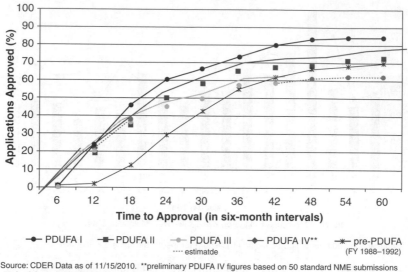

Source: CDER Data as of 11/15/2010. **preliminary PDUFA IV figures based on 50 standard NME submissions received through 9/30/2009

**Figure 7.3** Time to approval for standard new molecular entities by FDA under the Prescription Drug User Fee Act (PDUFA).

- PDUFA II (FY 1998 through FY 2002) – median: 24 months
- PDUFA III (FY 2003 through FY 2007) – median: 30 months
- PDUFA IV (FY 2008 through FY 9/2009) – median: 24 months.

Over the last four time periods, the median time to file ranged from 18 to 30 months, with a deterioration trend from 1993 to 2007 and a minor improvement in the beginning of the last period.

The next section presents the key challenges in drug development.

## 7.3 The challenges of drug development

The current medical product development path is becoming increasingly challenging, inefficient and costly. Although the number of medicinal product applications submitted has declined significantly, the number of innovative medical device applications has increased. In contrast, the cost of product development has soared over the last decade.

If the cost and difficulties of medicinal product development continue to grow, innovation will continue to stagnate and even decline, and the biomedical revolution may not deliver on its promise of better health. Basically, the bottleneck has shifted from discovery to clinical development. We focus next on various aspects of clinical trials and the critical path.

### 7.3.1 Clinical trials

Global expenditure on clinical trials exceeds $40 billion. More than 50% of Phase III clinical trials fail. The main causes of failure include safety problems and lack of effectiveness.

Inability to predict these failures before human testing or early in clinical trials dramatically escalates costs.

In the case of medical devices, the current capacity for technological innovation has outstripped the ability to assess performance in patients, resulting in prolonged delays between design and use.

## 7.3.2   The critical-path goals

Critical-path research needs to concentrate on developing new, publicly available scientific and technical tools, including assays, standards, computer modeling techniques, biomarkers and clinical endpoints. The objective is to make the development process itself more efficient and effective and more likely to result in safe products that benefit patients.

Such tools will make it easier to identify products that do not hold promise earlier in the process, thus reducing time and resource investments, and facilitating the process for development of medical products that hold promise for the patient.

## 7.3.3   Three dimensions of the critical path

The FDA document describing the critical-path challenges (FDA, 2006) identifies three dimensions summarized in Table 7.1. Many of the activities that are required to meet the critical-path challenges rely on proper statistical techniques, including design of experiments, multivariate methods, modeling, sequential methods and scale-up techniques. For a review of such techniques see Kenett and Stark (2008), Kenett and Kenett (2008) and Kenett (2009).

**Table 7.1**   Dimensions of the critical path.

| Dimension | Definition | Examples of activities |
| --- | --- | --- |
| Assessing safety | Show that the product is adequately safe for each stage of development | • Preclinical: show that product is safe enough for early human testing<br>• Eliminate products with safety problems early<br>• Clinical: show that product is safe enough for commercial distribution |
| Demonstrating medical utility | Show that the product benefits people | • Preclinical: select appropriate design (devices) or candidate (drugs) with high probability of effectiveness<br>• Clinical: show effectiveness in people |
| Industrialization | Go from lab concept or prototype to a manufacturable product | • Design a high-quality product<br>  • physical design<br>  • characterization<br>  • specifications<br>• Develop mass-production capacity<br>  • manufacturing scale-up<br>  • quality control |

### 7.3.4   A new-product development toolkit

The new-product development toolkit needs to both explain and provide insights on the mechanism of action and predict future outcomes. Exploratory power provides explanations on causality relationships and needs to be unbiased. Predictive models are evaluated by their prediction error (see Shmueli, 2010, and Kenett and Shmueli, 2011).

In summary, we need to develop:

- new predictive tools that improve predictability and efficiency along the critical path by:

  - early identification of a product candidate with the greatest efficacy

  - early evaluation of product safety;

- new evaluation tools that improve treatment choices and the performance of clinical trials.

### 7.3.5   Towards a better safety toolkit

There are currently significant needs and opportunities for developing better predictors of human responses to foreign antigens, methods to further enhance the safety of transplanted human tissues, new technology to assess drug liver toxicity, and identify gene therapy risks.

Specifically, proteomic and toxiogenomic approaches may ultimately provide sensitive and predictive safety assessment techniques. This is triggering targeted research aimed at specific toxicity problems.

Moreover, as biomedical knowledge increases and bioinformatics capability likewise grows, there is hope that greater predictive power may be obtained from *in silico* (computer modeling) analyses, such as in predictive toxicology.

For more on these topics see Chapter 3 on *Pharmacometrics in drug development*, Chapter 4 on *Interactive clinical trial design* and Chapter 5 on *Stage-wise clinical trial experiments in Phases I, II and III*.

### 7.3.6   Tools for demonstrating medical utility

Predicting and demonstrating medical utility (benefit or effectiveness) are the most difficult and important challenges in drug development.

Opportunities for targeted efforts in areas of effectiveness are, for example, statistical methods to control variability in trials of imaging devices and make analysis of software publicly available. The use of such methods can reduce sample size of imaging device trials, thereby reducing cost and improving the efficiency of clinical development.

The overall objective is to shift from *trial and error* with empirical testing, with patient-exposure-based assessment of efficacy and adverse events, to a *mechanistic approach* based on predictive evaluation using new molecular knowledge about the mechanism of disease and products (see Chapter 4).

The next section expands on aspects of modern clinical development.

## 7.4   A new era in clinical development

Clinical development in the modern era involves several paradigm shifts.

- **Learn/confirm structure:** implement exploration during early clinical development, rather than in conventional Phase I and II type design. The areas of relevant questions

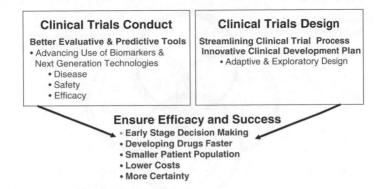

**Figure 7.4**   Innovative drug development to ensure efficacy and success.

include exploration of biological markers, the use of imaging technology confirmed by safety and efficacy and/or validation of surrogate markers wherever

- **Innovative drug development to ensure clinical development success** deals with the design and implementation of clinical trials, a better understanding of drug disease interactions, and improved synergies between various technologies. For a schematic description of these concepts see Figures 7.4–7.6.

## 7.4.1   Advancing new technologies in clinical development

One important advance in clinical research is the implementation of biomarkers followed by surrogate markers in the design of special studies. Biomarkers may be beneficial in evaluating dosing, selecting patient population, and assessing safety and/or efficacy, while exploring the drug's mechanism of action and understanding disease pathophysiology. This approach significantly enhances pharmacokinetic and pharmacodynamic assessments that are critical during clinical development (see Chapter 1).

Biomarkers may also be highly beneficial in assessing clinical outcome. The value of biomarkers is in optimizing the benefit/risk profiles of therapeutics by increasing biological knowledge, assessing more accurate dosing, optimizing patient population and helping in an early Go/No Go decision-making process.

## 7.4.2   Advancing new clinical trial designs

Microdosing is the administration of subpharmacological amounts (microdoses) of new chemical entities to humans to gain valuable information on human pharmacokinetics (PK)

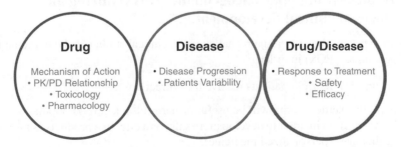

**Figure 7.5**   Implementation of new technologies in drug development.

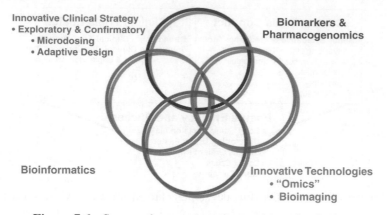

**Figure 7.6**    Synergy between new innovative technologies.

and pharmacodynamics (PD) and metabolism in early stages of drug product development. This approach should allow earlier first-in-man trials and improve the predictive capabilities of the study.

Potential benefits are to allow sponsors to stop futile development early. Some enabling technologies include accelerator mass spectrometry (AMS) and positron emission tomography (PET).

### 7.4.3    Advancing innovative trial designs

Innovative clinical trial designs involve the following.

- Seamless design: combining two phases of clinical development into one clinical trial.

- Adaptive design: using accumulating data to decide on how to modify aspects in a study without undermining validity and integrity, while maximizing the potential of success.

- Implementation of modern statistics by:

  - simulation experiments

  - Bayesian adaptive designs

  - data mining in the critical path of clinical research.

### 7.4.4    Implementing pharmacogenomics (PGx) during all stages of clinical development

Yet another aspect of the critical-path challenges in clinical studies is the implementation of pharmacogenomics (PGx) in order:

- to ensure that the right patients receive the correct dose;

- to explore whether a drug will be useful or harmful in a certain population and to use PGx information in order to develop more safer and effective products as individualized drug therapies (personalized medicine).

This section has reviewed various dimensions in new-era clinical development. The next section ties in Quality by Design (QbD) concepts presented in Chapter 1 and clinical research.

## 7.5    The QbD and clinical aspects

Quality by Design (QbD) is a systematic approach to development that begins with predefined objectives, emphasizes product and process understanding and sets up process control based on sound science and quality risk management. In the traditional approach, product quality and performance are achieved predominantly by restricting flexibility in the manufacturing process and by end product testing. Under the QbD paradigm, pharmaceutical quality is assured by understanding and controlling manufacturing and formulation variables. End product testing is used to confirm the quality of the product and is not part of the ongoing consistency assurance and/or process control. For a general introduction to QbD see Chapter 1 and Kenett (2009).

QbD can be described as a four-stage process addressing both design and control. The stages are as follows.

- **Design intent:** the active pharmaceutical ingredient (API) chemical and physical characteristics and drug product performance targets are identified for the commercial product.

- **Design selection:** the API manufacturing process and the drug product formulation and manufacturing process are selected to achieve the design intent for the commercial product.

- **Control definition:** the largest contributors to critical quality attribute (CQA) variability are established and controls defined to ensure process performance expectations are met.

- **Control verification:** the performance of the API and drug product processes in manufacturing are measured to verify that the controls are effective and the product performance acceptable.

For a comprehensive treatment of QbD and a description of implementation status see Nasr (2007, 2009) and Yu (2008); for applications of QbD to biological drug products see Kenett and Kenett (2008) and Rathore and Mhatre (2009); for statistical models applied in QbD see Peterson and Kenett (2011).

The main characteristics of QbD are:

- to ensure that the product is designed to meet the clinical performance;

- to establish a clear linkage between safety and efficacy of the product in the patients;

- to link the quality of the product back to the process of its preparation.

QbD requires the following.

- **Clinical understanding:** link between the product, the disease, the safety and efficacy in humans.

- **Process understanding:** link between the drug product and process attributes.

- **Product understanding:** product knowledge and product critical quality attributes.

### 7.5.1    Possible QbD clinical approach

QbD can help determine, systematically:

- target indication
- route of administration
- target patient population.

Specifically, it is anticipated that the future will see significant advances in reliable new methodologies to harness the potential of clinical development plans.

### 7.5.2    Defining clinical design space

The design space of a drug product is the multidimensional combination and interaction of input variables (e.g., material attributes) and process parameters that have been demonstrated to provide assurance of quality. Including a design space in a new drug application is a key element of the QbD initiative. Working within the design space is not considered a change requiring regulatory approval. Movement out of the design space is considered to be a change, and requires a regulatory post-approval change process. For statistical features of design spaces see Kenett and Kenett (2008), Rathore and Mhatre (2009) and Peterson and Kenett (2011).

The concept of *clinical design space* quantifies the clinical experience with the product. Like the product design space, the clinical design space is multidimensional in scope.

*The size of the clinical design space* for a given product depends on:

- the number of manufactured lots used in the clinical study
- process capability
- availability of applicable data from other similar products
- extent of product heterogeneity that has been introduced during clinical trials.

A clinical design space is expected to be limited in the early phases of clinical development, when only a few lots have been introduced into the study, but grows as the product reaches a more advanced stage of product development and more clinical data become available. Increased understanding of the linkage between product attributes and clinical performance via clinical and non-clinical studies results in a broader product design space.

### 7.5.3    Clinical deliverables to QbD

The components of a clinical study relevant to QbD include the following.

- Definition and design of clinical criteria that evaluate potential and biological relevance of the product early on in development.
- Exploration of alternatives to large clinical studies (including *in silico* patients).
- Design and implementation of innovative clinical design protocols during clinical development.
- Quality built in by design.
- Information from clinical development as the basis for quality risk management.

**Biomarkers Consortium Launches I-SPY 2 Breast Cancer Clinical Trial
(Bethesda, Maryland, USA, March 17, 2010)**

Groundbreaking
Public–Private
Collaboration
Combines
Personalized
Medicine &
Novel Trial
Design to
Develop
Potentially Life
Saving New
Breast Cancer
Drugs

The Biomarkers Consortium, a unique public-private partnership that includes the FDA, NIH and major pharmas, lead by the FNIH*, today announced the launch of a highly anticipated clinical trial to help screen promising new drugs being developed for women with high risk, fast-growing breast cancers, for whom an improvement over standard treatment could dramatically change the odds of survival.

- Janet Woodcock: "The I-SPY 2 trial explores a whole new way to rapidly screen new cancer treatments and match the therapy to specific markers"
- I-SPY 2 has the potential to significantly reduce the cost of drug development and speed the process of screening drugs with the goal of bringing safe and effective new drugs to market more efficiently.
- I-SPY 2 was developed to allow the activity of drugs to be assessed much earlier in the research process, potentially enabling drugs to be developed and approved using fewer patients, less time and far fewer resources.
- The goal is to shave several years and hundreds of millions of dollars off the current process.
- FNIH received IND approval to allow trial to graduate, drop and add drugs seamlessly during trial without having to stop to write new protocol.

*Foundation of National Institutes of Health

**Figure 7.7** Slide describing the activity of the biomarkers consortium (adapted from FNIH presentation).

Clinical QbD is a comprehensive approach that should involve industry, academia and regulatory bodies. The Biomarkers Consortium led by the Foundation for the National Institutes of Health (FNIH) is an example of such collaboration, where the National Institutes of Health (NIH), FDA and several major pharmaceutical companies work together (see Figure 7.7).

## 7.5.4 Quality by Design in clinical development

QbD in clinical development is necessary to increase our understanding by:

- speeding development of new drugs through focus on implementation of new technology;
- supporting development of innovative trial designs;
- advancing development of drugs also for rare diseases;
- providing clear information on benefits and risks;
- faster clinical development;
- maximizing success in clinical development;
- ensuring safety and effectiveness, making successful drugs available for unmet needs.

Such a QbD clinical strategy, which provides a systematic approach for improving product attributes and development, will maximize the success of bringing new products to the market, to the right patients **faster, safer, smarter, and with smaller budgets**.

# References

FDA (2004) Innovation or Stagnation: Challenge and Opportunity on the Critical Path to New Medical Products, Food and Drug Administration, Silver Spring, MD. www.fda.gov/ohrms/dockets/ac/07/briefing/2007-4329b_02_04_Critical%20Path%20Report%202004.pdf.

FDA (2006) Critical Path Opportunities Report, Food and Drug Administration, Silver Spring, MD.    www.fda.gov/downloads/ScienceResearch/SpecialTopics/CriticalPathInitiative/CriticalPath OpportunitiesReports/UCM077254.pdf.

Gilbert, J., Hauske, P. and Singh, A. (2001) *How New Drugs Move Through The Development and Approval Process*, Tufts Center for the Study of Drug Development, Background, Boston.

Kenett, R.S. (2009) By Design. Six Sigma Forum Magazine (November), pp. 27–29.

Kenett, R.S. and Kenett D.A. (2008) Quality by Design applications in biosimilar pharmaceutical products. *ACQUAL, Accreditation and Quality Assurance*, **13**(12), 681–690.

Kenett, R.S. and Shmueli, G. (2011) On Information Quality, ssrn.com/abstract=1464444 (accessed March 31, 2012).

Kenett, R.S. and Stark, Y. (2008) Drug Development Strategy: The Interface Between QbD and Statistical Methods. University of Wisconsin Global Pharmaceutical Conference, Practical Application of QbD in Accelerated Development: Laboratory, Quality and Regulatory Considerations, Frankfurt, Germany, April 2–4, 2008.

Kenett, R.S. and Steinberg, D. (2006, August) New frontiers in design of experiments. *Quality Progress*, 61–65.

Kenett, R.S. and Zacks, S. (1998) *Modern Industrial Statistics: Design and Control of Quality and Reliability*, 2nd edn, Chinese edition 2004, Duxbury Press, San Francisco.

Nasr, M. (2007) Quality by Design (QbD) – A Modern System Approach to Pharmaceutical Development and Manufacturing – FDA Perspective, FDA Quality Initiatives Workshop, North Bethesda, MD.

Nasr, M. (2009) Status and Implementation of ICH Q8, Q9, and Q10 Quality Guidelines: Topic Introduction and FDA Perspective, Pharmaceutical Science and Clinical Pharmacology Advisory Committee Meeting, Rockville, MD.

Rathore, A.S. and Mhatre, R. (2009) *Quality by Design for Biopharmaceuticals*, John Wiley & Sons, Inc., Hoboken, NJ.

Peterson, J. and Kenett, R.S. (2011) Modeling opportunities for statisticians supporting Quality by Design efforts for pharmaceutical development and manufacturing. *Biopharmaceutical Report*, **18**(2), 6–16.

Shmueli, G. (2010) To explain or to predict? *Statistical Science*, **25**(3), 289–310.

Yu, L. (2008) Pharmaceutical Quality by Design: product and process development, understanding, and control. *Pharmaceutical Research*, **25**(4), 781–791.

# Part Two

# STATISTICS IN OUTCOMES ANALYSIS

# 8

# The issue of bias in combined modelling and monitoring of health outcomes

**Olivia A. J. Grigg**
*CHICAS, School of Health and Medicine, Lancaster University, Lancaster, UK*

## Synopsis

The issue of bias in estimation of process parameters is discussed in relation to the combined activities of both modelling health outcomes and monitoring them. There are two motivating examples: six-monthly infection rates of MRSA in a UK NHS (National Health Service) Trust; patient length of stay following cardiac operations in a UK paediatric hospital. The first dataset is univariate in nature. Given a signal of a potential increase in the underlying infection rate, it is described and discussed how one might go about re-estimating the rate of infection and perhaps adjusting it for bias. Although the dataset as it is presented is univariate, some of the ways of correcting for bias that are described involve using external information from peer processes such as neighbouring or similar Trusts. The second dataset has a trivariate outcome measure relating to hospital length of stay, where this measure is assumed to depend on known risk factors. It is described how suspected erroneous data points can bias the signal of the combined chart statistic. Approaches to correcting for the bias caused by such data points are suggested, where these hinge on borrowing strength from information about the known risk factors and on the recent history of the outcome measures. Despite this second dataset presenting itself as seemingly more complex than the first, the extra information available means that bias affecting selected parts of the data can be dealt with more readily.

*Statistical Methods in Healthcare*, First Edition. Edited by Frederick W. Faltin, Ron S. Kenett and Fabrizio Ruggeri.
© 2012 John Wiley & Sons, Ltd. Published 2012 by John Wiley & Sons, Ltd.

# 8.1    Introduction

## 8.1.1    From the industrial setting to the health setting: Forms of bias and the flexibility of control charts

The issue of bias in control charting originated in the industrial setting, where the control chart was first used. Here, the term bias specifically referred to bias in the system or process being monitored. If a production process was somehow out of control, perhaps producing faulty goods or running abnormally, the process would be deemed to be biased from optimal conditions and not working to full capacity in some regard. This bias would ideally be corrected through the use of control charts, where they would be used as a diagnostic tool to hone in on system faults, malfunctions and any relevant anomalies. Once the system fault was isolated and identified, the damaged component could be replaced or the process re-tuned so that normal production and running of the system could resume. Control charts are designed so that they allow for timely intervention in relation to faults that might typically be seen in the process in question. Some systems might be more prone to sudden changes in the process parameter of interest, or gradual changes, and might be prone to increased volatility or variance in the parameter as well as a shift in the mean level. The control chart is a tool, then, that is adaptable to the monitoring problem at hand, whatever its particular facets might be.

Example contexts in the health setting where control charts are applicable, such as monitoring of surgical failures (Spiegelhalter *et al.*, 2003; Lovegrove *et al.*, 1999; DeLeval *et al.*, 1994), infectious disease rates (Grigg, Spiegelhalter and Jones, 2009; Kulldorff, Mostashari and Duczmal, 2007) or mortality rates in general practice (Shipman Inquiry, 2004; Marshall *et al.*, 2004; Aylin *et al.*, 2003) are broadly similar to the industrial processes that control charts were developed for, in that the care being provided may be biased away from best practice or an idealised standard, or there may be a developing epidemic in some infectious disease that leads to infection rates being biased away from normal background levels in a population (Woodall, 2006). However, data arising from health contexts differ dramatically from that seen in industrial applications in that the outcomes are typically markedly heterogeneous in comparison. Whereas an industrial process may be producing thousands of nearly identical loaves of bread, for example, surgical operations will be performed on patients with very different risk profiles; varying, say, in age, sex, weight, diabetes status, general health and, most importantly, severity of how they present with the disease in question. Much of the bias away from the mean parameter is caused sheerly by this patient heterogeneity, and, in order to detect changes of interest within the patient population as a whole, this heterogeneity needs to be modelled and adjusted for in any analysis of the data. This line of reasoning is essentially the theoretical basis for the statistical tools known as risk-adjusted control charts (Grigg and Farewell, 2004; Grigg, 2004; Steiner *et al.*, 2000; Poloniecki, Valencia and Littlejohns, 1998).

Though bias of the system away from idealised behaviour is of predominant interest when using control charts, in this chapter we are concerned mostly with statistical bias and not process bias. The term statistical bias specifically refers to bias that some measure calculated on observed data exhibits away from the true underlying value of the process parameter the data are being used to estimate. In the case of control charts, this bias usually arises from the fact that the chart is stopped whenever the chart statistic is large; that is, whenever the estimate of the process parameter differs significantly from the idealised value of that parameter. As the chart is only stopped at these times, estimates of the process parameter upon signal will necessarily be biased away from the true value. To see this, imagine the set of values collected upon stopping, over time. As the estimated values are always away from the idealised value, whether they reflect the state of the true underlying process or not, this set is a biased set in the sense that it is formed through a biased selection procedure where the domain of the estimated value is somehow restricted. The bias in the selection procedure and restricted domain of estimated values feeds through to the estimation side of monitoring, causing bias in the estimation of the true process parameter. This is the case even if the true process parameter changes dynamically with time – a fairly realistic assumption – though in that case the bias might then potentially be smaller. Obviously the question as to what measure we are considering the bias from is a pertinent one. That features of the measure, such as whether it changes with time, are essentially features of the assumed model for the process means that the question is also one that is inextricably linked to the adopted model and general approach to inference.

Another way that statistical bias can arise is through the inclusion of anomalous data points into estimates for the true underlying process parameter. The estimates are essentially contaminated with data that do not arise from the process of interest, but from some other process not of direct interest for the inference being carried out. The implications of this type of bias being present when monitoring or modelling health data are that making inferences could prove to be somewhat problematic. Data entry errors, for example, may be relatively easy to pick out in data sources if they are quantitatively large. However, small, insidious errors or process deviations may have very subtle effects on parameter estimation. Unfortunately, little can be done in practice about latent contaminations of the data that present only a small amount of physical evidence for the analyst to observe.

## 8.1.2   Specific types of control chart

Suppose we wish to monitor a particular health outcome in a specified population or health facility. There are a number of control charts that can be used, including Shewhart (Shewhart, 1931), cumulative sum (CUSUM) (Page, 1954; Hawkins and Olwell, 1997), exponentially weighted moving average (EWMA) (Roberts, 1959; Lucas and Saccucci, 1990) and variable life-adjusted display (VLAD) (Lovegrove *et al.*, 1997).

For charts such as the Shewhart chart, signals occur based on the extremity, or unusualness, of the most recent observation only. For other charts, such as the EWMA and CUSUM, where past data are taken into account, the occurrence of clusters of extreme events can also cause signals. The Shewhart chart can be adapted to also incorporate past data, by use of runs rules such as those suggested by the Western Electric Company (Western Electric Company, 1956).

Much focus is given here to the EWMA, its multivariate counterpart for multivariate responses, the multivariate EWMA (MEWMA) (Lowry *et al.*, 1992) and a version that allows for heterogeneity in the response, the risk-adjusted EWMA (Grigg and Spiegelhalter, 2007). This latter development of the EWMA is of especial importance in medical contexts, as observations typically vary through the inherent heterogeneity amongst the patient population of interest. All such developments also exist for other charts, notably the CUSUM (Steiner *et al.*, 2000; Pignatiello and Runger, 1990), but since the EWMA provides a direct estimate of the process parameter being monitored, this facilitates consideration of bias in the estimate as its effects would be immediately visible on an interpretable scale. The effects would also be visible on a CUSUM chart for example, but on a less interpretable scale.

The layout of the chapter is as follows: the first example is given in Section 8.2 and the second in Section 8.3; a discussion covering issues from both examples and general points is given in Section 8.4.

## 8.2 Example I: Re-estimating an infection rate following a signal

Consider a scenario where we wish to monitor the incidence of a disease in a population. At any point where a signal occurs on the control chart used, we would most likely want to revise our original estimate of the rate of infection, from which we were monitoring for change, so that the control chart could be recalibrated and monitoring continue anew. The question as to what is the new infection rate is part of the larger question: 'why was there a signal?'

### 8.2.1 Results from a Shewhart and an EWMA chart

Figure 8.1 shows infection rates of Methicillin-resistant *Staphylococcus Aureus* (MRSA) in a UK NHS Trust at six-monthly intervals in the period April 2001 to September 2005 (Department of Health, 2005). The observed rates are the number of blood samples taken that tested positive for MRSA divided by number of bed-days in thousands in a six-monthly interval. The observed rates are shown in black, accompanied by the wider pair of dashed lines, which are 99.8% Shewhart limits.

These Shewhart limits are calculated using the rate across the first four six-monthly intervals as a 'target' rate (central dotted line) and assuming counts follow a Poisson distribution where the denominator is bed-days in thousands. An exponentially weighted moving average (EWMA) of the data is shown in grey, as are the EWMA chart limits (the narrower pair of dashed lines). Specifically, we plot

$$\omega_0 = \mu_0$$
$$\omega_t = \kappa \omega_{t-1} + (1 - \kappa)Y_t, \quad t = 1, 2, \ldots, \quad 0 \le \kappa \le 1 \tag{8.1}$$

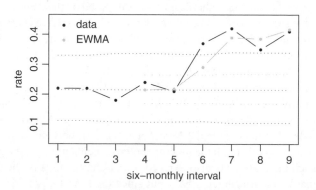

**Figure 8.1**   MRSA rates in a UK NHS Trust. Central dotted line – rate over first four periods; outer lines – transformed 99.8% Poisson limits, given bed-days; inner lines – 95% gamma limits, given bed-days.

where $\mu_0$ is a fixed starting value and $Y_t$ the process observation (or suitable function of) at time $t$. The value of the smoothing parameter, $\kappa$, used here is 0.5. The chart limits are 95% gamma limits centred on the target or null rate $\mu_0$, with precision (or effective number of observations) equal to $(1 - \kappa)^{-1} = 2$ (Grigg and Spiegelhalter, 2007). Note that this is a Bayesian formulation of the EWMA where the smoothing parameter represents prior information about the data; that is, how smoothly its mean changes with time.

In the quality control literature, the state of the process being monitored is often described as either 'in control' or 'out of control' at any one time, and signals indicating that the process has moved away from an in-control state, then, are described as either false or true. In practice, however, it may be difficult to know whether a signal was truly warranted. In Figure 8.1, suppose that we have just observed the signal in interval 6 (October 2003–March 2004). How might we go about re-estimating the true underlying infection rate at this juncture?

## 8.2.2    Results from a CUSUM, and general concerns about bias

Figure 8.2 shows a Poisson CUSUM for the same data, testing for a 20% increase in the rate from the level over the period April 2001–September 2002 (intervals 1–4), and so testing whether a rate of 0.26 is more plausible than a rate of 0.22. There is a signal in period six for this chart also. We might re-estimate the underlying rate following the signal using only the data since the chart was last at zero, since this is where the chart indicates that the process was last 'in control'. For the example, this gives an estimate of 0.37. Alternatively, we could use all the available data up to signal (giving an estimate of 0.24), but may be mixing data from different underlying sources and hence biasing the estimate of the rate from the 'true' source. We might attempt to exclude outlying data points. For instance, if it were decided that the observation in interval six were anomalous for some reason, the estimate would be equal to the original estimate, 0.22. In any case, it remains difficult to determine whether the underlying infection rate has changed, and likewise whether the original estimate was reasonable. In this example, the subsequent data points are consistent with the observed rate upon signal (the rate over the last four periods is 0.39) and the CUSUM continues to accumulate in favour of the alternative hypothesis with respect to the null.

Estimation following an early signal (one before the planned study end) of treatment benefit is of particular interest in the application of sequential clinical trials (Whitehead,

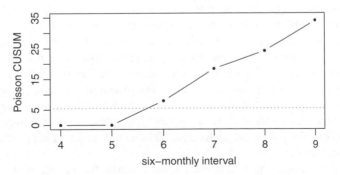

**Figure 8.2**  Poisson CUSUM testing for a 20% increase in MRSA infection rate in a UK NHS Trust from the level in April 2001–September 2002, with boundary set at $h = 5.5$.

1997; Emmerson and Fleming, 1990). A quick decision about whether the apparent benefit is real (that is, whether patients would benefit from future treatment) is desirable, but the estimate of the treatment effect may be biased if based on insufficient data, or a chance run of unlikely data under a null, or negligible effect. To be careful that the estimate of the treatment effect is not overstated, it might be bias-adjusted (Todd, Whitehead and Facey, 1996) or made more conservative according to some prior or external information (Pocock and Hughes, 1989).

### 8.2.3   More about the EWMA as both a chart and an estimator

In contrast to the CUSUM, which accumulates the log-likelihood ratio in favour of one hypothesis over another, the EWMA is a direct (Bayesian here) estimator for the rate (Grigg and Spiegelhalter, 2007). As illustrated in Figure 8.1, it is formed by a weighted average on all past data (in the dataset used), where the data are weighted exponentially according to their contemporaneity.

It appears as though the use of the EWMA or other estimators in a testing scheme provides a way of simultaneously estimating and testing. Charts based on smoothers like the EWMA have inertia (Woodall and Mahmoud, 2005), because they do not give full weight to the most recent observation, and so are robust to outliers, yet at the same time less adaptive to new process conditions. If we are primarily interested in estimating the rate directly after signals of a change in rate, then inertia, combined with the nature of the chart stopping rule, may bias the estimate.

In the event of the EWMA chart signalling, the chart statistic is necessarily larger than the threshold. So, for an endemic disease, EWMA values following signal may be upwardly biased in terms of predicting future typical behaviour of the disease if the signal is caused by an isolated cluster of observations that, in retrospect, is difficult to account for. However, this does not preclude the fact that if the underlying infection rate suddenly increases, the EWMA value just after signal may underestimate the increase. In the example, the EWMA value in period six (0.29), if biased, could be an overestimate of the rate if the true rate is closer to the observed rate over the first four periods (0.22), or an underestimate if it is closer to that over the last four periods (0.39). The type of bias that causes underestimation of the rate following signal might typically be seen in processes where step changes occur periodically; for example, from a baseline rate to an epidemic rate. If bias arises from a mechanism such as this, this gives us some foundation for taking it into account in analysis. Unsystematic sources of bias, conversely, are more difficult to treat.

Though the EWMA value is already smoothed (or, results from an assumption that the underlying true process is smooth), we might wish to adjust it towards the initial target or an external value from peer processes. In that way, the re-estimate of the infection rate would be conservative and protect against subsequent regression to the mean if the true underlying rate were unchanged. However, it may be that after adjustment the value is below the signalling threshold. For example, the EWMA value in period six in the example might be adjusted halfway towards the initial target if there were external information, with weight equal to the observed data, that the rate were unchanged. This would lead to a supported value for the rate, at that point, of 0.25.

If the adjusted value is taken to be the current estimate for the infection rate and is, as in our example, lower than the threshold for a signal (in the example, this is 0.26), we might ask whether we consider that a signal has still occurred. In both cases, inferences on the estimation and testing front would seem to contradict each other, because we either have a signal and an estimate lower than the pre-specified threshold, or do not have a signal but have an estimate higher than the threshold (if adjustment is only carried out given the presence of a signal). A solution would perhaps be to adjust the estimate no further than the threshold, but this would again present as a restriction on the parameter space of the estimate.

## 8.3    Example II: Correcting estimates of length-of-stay measures to protect against bias caused by data entry errors

### 8.3.1    The multivariate EWMA chart

The multivariate exponentially weighted moving average (MEWMA) was developed by Lowry et al. (1992) specifically for processes where the process parameter of interest is vector valued. A natural extension to the univariate procedure described in the previous example, a MEWMA chart plots the multivariate EWMA statistic $\omega_t$ where

$$\omega_0 = \mu_0$$
$$\omega_t = \kappa \omega_{t-1} + (1 - \kappa)Y_t, \quad t = 1, 2, \ldots \tag{8.2}$$

where $\mu_0$ is a vector-valued fixed starting value and $Y_t$ the vector-valued process observation at time $t$. In the example here, for simplicity, a common smoothing parameter $\kappa$ is assumed across the three elements of the MEWMA estimate $\omega_t$ for the trivariate length-of-stay measure. Specifically, a value of $\kappa = 0.7$ is chosen.

The chart is taken to signal when the size of the MEWMA statistic is greater than some positive value, $h$; that is, as soon as $(\omega_t - \mu_0)'\Sigma_\mu^{-1}(\omega_t - \mu_0) > h$, where $\Sigma_\mu$ is the asymptotic posterior covariance matrix for the trivariate process mean $\mu_t$ and satisfies the equation

$$\Sigma_\mu = (1 - \kappa)\Sigma. \tag{8.3}$$

The term $\Sigma$ in (8.3) is the covariance matrix describing the internal correlation structure of the vector-valued observation $Y_t$ at any given time, $t$. The relation (8.3) is the multivariate analogue of that used to specify the posterior variance for the mean for a univariate process (Grigg and Spiegelhalter, 2007). If a classical MEWMA chart (as in Lowry et al., 1992) is implemented, the statistic in (8.3) is multiplied by a factor of $1/(1 + \kappa)$, as it is based on the asymptotic variance of the MEWMA, treating it as a statistic and not as the posterior mean for the process mean, where that is considered to be a random variable as opposed to a determined yet unknown parameter.

Under 'in-control' or null conditions, the test statistic $(\omega_t - \mu_0)'\Sigma_\mu^{-1}(\omega_t - \mu_0)$ follows a $\chi_p^2$ distribution where $p$ is the dimension of the response vector. In this example, $p = 3$. The $\chi^2$ result follows from the fact that, under null conditions, $\mu_0$ is consistent with the posterior distribution for the process mean. The test statistic is the Mahalanobis distance in $p$ dimensions of the null target $\mu_0$ from the posterior distribution for the process mean. The control limit $h$, then, can be set at some upper percentage point of the $\chi_p^2$ distribution, so that signals have a known associated significance.

### 8.3.2    A risk model for length of stay given patient age and weight

In the example data used in this section, the response variable being modelled and monitored over time is a trivariate measure consisting of overall patient length of stay in days, bypass time in hours, and ventilation time following surgery in hours, for children undergoing cardiac operations at a UK paediatric hospital. In the calibration data, a period of approximately nine months here, a regression model can be fitted describing a log-linear relationship between the trivariate response measure and the age in months and weight in kg of the child. The regression model fitted is of the form

$$Y_t = \beta_0(s_t) + \beta_1(s_t)X_{1t} + \beta_2(s_t)X_{2t} + \beta_{12}X_{1t}X_{2t}, \quad t = 1, 2, \ldots, n, \tag{8.4}$$

where $t$ indexes operations in time order; $n$ is the number of operations carried out over the calibration period; $s$ denotes the type of operation, where this can fall into any of three strata; $Y_t$ is the logarithm of the trivariate length-of-stay measure; and $X_1$ and $X_2$ denote the logarithm of the age and weight patient measures, respectively. The vectors $\beta$ are model coefficients estimated when fitting the model. Some elements of the $\beta$ are zero if the model term is not significant or relevant in the part of the model relating to any particular element of the trivariate response. Hence, fitting a linear model of the form (8.4) returns a model whereby there is potentially a non-zero coefficient relating to each of age, weight and their interaction in any of the three parts or layers of the model. Also, in any of the three response layers, the first two of these three coefficients potentially differ depending on the operation type or stratum $s$, so that the fitted slopes for age and weight against each length-of-stay measure may vary with operation type (operation type is related to the severity of a patient's condition). The intercept vector $\beta_0$ may also differ for each operation type. The interaction between age and weight was not found to differ significantly by operation stratum for any of the three elements of the response vector, and hence $\beta_{12}$ is not defined as being dependent on $s$ in (8.4).

### 8.3.3    Risk adjustment

Given the fitted, calibrated model in (8.4) relating length of stay to patient 'risk' factors (i.e. age and weight), an 'in-control' or expected length of stay profile $\mu_{j0}$ can be estimated for various patient types $j = 1, 2, \ldots, J$. To clarify notation, as with the standard EWMA in Section 8.2.1, the zero subscript in the term $\mu_{j0}$ indicates that this is a calibrated, or null value.

The expected risk calculated from the calibration data, $\mu_{j0}$, can be used to adjust the observation vector $Y_t$, giving risk-adjusted observations $Z_t$ that can then be fed into the standard MEWMA; the resulting chart being a risk-adjusted MEWMA. By choosing some baseline patient type, say for which, without loss of generality, the set of (logged) covariate levels takes the mean population value, and calling the estimated in-control risk for that patient type $\mu_0$, a possible risk adjustment can be made by adjusting the outcome at time $t$ for a patient of type $j$, $Y_{jt}$, by $\mu_{j0} - \mu_0$. So, the risk-adjusted data can be denoted $Z_{jt}$, where

$$Z_{jt} = Y_{jt} - \mu_{j0} + \mu_0, \quad j = 1, 2, \ldots, J, \quad t = 1, 2, \ldots \tag{8.5}$$

A heuristic justification for this adjustment is that, under the null hypothesis that the risk for a patient with average covariates is $\mu_0$ given there is a fixed generalised linear model structure to patient risk given covariate levels,

$$g(\mu_j) = g(\mu) + \delta_j, \quad j = 1, 2, \ldots, J, \tag{8.6}$$

where $g(\cdot)$ is the canonical link function, and $\delta_j$ is the difference in risk on the natural scale from the baseline risk, $Z_{jt}$ is an unbiased estimator for $\mu_0$. More formally, the adjustment in (8.5) gives approximately the right likelihood contribution compared to the exact contribution from the full risk model consisting of an exponential family type model for $Y_{jt}$ given $\mu_j$ and a generalised linear model structure as in (8.6) for $\mu_j$ (Grigg and Spiegelhalter, 2007). In this particular example, the (logged) response is assumed to be linear in the covariates so that the function $g(\cdot)$ is the identity, as described by the model structure in (8.4). If this linearity is assumed to extend to Gaussianity of the error about the model, the adjustment in (8.5) would give exactly the right likelihood contribution to the MEWMA as it updates.

Using the risk-adjusted observations $Z_{jt}$, defined by (8.5), a risk-adjusted MEWMA chart monitoring the baseline trivariate process parameter $\mu$ can be described as

$$\begin{aligned} \omega_0 &= \mu_0 \\ \omega_t &= \kappa \omega_{t-1} + (1-\kappa)Z_{jt}, \quad j = 1, 2, \ldots, J, \quad t = 1, 2, \ldots, \quad 0 \le \kappa \le 1. \end{aligned} \tag{8.7}$$

If the estimated in-control risk for a patient of type $j$ is kept at that obtained from the calibration data, $\mu_{j0}$, then the asymptotic posterior covariance matrix for the baseline trivariate process mean $\mu_t$ remains the same as that for the standard MEWMA chart described in (8.2), and again satisfies the relation (8.3). The stopping rule for the risk-adjusted MEWMA is precisely the same as that for the standard MEWMA.

### 8.3.4   Results from a risk-adjusted multivariate EWMA chart

Figures 8.3–8.5 show estimates of each of the three elements of the length-of-stay measure (overall length of stay, bypass time, ventilation time) on the original scale of measurement, where these estimates are adjusted for patient age and weight through the risk model (8.4). In each figure there are three charts, each corresponding to a particular operation type (SAS, VSD, ASD) or stratum. The point estimates through time are given in black and are accompanied by 95% normal limits (given in grey), where the precision is taken to be the reciprocal of the relevant diagonal element in the posterior covariance matrix $\Sigma_\mu$. Figure 8.6 plots the combined chart statistic $(\omega_t - \mu_0)'\Sigma_\mu^{-1}(\omega_t - \mu_0)$, where this measures correlated change from the risk model. The dashed lines in Figure 8.6 mark out upper percentage points of the $\chi_p^2$ distribution.

On the plots relating to the operation type VSD, stratum 2, there are dotted lines displaying an alternative estimate and limits for the underlying process mean where a particular observation has been omitted from the chart. This observation is a suspected data entry error as the ventilation time in the follow-up after surgery is recorded as 1270 hours, corresponding to 53 days of assisted breathing through a ventilator. The overall length of stay for the patient is also exceptionally large at 67 days. Given that this observation may be erroneous, how would we correct the estimate of the underlying process mean for the bias induced? Moreover, what is the effect upon the chart statistic monitoring change from the calibrated risk model?

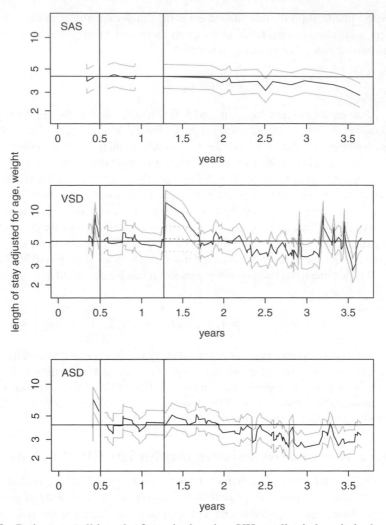

**Figure 8.3**   Patient overall length of stay in days in a UK paediatric hospital where patients undergo cardiac surgery, stratified by operation type (SAS, VSD, ASD). Black – estimate from a risk-adjusted multivariate EWMA with $\kappa = 0.7$; grey – 95% normal limits. Vertical lines demarcate the calibration period of approximately nine months.

### 8.3.5   Correcting for bias in estimation through regression

When the observed value of the response variable is erroneous, or essentially missing, a regression model relating the response to covariates allows the missing response variable to be imputed. By doing this we borrow strength from the covariates, using the structure of the regression to transfer information across to the response variable. In this example, to impute the potentially erroneous data point in both the ventilation time series and the overall length of stay series, the patient age and weight can be plugged into the multivariate regression model (8.4) as follows.

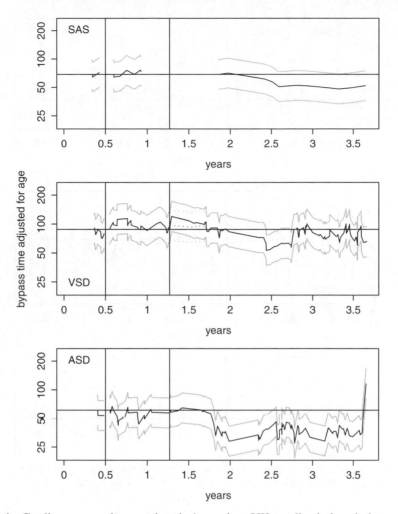

**Figure 8.4** Cardiac surgery bypass time in hours in a UK paediatric hospital, stratified by operation type (SAS, VSD, ASD). Black – estimate from a risk-adjusted multivariate EWMA with $\kappa = 0.7$; grey – 95% normal limits.

The precise risk equation for (logged) ventilation time conditional on patient age in days and weight in kg, and conditional on being in stratum 2 (VSD) is given by

$$Y_t^{(3)} = 3.48 - 0.10X_{1t} - 0.21X_{2t}, \quad t = 1, 2, \ldots, n, \tag{8.8}$$

where $X_{1t}$ is log patient age and $X_{2t}$ is log weight. For (logged) patient overall length of stay, the risk equation conditional on covariates and membership of stratum 2 is given by

$$Y_t^{(1)} = 3.01 - 0.14X_{1t} - 0.80X_{2t} + 0.08X_{1t}X_{2t}, \quad t = 1, 2, \ldots, n. \tag{8.9}$$

Inputting the patient age and weight for the erroneous data point, namely 438 days and 8.1 kg, gives predicted values for the ventilation time and overall length of stay of 12 hours

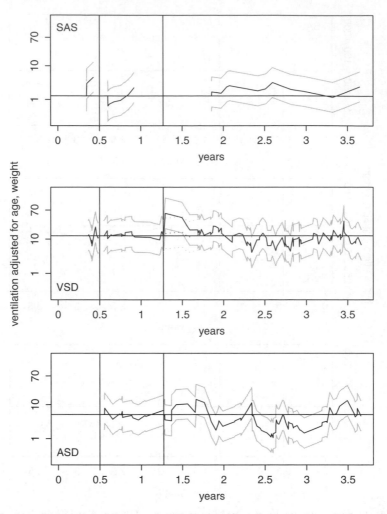

**Figure 8.5** Ventilation time in hours following cardiac operations in a UK paediatric hospital, stratified by operation type (SAS, VSD, ASD). Black – estimate from a risk-adjusted multivariate EWMA with $\kappa = 0.7$; grey – 95% normal limits.

and 5 days respectively. These values differ greatly in magnitude compared to the recorded values. To obtain an estimate of the baseline ventilation time, or baseline overall length of stay from the risk-adjusted EWMA, we can enter the imputed responses as though they were observed. The imputed risk-adjusted response is then equal to the calibrated baseline risk, as it agrees exactly with the risk model, and the predicted baseline measure is simply a weighted mean of the previous EWMA value and the calibrated baseline risk $\mu_0$ with weight $\kappa$. This gives a predicted baseline mean ventilation time of 13.5 hours and mean overall length of stay of 5 days. Here we assume, without loss of generality, that baseline patients are those who have average response, where the baseline is stratified by operation type. Since the models are linear, we would expect baseline patients defined in this way to have covariate values close to the population mean (measured on the log scale).

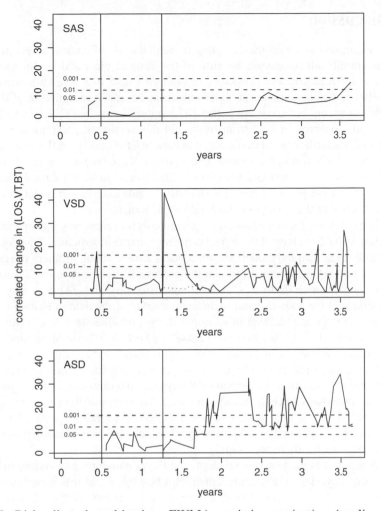

**Figure 8.6** Risk-adjusted multivariate EWMA statistic monitoring baseline trivariate length-of-stay measure (stratified by operation type) in a UK paediatric hospital where patients undergo cardiac surgery. The dashed lines indicate upper percentage points of a $\chi_3^2$ distribution. LOS – overall length of stay; VT – ventilation time; BT – bypass time.

Action following the potential signal caused by the erroneous data point here is more straightforward than that from general signals where the cause is unknown, as described in relation to Example I. There we would need more information from external sources, such as peer processes, to get some idea regarding the magnitude of potential biases, especially that due to signals. If, as in Example II, it is decided that the data point is an anomaly, the estimation of the current process level can essentially be treated as a missing data problem. The EWMA allows us to borrow information from previous observations through smoothing, and this is further helped by also borrowing information through regression from relevant covariates. It is seen then that, although the data here present themselves as more complex than those in Example I, the issues regarding bias and action following signal are not as subtle.

## 8.4   Discussion

Combined estimation and hypothesis testing through the use of control charts may produce results that are difficult to analyse because of the issue of bias, and lead to possible contradictions in inferences made. Hawkins' and Olwell's note that 'even a somewhat biased estimate is better than no estimate at all' is reassuring here, and reminiscent of Box's words 'All models are wrong, but some are useful'. The suggestion is that faith in tangible models should override concerns of bias from truth, and this sentiment gains more weight when the model extends further, across covariates, where 'useful' models help us make practical assertions about large and often complicated systems. There is the danger, though, that as the model increases in complexity with increasing dimension of the data, improvement in strength and predictive power is paid for through a weakening of our understanding of the fundamental nature of the system in clear and simple terms.

In sufficiently complex models, we have a firm basis for recovering misrecorded observations which we would not have if the model were very simple in structure. This does of course rest upon faith in the adopted model, and presents as a more subtle problem if a data point is borderline suspect or has unseen effects on the process. If the response itself is multivariate, we may then be faced with Bellman's 'curse of dimensionality', where biases may affect more than one element of the response and to different extents: if the data in Example I consisted of a multivariate response like that in Example II, the problems associated with diagnosing the signal and adjusting for any biases discussed in Section 8.2 would be magnified many times. Also due to dimensionality, a signal on a multivariate chart is naturally more difficult to diagnose than that on a univariate chart, since the change in response may be in any direction in the multivariate domain of the responses. Only once the direction of the signal has been assessed can we perhaps begin to understand what the causes of the signal might be. Only once equipped with some idea of the cause of a signal can we best approach the problem of estimating the process parameter following signal, taking into consideration possible sources of bias and adjusting for them accordingly.

The EWMA as it is presented here adopts the Bayes paradigm as a framework for inference. Typically, Bayesians are not concerned with bias *per se*, as it is inherently a classical concept that is readily associated with hypothetical repetitions of the observed data: we can envisage some mechanism for bias that systematically affects observations upon (hypothetical) repeat. A Bayesian would, however, be concerned about mixing incompatible data sources in an inappropriate way. In particular, in Bayesian analysis maintaining interpretability of estimates for quantities of interest is paramount. If the estimate does not represent whatever the analyst believes it represents, then results obtained will not match the scientific question asked.

## References

Aylin, P., Best, N., Bottle, A. and Marshall, C. (2003) Following Shipman: a pilot system for monitoring mortality rates in primary care. *Lancet*, **362**(9382), 485–491.

DeLeval, M.R., François, K., Bull, C. *et al*. (1994) Analysis of a cluster of surgical failures. *The Journal of Thoracic and Cardiovascular Surgery*, **104**, 914–924.

Department of Health (2005) MRSA Surveillance Data April 2001–September 2005. www.dh.gov.uk/assetRoot/04/12/79/13/04127913.pdf (accessed December 8, 2006).

Emmerson, S.S. and Fleming, T.R. (1990) Parameter estimation following group sequential hypothesis testing. *Biometrika*, **77**, 875–892.

Grigg, O. and Farewell, V. (2004) An overview of risk-adjusted charts. *Journal of the Royal Statistical Society, Series A*, **167**(3), 523–539.

Grigg, O.A. (2004) Risk-adjusted Monitoring and Smoothing in Medical Contexts. PhD thesis, King's College, Cambridge.

Grigg, O.A. and Spiegelhalter, D.J. (2007) A simple risk-adjusted exponentially weighted moving average. *Journal of the American Statistical Association*, **102**(477), 140–152.

Grigg, O.A., Spiegelhalter, D.J. and Jones, H.E. (2009) Local and marginal control charts for MRSA bacteraemia reports in UK acute NHS Trusts. *Journal of the Royal Statistical Society, Series A*, **172**, 49–66.

Hawkins, D.M. and Olwell, D.H. (1997) *Cumulative Sum Charts and Charting for Quality Improvement*, Springer, New York.

Kulldorff, M., Mostashari, F., Duczmal, L. *et al.* (2007) Multivariate scan statistics for disease surveillance. *Statistics in Medicine*, **26**, 1824–1833.

Lovegrove, J., Sherlaw-Johnson, C., Valencia, O. *et al.* (1999) Monitoring the performance of cardiac surgeons. *Journal of the Operational Research Society*, **50**, 684–689.

Lovegrove, J., Valencia, O., Treasure, T. *et al.* (1997) Monitoring the results of cardiac surgery by variable life-adjusted display. *Lancet*, **350**, 1128–1130.

Lowry, C.A., Woodall, W.H., Champ, C.W. and Rigdon, S.E. (1992) A multivariate exponentially weighted moving average control chart. *Technometrics*, **34**, 46–53.

Lucas, J.M. and Saccucci, M.S. (1990) Exponentially weighted moving average control schemes: properties and enhancements. *Technometrics*, **32**(1), 1–12.

Marshall, C., Best, N., Bottle, A. and Aylin, P. (2004) Statistical issues in the prospective monitoring of health outcomes across multiple units. *Journal of the Royal Statistical Society, Series A*, **167**(3), 541–559.

Page, E.S. (1954) Continuous inspection schemes. *Biometrika*, **41**, 100–115.

Pignatiello, J.J. and Runger, G.C. (1990) Comparisons of multivariate CUSUM charts. *Journal of Quality Technology*, **22**, 173–186.

Pocock, S.J. and Hughes, M.D. (1989) Practical problems in interim analyses, with particular regard to estimation. *Controlled Clinical Trials*, **10**, 209–221.

Poloniecki, J., Valencia, O. and Littlejohns, P. (1998) Cumulative risk adjusted mortality chart for detecting changes in death rate: observational study of heart surgery. *British Medical Journal*, **316**, 1697–1700.

Roberts, S.W. (1959) Control chart tests based on geometric moving averages. *Technometrics*, **1**, 239–250.

Shewhart, W.A. (1931) *Economic Control of Quality of Manufactured Product*, Van Nostrand, New York.

Shipman Inquiry (2004) *Shipman Inquiry Fifth Report – Safeguarding Patients: Lessons from the Past, Proposals for the Future*, HMSO, London. Available from http://www.shipman-inquiry.org.uk/fifthreport.asp.

Spiegelhalter, D.J., Grigg, O.A.J., Kinsman, R. and Treasure, T. (2003) Risk-adjusted sequential probability ratio tests: applications to Bristol, Shipman and adult cardiac surgery. *International Journal for Quality in Health Care*, **15**(1), 7–13.

Steiner, S.H., Cook, R.J., Farewell, V.T. and Treasure, T. (2000) Monitoring surgical performance using risk-adjusted cumulative sum charts. *Biostatistics*, **1**, 441–452.

Todd, S., Whitehead, J. and Facey, K.M. (1996) Point and interval estimation following a sequential clinical trial. *Biometrika*, **83**, 453–461.

Western Electric Company (1956) *Statistical Quality Control Handbook*, Western Electric Corporation, Indianapolis.

Whitehead, J. (1997) *The Design and Analysis of Sequential Clinical Trials*, 3rd edn, Ellis Horwood, Chichester.

Woodall, W.H. (2006) The use of control charts in health-care and public-health surveillance (with discussion). *Journal of Quality Technology*, **38**, 89–134.

Woodall, W.H. and Mahmoud, M.A. (2005) The inertial properties of quality control charts. *Technometrics*, **47**, 425–436.

# 9

# Disease mapping

## Annibale Biggeri[1,2] and Dolores Catelan[1,2]

[1]Department of Statistics 'G. Parenti', University of Florence,
Florence, Italy
[2]Biostatistics Unit, ISPO Cancer Prevention and Research Institute,
Florence, Italy

## Synopsis

This chapter introduces basic issues regarding the production and use of maps in healthcare research. Data sources, design issues and characteristics of spatial data are illustrated. Specific aspects in the production of maps, like pattern or color choices, are presented. The main part of the chapter is dedicated to statistical approaches to mapping. The most popular models are considered in detail. In particular Bayesian hierarchical models and conditional autoregressive models for counts are discussed and prior choices and model checking are reviewed. Specific topics are then addressed, being illustrative of realistic applications in healthcare research. Disease mapping is useful to report in a compact way − a map − the spatial variability of health needs, utilization and outcome. Usually the data are in the form of event counts for administrative areas, and spatial autoregressive models are commonly used. Bayesian approaches proved to be a flexible and powerful way to filter out random variability which can be troublesome when the population size of the areas is small. However posterior inference may be strongly dependent on prior choices when the amount of information in the data is scanty. Bayesian models may have identifiability problems for some parameters which could be of applied interest. These issues are discussed in the chapter and some account of recent literature is given.

*Statistical Methods in Healthcare*, First Edition. Edited by Frederick W. Faltin, Ron S. Kenett and Fabrizio Ruggeri.
© 2012 John Wiley & Sons, Ltd. Published 2012 by John Wiley & Sons, Ltd.

## 9.1    Introduction

The description of the spatial variability of occurrence of health events is commonly used to summarize information on populations health needs.[1] It is useful in planning resource allocation among populations resident within a large region. Maps report, in a single picture, estimates of a given health indicator over space, and they are widely used in lay documents. The increasing power in analyzing geo-referenced data provided by Geographic Information Systems (GIS) results in a large demand for appropriate statistical data analysis (Lawson *et al.*, 2010). The GIS diffusion reflects in a growing utilization of them in decision processes (McLafferty, 2003; Graves, 2008).

In this chapter we briefly introduce basic notions on epidemiologic design and disease tracking, type of spatial data, maps and related issues on visualization and image perception. We then present the main statistical models used to filter out random variability and to analyze and report spatial phenomena, in particular hierarchical Bayesian models which are commonly used in this field. The second part of the chapter is dedicated to special topics of interest in healthcare research.

## 9.2    Epidemiological design issues

Currently, routine data from mortality records, hospital discharge forms, out-patient clinics, specialized care visits and pharmaceutical prescriptions are geo-referenced. Record linkage technology is rapidly evolving and it is expected to efficiently trace patient histories throughout the health system. Confidentiality issues are important but can be managed by *pseudonymization* and related approaches (Pfitzmann and Hansen, 2010). Geomasking methods are also important in spatial analysis, particularly to protect privacy when performing clustering analysis (Hampton *et al.*, 2010). Leaving these issues as solved, as less pertinent here, we stress the difficulties in interpreting the analysis of geo-referenced data when collected without taking into consideration the causal mechanism implied in the phenomenon under study. A mere description of routine data is scarcely informative and can lead to erroneous conclusions.

Mortality statistics provide clues on severe diseases and represent the more important source of information on health needs of a given population. However, misclassification and selection biases may affect such results. The underlying cause of death can be difficult to recognize, and the proportion of ill-defined causes of death must be monitored in any spatial comparison. Notice that we should analyze the proportion of ill-defined deaths and not inspect the rate of ill-defined causes of death. In fact, this is misleading because it depends on the underlying death rate (Mathers, Ma Fat and Inoue, 2005). The assumption of a dynamic stable population may not be fulfilled: the presence of birth cohort effects and population mixing due to migratory flows are important aspects to be considered when interpreting the results (MacMahon and Pugh, 1970).

Morbidity data arise from record linkage of hospital discharge forms. Linking all health records of a given subject may approximate prevalence data or even incidence data for a

---

[1] Here the assumption is that populations are completely defined by the geographical space. It is likely that this assumption will be relaxed as far as connections among individuals are established in a different space (e.g. social networks).

stable population. Indeed, if we can collect data for a long calendar time period, we could discriminate a new health event (e.g. a new diagnosis) from a health contact (e.g. a hospital admission) during the course of a disease for a given subject. Such incidence data are more difficult to obtain and their validity is menaced by several biases (Acheson, 1967; Brameld *et al.*, 2003; Biggeri *et al.*, 2006; Wiréhn, Karlsson and Carstensen, 2007) Some examples are in Short, Carlin and Bushhouse (2002).

Health utilization data (e.g. hospital discharge forms, out-patient clinics, specialized care visits) are sometimes erroneously used as proxy of morbidity data. They quantify the volume of healthcare provided to the population. Spatial analysis of these data is useful to study appropriateness of resource allocation in a given region or country. The reader should remember that equity analysis can be worthwhile: for example a uniform spatial resource allocation can be very unfair if the health need differs greatly among areas (Kjellstrom, 2008; Mackenbach *et al.*, 2008). Population mobility for health reasons is also important, and attraction models were used to study hospitals' location or to plan their re-location (Bailey and Gatrell, 1995; Lowe and Sen, 1996; Congdon, 2001, 2010; Dreassi and Biggeri, 2003).

Health consumption data (e.g. prescriptions) are the results of a trade-off between needs and supply. The analysis may help to detect areas of inappropriateness, wasting of resources and surrogacy. It addresses the evaluation of inefficiencies in the health system and the identification of areas requiring specific interventions (Oleske, 2009; Jatrana, Crampton and Norris, 2011).

Time-course data are important to monitor the health process also in terms of efficacy and equity (for example when analyzing specific health outcomes). Within-hospital mortality or mortality in the short-term period after a hospital discharge may highlight inappropriateness of care for given diseases like myocardial infarction or femur fracture. The efficacy of a given treatment may vary by socio-demographic characteristics of the patient. Again, mapping these statistics will show phenomena of population segregation and marginalization (MacNab, 2003; MacNab *et al.*, 2006; Agabiti *et al.*, 2011).

In conclusion, the definition of the health event to be studied depends on the purpose of the analysis, varying from etiology (health needs) to performance indicators (health utilization) or efficacy indicators (health outcomes). For each of them a specific causal mechanism is implied (Dowd, 2010). For mortality data, the assumption of a dynamic stable population is required to study the geographical variability of risk of death. In fact there is a long latency time period between exposure to the etiologic agent(s), occurrence of the disease and subsequent death. If we use the residence at death – as usual in routine geo-referenced mortality records – we may strongly misclassify our data, depending on the extent of migration and population mixing. Health needs are the effect of phenomena acting over a long period; we cannot modify the natural history of the disease in a short time-span. On the contrary, healthcare utilization and healthcare services offered are subject to rapid changes, and decision makers and health managers may efficiently interfere in the process.

## 9.3   Disease tracking

The identification of disease cases occurring in large populations is the aim of epidemiological surveillance. In the case of infectious diseases, the short latency and the biological characteristics of the pathological agents require an epidemiological investigation on the incident cases and their contacts. Space, time or space-time analyses are used to detect disease outbreaks and epidemics (see for example the journal *Spatial and Spatio-temporal Epidemiology*). Syndromic surveillance aims to screen huge amounts of routine health data to detect unusual patterns to be further investigated (May, Chretien and Pavlin, 2009; Shmueli and Burkom, 2010). Such a data-mining approach has to be considered with caution since several biases (misclassification and selection) may affect the data. Routine data are recorded for administrative purposes, and the quality and completeness of the information on the disease may be poor. Disease cases may not be recorded in a routine data archive because of under diagnosis, or because private healthcare is not covered by the health information system, or because of elusiveness of the case population (for example in the case of drug addiction or some infectious diseases more prevalent among illegally immigrated people) (Sweeting *et al.*, 2009).

## 9.4   Spatial data

Spatial data arise from two distinct stochastic mechanisms: a continuous process in the plane, which can be measured at fixed sampling point locations, and a discrete point process, in which the measure locations are themselves part of the process (Banerjee, Carlin and Gelfand, 2004). Sometimes the data are aggregate summaries by area, on a predefined regular grid or irregular administrative partition of the region of interest. Areal data can be generated by the researcher from point-referenced data or they can be only available in such form. Particular care should be taken in interpreting results from areal data because of the size of the areas. If the areas are too large the phenomenon under study may be diluted; while if they are too narrow additional noise may be introduced (Lawson *et al.*, 1999; Elliott *et al.*, 2000). The spatial pattern can be evident at one given scale of aggregation but not at others – the so-called *modifiable area unit* problem (Gehlke and Biehl, 1934; Openshaw, 1984).[2]

Again we want to stress the causal data-generating mechanism, which characterizes each particular field of application and that can help in clarifying the appropriate scale to be chosen. Using individual geo-referenced data may have paradoxical results, introducing additional sources of variability and misclassification, while aggregate data on an appropriate scale may have balanced a Berksonian measurement error (Diggle and Elliott, 1995; Zeger, Thomas and Dominici, 2000).

## 9.5   Maps

Graphical objects are vulnerable to subjective interpretation, which is influenced by psychological factors. Since graphical objects convey several points of information in only one picture, we cannot properly control what aspect receives more attention by the reader, and misunderstandings are common (Walter, 1993; Lawson and Williams, 2001).[3]

Tom Koch (2011, 2012) acutely noted that 'Maps are the workbench on which ideas are fashioned in a manner that permits them to be argued and, often, tested... A map is not a representation of work that has been completed but the presentation of *arguments* about the

---

[2]Zhu and Carlin (2000) addressed the analysis of areal data which are spatially misaligned; that is, involving variables (typically counts or rates) which are aggregated over differing sets of regional boundaries.

[3]*How to Lie with Statistics* has a chapter dedicated to graphs (Huff, 1991).

relationships between things' [italics used by us]. There is subjectivity also in the creator of the map.

From a purely statistical point of view Gelman and Price (1999) were also very skeptical of maps. They show why 'all maps of parameter estimates are misleading', when reporting rates or statistical significance but also when reporting parameter estimates from hierarchical models. Rates or maximum likelihood estimates tend to have extreme values (highest or lowest) for the less populated areas; that is the more imprecise estimates dominate the map. Plotting statistical significance produces the opposite effect: large areas tend to be statistically significantly different from average even if their rates are only slightly different, because of large sample size. These problems are only partially solved by smoothing estimators; in fact areas with imprecise estimates are subjected to strong smoothing, a situation in which absence of information on the risk of a given area is confused with evidence on absence of divergent risk from the average.

In the following we restrict our attention to statistical modeling of areal data. A map is the simplest way to report the results of a statistical analysis of areal data. Estimates are produced for each area and the graphical representation needs scale and palette to be defined.

The adoption of a relative scale with respect to an absolute scale has to be considered with caution. In fact a relative scale reports the order statistics and therefore is measurement free. It masks the magnitude of the observed variability, and a given spatial pattern shown in the map can be either important or irrelevant on a subject-specific basis. We want to underline the importance of using a measurement scale and a parameterization that is relevant to the field of application and the subject-specific model of the phenomenon under study.

Maps are usually reported in grey or one-color scale, using different degrees of brightness or saturation. However sometimes multicolor scales are used. This is dangerous because the perception of colors is on a circular scale and it is not immediately obvious which hue you associate to a high/low level in the scale. See Figure 9.1 (color version available at the book companion website www.wiley.com/go/statistical_methods_healthcare) the hue-brightness circle. The hue circle is based on opponent colors which are called *psychological primaries* because of the way we experience color. Therefore the opposing colors on the hue circle are experienced as having nothing in common. The radii in

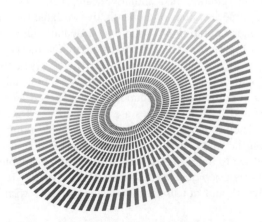

**Figure 9.1** The hue-brightness circle. Each angle shows a hue (opponent colors are red–green and yellow–blue). The radii show varying brightness for fixed hue.

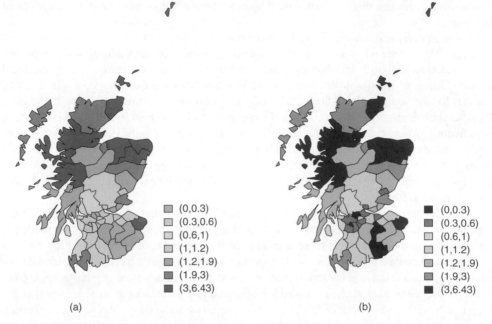

**Figure 9.2** Which colors to use for the map? Standardized mortality ratio, lip cancer, Scotland (Clayton and Kaldor, 1987). (a) color map not understandable for a red-green colorblind person; (b) map using a more appropriate color palette.

the figure are obtained varying the relative brightness (which measures the perceived intensity of a color compared to the maximum possible for a color of the same hue and saturation). A third dimension can be considered the relative saturation (which measures the perceived purity of color compared to the maximum possible) (Briggs, 2007). The solution in disease-mapping exercises is therefore to use only two of the three basic colors (red–green–blue), and never use white – which is not a color (Smans and Esteve, 1992). Once having selected a color palette, different degrees of brightness or saturation can be used. Remember that colors (hues) are not perceived in a continuum quantitative scale, even if they are opponent: therefore be careful to associate numeric values of a quantitative variable to different colors. Varying the degree of brightness or saturation is a solution, particularly simple if we fix hue (i.e. we move along a radius in Figure 9.1 [color version available at the book companion website `www.wiley.com/go/statistical_methods_healthcare`]). Two further observations are necessary with regard to this point. First, we should take care of people who have colorblindness, a condition more common then supposed (for example in the USA around 7.0% of males and 0.4% of females are affected by red-green colorblindness, the most common form). Therefore we should never use a scale ranging from green to red, which are perceived on the same degree of grey by colorblind subjects. A better choice is a scale from yellow/brown to blue (Figure 9.2 [color version available at the book companion website `www.wiley.com/go/statistical_methods_healthcare`]) (Pickle *et al.*, 1999).[4] Last, we should not use a three-category scale with white for the central

---

[4] Remember always to specify in words if the map is in grey tones or color. Colorblind people cannot know this by looking at the map.

category: this resembles the traditional, but inappropriate, way to classify results by statistical significance.

## 9.6   Statistical models

We will start by showing how aggregate (areal) data can be generated from discrete point-process data. We then address statistical modeling of areal data. In doing so, we will consider, briefly, geostatistical models. These are appropriate for point-referenced data but may be useful to overcome some difficulties with areal data. We will not cover statistical modeling and analysis of point process data (Diggle, 2000).

Binomial or Poisson models are usually assumed for areal data. Without loss of generality we assume the observed health event count $Y_i$ for the $i$th area follows a Poisson law with parameter given by $\theta_i \times D_i$, the risk parameter times a population denominator. Often a dimension reduction is achieved collapsing over strata of a confounder (e.g. age) by direct or indirect standardization. When using indirect standardization, an internal set of reference rates is recommended to by-pass the comparability problem (Breslow and Day, 1987; Armstrong, 1995; and Ocaña-Riola, 2010 for a discussion of potential errors in disease mapping). When space-time models are considered, the relevant time axis for the phenomenon under study should be discussed; for example, in analyzing mortality, the birth-cohort time axis may be more important then calendar time (MacMahon and Pugh, 1970; Lilienfeld, Stolley and Lilienfeld, 1994).

The Poisson model arises as follows. Denote R the study region, A an area within R, $x$ a vector of generic coordinates (e.g. latitude and longitude) of a case location in R. The spatial distribution of a set of points at locations $\{x_i; \ i-1, \ldots, n\}$ in R is the realization of a two-dimensional point process, which can be described using a counting measure $\phi$ on R; $\phi(A)$ denotes the number of case events in A (Cox and Isham, 1980). The first- and second-order intensity functions are:

$$\lambda(x) = \lim_{|dx|\to 0} \left\{ \frac{E[\phi(dx)]}{|dx|} \right\}$$

$$\lambda_2(x, y) = \lim_{|dx|\,|dy|\to 0} \left\{ \frac{E[\varphi(dx)\,\varphi(dy)]}{|dx|\,|dy|} \right\}$$

in given infinitesimal areas $dx$ and $dy$ in R ($|A|$ being the area of A). Stationarity implies invariance under translation ($\lambda(x) = \lambda$ and $\lambda_2(x, y) = \lambda_2(x - y)$); isotropy implies invariance under rotation ($\lambda_2(x, y) = \lambda_2(\|x - y\|)$) (Diggle, 1983). The simple homogeneous Poisson point process assumes the probability of two points occurring at the same location $x$ to be negligible, and the counts of points on two disjoint areas $A_1$ and $A_2$ to be independent. Then:

$$\lambda(x) = \lim_{|dx|\to 0} \left\{ \frac{E[\phi(dx)]}{|dx|} \right\} = \lim_{|dx|\to 0} \left\{ \frac{Pr[\phi(dx) = 1]}{|dx|} \right\}$$

$$\lambda_2(x, y) = \lim_{|dx||dy|\to 0} \left\{ \frac{E[\phi(dx)\phi(dy)]}{|dx||dy|} \right\} = \lim_{|dx||dy|\to 0} \left\{ \frac{E[\phi(dx)]\,E[\phi(dy)]}{|dx||dy|} \right\} = \lambda^2.$$

The case event count (i.e. the number of points) in a given area follows a Poisson law with expected value $\int_A \lambda(u)du$, $(\lambda|A|$ under stationarity).

However this is not the most common situation because the case intensity depends on the population intensity which is not uniform in space.

The inhomogeneous Poisson process can be derived considering that the intensity of the population at location $x$ again follows the Poisson assumptions:

$$\lambda_P(x) \cong \frac{\Pr[\varphi_P(dx) = 1]}{|dx|}.$$

A case of disease can be observed, at a given time at location $x$, only if the person was healthy and present at the same location an instant before she got ill. Let $\mu(x)$ denote the probability of being a case for a subject resident at $x$. Then, the spatial point process that generates disease cases is again a Poisson process but with intensity function $\lambda_{CS}(x) = \mu(x)\lambda_P(x)$ (Diggle, 1983; Cressie, 1991). Notice that the intensity of the case disease process factorizes into two terms: the first is the probability function of having the disease being at $x$, and the second is the number at risk at $x$. The expected number of cases in area A is:

$$E[\varphi_{CS}(A)] = \int_A \mu(u)\lambda_P(u)du.$$

Areal data come from aggregating counts. The underlying stochastic mechanism is an inhomogeneous Poisson process, but information on case/population locations is lost. The total amount of person-area at risk is known for each area, and usually this is largely variable. Remember that in the present context, disease mapping is useful at fine spatial resolution. The aggregate areal data are small areas which suffer from substantial variability in population size. As a consequence extreme rates or relative risks are observed in areas with small population size; for example it can be possible to have zero or one observed case event in such small areas, corresponding to an estimate of zero or a value much larger than the average risk parameter. Using a p-value metric does not help here because only areas with large population size may achieve sufficient power to be detected; a picture not consistent with the observed data or the maximum likelihood estimates (Figure 9.3).

Several statistical approaches have been proposed to 'stabilize' such (relative) risk estimates. Shrinkage estimators are currently applied (Lawson et al., 1999; Elliott et al., 2000; and the special issue of *Statistical Methods in Medical Research* 14, 2005). In healthcare research, exploratory nonparametric approaches are proposed by MacNab and Gustafson (2007) and Silva *et al.* (2008). These authors used hierarchical Bayesian representations of regression splines to smooth spatially or spatiotemporal correlated data in disease mapping of healthcare indicators.

## 9.7    Hierarchical models for disease mapping

We describe the two most common Bayesian hierarchical models used to smooth risk estimates in disease mapping: the Poisson-Gamma model (hereafter denoted as PG model; Clayton and Kaldor, 1987), and the Besag–York–Mollié (BYM) model (Besag *et al.*, 1991).

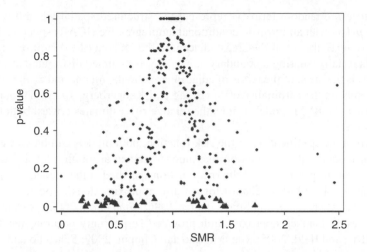

**Figure 9.3** Lung cancer at municipality level: males, Tuscany, 1995–1999. Volcano plot: standardized mortality ratios (SMR: $y$-axis) vs. p-values ($x$-axis). Triangles: areas with p-value $\leq 0.05$.

The likelihood for the disease counts $Y_i$ is assumed to be Poisson with parameters $\theta_i \times D_i$, where $D_i$ is a function of population denominators for the $i$th area and $\theta_i$ is the (relative) risk parameter (RR).

The maximum likelihood estimator of $\theta_i$ is $\hat{\theta}_i = Y_i/D_i$. When the denominator comes from indirect age-standardization, this estimator is the ratio between the observed and expected number of cases in the $i$th area, the well-known standardized mortality ratio (SMR) when we have death counts. The precision (inverse of the variance) of the RR estimate is proportional to $D_i$ since the variance of RR is $1/D_i$. The precision is lower in the small areas with a low number of expected counts ($D_i$) and less information for the estimation of the risk.

Bayesian inference requires the specification of appropriate prior distributions on model parameters ($\theta_i$) and hyperparameters. Clayton and Kaldor (1987) assumed a conjugate Gamma($k,\nu$) prior distribution for $\theta_i$.

The posterior for the relative risk parameter $\theta_i$ is still Gamma($k + D_i$, $\nu + Y_i$) with posterior mean $(\nu + Y_i)/(k + D_i)$. It is easy to show that it is a weighted average between the maximum likelihood estimate and the prior mean. In this model, Poisson random variability is filtered out and relative risk estimates are shrunken toward the general mean (see Wakefield (2007) for a discussion and a slightly different parameterization of the Gamma prior).

Empirical Bayes and full Bayes methods have been proposed for the estimation of the relative risks $\{\theta_i\}$. The empirical Bayes approach uses the method of moment or the marginal Negative Binomial distribution to estimate the prior parameters $k$ and $\nu$ from the same data. Full Bayesian inference requires one to specify a distribution for the hyperparameters $k$ and $\nu$, for example assuming them to be exponentially distributed.

Besag, York and Mollié (1991) specified a random-effect loglinear model for the relative risk: $\log(\theta_i) = u_i + v_i$. The *heterogeneity* random terms $u_i$ represent an unstructured spatial variability component assumed *a priori* distributed as Normal $(0, \tau_u)$, where $\tau_u$ is the precision parameter, modeled as Gamma.

The *clustering* random terms $v_i$ represent the structured spatial variability component, assumed *a priori* with an intrinsic conditional autoregressive (ICAR) specification. In other words, denoting $S_i$ the set of the areas adjacent to the $i$th area (the definition of adjacent for two areas is usually 'sharing a boundary'), $v_i|v_j \in S_i$ is assumed distributed as Normal($\bar{v}_i$, $\tau_v$ $n_i$), where $\bar{v}_i$ is the mean of the terms of adjacent areas to the $i$th one and $\tau_v\, n_i$ is the precision, which depends on the cardinality of $S_i$ (Besag and Kooperberg, 1995). Through these two random terms, the BYM model shrinks the relative risk estimates toward both the local and the general mean.

Apart from the specification of the risk function, both models can be viewed as bi-level hierarchical models with the Poisson likelihood specified at the first level and the *a priori* distributions for the parameters of the risk function specified at the second.

Computationally, Markov chain Monte Carlo approximations to posterior distributions are used (Gilks, Richardson and Spiegelhalter, 1996; Lunn *et al.*, 2000). Recently, a doubly-integrated nested Laplace approximation provided surprisingly accurate results in spatial problems (Rue and Held, 2005; Rue, Martino and Chopin, 2009; Schrödle and Held, 2011).

### 9.7.1   How to choose priors in disease mapping?

The choice of hyperpriors and related parameters for PG and BYM models was discussed, among others, in Bernardinelli, Clayton and Montomoli (1995) and Wakefield (2007). In any case it is recommended to report at least two maps: the crude map of maximum likelihood estimates and the map of the smoothed estimates (Figure 9.4).

In the hierarchical model, the adoption of hyperpriors with large variances for precision parameters may be inappropriate because the resulting *a priori* probability of large parameter

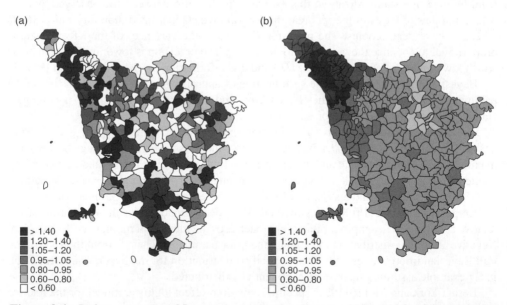

(a)    (b)

> 1.40
1.20–1.40
1.05–1.20
0.95–1.05
0.80–0.95
0.60–0.80
< 0.60

**Figure 9.4**   Is there a true map? Larynx cancer, males, Tuscany 2001–2006. (a) Standardized mortality ratio (SMR); (b) smoothed Bayesian relative risk from the BYM model (see text). Absolute scale.

values may not be negligible. A more informative approach is recommended. For example the range of plausible relative risks for a given disease among areas in a given region and calendar time period can be easily elicited from experts. Then priors can be re-parameterized as follows. Let us consider the non-spatial PG model. We can specify informative Gamma priors by fixing the *a priori* RR ratio $\theta_{(1-\alpha/2)}/\theta_{(\alpha/2)} = K$, where $\theta_{(.)}$ are the centiles of the Gamma prior. Suitable choices may be $1.8 - 1.4 - 1.2$, corresponding to 90% centile ranges of $0.7$–$1.3$; $0.8$–$1.2$; $0.9$–$1.1$. A more sophisticated strategy would be to model the prior parameters by appropriate hyperpriors. This is facilitated under a Poisson-lognormal model, where we specify a prior for the precision parameter. Let us assume a loglinear random-effects model for the relative risk $\log(\theta_i) = \beta_0 + u_i$, with $u_i$ distributed as Normal with zero mean and a precision parameter $\tau_u$. Then, letting $\sigma = \tau_u^{-2}$, the *a priori* log RR ratio is log $[\theta_{(1-\alpha/2)}/\theta_{(\alpha/2)}] = 2 z_{1-\alpha/2} \times \sigma$. For example, for a ratio of 2 and 90% probability level we obtain $\sigma = 0.2$. Bernardinelli, Clayton and Montomoli (1995) proposed a series of chi-square distributions for $\tau_u = \sigma^{-2}$ with different scale and degrees-of-freedom parameters. Wakefield (2007) calibrated the hyperprior parameters for the $\tau_u$ density using the marginal distribution of RR, which is a Student's $t$-distribution with $2a$ degrees of freedom under a Gamma($a,b$) density for $\tau_u$. Therefore, fixing on the marginal distribution $\log[\theta_{1-\alpha/2}/\theta_{\alpha/2}] = 2t(2a)_{1-\alpha/2} \times \sqrt{b/a}$, and specifying a Student's $t$ with 2 (or 4) degrees of freedom, a ratio of 2 and 90% probability, we obtained $b = 0.014$ (or $0.026$) and a prior Gamma($1,0.014$ (or $0.026$)) for $\tau_u$.

For the spatial random components, the difficulty lies in the interpretation of the precision parameter of the ICAR prior. In fact it refers to the conditional distribution. Bernardinelli, Clayton and Montomoli (1995) explored the relationship between the conditional parameter and the marginal variability of the random terms. This depends on the adjacency structure of the map. An average marginal variance is derived as a function of the conditional variance parameter and a constant, $c$. A prior is then specified according to:

$$\frac{\theta_{(1-\alpha/2)}}{\theta_{(\alpha/2)}} = \exp\left(2z_{1-\alpha/2}\sqrt{\sigma_u^2 + c\sigma_v^2}\right),$$

as before assuming chi-square priors for the precision parameters. Wakefield (2007) calibrated the prior parameters for the total precision $\tau_T = \left(\sigma_u^2 + c'\sigma_v^2\right)^{-1}$ assuming a marginal Student's $t$-distribution. The total precision is then split into the two components specifying a model for the proportion of the total RR variability that is attributable to the spatial component. A prior Gamma($1,b$) for $\tau_T$ and a Beta($c,d$) for the proportion of spatial variability is then specified.

Both approaches are approximate; the constant expressing the adjacency structure is different.

It is important also to note that informative priors are necessary with sparse data, and in practical applications a sensitivity analysis specifying a wide range of prior choices should be addressed and discussed. A graphical approach exploring the degree of conflict between prior and likelihood has been proposed (Scheel, Green and Rougier, 2011).

## 9.7.2    More on the BYM model and the clustering term

The BYM model described so far has several aspects which must be discussed: (1) the conditional autoregressive model leads to a singular precision matrix in the joint distribution, even if this is not a problem since the posterior is proper; (2) only the sum of the two random terms is strictly identifiable, and the random terms are constrained to sum to zero to allow identifiable intercept.

*(1)* Let us concentrate on the clustering random components, the set of area-specific spatially structured random effects $v = (v_1, \ldots, v_n)'$. Their joint distribution may be expressed as $v \sim \text{MVN}(\mu, \sigma^2_v \Sigma)$, where MVN denotes Multivariate Normal distribution, $\mu$ is the mean vector, $\sigma^2_v > 0$ controls the overall variability of the $v_i$ and $\Sigma$ is an $n \times n$ positive definite matrix. Different specifications are possible for $\Sigma$.

A convenient *parametric* form for the elements of the matrix $\Sigma$ is the exponential one, in which $\Sigma_{ij} = \exp[-(\varphi \, d_{ij})^\xi]$ where $d_{ij}$ is the distance between the centroids of areas $i$ and $j$, $\varphi > 0$ controls the rate of decline of correlation by distance and $\xi \in (0, 2]$ controls the amount of spatial smoothing (Diggle, Tawn and Moyeed, 1998). This specification comes from Geostatistics, where the covariance matrix is a function of the distance between pairs of points. Strictly speaking this specification seems inappropriate for areal data such as disease counts, which are generated by a discrete point process. However it is a mathematically convenient parametric form of the correlation between area counts (see Cook and Pocock, 1983; a similar approach was developed by Kelsall and Wakefield, 2002).

The nonparametric (usually called *conditional*) form consists in specifying the between-area covariance matrix as $\sigma^2_v \Sigma = \sigma^2_v (I - \rho W)^{-1} M$ where $I$ is the identity matrix, $W$ is a weight matrix with elements $W_{ij}$ reflecting the spatial association between areas $i$ and $j$, $M$ is a diagonal matrix with elements $M_{ii}$ proportional to the conditional variance of $v_i | v_j \in S_i$ and $\rho$ controls the amount of spatial dependence.

In the formulation of Besag (1974), we do not need to specify the elements of the co-variance matrix $\Sigma$ but work just on $W$, $M$ and $\rho$. Let $n_i$ be the number of adjacent areas to the $i$th, and denote by $j \in S_i$ that areas $i$ and $j$ are adjacent (i.e. share part of the boundary, $S_i$ being the set of adjacencies as before). The ICAR model used in disease mapping (Besag et al., 1991) corresponds to choosing $W_{ij} = 1/n_i$ if $j \in S_i$ and 0 otherwise; $M_{ii} = 1/n_i$ and $\rho = 1$. These assumptions lead to the normal conditional distribution for the spatially struc-tured terms with mean given by the average of adjacent terms. As said before, the resulting ICAR model has $\Sigma$ not positive definite.

When the parameter $\rho$ is not constrained to be equal to 1 (Cressie and Chan (1989); see also Cressie (1993) with an example on health service research), then the variance–covariance matrix is positive definite if $\rho \in (\rho_{min}, \rho_{max})$, where $\rho_{min} < 0$ and $\rho_{max} = 1$ are the smallest and largest eigenvalues of matrix $W$. As we said, $\rho$ controls the strength of spatial dependence. This model is denoted as proper CAR (conditional autoregressive).

Stern and Cressie (1999) defined $M_{ii} = 1/D_i$, $W_{ij} = (D_j/D_i)^{1/2}$, where $D_i$ is the expected number of cases under indirect standardization in the $i$th area. A suitable prior distribution for $\rho$ may be uniform in $(\rho_{min}, \rho_{max})$.

Latouche *et al.* (2007) and Catelan, Biggeri and Lagazio (2009) noted that spatially structured variability in the model fitted to the data may bias the estimation of the ecological association between covariates and relative risks toward the null. Catelan, Biggeri and Lagazio (2009) discussed the role of proper vs. improper CAR specification and the sensitivity to spatial concurvity of the ICAR model (see Table 9.1). Reich, Hodges and Zadnik (2006) explored the effect of spatial concurvity between covariates and the underlying CAR random effects. Their approach is directed to detect influential observations and to provide a restricted model in which some CAR random terms are removed.

To overcome such difficulties, there are other alternatives in the literature.

**Table 9.1**  Ecological regression analysis of the association between material deprivation and mortality for lung cancer in Tuscany in different calendar time periods. We report the regression coefficients (95% credible interval) under different specifications of the clustering component: improper conditional autoregressive ICAR, proper CAR specification (Stern and Cressie, 1999), parametric geostatistical model.

| Time period | ICAR | Proper CAR | Geostatistical model |
| --- | --- | --- | --- |
| 1971–1974 | −0.17 (−0.22, −0.13) | 0.18 (0.13, 0.24) | 0.19 (0.14, 0.25) |
| 1975–1979 | −0.15 (−0.19, −0.11) | 0.13 (0.09, 0.18) | 0.15 (0.10, 0.20) |
| 1980–1984 | −0.08 (−0.11, −0.50) | 0.10 (0.06, 0.14) | 0.13 (0.08, 0.17) |
| 1985–1989 | −0.07 (−0.11, −0.03) | 0.05 (0.01, 0.05) | 0.07 (0.04, 0.11) |
| 1990–1994 | −0.08 (−0.13, −0.03) | 0.03 (0.00, 0.07) | 0.06 (0.03, 0.09) |
| 1995–1999 | −0.04 (−0.10, 0.01) | 0.07 (0.04, 0.11) | 0.09 (0.06, 0.12) |

Our elaboration from Catelan, Biggeri and Lagazio (2009). Details of the models and other alternatives for the clustering component can be found there.

This example underlines that, in the presence of strong association between the covariate spatial pattern and the clustering random effects, estimates of the ecological regression coefficient can be very unstable – we can even observe a change in sign of the association. The ICAR model assumes a strong spatial interaction; the parameter $\rho$ is set to its maximum value of 1.

Giudici, Knorr-Held and Rasser (2000), and Denison and Holmes (2001), proposed spatial partition models. Such models aim to detect clusters of areas at different risk (see also Gangnon and Clayton, 2003). Several extensions to these approaches appeared; a recent one was proposed by Hegarty and Barry (2008). They used a product partition model (PPM) in which they assume that the true relative risks can be partitioned into a number of components or sets of areas where the relative risks are equal.

Kottas, Duan and Gelfand (2008) proposed Bayesian nonparametric spatial modeling approaches to disease mapping. Their formulation is based on spatial random effects modeled via a Dirichlet process prior. The novelty lies in the Dirichlet process being centered around a multivariate normal distribution with a parametric spatial covariance function (see also the review in Best, Richardson and Thomson (2005) and the related special issue 14 of *Statistical Methods in Medical Research*, 2005).

*(2)* The identifiability issue between the two random terms in the BYM model is also related to the assessment of the relative role of the global or local rates.

Leroux, Lei and Breslow (1999) proposed to specify a Spatial Gaussian Random Field as (a model later also used in health service research by MacNab, 2003):

$$\log \theta_i = a + b_i$$
$$b_i \propto \mathrm{MVG}\left(0, \Sigma(\omega, \sigma^2)\right)$$
$$\Sigma(\omega, \sigma^2) = \sigma^2 D^{-1}$$
$$D = \omega W + (1 - \omega) \times I,$$

which is a weighted function of the matrix $W$ (the neighborhood matrix in the CAR formulation) and the identity matrix $I$ (see also Assunção and Krainski, 2009). In this model only one set of random terms is considered, their joint multivariate distribution is specified with

**Table 9.2**    Heterogeneity/clustering ratio and spatial pattern of disease.

|  | Heterogeneity | Clustering | Ratio |
| --- | --- | --- | --- |
| Lung cancer, male | 0.28 | 0.04 | 7 : 1 |
| Lung cancer, female | 0.04 | 0.26 | 1 : 6.5 |
| Breast cancer | 0.10 | 0.10 | 1 : 1 |

Standard deviation of the posterior distributions of the clustering and heterogeneity random terms. Lung cancer in male and female, and breast cancer, Emilia Romagna region, 1982–1988 (modified from Biggeri *et al.*, 2000).

a variance–covariance matrix which is a function of the weighted sum of spatially and not spatially structured components. The identifiability of the $u_i$ and $v_i$ terms is resolved.

Eberly and Carlin (2000) discussed in detail the identifiability in the context of the spatial models used in disease mapping. The BYM model is overparametrized, being larger than the data support, indeed for each area only one observation is used for the identification of the two random terms, heterogeneity and spatial clustering. As highlighted also by Wakefield (2007), only their sum is well identified. Of course, identifiability is a non-issue for Bayesian analyses, since given proper prior distributions the corresponding posteriors must be proper as well; hence every parameter can be well estimated. But this opens the question about the choice of the prior distributions (see the paragraph on prior choice, above).

Some authors (for example Biggeri *et al.*, 2000) used descriptively the estimated marginal standard deviation of the two random effects. Their posterior ratio may suggest if most of the excess variation is attributable to spatial clustering, or to unstructured heterogeneity (Wakefield, 2007). For modeling, the interest in the trade-off between these two sources of variability (unstructured vs. spatially structured) demands proper yet vague priors (Table 9.2 and Figure 9.5). Eberly and Carlin (2000) concluded that Bayesian learning is effective for the ratio of the marginal standard deviations, and a prior ratio 1 : 1 seems a plausible choice. To achieve this, the formula given by Bernardinelli, Clayton and Montomoli (1995) can be used. However, the reader should be warned about simplistic interpretation on the relative magnitude of the spatially structured vs. unstructured variability.

MacNab (2003) followed the model specification of Leroux, Lei and Breslow (1999) in which the two random effects (the spatially structured and the unstructured terms) are combined in a weighted average. The advantage is being able to avoid the identifiability problem and to make inferences on the weight parameter. Computationally, MacNab adopted a hybrid Markov chain Monte Carlo algorithm.

How to choose between all these different model specifications is not an easy task, since there is not a unique model that better represents the data. In disease mapping it is therefore common to perform a sensitivity analysis, reporting results from several model assumptions. Gelman and Price (1999) remembered that mapping observed rates (i.e. maximum likelihood estimates) can have serious drawbacks when population sizes vary by area, since very high (and low) rates are found disproportionately in less populated areas. Unfortunately, even model-based smoothed rates can introduce a bias, in which the highest rates tend to be found disproportionately in more populated areas. The map is still confounded by spatial variation in population sizes. Spatial patterns occur even if there is no spatial structure in the underlying parameters of interest, and smoothed rates tend to look too uniform in areas with

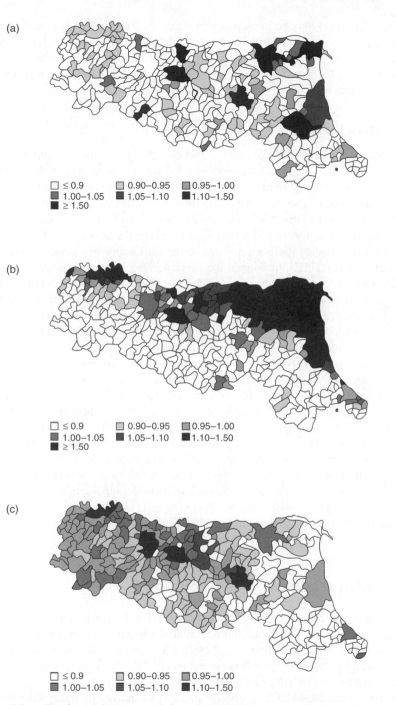

**Figure 9.5** Mortality for (a) lung cancer, females ; (b) lung cancer, males; (c) breast cancer, females. Emilia Romagna region, 1982–1988. Smoothed Bayesian relative risks BYM model (see text). Absolute scale. The three different spatial patterns correspond to a specific ratio of heterogeneity/clustering standard deviation.

little data. This effect may be particularly evident when using inappropriately a model with spatially structured random terms (Lawson *et al.*, 2000). A similar problem was noted by Scheel, Green and Rougier (2011) analyzing the spatial distribution of risk of larynx cancer in females among the French Departments. A safe approach would be to report a map of PG estimates together with a map of BYM estimates.

### 9.7.3    Model checking

Much work has been done on Bayesian model checking in the disease-mapping framework. The motivation lies in the difficulties encountered when analyzing such data. The empirical information can be very little in some areas with low population size, and the risk of strong prior influence is high. This is why we recommend reporting a series of maps or at least two maps, the rough and the smoothed, and sensitivity analysis on prior choices.

Bernardinelli, Clayton and Montomoli (1995) cast the problem and Stern and Cressie (2000) used cross-validation posterior predictive distributions to assess model departures. Spiegelhalter *et al.* (2002) introduced the Deviance Information Criterion (DIC) to assess model fit of hierarchical Bayesian models. This measure takes into account the goodness of fit and the model complexity, which is particularly difficult to assess in Bayesian random-effects models. Plummer (2008) reviewed the issue and showed that the DIC is an approximation to a penalized loss function. When the effective number of model parameters is much smaller than the number of observations, the approximation is not valid.

This result is extremely relevant for disease mapping because this condition is the rule. The consequence is that we will select more complex models than necessary using DIC. A better approach is to follow a leave-one-out cross-validation. In a sort of residual analysis, Marshall and Spiegelhalter (2003) proposed a computationally easy approach using Markov chain Monte Carlo techniques and addressed the identification of divergent observations. Their approach is coherent with the proposed use of the posterior predictive distributions for model checking (Gelfand and Ghosh, 1998). The excess in optimism due to using the data twice, for getting estimates of model parameters and for predicting new observations, is controlled by cross-validation. On this same line, a correction of DIC was given by Plummer (2008); alternatively the Conditional Predictive Ordinate or the Probability Integral Transform can be used for model checking (Geisser, 1980; Dawid, 1984; see also Held, Schrödle and Rue, 2010).

## 9.8    Multivariate disease mapping

More recent literature focused on statistical approaches for joint analysis of more than one disease. The idea is to study the common spatial pattern of different diseases that could be attributable to some common risk factors (i.e. smoking, for an example in etiologic research). Among others the share component model (SCM) and the multivariate conditional autoregressive model (MCAR) have found a wide consensus in the epidemiological literature.

Knorr-Held and Best (2001) proposed an SCM to analyze mortality data on oral cavity and esophageal cancer in Germany. The basic idea is to decompose the risk surface into a shared and disease-specific terms.

Let's assume that $Y_{ik}$ is the number of events in the $i$th area ($i = 1, \ldots, N$) and $k$th disease ($k = 1, \ldots, K$), which follows a Poisson distribution with mean $\theta_{ik}$. The logarithm of the relative risk could be decomposed as $\log(\theta_{ik}) = \alpha_k + u_i\delta_k + I(1 \in \Gamma)\psi_{ik}$, where $\alpha_k$ is the disease-specific baseline log risk of disease in the region (*a priori* independent improper, uniformly distributed), $u_i$ is a shared clustering term between diseases modeled as CAR; $\psi_{ik}$ represents a specific clustering term by $\Gamma$, an appropriate subset of $K$. Fixing, for example, $K=4$, the terms $\log\delta_1, \ldots, \log\delta_4$, constrained to $\sum_{k=1}^{4} \log \delta_k = 0$, are assumed to be multivariate normal distributed with zero mean and variance–covariance matrix respectively:

$$\Sigma_\delta = \sigma_\delta^2 \begin{pmatrix} 1 & -1/3 & -1/3 & -1/3 \\ -1/3 & 1 & -1/3 & -1/3 \\ -1/3 & -1/3 & 1 & -1/3 \\ -1/3 & -1/3 & -1/3 & 1 \end{pmatrix}$$

and represent the scaling factors which allow the risk gradient related to the shared term to be different for each one of the $k$th diseases (Held *et al.*, 2005). An extension of this model restricts the shared component to a subset of $K$. An example of this model for normally distributed data in the context of spatial veterinary epidemiology is in Biggeri *et al.* (2007).

In the MCAR model we assume that $\log(\theta_{ik}) = \alpha_k + \psi_{ik}$ where $\alpha_k$ is, again, a disease-specific intercept, and $\psi_{ik}$ is the area and disease-specific log relative risk. The random terms $\psi_{ik}$ are now modeled as multivariate conditionally autoregressive MCAR (Jin, Carlin and Banerjee, 2005), a generalization of the univariate CAR model (Besag, 1974). It can be viewed as a flexible nonparametric way to take into account hidden, long-range spatially structured confounders (Clayton, Bernardinelli and Montomoli, 1993).

In detail, let us define $\boldsymbol{\psi}_i = (\psi_{1i}, \psi_{2i}, \ldots, \psi_{ki})'$ $i = 1, \ldots, n$ to be the multivariate $k$-dimensional vector of spatially correlated random effects in each area. Then, $\boldsymbol{\psi}_i | \boldsymbol{\psi}_{j \in S_i} \text{dist MVN}(\bar{\boldsymbol{\psi}}_{j \in S_i}, \boldsymbol{\Sigma}_i / n_{j \in S_i})$; that is the conditional distribution of $\boldsymbol{\psi}_i$ given $\boldsymbol{\psi}_{j \in S_i}$, where $S_i$ represents the set of areas adjacent to the $i$th one, is Multivariate Normal with a vector mean $\bar{\boldsymbol{\psi}}_{j \in S_i} = \sum_{j \in S_i} \boldsymbol{\psi}_j / n_{j \in S_i}$, and precision matrix $\boldsymbol{\Sigma}_i / n_{j \in S_i}$, proportional to the number of areas in $S_i$. In other words, for each $k$th disease we are assuming that the relative risks are spatially correlated across areas and also that the relative risks for the $k$ diseases are correlated for the presence of shared area-level unmeasured confounders.

The multivariate joint distribution and the between-area covariance matrix are obtained analogously to the univariate CAR. From the identity $\sigma^2_v (\mathbf{I} - \rho W)^{-1} M = [\tau^2_v (\text{Diag}(w_i) - \rho B)]^{-1}$ we can use the Kronecker product notation and obtain $[\mathbf{T} \otimes (\text{Diag}(w_i) - \rho B)]^{-1}$. Again the joint covariance matrix is not positive definite if the adjacency matrix is specified and $\rho = 1$. Gelfand and Vounatsou (2003) showed that the variance–covariance matrix is positive definite when $\boldsymbol{\Sigma}' = R\boldsymbol{\Sigma}$. A simple solution is $R = \rho \mathbf{I}$ with $\rho \in (\varphi_{\min}, \varphi_{\max})$, where $\varphi_{\min} < 0$ and $\varphi_{\max} = 1$ are the smallest and largest eigenvalues of the adjacency matrix as in the univariate case. Carlin and Banerjee (2003) observed that the above MCAR distribution imposes some rather unnatural symmetry properties on the joint covariance matrix. Jin, Carlin and Banerjee (2005) discussed several alternative MCAR models.

MacNab (2007) used the shared component model in the context of Bayesian disability-adjusted life year (DALY) methodology for spatial and spatiotemporal analyses of disease and/or injury burden. In particular, she defined a model framework that enables SCM as well as multivariate CAR modeling of non-fatal and fatal disease or injury rates and included spline smoothing for non-linear time trends.

MacNab (2009, 2010) adopted the proper MCAR model as part of a Bayesian DALY analysis of multivariate disease or injury data and associated ecological risk factors. She derived the multivariate CAR from the Leroux, Lei and Breslow (1999) model, interpreting the spatial smoothness parameter as the weighting factor between the spatially structured and unstructured terms. Extensions to non-Gaussian random fields are discussed in Chagneau *et al.* (2011).

## 9.9    Special issues

### 9.9.1    Gravitational models

An important aspect in health services research is the study of allocation and accessibility of healthcare units. The hospitalization rate, or other equivalent measure, is modeled as a function of the attraction exercised by each single healthcare provider. Geographical differences in hospitalization rates could then reflect not only ecological and socio-economic determinants of disease status but also the availability of diagnostic examinations or treatments, the access to them and selection processes among potential users (see for example Dreassi and Biggeri, 2003).

The attraction effects of healthcare providers are considered by introducing a specific term in a disease-mapping model (for example the BYM model).

Suppose we have information on the $k$th provider location ($k = 1, \ldots, K$); the BYM random-effect loglinear model becomes $\log(\theta_i) = u_i + v_i - \beta_k \ln(d_{ik})$, where $d_{ik}$ represents the distance between the $k$th provider and the $i$th area centroid. The terms $\beta_k$ are usually considered fixed effects and are modeled using non-informative normal distributions. They represent the decay by unit distance of the power of attraction of each $k$th provider.

When hospitalization records contain information on origin ($i$th subject's residence) and destination ($k$th location of the subject's admission hospital), the disease counts $Y_{ik}$ are cross-classified and the model becomes $\log(\theta_{ik}) = u_i + v_i - \beta_k \ln(d_{ik}) - \beta_0 \ln(C_k)$. Here $C_k$ represents a measure of the $k$th provider's *capacity* and $\beta_k$, as before, the decay by unit distance of its power of attraction (Bailey and Gatrell, 1995; Congdon, 2001, 2010).

### 9.9.2    Wombling

The adjacency structure in the spatial models is arbitrary and usually is defined by an administrative partition of the region of interest. Assunção and Krainski (2009) showed some impractical or counterintuitive consequences of these specifications either on the prior covariance matrix or on the posterior covariance matrix of the CAR spatial random-effects model. The reason lies in the neighborhood graph structure, synthesized in the eigenvalues and eigenvector structure of a matrix associated to the adjacency matrix.

To overcome such difficulties some authors proposed the definition of a spatial neighborhood function, the parameters of which are used in the selection of a neighborhood structure.

White and Ghosh (2009) proposed an extension of the CAR model where the selection of the neighborhood depends on unknown parameter(s) – the Stochastic Neighborhood CAR 'SNCAR' model. A different approach called *wombling* was used in Liang, Banerjee and Carlin (2009) and Ma, Carlin and Banerjee (2010).

Wombling, from Womble (1951), is the detection of discontinuities – boundaries of rapid change on the surface. In such cases, we aim to detect areas of high gradient which can occur due to hidden spatial variables representing local disparities – disparities in income/access to healthcare. This may help decision markers to better allocate resources.

Consider a set of random locations $S = \{s_i\}_{i=1}^n$ where the health event process is observed over the region $R$. Recall that the data are a realization of a inhomogeneous Poisson process with intensity $\lambda(s)$ over the space $R$, with likelihood

$$L = \exp\left\{ -\int_R \lambda(s)\, ds \right\} \times \prod_i \lambda(s_i).$$

The spatial intensity factorizes as $\lambda(s) = \lambda_p(s)\,\mu(s)$, the first factor being the population intensity surface – remember $\lambda_p(s) = \phi(R)/|R|$ for a counting measure $\phi$ and the total area $|R|$ of $R$. A loglinear model is specified for $\log\mu(s) = \beta_0 + X(s)\beta + \varepsilon(s)$. When we aggregate to areas (e.g. census blocks), $\varepsilon(s) = \varepsilon_i$ if $s \in i$th area. Conditional autoregressive models are natural to this case. Now let's allow the areal adjacencies to be random and subject to the influence of such covariate information. Ma, Carlin and Banerjee (2010) presented an application to the Medicare Hospice Service Region. A boundary likelihood value (BLV) is defined as $\Delta_{i,j} = |\varepsilon_i - \varepsilon_j|$ for any two adjacent areas. Crispy (a given edge is part of a boundary if one or the other condition is satisfied: $E(\Delta_{i,j}|\text{Data}) > c$ or $Pr(\Delta_{i,j} > c|\text{Data}) > c^*$) and fuzzy (a given edge is shaded according to $Pr(\Delta_{i,j} > c|\text{Data}) > c^*$) wombling boundaries are then obtained from the posterior distributions of the BLVs. Alternatively we can use the relative intensity surface $\mu(s)$ to define a boundary likelihood value. Point-referenced wombling requires one to specify a wombling measure with directional derivatives (Banerjee and Gelfand, 2006).

### 9.9.3    Some specific statistical modeling examples

There are several disease-mapping examples pertinent to healthcare research.

When facing administrative datasets on the health service, a large number of covariates are available and there may be interest in exploring joint association structures. Tassone, Miranda and Gelfand (2010) screened a set of contingency tables, one for each area, with a spatially structured random-effects specification. The usual Poisson assumption for area counts was then extended to the vector of cell counts. The cell parameters of a parsimonious loglinear model are then modeled at Stage two on area-specific covariates and spatially structured random terms. The application highlights the extent and distribution of racial disparity with regard to low birthweight in the region of interest and its decomposition by each subgroup of interest (the eight combinations of race $\times$ infant sex $\times$ mother's tobacco use). In summary, at Stage 1 subjects in area $s$ are cross-classified by $M$ categorical covariates into $L$ classification cells. Let $n_l^s$ be the count for area $s$ in cell $l$:

$$n_l^s \propto Poisson\left(\lambda_l^s\right)$$
$$\log \lambda_l^s = X_l \beta_s.$$

At Stage 2, the spatial random components are specified:

$$\beta_{st} = \eta_t w_s + \varphi_t^s$$
$$\varphi \propto \text{CAR}.$$

Other interesting examples of uses of spatial disease-mapping models are in Souza *et al.* (2007) with regard to socio-economic factors and disease prevalence. Kazembe and

Namangale (2007) present an application of a conditionally autoregressive model to self-reported illness data. There, a random-effects multinomial model was specified to assess risk factors of childhood co-morbidity of fever, diarrhea and pneumonia, and quantify area-specific spatial effects.

Wang, Luo and McLafferty (2009) studied possible associations between several risk factors and late-stage diagnosis for four types of cancer. Potential risk factors are composed of spatial and non-spatial covariates. The spatial factors include accessibility to primary healthcare and distance or travel time to the nearest cancer screening facility. The Bayesian model with convolution priors is utilized to analyze the relationship between the above risk factors and each type of late-stage cancer while controlling for spatial autocorrelation.

In Rasmussen (2004), models for analysis of trends in hospitals and small-area variation in case fatality after acute myocardial infarction are presented. The data are from administrative registries in Denmark. Hierarchical modeling in a logistic regression with a Bayesian approach is used.

Knorr-Held, Rasser and Becker (2002) proposed an elegant approach to the spatial analysis of cancer incidence data with additional information on the stage of the disease at time of diagnosis. The methods are useful in monitoring the effectiveness of mass cancer screening. They embedded the cumulative odds and the continuation ratio models for ordinal response in a disease- mapping framework. The category-specific intercepts for the two models are considered spatially structured random terms, using independent CAR formulations or a multivariate CAR model. Zhou et al. (2008) extended this approach to cancer registry data and compared baseline-category logit, proportional odds and adjacent odds models.

Zhang et al. (2006) proposed to capture the interaction among demographic effects (age and gender), spatial effects (county) and temporal effects of colorectal cancer incidences simultaneously.

Mugglin, Cressie and Gemmell (2002) present an example on infectious disease surveillance. When small-scale movements and contacts between people are not recorded, we rely on small-area counts of the numbers infected during successive, regular time intervals. The authors develop a spatially descriptive, temporally dynamic hierarchical model to be fitted to such data. A proper CAR model is specified for the spatial component.

Spatiotemporal models are a specific research field. Here we simply recall some basic concepts. Time profiles can be modeled independently from spatial patterns, and simple autoregressive assumptions of order one were suggested. Proposed priors for the time parameters are random walk with independent Gaussian increments or second-order random walk (with independent second differences) (Schmid and Held, 2004).

Space-time interactions are however plausible because time trends can be shared by spatially contiguous areas (e.g. Waller et al., 1997). A definition of different kinds of space-time patterns is given in Knorr-Held (2000). Other examples are also given in Assunção, Reis and Oliveira (2001).

Lagazio, Dreassi and Biggeri (2001) introduced the birth-cohort dimension in space-time disease mapping. Eventually, a complete age-period-cohort modeling was considered in Lagazio, Biggeri and Dreassi (2003) and recently by Riebler and Held (2010) in a multivariate framework (Figure 9.6).

Buenconsejo et al. (2008) introduced a spatial random-effects model in a capture-recapture loglinear model. They analyzed two incomplete disease surveillance datasets which consist of case counts, each originating from a specific geographical area.

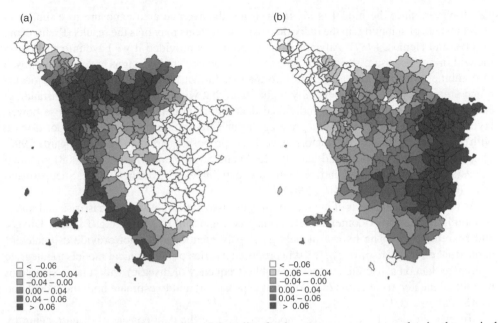

**Figure 9.6**  Space-time interactions. Mortality for lung cancer among males in the period 1971–1999, Tuscany (Italy). Maps of the space-time interaction parameters for the birth cohort 1901–09 (a) and 1921–29 (b). (for a complete discussion of this example see Biggeri, Catelan and Dreassi, 2009).

Sun and Clayton (2008) addressed the analysis of cross-classified categorical data that are spatially autocorrelated. We first extend the autologistic model to accommodate two variables. Two bivariate autologistic models are constructed, namely a two-step model and a symmetric model.

Banerjee, Wall and Carlin (2003); Banerjee and Carlin (2004); Banerjee and Dey (2005); Jin, Carlin and Banerjee (2005); Cooner, Banerjee and McBean (2006); and Diva, Dey and Banerjee (2008) proposed Bayesian hierarchical survival models for capturing spatial correlations within the proportional hazards (PH) and proportional odds (PO) frameworks.

Seppä *et al.* (2010) applied a mixture cure-fraction model with random effects to cause-specific survival data from the Finnish Cancer Registry. Two sets of random effects were used to capture the regional variation in the cure fraction and in the survival of the non-cured patients, respectively.

### 9.9.4  Ecological bias

Ecological bias menaces the validity of association studies based on aggregate data. Results from ecological regression performed after a disease-mapping exercise are therefore to be interpreted with caution. Conditions for absence of ecological bias are usually impossible to check. The basic assumption of homogeneity of exposure within areas is rarely fulfilled. If the area size is sufficiently small in terms of population and physical characteristics of the exposure, we can assume the homogeneity assumption approximately holds. Random-effects models, eventually spatially structured, are then fitted to account for unobserved confounders.

However, since the model is loglinear, using the average area exposure to estimate its effect instead of summing up the individual exposure effects may bias the results (Richardson, Stücker and Hemon, 1987). An approximate solution is provided if we have information on the within-area exposure variability. As a corollary, several study designs have been proposed to combine individual and aggregate information. In fact, the variability of disease occurrence among populations is generally higher than that within population. Notwithstanding, epidemiological studies rely on individual data within populations and may loose power. Hybrid ecological models that integrate aggregate information on the frequency of disease with individual data on risk factors have been proposed (Prentice and Sheppard, 1995; Sheppard, 2003). Wakefield and Salway (2001) and Salway and Wakefield (2008) provided Bayesian solutions, and applications to disease mapping were given in Guthrie, Sheppard and Wakefield (2002) and Best et al. (2001).

In healthcare studies it is of interest to study the association between disease risk and socio-economic indicators. A contextual effect may be important to assess (e.g. Biggeri, Dreassi and Marchi, 2004). The hybrid models previously mentioned do not provide estimates of contextual effects. Grisotto et al. (2011) proposed a series of hierarchical models to integrate aggregate data on a discrete response variable (frequency of disease) with a large sample of individual data on risk factors (e.g. material deprivation) and to estimate both individual and contextual effects.

To give an idea of the statistical modeling, assume the data consist of disease count by area, $Y_j$, and a sample of $n_j$ subjects for each area with information on individual covariate (e.g. material deprivation index), $X_{ij}$ for the $i$th individual in the $j$th area.

Now, $Y_j$ follows a Poisson distribution with parameters $D_j \times \theta_j$, where $D_j$ represents the expected counts or population denominators fixed by design, and $\theta_j$ the unknown relative risk.

Denote $\mu_{xj}$ and $\sigma^2_{xj}$ the mean and variance of the distribution of the covariate for the generic $j$th area. The parametric ecological model of Salway and Wakefield (2008) is

$$\log(\theta_j) = \alpha + \beta\mu_{xj} + \beta^2/2\sigma^2_{xj}.$$

In absence of ecological bias, the aggregate effect is given by the sum of two effects, the individual and the contextual (Cronbach and Webb, 1975; Firebaugh, 1978). Simple algebra gives:

$$\log(\theta_j) = \alpha + \beta_A\mu_{xj} + \beta_I^2/2\sigma^2_{xj},$$

with $\beta_A = \beta_C + \beta_I$, $\beta_A$ the aggregate, $\beta_C$ the contextual and $\beta_I$ the individual effect.

A BYM model can be specified replacing the intercept term with spatially structured and unstructured random terms (Best et al., 2001; Guthrie, Sheppard and Wakefield, 2002).

A fully Bayesian model specifies a covariate measurement error model. We get information on $\mu_{xj}$ and $\sigma^2{}_{xj}$ from a sample of $n_j$ individuals (Best et al., 2001). A simpler alternative is to specify the following priors:

$$\mu_{xj} \sim \text{Normal}(x_j, \sigma^2_j/n_j)$$

$$\sigma^2_{xj} \sim \chi_{vj}(s^2_j/n_j),$$

where $x_j$ and $s^2_j$ are the sample mean and variance.

A final warning on estimation of contextual effects: associations are not causation. To address causal effect in neighborhood research, special approaches are necessary (VanderWeele, 2008).

## 9.9.5   Area profiling

In the framework of healthcare, whenever we look at Atlases of health events the interest relies on the scrutiny of long lists of relative risks and associated hypothesis tests. The purpose is to detect divergences from local or national averages.

There are some examples in the literature. First Carpenter *et al.* (1997) and Law *et al.* (2001) in the context of surveillance for new occupational risks proposed a q-q plot of standardized statistics with guiderails; Goldstein and Spiegelhalter (1996) introduced the idea of ranking in educational and health provider assessment. Recently Ohlssen, Sharples and Spiegelhalter (2007) introduced more complex hierarchical models to health provider profiling.

All these approaches are justified in terms of control for multiple comparisons.

In the disease-mapping context relative risk estimates and p-values may be reported for a set of areas by a given disease or for a whole spectrum of diseases by a single given area. In any case we are interested in assessing departure from a set of reference rates.

Bayesian approaches to smooth relative risk estimates may be erroneously interpreted as a solution to the multiple comparison problem (Richardson *et al.*, 2004). In fact, Bayesian posterior estimators minimize a squared loss function over the whole set of areas, and it can be shown that they are better than maximum likelihood estimates (Efron and Morris, 1973). But this does not imply that posterior probabilities of RR > cut-off are adjusted for multiple comparisons.

The same argument applies to corrected empirical Bayes confidence intervals. Escaramís, Carrasco and Ascaso (2008) presented an analytical adjustment for disease risk inference that provides accurate interval predictions by using the penalized quasilikelihood (PQL) technique to obtain model parameter estimates. The method is a first-order approximation of the naive standard error based on a Taylor expansion, and is interpreted as a conditional measure of variability providing conditional calibrated prediction intervals, given the data.

MacNab *et al.* (2004) proposed an extension of the Carlin and Gelfand (1990, 1991) bootstrap procedure for deriving Empirical Bayes confidence intervals in the case of a CAR model (see also Biggeri, Braga and Marchi (1995) for an early application of the same approach).

Shen and Louis (1998) identified different inferential goals: estimating relative risks, their distribution, and their ranks. They proposed several estimators and discussed in depth posterior rank estimates. A multivariate CAR prior was used by Catelan and Biggeri (2008) to borrow strength and to estimate disease profiles and area signatures in disease mapping. The use of ranks is very immediate and simple for decision makers, allowing an easy appreciation of classification uncertainty. Marginalizing joint posterior rank distributions over disease or over areas permits one to appreciate uncertainty and identify priorities (Figure 9.7).

An appropriate Bayesian approach to multiple inference would consist of a tri-level hierarchical Bayesian model for the estimation of the posterior probability of a given disease/area belonging to the set of null or alternative hypotheses (Müller, Parmigiani and Rice, 2006; Catelan, Lagazio and Biggeri, 2010).

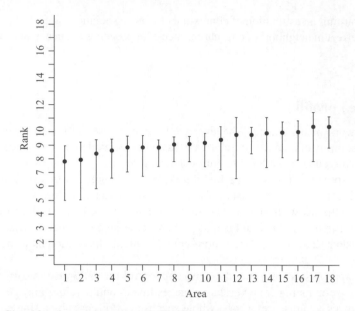

**Figure 9.7** Classification uncertainty. Mortality among males in the period 1997–2001. Marginal posterior rank estimates and 80% credibility interval for 18 high-risk areas of Sardinia Region (Italy). The posterior distributions are integrated over 29 mutually exclusive causes of death (see text).

Multiple comparison is considered in cluster detection and spatial and spatiotemporal surveillance. However, mostly control of the family wise error rate (FWER) is applied (Kulldorff, 2001; Frisén, 2003). Rolka, Burkom and Cooper (2007) proposed False Discovery Rate (FDR) control in syndromic surveillance. FDR is the expected value of the rate of false positives among all rejected hypotheses. FDR control has also been proposed for the screening of 'hot spots' (Castro and Singer, 2006), for profiling healthcare providers (Jones, Ohlssen and Spiegelhalter, 2008; Ohlssen, Sharples and Spiegelhalter, 2007) and in disease mapping (Catelan and Biggeri, 2010).

### 9.9.5.1    Multiple testing in disease mapping

The traditional strategy to account for multiple comparisons when $m$ tests of hypothesis are performed is to control the error rate at a desired level while maintaining the power of each test as much as possible. The commonly controlled quantity is the FWER, for example via the Bonferroni correction. Setting the probability of type I error at $\alpha$ when performing $m$ tests, each test is controlled at the level $\alpha^* = \alpha/m$ (Bonferroni, 1936). This guarantees that the probability of a false positive is at maximum equal to $\alpha$.

This procedure is not of real interest when we are interested in testing multiple hypotheses; that is, the consequences of rejecting one hypothesis are different from those related to rejection of other hypotheses. Benjamini and Hochberg (1995) proposed to control the expected proportion of error among all rejected hypotheses and called it the false discovery rate (FDR).

Without entering into details let's define $I_i$ an indicator for rejecting $H_0$ for the $i$th area, $R = \sum I_i$ is the total number of rejections and $r_i \in \{0,1\}$ the indicator of the unknown true status; that is, the indicator that the $i$th area is truly not divergent from the reference. The false discovery proportion (FDP) can be derived as $\sum (r_i \times I_i)/R$, the fraction of false rejections over the total number of rejections (Genovese and Wasserman, 2006). Benjamini and Hochberg (1995) proposed to control the expected value of FDP, taking the expectation over repeated experiments.

Storey (2003) considered modeling the positive FDR (pFDR), conditioning on at least one 'positive' result occurred (one rejection). Under certain conditions holding, the pFDR can be shown to be a posterior Bayesian probability, the posterior probability of the null given that the test statistics fall in the rejection region. This derivation depends on the validity of the assumption that the tests are i.i.d. and exchangeable; in other words we have no *a priori* reason to believe that the probability of the null should be greater for some tests. pFDR led to the definition of the *q-value* which represents the Bayesian analogue of the p-value. The q-value is the minimum pFDR that can occur rejecting the null hypothesis on the basis of the observed or more extreme values of the test statistic; that is $\text{Prob}(H_0 \mid Y \geq Y_{obs})$, $Y$ being a test statistic and $Y_{obs}$ the observed value, for a generic $i$th test. Efron (2005, 2007) focused on $\text{Prob}(H_0 \mid Y = Y_i; Y, \xi) = \text{Prob}(r_i = 1 \mid Y = Y_i; Y, \xi)$ and called it the local FDR, the posterior probability of the null hypothesis conditional on observed vector $Y$ and hyperparameter vector $\xi$.

A full Bayes approach would provide $\text{Prob}(H_0 \mid Y = Y_i; Y) = \text{Prob}(r_i = 1 \mid Y = Y_i; Y)$, the marginal posterior probabilities, having defined a density for $\xi$ (Müller, Parmigiani and Rice, 2006).

Jones, Ohlssen and Spiegelhalter (2008) discussed this approach in the context of healthcare provider profiling and noted that q-values can be screened in an exploratory manner without having a fixed significance level in advance. In simple problems, the computation of a q-value is easy and can be based on observed p-values. A frequentist procedure was proposed by Benjamini, Krieger and Yekutieli (2006) and an empirical Bayes procedure by Storey (2002).

In the disease-mapping context, the problem is complicated by the spatial autocorrelation among responses. A full Bayesian approach consists in a tri-level hierarchical Bayesian model with spatially structured priors to estimate the posterior probability of a given disease/ area belonging to the set of the null hypothesis or alternative sets (Catelan, Lagazio and Biggeri, 2010).

We already noted that using posterior probabilities for each area of having a risk higher than a predefined cut-off (Bernardinelli and Montomoli, 1992; Richardson *et al.*, 2004) is not sufficient to adjust for multiple testing. The probability model needs to include a null prior and related hyperparameters that define the prior probability mass for non-*divergent* areas (Scott and Berger, 2006).

The standard hierarchical Bayesian models for disease mapping are extended to obtain fully Bayesian estimates of $\text{Prob}(r_i = 1 \mid Y = Y_i; Y)$. This can be done assuming a mixture model for the unknown relative risks $\theta_i$. At the first level of the hierarchy we have the Poisson likelihood for the count of disease in the $i$th area, $Y_i \sim \text{Poisson}(D_i \theta_i)$. The mixture is introduced at the second level of the hierarchy. In particular we assume that $\log(\theta_i) = r_i \mu_{0i} + (1 - r_i)\mu_{1i}$, which means that the logarithm of the relative risk $\theta_i$ is modeled as the mixture of $\mu_{0i}$, the value of the log relative risk under the null hypothesis, and $\mu_{1i}$ the corresponding value under the alternative. The $r_i$ indicator denotes group membership.

Under the null, all the probability mass is concentrated at one point; that is, $\mu_{0i} = 0$, leaving only a Poisson random variability modeled at the first level. Under the alternative, extra Poisson variability, which reflects the heterogeneity of relative risk among areas, should be modeled following, for example, the PG or the BYM specifications.

The third level of the hierarchy consists in the definition of the prior distribution for the indicator of the unknown true status, $r_i$. In Catelan, Lagazio and Biggeri (2010) it is assumed to be Bernoulli distributed with parameter $\pi_i$, which, in turn, is modeled as a Beta$(c,d)$ distribution. The parameters of the Beta distribution define the *a priori* belief on the null hypothesis, and a sensitivity analysis is suggested changing the $c$, $d$ parameters, since there is a strong sensitivity to hyperprior choice for $\pi$. A naive choice of a uniform distribution for $\pi$ is strongly expected to be in error. However, the amount of information about $\pi$ in the data could be low when the number of tests is not large enough. In the disease-mapping context the number of tests is typically between 100 and 1000, and therefore eliciting appropriate informative hyperprior inference on $\pi$ is important.

The quantity of interest for each $i$th area is some appropriate summary measure over the posterior distribution of $\pi_i$; that is, the posterior classification probability of belonging to the set of the null hypothesis (Scott and Berger, 2006).

## 9.10    Summary

In this chapter we discussed statistical aspects of the analysis of spatial data, in particular aggregated areal data, which are commonly available from routine sources (as mortality of hospital discharge records). We did not review all the relevant statistical issues in the context of disease mapping but we focused on the literature of the last 10 years which has a direct connection with healthcare research, and we highlighted some related statistical aspects which are not usually considered by applied researchers in those subject-specific fields. Indeed, the diffusion of free statistical software that allows one to perform Bayesian analysis in a very easy way, together with GIS software packages that allow several simple geographical analyses and building of a *standardized map* of risk indicators, have increased the number of geographical analyses done by 'non-experts'. If, on one hand, this is making headway for people who work in healthcare research, on the other, we want to stress the complexity of the assumptions underlying the statistical models used for analyzing geographical data and the danger of simple automatic approaches to this task.

Mapping disease occurrence is useful in identification of health needs and it is one basic input in healthcare planning; mapping healthcare contacts allows the estimation of disease prevalence and health services utilization and it is one fundamental input for decisions on the delivering of healthcare; and last, the performance of healthcare providers can be evaluated by mapping appropriate random-effect terms. Monitoring healthcare is then complemented by this kind of spatial analysis.

## References

Acheson, E.D. (1967) *Medical Record Linkage*, Oxford University Press, London.

Agabiti, N., Davoli, M., Fusco, D. *et al.* (2011) Comparative evaluation of health services outcomes. *Epidemiol Prev*, **35**, S1–S80.

Armstrong, B.G. (1995) Comparing standardized mortality ratios. *Ann Epidemiol*, **5**, 60–64.

Assunção, R.M. and Krainski, E. (2009) Neighborhood dependence in Bayesian spatial models. *Biom J*, **51**, 851–869.

Assunção, R.M., Reis, I.A. and Oliveira, C.D. (2001) Diffusion and prediction of Leishmaniasis in a large metropolitan area in Brazil with a Bayesian space-time model. *Stat Med*, **20**, 2319–2335.

Bailey, T. and Gatrell, A. (1995) *Interactive Spatial Data Analysis*, Longman, London.

Banerjee, S. and Carlin, B.P. (2004) Parametric spatial cure rate models for interval-censored time-to-relapse data. *Biometrics*, **60**, 268–275.

Banerjee, S. and Dey, D.K. (2005) Semiparametric proportional odds models for spatially correlated survival data, *Lifetime Data Anal*, **11**, 175–191.

Banerjee, S. and Gelfand, A.E. (2006) Bayesian wombling: curvilinear gradient assessment under spatial process models. *J Amer Stat Assoc*, **101**, 1487–1501.

Banerjee, S., Carlin, B.P. and Gelfand, A.E. (2004) *Hierarchical Modeling and Analysis of Spatial Data*, Chapman & Hall/CRC, Boca Raton, FL.

Banerjee, S., Wall, M.M. and Carlin, B.P. (2003) Frailty modeling for spatially correlated survival data, with application to infant mortality in Minnesota. *Biostatistics*, **4**, 123–142.

Benjamini, Y. and Hochberg, Y. (1995) Controlling the false discovery rate: a practical and powerful approach to multiple testing. *J R Stat Soc B*, **57**, 289–300.

Benjamini, Y., Krieger, A.M. and Yekutieli, D. (2006) Adaptive linear step-up procedures that control the false discovery rate. *Biometrika*, **93**, 491–507.

Bernardinelli, L. and Montomoli, C. (1992) Empirical Bayes versus fully Bayesian analysis of geographical variation in disease risk. *Stat Med*, **11**, 983–1007.

Bernardinelli, L., Clayton, D. and Montomoli, C. (1995) Bayesian estimates of disease maps: how important are priors? *Stat Med*, **14**, 2411–2431.

Besag, J. (1974) Spatial interaction and the statistical analysis of lattice systems. *J R Stat Soc B*, **36**, 192–236.

Besag, J. and Kooperberg, C. (1995) On conditional and intrinsic auto-regressions. *Biometrika*, **82**, 733–746.

Besag, J., York, J. and Mollié, A. (1991) Bayesian image restoration, with two applications in spatial statistics. *Ann I Stat Math*, **43**, 1–59.

Best, N., Cocking, S., Bennett, J. *et al.* (2001) Ecological regression analysis of environmental benzene exposure and childhood leukaemia: sensitivity to data inaccuracies, geographical scale and ecological bias. *J R Stat Soc A*, **164**, 155–174.

Best, N., Richardson, S. and Thomson, A. (2005) A comparison of Bayesian spatial models for disease mapping. *Stat Methods Med Res*, **14**, 35–59.

Biggeri, A., Braga, M. and Marchi, M. (1995) Empirical Bayes confidence intervals: an application to geographical epidemiology. *J Ital Stat Soc*, **3**, 251–268.

Biggeri, A., Catelan, D. and Dreassi, E. (2009) The epidemic of lung cancer in Tuscany (Italy): a joint analysis of male and female mortality by birth cohort. *Spat Spatiotemporal Epidemiol*, **1**, 31–40.

Biggeri, A., Catelan, D., Dreassi, E. *et al.* (2007) Multivariate spatially-structured variability of ovine helminth infections. *Geospat Health*, **2**, 97–104.

Biggeri, A., Dreassi, E. and Marchi, M. (2004) A multilevel Bayesian model for contextual effect of material deprivation. *Stat Meth Appl*, **13**, 87–101.

Biggeri, A., Lagazio, C., Catelan, D. *et al.* (2006) Rapporto sullo stato di salute delle popolazioni residenti in aree interessate da poli industriali, minerari o militari della Regione Sardegna. *Epidemiol Prev*, **30**, S1–S96.

Biggeri, A., Marchi, M., Lagazio, C. *et al.* (2000) Non-parametric maximum likelihood estimators for disease mapping. *Stat Med*, **19**, 2539–2554.

Bonferroni, C. (1936) Teoria statistica delle classi e calcolo delle probabilità. *Pubblicazioni del Regio Istituto Superiore di Scienze Economiche e Commerciali di Firenze*, **8**, 3–62.

Brameld, K.J., Holman, C.D., Lawrence, D.M. and Hobbs, M.S. (2003) Improved methods for estimating incidence from linked hospital morbidity data. *Int J Epidemiol*, **32**, 617–24.

Breslow, N. and Day, N.E. (1987) Statistical Methods in Cancer Research, Vol. II, *The Design and Analysis of Cohort Studies*, IARC Scientific Publications No. 82, International Agency for Research on Cancer, Lyon.

Briggs, D. (2007) The Dimensions of Colour. www.huevaluechroma.com (accessed April 2, 2012).

Buenconsejo, J., Fish, D., Childs, J.E. and Holford, T.R. (2008) A Bayesian hierarchical model for the estimation of two incomplete surveillance data sets. *Stat Med*, **27**, 3269–3285.

Carlin, B. and Banerjee, S. (2003) Hierarchical multivariate CAR models for spatio-temporally correlated survival data, in *Bayesian Statistics 7* (eds J.M. Bernardo, M.J. Bayarri, O. Berger *et al.*), Oxford University Press, Oxford, pp. 45–63.

Carlin, B. and Gelfand, A.E. (1990) Approaches for empirical Bayes confidence intervals. *J Amer Stat Assoc*, **85**, 105–115.

Carlin, B. and Gelfand, A.E. (1991) Approaches for empirical Bayes confidence intervals. *J R Stat Soc B*, **53**, 189–200.

Carpenter, L.M., Maconochie, N.E.S., Roman, E. and Cox, D.R. (1997) Examining associations between occupation and health by using routinely collected data. *J R Stat Soc A*, **160**, 507–521.

Castro, M.C. and Singer, B.H. (2006) Controlling the false discovery rate: a new application to account for multiple and dependent tests in local statistics of spatial association. *Geogr Anal*, **38**, 180–208.

Catelan, D. and Biggeri, A. (2008) A statistical approach to rank multiple priorities in environmental epidemiology: an example from high-risk areas in Sardinia, Italy. *Geospat Health*, **3**, 81–89.

Catelan, D. and Biggeri, A. (2010) Multiple testing in disease mapping and descriptive epidemiology. *Geospat Health*, **4**, 219–229.

Catelan, D., Biggeri, A. and Lagazio, C. (2009) On the clustering term in ecological analysis: how do different prior specifications affect results? *Stat Meth Appl*, **18**, 49–61.

Catelan, D., Lagazio, C. and Biggeri, A. (2010) A hierarchical Bayesian approach to multiple testing in disease mapping. *Biom J*, **52**, 784–797.

Chagneau, P., Mortier, F., Picard, N. and Bacro, J.N. (2011) A hierarchical Bayesian model for spatial prediction of multivariate non-Gaussian random fields. *Biometrics*, **67**, 97–105.

Clayton, D. and Kaldor, J. (1987) Empirical Bayes estimates of age-standardized relative risks for use in disease mapping. *Biometrics*, **43**, 671–681.

Clayton, D., Bernardinelli, L. and Montomoli, C. (1993) Spatial correlation in ecological analysis. *Int J Epidemiol*, **22**, 1193–1202.

Congdon, P. (2001) The development of gravity models for hospital patient flows under system change: a Bayesian modelling approach. *Health Care Manag Sci*, **4**, 289–304.

Congdon, P. (2010) Random-effects models for migration attractivity and retentivity: a Bayesian methodology. *J R Stat Soc A*, **173**, 755–774.

Cook, D.G. and Pocock, S.J. (1983) Multiple regression in geographic mortality studies with allowance for spatially correlated errors. *Biometrics*, **39**, 361–371.

Cooner, F., Banerjee, S. and McBean, A.M. (2006) Modelling geographically referenced survival data with a cure fraction. *Stat Methods Med Res*, **15**, 307–324.

Cox, D.R. and Isham, V. (1980) *Point Processes*, Chapman and Hall, London.

Cressie, N. (1991) *Statistics for Spatial Data*, John Wiley & Sons, Inc., New York.

Cressie, N. (1993) Regional mapping of incidence rates using spatial Bayesian models. *Med Care*, **31**, YS60–YS65.

Cressie, N. and Chan, N.H. (1989) Spatial modelling of regional variables. *J Amer Stat Assoc*, **84**, 393–401.

Cronbach, L.J. and Webb, J. (1975) Between-class and within-class effects in a reported aptitude X treatment interaction. *J Educ Psychol*, **67**, 717–724.

Dawid, A.P. (1984) Statistical theory: the prequential approach. *J R Stat Soc A*, **147**, 278–292.

Denison, D.G. and Holmes, C.C. (2001) Bayesian partitioning for estimating disease risk. *Biometrics*, **57**, 143–149.

Diggle, P. and Elliott, P. (1995) Disease risk near point sources: statistical issues for analyses using individual or spatially aggregated data. *J Epidemiol Commun H*, **49**, S20–S27.

Diggle, P.J. (1983) *Statistical Analysis of Spatial Point Patterns*, Academic Press, London.

Diggle, P.J. (2000) Overview of statistical methods for disease mapping and its relationship to cluster detection, in *Spatial Epidemiology* (eds P. Elliott, J. Wakefield, N. Best, and D. Briggs), Oxford University Press, Oxford.

Diggle, P.J., Tawn, J.A. and Moyeed, R.A. (1998) Model-based geostatistics (with discussion). *Appl Stat*, **47**, 299–350.

Diva, U., Dey, D.K. and Banerjee, S. (2008) Parametric models for spatially correlated survival data for individuals with multiple cancers. *Stat Med*, **27**, 2127–2144.

Dowd, B. (2010) Separated at birth: statisticians, social scientists, and causality in health services research. *Health Serv Res*, **46**, 397–420.

Dreassi, E. and Biggeri, A. (2003) Disease mapping and attraction models for health planning. *Biom J*, **45**, 207–217.

Eberly, L.E. and Carlin, B.P. (2000) Identifiability and convergence issues for Markov chain Monte Carlo fitting of spatial models. *Stat Med*, **19**, 2279–2294.

Efron, B. (2005) Local False Discovery Rates, Technical Report 2005–20B/234, Standford University.

Efron, B. (2007) Size, power and false discovery rates. *Ann of Stat*, **35**, 1351–1377.

Efron, B. and Morris, C. (1973) Stein's estimation rule and its competitors: an empirical Bayes approach. *J Amer Stat Assoc*, **68**, 117–130.

Elliott, P., Wakefield, J., Best, N. and Briggs, D. (2000) *Spatial Epidemiology*, Oxford University Press, Oxford.

Escaramís, G., Carrasco, J.L. and Ascaso, C. (2008) Detection of significant disease risks using a spatial conditional autoregressive model. *Biometrics*, **64**, 1043–1053.

Firebaugh, G. (1978) A rule for inferring individual-level relationships from aggregate data. *Am Sociol Rev*, **43**, 557–572.

Frisén, M. (2003) Statistical surveillance. Optimality and methods. *Int Stat Rev*, **71**, 403–434.

Gangnon, R.E. and Clayton, M.K. (2003) A hierarchical model for spatially clustered disease rates. *Stat Med*, **22**, 3213–3228.

Gehlke, C. and Biehl, H. (1934) Certain effects of grouping upon the size of the correlation coefficient in census tract material. *J Amer Stat Assoc*, **29**, S169–S170.

Geisser, S. (1980) Discussion on Sampling and Bayes' inference in scientific modelling and robustness (by G. E. P. Box). *J R Stat Soc A*, **143**, 416–417.

Gelfand, A.E. and Ghosh, S.K. (1998) Model choice: a minimum posterior predictive loss approach. *Biometrika*, **85**, 1–11.

Gelfand, A.E. and Vounatsou, P. (2003) Proper multivariate conditional autoregressive models for spatial data analysis. *Biostatistics*, **4**, 11–25.

Gelman, A. and Price, P.N. (1999) All maps of parameter estimates are misleading. *Stat Med*, **18**, 3221–3234.

Genovese, C.R. and Wasserman, L. (2006) Exceedance control of the false discovery proportion. *J Amer Stat Assoc*, **101**, 1408–1417.

Gilks, W.R., Richardson, S. and Spiegelhalter, D.J. (1996) *Markov Chain Monte Carlo in Practice*, Chapman & Hall/CRC, Boca Raton.

Giudici, P., Knorr-Held, L. and Rasser, G. (2000) Modelling categorical covariates in Bayesian disease mapping by partition structures. *Stat Med*, **19**, 2579–2593.

Goldstein, H. and Spiegelhalter, D.J. (1996) League tables and their limitations: statistical issues in comparisons of institutional performance. *J R Stat Soc A*, **159**, 385–443.

Graves, B.A. (2008) Integrative literature review: a review of literature related to geographical information systems, healthcare access, and health outcomes. *Perspect Health Inf Manag*, **5**, 11.

Grisotto, L., Catelan, D., Saez, M. and Biggeri, A. (2011) Empirical Bayes models to estimate contextual effects, in *Proceedings of the 26th International Workshop on Statistical Modelling. Valencia, Italy, 11–15 July 2011* (eds D. Conesa, A. Forte, A. Lopez-Quilez and F. Munoz), Statistical Modelling Society.

Guthrie, K.A., Sheppard, L. and Wakefield, J. (2002) A hierarchical aggregate data model with spatially correlated disease rates. *Biometrics*, **58**, 898–905.

Hampton, K.H., Fitch, M.K., Allshouse, W.B. *et al.* (2010) Mapping health data: improved privacy protection with donut method geomasking. *Am J Epidemiol*, **172**, 1062–1069.

Hegarty, A. and Barry, D. (2008) Bayesian disease mapping using product partition models. *Stat Med*, **27**, 3868–3893.

Held, L., Natario, I., Fenton, S.E. *et al.* (2005) Towards joint disease mapping. *Stat Methods Med Res*, **14**, 61–82.

Held, L., Schrödle, B. and Rue, H. (2010) Posterior and cross-validatory predictive checks: a comparison of MCMC and INLA, in *Statistical Modelling and Regression Structures - Festschrift in Honour of Ludwig Fahrmeir* (eds G. Tutz and T. Kneib), Physica-Verlag, Heidelberg, pp. 91–110.

Huff, D. (1991) *How to Lie with Statistics*, New Ed edn, Penguin, New York.

Jatrana, S., Crampton, P. and Norris, P. (2011) Ethnic differences in access to prescription medication because of cost in New Zealand. *J Epidemiol Commun H*, **5**, 454–460.

Jin, X., Carlin, B. and Banerjee, S. (2005) Generalized hierarchical multivariate CAR models for areal data. *Biometrics*, **61**, 950–961.

Jones, H.E., Ohlssen, D.I. and Spiegelhalter, D.J. (2008) Use of the false discovery rate when comparing multiple health care providers. *J Clin Epidemiol*, **61**, 232–240.

Kazembe, L.N. and Namangale, J.J. (2007) A Bayesian multinomial model to analyse spatial patterns of childhood co-morbidity in Malawi. *Eur J Epidemiol*, **22**, 545–556.

Kelsall, J.E. and Wakefield, J. (2002) Modeling spatial variation in disease risk: a geostatistical approach. *J Amer Stat Assoc*, **97**, 692–701.

Kjellstrom, T. (2008) *Our Cities, Our Health, Our Future. Acting on Social Determinants for Health Equity in Urban Settings. Report to the WHO Commission on Social Determinants of Health from the Knowledge Network on Urban Settings*. WHO Centre for Health Development, Kobe City, Japan.

Knorr-Held, L. (2000) Bayesian modelling of inseparable space-time variation in disease risk. *Stat Med*, **19**, 2555–2568.

Knorr-Held, L. and Best, N.G. (2001) A shared component model for detecting joint and selective clustering of two diseases. *J R Stat Soc A*, **164**, 73–85.

Knorr-Held, L., Rasser, G. and Becker, N. (2002) Disease mapping of stage-specific cancer incidence data. *Biometrics*, **58**, 492–501.

Koch, T. (2011) Visualizing Disease, ESRI.COM, www.esri.com/news/arcuser/0311/files/diseasemap .pdf (accessed March 3, 2012).

Koch, T. (2012) *Disease Maps: Epidemics on the Ground*, University of Chicago Press, Chicago.

Kottas, A., Duan, J.A. and Gelfand, A.E. (2008) Modeling disease incidence data with spatial and spatio temporal Dirichlet process mixtures. *Biom J*, **50**, 29–42.

Kulldorff, M. (2001) Prospective time-periodic geographical disease surveillance using a Scan Statistic. *J R Stat Soc A* **164**, 61–72.

Lagazio, C., Biggeri, A. and Dreassi, E. (2003) Age-period-cohort models and disease mapping. *Environmetrics*, **14**, 475–490.

Lagazio, C., Dreassi, E. and Biggeri, A. (2001) A hierarchical Bayesian model for the analysis of spatio-temporal variation in disease risk. *Statistical Modelling*, **1**, 17–29.

Latouche, A., Guihenneuc-Jouyaux, C., Girard, C. and Hémon, D. (2007) Robustness of the BYM model in absence of spatial variation in the residuals. *Int J Health Geogr*, **6**, 39.

Law, G., Cox, D.R., Machonochie, N. *et al.* (2001) Large tables. *Biostatistics*, **2**, 163–171.

Lawson, A.B. and Williams, F.L.R. (2001) *An Introductory Guide to Disease Mapping*, John Wiley & Sons, Ltd, Chichester.

Lawson, A.B., Biggeri, A., Böhning, D. *et al.* (eds) (1999) *Disease Mapping and Risk Assessment for Public Health*, John Wiley & Sons, Ltd, Chichester.

Lawson, A.B., Biggeri, A., Böhning, D. *et al.* (2000) Disease mapping models: an empirical evaluation. *Stat Med*, **19**, 2217–2242.

Lawson, A.B., Song, H.R., Cai, B. *et al.* (2010) Space-time latent component modeling of geo-referenced health data. *Stat Med*, **29**, 2012–2027.

Leroux, B.G., Lei, X. and Breslow, N. (1999) Estimation of disease rates in small areas: a new mixed model for spatial dependence, in *Statistical models in Epidemiology, the Environment and Clinical Trials* (eds M.E. Halloran and D. Berry), Springer, New York, pp. 135–178.

Liang, S., Banerjee, S. and Carlin, B.P. (2009) Bayesian wombling for spatial point processes. *Biometrics*, **65**, 1243–1253.

Lilienfeld, D.E., Stolley, P.D. and Lilienfeld, A.M. (1994) *Foundations of Epidemiology*, Oxford University Press, Oxford.

Lowe, J.M. and Sen, A.S. (1996) Gravity model applications in health planning. Analysis of an urban hospital market. *J Regional Sci*, **36**, 437–461.

Lunn, D.J., Thomas, A., Best, N. and Spiegelhalter, D. (2000) WinBUGS – a Bayesian modelling framework: concepts, structure, and extensibility. *Stat Comput*, **10**, 325–337.

Ma, H., Carlin, B.P. and Banerjee, S. (2010) Hierarchical and joint site-edge methods for Medicare hospice service region boundary analysis. *Biometrics*, **66**, 355–364.

Mackenbach, J.P., Stirbu, I., Roskam, A.J. *et al.* (2008) European union working group on socioeconomic inequalities in health. Socioeconomic inequalities in health in 22 European countries. *N Engl J Med*, **358**, 2468–2481. Erratum in *N Engl J Med*, **359**.

MacMahon, B. and Pugh, T.F. (1970) *Epidemiology*, Little Brown and Co, Boston.

MacNab, Y.C. (2003) Hierarchical Bayesian modeling of spatially correlated health service outcome and utilization rates. *Biometrics*, **59**, 305–316.

MacNab, Y.C. (2007) Mapping disability-adjusted life years: a Bayesian hierarchical model framework for burden of disease and injury assessment. *Stat Med*, **26**, 4746–4769.

MacNab, Y.C. (2009) Bayesian multivariate disease mapping and ecological regression with errors in covariates: Bayesian estimation of DALYs and 'preventable' DALYs. *Stat Med*, **28**, 1369–1385.

MacNab, Y.C. (2010) On Bayesian shared component disease mapping and ecological regression with errors in covariates. *Stat Med*, **29**, 1239–1249.

MacNab, Y.C. and Gustafson, P. (2007) Regression B-spline smoothing in Bayesian disease mapping: with an application to patient safety surveillance. *Stat Med*, **26**, 4455–4474.

MacNab, Y.C., Farrell, P.J., Gustafson, P. and Wen, S. (2004) Estimation in Bayesian disease mapping. *Biometrics*, **60**, 865–873.

MacNab, Y.C., Kmetic, A., Gustafson, P. and Sheps, S. (2006) An innovative application of Bayesian disease mapping methods to patient safety research: a Canadian adverse medical event study. *Stat Med*, **25**, 3960–3980.

Marshall, E. and Spiegelhalter, D. (2003) Approximate cross-validatory predictive checks in disease mapping models. *Stat Med*, **22**, 1649–1660.

Mathers, C.D., Ma Fat, D., Inoue, M. *et al.* (2005) Counting the dead and what they died from: an assessment of the global status of cause of death data. *WHO Bull*, **83**, 171–177.

May, L., Chretien, J.P. and Pavlin, J.A. (2009) Beyond traditional surveillance: applying syndromic surveillance to developing settings –opportunities and challenges. *BMC Public Health*, **9**, 242.

McLafferty, S.L. (2003) GIS and health care. *Annu Rev Public Health*, **24**, 25–42.

Mugglin, A.S., Cressie, N. and Gemmell, I. (2002) Hierarchical statistical modelling of influenza epidemic dynamics in space and time. *Stat Med*, **21**, 2703–2721.

Müller, P., Parmigiani, G. and Rice, K. (2006, July) FDR and Bayesian Multiple Comparisons Rules, Working Paper 115, Johns Hopkins University, Dept. of Biostatistics Working Papers, http://biostats.bepress.com/jhubiostat/paper115 (accessed April 18, 2012).

Ocaña-Riola, R. (2010) Common errors in disease mapping. *Geospat Health*, **4**, 139–154.

Ohlssen, D.I., Sharples, L.D. and Spiegelhalter, D.J. (2007) A hierarchical modelling framework for identifying unusual performance in health care providers. *J R Stat Soc A*, **170**, 865–890.

Oleske, D. (2009) *Epidemiology and the Delivery of Health Care Services: Methods and Applications*, 3rd edn, Springer, New York, NY.

Openshaw, S. (1984) *The Modifiable Areal Unit Problem*, Geo Books, Norwich.

Pfitzmann, A. and Hansen, M. (2010, August 10) A Terminology for Talking about Privacy by Data Minimization: Anonymity, Unlinkability, Undetectability, Unobservability, Pseudonymity, and Identity Management, Version v0.34, TU Dresden ULD, Kiel. Available at: http://dud.inf.tu-dresden.de/Anon_Terminology.shtml.

Pickle, L.W., Mungiole, M., Jones, G.K. and White, A.A. (1999) Exploring spatial patterns of mortality: the new atlas of United States mortality. *Stat Med*, **18**, 3211–3220.

Plummer, M. (2008) Penalized loss functions for Bayesian model comparison. *Biostatistics*, **9**, 523–539.

Prentice, R.L. and Sheppard, L. (1995) Aggregate data studies of disease risk factors. *Biometrika*, **82**, 113–125.

Rasmussen, S. (2004) Hierarchical modelling of small area and hospital variation in short-term prognosis after acute myocardial infarction. A longitudinal study of 35- to 74-year-old men in Denmark between 1978 and 1997. *Stat Med*, **23**, 2599–2621.

Reich, B.J., Hodges, J.S. and Zadnik, V. (2006) Effects of residual smoothing on the posterior of the fixed effects in disease-mapping models. *Biometrics*, **62**, 1197–1206.

Richardson, S., Stücker, I. and Hemon, D. (1987) Comparison of relative risks obtained in ecological and individual studies: some methodological considerations. *Int J Epidemiol*, **16**, 111–120.

Richardson, S., Thomson, A., Best, N. and Elliott, P. (2004) Interpreting posterior relative risk estimates in disease-mapping studies. *Environ Health Pers*, **112**, 1016–1025.

Riebler, A. and Held, L. (2010) The analysis of heterogeneous time trends in multivariate age–period–cohort models. *Biostatistics*, **11**, 57–69.

Rolka, H., Burkom, H., Cooper, G. *et al.* (2007) Issues in applied statistics for public health bioterrorism surveillance using multiple data streams: research need. *Stat Med*, **26**, 1834–1856.

Rue, H. and Held, L. (2005) *Gaussian Markov Random Fields: Theory and Applications*, Chapman & Hall, London.

Rue, H., Martino, S. and Chopin, N. (2009) Approximate Bayesian inference for latent Gaussian models by using integrated nested Laplace approximations (with discussion). *J R Stat Soc B*, **71**, 319–392.

Salway, R. and Wakefield, J. (2008) A hybrid model for reducing ecological bias. *Biostatistics*, **9**, 1–17.

Scheel, I., Green, P.J. and Rougier, J. (2011) Identifying influential model choices in Bayesian hierarchical models. *Scand J Stat*, **38**, 529–550.

Schmid, V. and Held, L. (2004) Bayesian extrapolation of space-time trends in cancer registry data. *Biometrics*, **60**, 1034–1042.

Schrödle, B. and Held, L. (2011) A primer on disease mapping and ecological regression using INLA. *Comput Stat*, **26**, 241–258.

Scott, J.G. and Berger, J.O. (2006) An exploration of aspects of Bayesian multiple testing. *J Stat Plan Infer*, **136**, 2144–2162.

Seppä, K., Hakulinen, T., Kim, H.L. and Läärä, E. (2010) Cure fraction model with random effects for regional variation in cancer survival. *Stat Med*, **29**, 2781–2793.

Shen, W. and Louis, T.A. (1998) Triple-goal estimates in two-stage hierarchical models. *J R Stat Soc B*, **60**, 455–471.

Sheppard, L. (2003) Insight on bias and information in group-level studies. *Biostatistics*, **4**, 265–278.

Shmueli, G. and Burkom, H. (2010) Statistical challenges facing early outbreak detection in biosurveillance. *Technometrics*, **52**, 39–51.

Short, M., Carlin, B.P. and Bushhouse, S. (2002) Using hierarchical spatial models for cancer control planning in Minnesota (United States). *Cancer Causes Control*, **13**, 903–916.

Silva, G.L., Dean, C.B., Niyonsenga, T. and Vanasse, A. (2008) Hierarchical Bayesian spatiotemporal analysis of revascularization odds using smoothing splines. *Stat Med*, **27**, 2381–2401.

Smans, M. and Esteve, J. (1992) Practical approaches to disease mapping, in *Geographical and Environmental Epidemiology: Methods for Small-Area Studies* (eds P. Elliot, J. Cuzick, D. English and R. Stern), Oxford University Press, Oxford, pp. 141–157.

Souza, W.V., Carvalho, M.S., Albuquerque, M.F. *et al.* (2007) Tuberculosis in intra-urban settings: a Bayesian approach. *Trop Med Int Health*, **12**, 323–330.

Spiegelhalter, D., Best, N., Carlin, B. and van der Linde, A. (2002) Bayesian measures of model complexity and fit (with discussion). *J R Stat Soc B*, **64**, 583–639.

Stern, H.S. and Cressie, N. (1999) Inference for extremes in disease mapping, in *Disease Mapping and Risk Assessment for Public Health* (eds A. Lawson, A. Biggeri, D. Boehning *et al.*), John Wiley & Sons, Ltd, Chichester.

Stern, H. and Cressie, N. (2000) Posterior predictive model checks for disease mapping models. *Stat Med*, **19**, 2377–2397.

Storey, J.D. (2002) A direct approach to false discovery rates. *J R Stat Soc B*, **64**, 479–498.

Storey, J.D. (2003) The positive false discovery rate: a Bayesian interpretation and the q-value. *Ann Stat*, **31**, 2013–2035.

Sun, L. and Clayton, M.K. (2008) Bayesian analysis of crossclassified spatial data with autocorrelation. *Biometrics*, **64**, 74–84.

Sweeting, M., De Angelis, D., Ades, A. and Hickman, M. (2009) Estimating the prevalence of ex-injecting drug use in the population. *Stat Methods Med Res*, **18**, 381–395.

Tassone, E.C., Miranda, M.L. and Gelfand, A.E. (2010) Disaggregate spatial modelling for areal unit categorical data. *Appl Statist*, **59**, 175–190.

VanderWeele, T.J. (2008) Ignorability and stability assumptions in neighbourhood effects research. *Stat Med*, **27**, 1934–1943.

Wakefield, J. (2007) Disease mapping and spatial regression with count data. *Biostatistics*, **8**, 158–183.

Wakefield, J. and Salway, R. (2001) A statistical framework for ecological and aggregate studies. *J R Stat Soc A*, **164**, 119–137.

Waller, L.A., Carlin, B.P., Xia, H. and Gelfand, A.E. (1997) Hierarchical spatio-temporal mapping of disease rates. *J Amer Stat Assoc*, **92**, 607–617.

Walter, S.D. (1993) Visual and statistical assessment of spatial clustering in mapping data. *Stat Med*, **12**, 1275–1291.

Wang, F., Luo, L. and McLafferty, S. (2009) Healthcare access, socioeconomic factors and late-stage cancer diagnosis: an exploratory spatial analysis and public policy implication. *Int J Public Policy*, **5**, 237–258.

White, G. and Ghosh, S.K. (2009) A stochastic neighborhood conditional autoregressive model for spatial data. *Comput Stat Data An*, **53**, 3033–3046.

Wiréhn, A.B., Karlsson, H.M. and Carstensen, J.M. (2007) Estimating disease prevalence using a population-based administrative healthcare database. *Scand J Public Health*, **35**, 424–431.

Womble, W.H. (1951) Differential systematics. *Science*, **114**, 315–322.

Zeger, S.L., Thomas, D., Dominici, F. *et al.* (2000) Exposure measurement error in time-series studies of air pollution: concepts and consequences. *Environ Health Persp*, **108**, 419–426.

Zhang, S., Sun, D., He, C.Z. and Schootman, M. (2006) A Bayesian semi-parametric model for colorectal cancer incidences. *Stat Med*, **25**, 285–309.

Zhou, H., Lawson, A.B., Hebert, J.R. *et al.* (2008) A Bayesian hierarchical modeling approach for studying the factors affecting the stage at diagnosis of prostate cancer. *Stat Med*, **27**, 1468–89.

Zhu, L. and Carlin, B.P. (2000) Comparing hierarchical models for spatio-temporally misaligned data using the deviance information criterion. *Stat Med*, **19**, 2265–2278.

# 10

# Process indicators and outcome measures in the treatment of acute myocardial infarction patients

Alessandra Guglielmi[1], Francesca Ieva[1],
Anna Maria Paganoni[1] and Fabrizio Ruggeri[2]
[1]*Department of Mathematics, Politecnico di Milano, Milan, Italy*
[2]*CNR IMATI, Milan, Italy*

## Synopsis

Studies of variations in healthcare utilization and outcome involve the analysis of multilevel, clustered data, considering in particular the estimation of a cluster-specific adjusted response, covariate effects and components of variance. Besides reporting on the extent of observed variations, these studies quantify the role of contributing factors including patients' and providers' characteristics. In addition, they may assess the relationship between healthcare process and outcomes. We consider Bayesian generalized linear mixed models to analyze MOMI$^2$ (Month MOnitoring Myocardial Infarction in MIlan) data on patients admitted with ST-elevation myocardial infarction (STEMI) diagnosis in the hospitals belonging to the Milano Cardiological Network. Both clinical registries and administrative databanks were used to predict survival probabilities. We fit a logit model for the survival probability with one random effect (the hospital), under a semiparametric prior. We take advantage of the in-built clustering property of the Dirichlet process prior assumed for the random-effects parameters to obtain a classification of providers.

*Statistical Methods in Healthcare*, First Edition. Edited by Frederick W. Faltin, Ron S. Kenett and Fabrizio Ruggeri.
© 2012 John Wiley & Sons, Ltd. Published 2012 by John Wiley & Sons, Ltd.

## 10.1    Introduction

Performance indicators for assessing quality in healthcare research have drawn more and more attention over recent years, since they can evaluate some aspects of the healthcare process, clinical outcomes and disease incidence. At the same time, questions about the right use of such indicators as a measure of quality of care have emerged.

Several examples, available in clinical literature (see, for instance, Hasday, Behar and Wallentin, 2002, and Saia, Marzocchi and Manari, 2009), make use of clinical registries to evaluate performance of medical institutions, because they enable people concerned with the healthcare governance to plan activities on real epidemiological evidence and needs; moreover clinical registries help in evaluating performance of structures they manage, providing knowledge about the number of cases, incidence, prevalence and survival concerning a specific disease.

In this work, clinical registries are used to model in-hospital survival of acute myocardial infarction patients, in order to classify providers' performances and to enable healthcare governance to better manage resources.

The disease we are interested in is the ST-segment Elevation acute Myocardial Infarction (STEMI): it consists of a stenotic plaque detachment, which causes a coronary thrombosis and a sudden critical reduction of blood flow in coronary vessels, leading to an inadequate feeding of myocardial muscle itself. STEMI is characterized by a very high incidence (650–700 events per month have been estimated in just the Lombardia Region, the inhabitants of which number approximately 10 million) and serious mortality (in Italy, about 8% in adults aged between 35 and 74 years). A case of STEMI is usually treated by percutaneous transluminal coronary angioplasty (PTCA): an empty and collapsed *balloon* on a guide wire, known as a balloon catheter, is passed into the narrowed or obstructed vessels and then inflated to a fixed size.

The balloon crushes the fatty deposit, so opening up the blood vessel to improved flow, and is then collapsed and withdrawn. Good results for the treatment can be evaluated for instance by observing, first, the in-hospital survival of inpatients.

For heart attacks, survival strongly depends on time saved during the process and, therefore, in this work we focus on the survival outcome. In any case, time indeed has a fundamental role in the overall STEMI healthcare process. By *Symptom Onset to Door time* we mean the time since symptom onset up to the arrival at the Emergency Room (ER); and *Door to Balloon time* (DB time) is the time from the arrival at the ER up to the surgical practice of PTCA. Clinical literature strongly stresses the connection between in-hospital survival and procedure time (Cannon, Gibson and Lambrew, 2000; Jneid, Fonarow and Cannon, 2008; MacNamara *et al.*, 2006): 90 minutes for DB time in the case of primary PTCA (i.e. PTCA without any previous pharmacological treatment) is the actual gold standard limit suggested by the American Heart Association (AHA)/American College of Cardiology (ACC) guidelines; see Antman, Hand and Amstrong, 2008.

The presence of differences in the outcomes of healthcare has been documented extensively in recent years. In order to design regulatory interventions by institutions, for instance, it is interesting to study the effects of variations in healthcare utilization on patients' outcomes, in particular examining the relationship between process indicators, which define regional or hospital practice patterns, and outcome measures, such as patients' survival or a treatment's efficacy.

Analyses of variations concerning the comparison of the performance of healthcare providers are commonly referred to as *provider profiling* (Normand, Glickman and Gatsonis, 1997; Racz and Sedransk, 2010).

The results of profiling analyses often have far-reaching implications. They are used to generate feedback for healthcare providers, to design educational and regulatory interventions by institutions and government agencies, to design marketing campaigns by hospitals and managed-care organizations, and, ultimately, used by individuals and managed-care groups to select healthcare providers.

The aim of this work is twofold: on one hand we want to quantify the magnitude of the variations in healthcare providers and to assess the role of contributing factors, including patients' and providers' characteristics, on survival outcome. Data on healthcare utilization have a 'natural' multilevel structure, usually with patients at the lower level and hospitals forming the upper-level clusters. Within this formulation, the main goal is to derive estimates of providers' effects; that is, differences between hospitals. On the other hand, we want to cluster hospitals according to their performance in patients' care.

Hierarchical regression modelling from a Bayesian non-parametric perspective provides a framework that can accomplish both these goals.

Here, this article considers a Bayesian generalized linear mixed model (Zeger and Karim, 1991) to predict the binary survival outcome by means of relevant covariates, taking into account overdispersion induced by the grouping factor, and modelling the random effects non-parametrically.

In particular, as in Kleinman and Ibrahim (1998), the random-effects parameters are a sample from a Dirichlet process prior (Ferguson, 1973), which provides a natural setting for the classification of hospitals thanks to the discreteness property of its trajectories. We illustrate the analysis on data coming from a survey on patients admitted with STEMI diagnosis in one of the structures belonging to the Milano Cardiological Network, using a logit model for the survival probability and a Dirichlet process for the distribution of the random effect.

For this analysis, patients are grouped by the hospital they have been admitted to for their infarction. A Markov chain Monte Carlo (MCMC) algorithm is necessary to compute the posterior distributions of parameters and predictive distributions of outcomes. The choice of covariates and link functions was suggested first in Ieva and Paganoni (2011), according to frequentist selection procedures and clinical know-how, and was confirmed in Guglielmi *et al.* (2012) using Bayesian tools.

Concerning modelling of provider's variability, we take advantage of in-built clustering provided by the Dirichlet process, jointly with the partitioning around medoids (PAM) algorithm (see Kaufman and Rousseeuw, 1987) to obtain classification of providers and estimation of their effects on survival outcome adjusted for case mix.

The advantages of a Bayesian non-parametric approach to this problem are more than one: the providers' profiling or patients' classification can be guided not only by statistical but also by clinical knowledge, hospitals with low exposure can be automatically included in the analysis, providers' profiling can be simply achieved through the posterior distribution of the hospital-effects parameters and in-built clustering is naturally provided by the non-parametric setting. In the following sections, dataset, performed analyses and results are discussed and future work is presented.

All the analyses have been performed with the R (version 2.10.1, R Development Core Team, 2009) program.

## 10.2   A semiparametric Bayesian generalized linear mixed model

We fit a generalized mixed-effects model for binary data from a Bayesian viewpoint. For patient $i = 1, \ldots, n_j$ in each hospital $j = 1, \ldots, J$, let $Y_{ij}$ be a Bernoulli random variable with mean $p_{ij}$, which represents the probability that the patient survived after STEMI.

The $p_{ij}$s are modelled through a logit regression with covariates $x := x_{ij}$, $x_{ij} \in \mathbb{R}^p$; that is,

$$Y_{ij} \mid p_{ij} \overset{ind}{\sim} \mathrm{Be}(p_{ij}), \quad j = 1, \ldots, J, \quad i = 1, \ldots, n_j \tag{10.1}$$

and

$$\mathrm{logit}(p_{ij}) = \log \frac{p_{ij}}{1 - p_{ij}} = \beta_0 + \sum_{h=1}^{p} \beta_h x_{ijh} + \sum_{l=1}^{J} b_l z_{il}, \tag{10.2}$$

where $b_j$ represents the $j$th hospital effect, and $z_{ij} = 1$, $z_{il} = 0$ for $l \neq j$.

We will denote by $\boldsymbol{\beta}$ the vector of regression parameters $(\beta_0, \beta_1, \ldots, \beta_p)$, which are called fixed effects, while $\boldsymbol{b} = (b_1, \ldots, b_j)$ are the random-effects parameters.

Note that (10.1)–(10.2) is a generalized linear mixed model with $(p + 1)$ regression coefficients and one random effect (the random intercept taking into account the grouping structure of hospitals).

Traditionally, $\boldsymbol{\beta}$ and $\boldsymbol{b}$ are assumed *a priori* independent, $\boldsymbol{\beta}$ is Gaussian distributed, and the random variables $b_j$, conditionally on $\sigma^2$, are independent identically Gaussian distributed, with random variance $\sigma^2$. Here, according to Kleinman and Ibrahim (1998), we assume a nonparametric prior for $\boldsymbol{b}$, namely the $b_j$s will be i.i.d. as a Dirichlet process, to include robustness to misspecification of the prior at this stage, since it is known that the regression parameters can be sensitive to the assumption of normality about the random effects.

Generally, nonparametric Bayesian models are assumed to avoid critical dependence on parametric assumptions, to robustify parametric models, or to perform sensitivity analysis for parametric models by embedding them in a larger encompassing nonparametric model. Priors under a nonparametric Bayesian perspective consist in probabilities on probability spaces: instead of considering models that can be indexed by a finite-dimensional parameter, we consider a prior probability $q$ for the unknown population distribution $G$, which, in the case considered here, represents the probability distribution of the random-effect parameter $b_j$. In particular, we will assume that $q$ is a Dirichlet prior, or, equivalently, that $G$ is a Dirichlet process. For a more formal definition of the Dirichlet process and a review of Bayesian nonparametric inference, see Müller and Quintana (2004). Here we would like to mention two properties only.

First, the Dirichlet process is indexed by two 'parameters', a positive parameter $\alpha$ and a distribution $G_0$ on $\mathbb{R}$. This latter represents the mean trajectory of $G$; that is, $\mathrm{E}(G(A)) = G_0(A)$ for each measurable subset $A$ of $\mathbb{R}$; in this way, the parametric model $G_0(\vartheta)$ could be embedded in a larger encompassing nonparametric model $G$. The parameter $\alpha$ is a precision parameter that defines variance: when $\alpha$ increases, the prior $q$ will concentrate more and more mass on the mean distribution $G_0$.

The second property we refer to is the discreteness of the trajectories of $G$: realizations of the Dirichlet process are infinite mixtures of point masses.

This feature of $G$ will provide a natural setting for the classification of the hospitals. In fact, if, conditionally on $G$, $b_1, \ldots, b_J$ are i.i.d. according to $G$, there is a positive probability, depending on $\alpha$ and the sample size $J$, of having coincident values among the $b_j$s, since the next observation $b_j$ in the sample will be a new sampled value from $G_0$ with probability $\alpha/(\alpha + j - 1)$, or one of the previously sampled $(b_1, b_2, \ldots, b_{j-1})$, with probability $1/(\alpha + j - 1)$; that is,

$$b_j \sim \frac{\alpha}{\alpha + j - 1} G_0 + \frac{1}{\alpha + j - 1} \sum_{i=1}^{j-1} \delta_{b_i}.$$

The joint posterior distribution of the random effects will preserve a similar clustering structure as well, so that this will prompt a natural classification among random effects, and consequently among hospitals (*a posteriori*). See the next section.

With more details, the prior we assume is

$$\beta \perp b, \ \beta \sim N_{p+1}(0, \Sigma_0)$$
$$b_1, \ldots, b_J \mid G \sim iid\, G,$$
$$G \sim Dir(\alpha N(\mu, \sigma^2)), \quad \mu \sim N(\mu_b, S_b), \quad \frac{1}{\sigma^2} \sim gamma\left(\frac{v_0}{2}, \frac{t_0^{-1}}{2}\right). \tag{10.3}$$

Integrating out $G$, this prior yields a prior marginal for $b_j$ which, conditionally on $(\mu, \sigma^2)$, is $N(\mu, \sigma^2)$, but hyperparameters are not fixed, and, to decrease sensitivity of the inferences, we assume them random, as in (10.3).

Moreover, as in the parametric case (Guglielmi *et al.*, 2012), the random-effects parameters are assumed dependent (this is a sensible assumption), and we will be able to use the whole dataset to make inferences on hospitals which have few or no patients in the study, borrowing strength across hospitals.

Of course, model (10.1)–(10.2) under prior (10.3) cannot be fit without resorting to an MCMC scheme to compute the joint posterior distribution of all parameters, which will be used to compute the Bayesian estimates of interest.

The joint posterior of the random-effect parameters can be expressed via the full conditionals of a Gibbs sampler algorithm: a 'new' value for $b_j$, given the data, the other random-effects parameters $b_{-j} = (b_1, \ldots, b_{j-1}, b_{j+1}, \ldots, b_J)$, and all the 'rest', is sampled either from a Gaussian distribution with some probability, or it is equal to one of the component $b_i$s of the vector $b_{-j}$ (with appropriate weight).

See Kleinman and Ibrahim (1998) for the expressions of the full conditionals of a Gibbs sampler algorithm in this case.

## 10.3   Hospitals' clustering

As we mentioned before, there will be coincident values among the MCMC-sampled random-effects parameters $b$.

Here we propose how to use the sample's bias of the posterior distribution of $b$, in order to detect a clustering structure between hospitals in affecting in-hospital survival.

Let us denote by $D(b_1, \ldots, b_J)$ a $J \times J$ symmetric matrix such that the $(i, j)$th element $[D(b_1, \ldots, b_J)]_{ij} = 1$ if $b_i \neq b_j$ and 0 otherwise.

Then we compute the matrix $D$ of the posterior means of $[D(b_1, \ldots, b_J)]_{ij}$; in short,

$$D = E[D(b_1, \ldots, b_J) \mid y]. \tag{10.4}$$

It is easy to prove that $D$ is a pseudo-metric which represents a mean dissimilarity measure between hospitals and can be computed via the MCMC samples of $(b_1, \ldots, b_J)$; a PAM algorithm is then applied to hospitals. A PAM algorithm is based on the search for $k$ representative objects, called *medoids*, among objects of the dataset (in our case hospitals).

These medoids are computed such that the total dissimilarity of all objects to their nearest medoid is minimal. In this case our goal is to find a subset $\{m_1, \ldots, m_k\} \subset \{1, \ldots, J\}$ which minimizes the objective function

$$\sum_{j=1}^{J} \min_{t=1,\ldots,k} D_{jm_t}$$

where $D_{ij}$ is the $(i, j)$th element of the matrix $D$.

A critical point is the choice of $k$, the number of groups: a helpful method is the computation of the average silhouette width, and the inspection of the silhouette plot of PAM. For each hospital $j$, we denote by $A$ the cluster to which it belongs and compute $a(j)$, the average dissimilarity of $j$ to all other objects of $A$:

$$a(j) = \frac{1}{|A| - 1} \sum_{i \in A, i \neq j} D_{ij}.$$

Now let us consider any cluster $C$ different from $A$ and denote by

$$d(j, C) = \frac{1}{|C| - 1} \sum_{i \in A} D_{ij}$$

the average dissimilarity of $j$ to all objects of $C$; we define $c(j)$ as the smallest value of all $d(j, C)$ for all clusters $C$ different from $A$. The *silhouette value* $s(j)$ of an object $j$ is defined as:

$$s(j) = \frac{c(j) - a(j)}{\max\{a(j), c(j)\}}.$$

The silhouette value $s(j)$ of each object $j$, the entire silhouette plot, that is, the plot of all $s(j)$, and the average of all silhouette values are qualitative indexes to judge and compare the results of different PAM procedures (see Struyf, Hubert and Rousseeuw, 1997 for more details).

## 10.4    Applications to AMI patients

The dataset we are interested in is about patients admitted with STEMI diagnosis in one of the hospitals belonging to the Milano Cardiological Network.

For these units, information concerning mode of admission (on his/her own or by three different types of 118 rescue units), demographic features (sex, age), clinical appearance (presenting symptoms and Killip class at admittance), Symptom Onset to Door time, in-hospital times (first ECG time, DB time), hospital organization (for example, admission during on/off hours) and clinical outcome (in-hospital survival) have been collected.

The Killip classification is a system used in individuals with an acute myocardial infarction, in order to risk stratify them into four severity classes. Individuals with a low Killip class are less likely to die within the first 30 days after their myocardial infarction than individuals with a high Killip class.

Previous frequentist and Bayesian analyses (for further details see Ieva and Paganoni, 2011; Guglielmi et al., 2012) pointed out that age, total ischemic time (Symptom Onset to Balloon time, denoted by OB) in the logarithmic scale and Killip of the patient, categorized as a binary variable, corresponding to 0 for less severe (Killip class equal to 1 or 2) and 1 for more severe (Killip class equal to 3 or 4) infarction, are the most significant factors in order to explain survival probability from a statistical and clinical point of view.

There are $n = n_1 + \cdots + n_J = 240$ patients, in $J = 17$ hospitals in the dataset; the number of patients per hospital ranges from 1 to 32, with a mean of 14.12. Each observation $y_i = 1$ if the $i$th patient survived; $y_i = 0$ otherwise.

In this study we fitted model (10.1)–(10.2) with $p = 3$, under (10.3), with the help of an R package called *DPpackage* (Jara, 2007).

In particular, we ran the function *DPglmm*, which adopts a slightly different parameterization from (10.3); however it is only the prior of $\beta_0$ which changes (Jara et al., 2011).

After some preliminary robustness analysis, the prior was fixed so that $\beta_1$, $\beta_2$, $\beta_3$ are i.i.d. according to $N(0,100)$, $\mu_b = 0$, $S_b = 100$, $\nu_0 = 5$, $t_0^{-1} = 30$, $a_0 = b_0 = 1$. We assumed such values since, in this case, the prior expected number of distinct values among the $b_j$s is 3 (which seems a sensible choice), however letting $\alpha$ be not too informative, while the prior expectation and variance of the conditional variance parameter $\Sigma$ are 10 and 200, respectively, so that the marginal prior variance of each $b_j$ is 110. Moreover, the robustness analysis showed that the inferences are not sensitive to different choices of $\mu_b$ and $\Sigma_0$.

Summary inferences about regression parameters can be found in Table 10.1.

A look at the posterior distributions of $\beta_i$, for $i = 1, 2, 3$ (not included here for brevity) shows that Killip and age have a negative effect on the survival probability, while log(OB) has a lighter influence on it.

Summary inferences about random-effects parameters can be found in Table 10.2. Their posterior means range from 3.058 to 4.783.

The marginal posterior densities of all the random-effects parameters, clustered in $k = 3$ groups, are depicted in Figure 10.1; while in Figure 10.2 the corresponding dissimilarity matrix $D$ is showed.

**Table 10.1**  Posterior means and standard deviations of the fixed-effects regression parameters.

|           |            | Mean      | sd      |
|-----------|------------|-----------|---------|
| Age       | $\beta_1$  | −0.0804   | 0.0339  |
| log(OB)   | $\beta_2$  | −0.1758   | 0.3733  |
| Killip    | $\beta_3$  | −1.6979   | 0.8747  |

**Table 10.2**  Posterior means and standard deviations of the random-effect regression parameters.

| $\beta_0 + b_j$ | $j = 1$ | $j = 2$ | $j = 3$ | $j = 4$ | $j = 5$ | $j = 6$ | $j = 7$ | $j = 8$ | $j = 9$ |
|---|---|---|---|---|---|---|---|---|---|
| Mean | 4.5472 | 4.1969 | 4.4122 | 4.6339 | 3.7119 | 3.9503 | 3.8226 | 4.0220 | 4.7827 |
| sd | 1.7269 | 1.5591 | 1.6909 | 1.7698 | 0.8452 | 0.9141 | 0.8585 | 1.5808 | 1.8754 |

| $\beta_0 + b_j$ | $j = 10$ | $j = 11$ | $j = 12$ | $j = 13$ | $j = 14$ | $j = 15$ | $j = 16$ | $j = 17$ |
|---|---|---|---|---|---|---|---|---|
| Mean | 3.1948 | 3.0584 | 4.4685 | 3.3995 | 3.9017 | 3.1969 | 3.3625 | 4.5776 |
| sd | 0.8174 | 0.8824 | 1.6423 | 0.8809 | 0.8816 | 0.8735 | 0.8854 | 1.7906 |

The PAM algorithm assigns hospitals 1, 4, 9, 12, 17 to the first group, hospitals 2, 3, 5, 6, 7, 8, 14 to the second and hospitals 10, 11, 13, 15, 16 to the third group.

According to the values of the posterior means of the $b_j$s, the related medoids (hospitals 4, 14 and 10) represent 'good', 'medium' and 'poor' performances, respectively. This classification is also in agreement with results in Guglielmi et al. (2012).

The clustering structure in three groups has been selected inspecting the boxplots of the dissimilarity between hospitals and the medoid of the cluster they belong to, obtained for different values of the number $k$ of clusters, and evaluating average silhouette widths. From this inspection, the presence of either $k = 2$ or $k = 3$ clusters can be supported; however we decided to propose a three-group clustering structure which distinguishes strongly good, or strongly poor hospitals from the medium ones.

In Table 10.3 the estimated in-hospital survival probabilities for different case-mixes, in 'poor', 'medium' and 'good' medoids are shown.

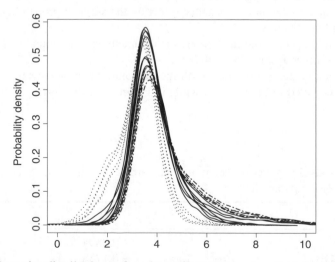

**Figure 10.1**  Posterior distributions of random-effects parameters $\beta_0 + b_j$, clustered in three groups: 'poor' (dotted), 'medium' (solid) and 'good' (dashed) hospitals.

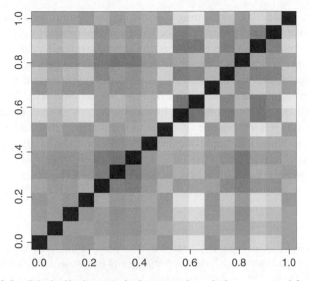

**Figure 10.2**  Dissimilarity matrix between hospitals, computed from (10.4).

In particular, when moving from a 'poor' hospital to a 'good' one, the in-hospital survival probability gain ranges from 1.5%, for a young patient with less severe infarction, to 32% in the case of an old patient with more severe infarction.

## 10.5   Summary

One of the major aims of this work is to measure the magnitude of the variations of healthcare providers and to assess the role of contributing factors, including patients' and providers' characteristics, on survival outcome.

Concerning patient features, we found out that Killip and age have a sharp negative effect on the survival probability, while the Symptom Onset to Balloon time has a lighter influence on it.

Moreover, the PAM algorithm applied to the posterior distributions of the hospitals' random effect enabled us to identify three clusters of providers: a group (hospitals 1, 4, 9, 12, 17) performing better than a medium group (hospitals 2, 3, 5, 6, 7, 8, 14) and a third group

**Table 10.3**   Estimated in-hospital survival probabilities for different case-mix, with average OB time 553 minutes in 'poor', 'medium' and 'good' medoids.

| Patient | | Estimated survival probability | | |
|---|---|---|---|---|
| Age | Killip | Poor | Medium | Good |
| 55 | 0 | 0.9805 | 0.9903 | 0.9953 |
| 85 | 0 | 0.8185 | 0.9014 | 0.9501 |
| 55 | 1 | 0.9021 | 0.9492 | 0.9749 |
| 85 | 1 | 0.4522 | 0.6260 | 0.7768 |

(hospitals 10, 11, 13, 15, 16) performing worse than the central one. Finally we estimated the effect of medoids for each group on in-hospital survival probability, to quantify loss/gain on survival due to provider's behaviour. This could be considered by healthcare governance as an instrument supporting healthcare decisions on optimizing network resources. Since the joint use of clinical registries and administrative databases proposed in this and previous analyses (see Ieva and Paganoni, 2010 and Barbieri, Grieco and Ieva, 2010) produced such useful results, a wider and more complete clinical register on STEMI, extended to the whole territory of Lombardia Region, has been planned and activated in 2010, called STEMI Archive.

As a future work we will apply the methodology and the models illustrated here to this larger dataset, to enable healthcare governance to establish benchmarks and to evaluate hospital network performances, then to offer better services to healthcare users.

# References

Antman, E.M., Hand, M., Amstrong, P.W. *et al.* (2008) Update of the ACC/AHA 2004 guidelines for the management of patients with ST elevation myocardial infarction. *Circulation*, **117**, 269–329.

Barbieri, P., Grieco, N., Ieva, F. *et al.* (2010) Exploitation, integration and statistical analysis of Public Health Database and STEMI Archive in the Lombardia region, in *Complex Data Modeling and Computationally Intensive Statistical Methods* (eds P. Mantovan and P. Secchi), Contributions to Statistics, Springer, pp. 41–56.

Cannon, C.P., Gibson, C.M., Lambrew, C.T. *et al.* (2000) Relationship of symptom-onset-to-balloon time and door-to-balloon time with mortality in patients undergoing angioplasty for acute myocardial infarction. *Journal of American Medical Association*, **283**(22), 2941–2947.

Ferguson, T.S. (1973) A Bayesian analysis of some nonparametric problems. *The Annals of Statistics*, **1**, 209–230.

Guglielmi, A., Ieva, F., Paganoni, A.M. and Ruggeri, F. (2012) A Bayesian random-effects model for survival probabilities after acute myocardial infarction. Chilean Journal of Statistics, **3**, 15–29.

Hasday, D., Behar, S., Wallentin, L. *et al.* (2002) A prospective survey of the characteristics, treatments and outcomes of patients with acute coronary syndromes in Europe and the Mediterranean basin. The Euro heart survey of acute coronary syndromes. *European Heart Journal*, **23**, 1190–1210.

Ieva, F. and Paganoni, A.M. (2010) Multilevel models for clinical registers concerning STEMI patients in a complex urban reality: a statistical analysis of MOMI$^2$ survey. *Communications in Applied and Industrial Mathematics*, **1**(1), 128–147.

Ieva, F. and Paganoni, A.M. (2011) Process indicators for assessing quality of hospitals care: a case study on STEM1 patients. *JP Journal of Biostatistics*, **6**(1), 53–75.

Jara, A. (2007) Applied Bayesian non- and semi-parametric inference using DPpackage. *Rnews*, **7**, 17–26.

Jara, A., Hanson, T., Quintana, F. *et al.* (2011) DPpackage: Bayesian non- and semi-parametric modelling in R. *Journal of Statistical Software*, **40**(5), 1–30.

Jneid, H., Fonarow, G., Cannon, C. *et al.* (2008) Impact of time of presentation on the care and outcomes of acute myocardial infarction. *Circulation*, **117**, 2502–2509.

Kaufman, L. and Rousseeuw, P.J. (1987) *Finding Groups in Data*, John Wiley & Sons, Inc., New York.

Kleinman, K.P. and Ibrahimm, J.G. (1998) A semi-parametric Bayesian approach to generalized linear mixed models. *Statistics in Medicine*, **17**, 2579–2596.

MacNamara, R.L., Wang, Y., Herrin, J. *et al.* (2006) Effect of door to balloon time on mortality in patients with ST-segment elevation myocardial infarction. *Journal of American College of Cardiology*, **47**, 2180–2186.

Müller, P. and Quintana, F.A. (2004) Nonparametric Bayesian data analysis. *Statistical Science*, **19**, 95–110.

Normand, S.T., Glickman, M.E. and Gatsonis, C.A. (1997) Statistical methods for profiling providers of medical care: issues and applications. *Journal of the American Statistical Association*, **92**, 803–814.

R Development Core Team (2009) *R: A Language and Environment for Statistical Computing*. R Foundation for Statistical Computing, Vienna, Austria.

Racz, J. and Sedransk, J. (2010) Bayesian and frequentist methods for provider profiling using risk-adjusted assessments of medical outcomes. *Journal of the American Statistical Association*, **105**(489), 48–58.

Saia, F., Marzocchi, A., Manari, G. *et al.* (2009) Patient selection to enhance the long-term benefit of first generation drug-eluting stents for coronary revascularization procedures: insights from a large multicenter registry. *Eurointervention*, **5**(1), 57–66.

Struyf, A., Hubert, M. and Rousseeuw, P.J. (1997) Clustering in an object-oriented environment. *Journal of Statistical Software*, **1**(4), 1–30.

Zeger, S.L. and Karim, M.R. (1991) Generalized linear models with random effects: a Gibbs Sampling approach. *Journal of the American Statistical Association*, **86**, 79–86.

# 11

# Meta-analysis

## Eva Negri

*Department of Epidemiology, Istituto di Ricerche Farmacologiche 'Mario Negri',
Milan, Italy*

## Synopsis

Systematic reviews were developed in order to provide a rigorous tool to summarize available evidence in a systematic, transparent and objective way. Meta-analysis is the statistical methodology that has been developed in order to summarize and compare results across studies. It consists of a large battery of tools where the individual study is the experimental unit. Although this chapter focuses mainly on the statistical tools, other aspects of a systematic review are also briefly discussed.

The choice of the effect measure that represents the results for each individual study depends on which data are available in these studies, on the research question investigated and on the properties of the possible measures, evaluated in the context of the specific study setting.

The methods for obtaining a summary estimate are broadly divided into two models: fixed-effects and random-effects models. The former assume that all studies measure the same effect, while the latter assume that studies measure different effects, and take between-studies variation into account. Among the fixed-effects methods, widely used are the inverse variance method and, for binary outcomes, the Mantel–Haenszel and the Peto method. The most commonly used random-effects model is the one developed by DerSimonian and Laird.

A fundamental component in meta-analyses is quantifying heterogeneity across studies and investigating its sources. This can be accomplished by forming groups of studies according to some given characteristic, and comparing the variance within and between groups. Meta-regression investigates whether a linear relationship exists between the outcome measure and one or more covariates.

*Statistical Methods in Healthcare*, First Edition. Edited by Frederick W. Faltin, Ron S. Kenett and Fabrizio Ruggeri.
© 2012 John Wiley & Sons, Ltd. Published 2012 by John Wiley & Sons, Ltd.

Besides sources of bias in the individual studies, biases pertaining to the reviewing process (e.g., publication bias, outcome bias) must also be investigated.

## 11.1   Introduction

In healthcare, there are generally several studies that investigate the same issue, with results that are not always consistent, either in the direction or in the strength of the association. In the past, in order to summarize the accumulated evidence on a given topic, narrative reviews were published, where one or more experts presented and commented on the available studies, drawing conclusions on the nature and strength of the association.

Meta-analysis, in the context of systematic reviews, was developed in order to provide a more rigorous tool to summarize available evidence in a systematic, transparent and objective way (Normand, 1999; Egger, Smith and Altman, 2001; Higgins and Green, 2011). The development of the meta-analytic approach has gone in parallel with the increasing popularity, in the scientific and medical community, of the concept of evidence-based medicine; that is, the 'conscientious, explicit, and judicious use of current best evidence in making decisions about the care of individual patients' (Sackett *et al.*, 1996).

Although the term meta-analysis has sometimes been used to indicate the whole reviewing process, the definitions of the Cochrane Collaboration for 'systematic review' and 'meta-analysis' are generally accepted. According to their online glossary, a systematic review is 'A review of a clearly formulated question that uses systematic and explicit methods to identify, select, and critically appraise relevant research, and to collect and analyse data from the studies that are included in the review. Statistical methods (*meta-analysis*) may or may not be used to analyse and summarise the results of the included studies.' Thus, meta-analysis is often part of a systematic review and is 'The use of statistical techniques in *a systematic review* to integrate the results of included studies'. Thus, the term meta-analysis refers to a number of quantitative methods used to compare and combine results of independent studies, where the experimental units are the studies.

Briefly, meta-analysis consists in identifying all the evidence on a given topic, and combining the results of the single studies in order to provide a summary quantitative estimate of the association of interest, which is generally a weighted average of the estimates from individual studies. Quantification and investigation of sources of heterogeneity is also part of the process.

Meta-analysis was first developed for the purpose of summarizing results from clinical trials in order to assess the efficacy/effectiveness of a given treatment. Its use has however extended to observational epidemiology and other settings, and meta-analysis of qualitative data has also been proposed (Dixon-Woods *et al.*, 2005).

The term meta-analysis is used both for the combination of results extracted from published articles and for the pooling of data from original studies at the individual patient level. Here we will mainly refer to meta-analyses of published articles. Many issues, however, apply to both types of meta-analysis.

When conducting a meta-analysis, the objective is not merely the computing of a combined estimate. Several other aspects of the evidence available for evaluation should be considered, like the quality of the studies included and hence their adequacy to provide information on the investigated issue, the consistency of results across studies and the evidence of publication bias.

In the following sections the steps needed to conduct a systematic review with meta-analysis will be described:

- formulation of the research question and definition of inclusion/exclusion criteria

- identification of relevant studies

- data extraction

- obtaining a common summary estimate

- measuring and investigation of heterogeneity

- other statistical issues

- presentation and interpretation of results.

Although a systematic review is an iterative process, because how to proceed depends heavily on what evidence is retrieved, it is good practice to prepare a protocol from the beginning, and amend it en route, according to what emerges during the process. These changes to the original protocol should be documented, motivated and described in the final report.

## 11.2    Formulation of the research question and definition of inclusion/exclusion criteria

The objective of the analysis must be formulated clearly and unambiguously. First the research question must be defined. The following step is to evaluate which studies can give an answer to this question. Thus, the inclusion and exclusion criteria for the potentially eligible studies must be set. One important issue when combining results of different studies is that they must be similar enough to be combined. One can also include different sets of studies in the same systematic review, and combine them by group, in order to investigate different aspects of a research question.

In order to define the inclusion/exclusion criteria, several aspects of the eligible studies must be considered. Among the issues to be considered when setting inclusion/exclusion criteria there are the following.

- **Study design.** One important issue is to decide whether to include controlled trials only or observational studies as well (Shrier *et al.*, 2007). This clearly depends on what kind of studies is available. Given that randomized controlled trials (RCTs) are in general less affected by bias than observational studies, these are generally preferred. Systematic reviews of the effects of treatments often are based on RCTs. However, not always is a meaningful mass of information available from RCTs. Often a meta-analysis of the available evidence from observational studies and/or from non-randomized clinical trials is performed to determine whether there is scope to conduct an RCT. Furthermore, where RCTs cannot be conducted, for example in the investigation of the effects of lifestyle habits such as tobacco smoking or alcohol drinking, the evidence relies on observational studies alone. Even among RCTs, some characteristics like duration or dose of the treatment or of the follow-up, blinding, and so on, may be part of the criteria for study selection.

- **Study population.** Even studies investigating the same exposure/treatment and the same outcome cannot be reasonably combined if the study populations are too different. For example, the ability of influenza vaccine to prevent influenza has been investigated in a huge number of studies, and several systematic reviews have been performed. These however, have generally focused on a specific study population, for example healthy children, healthy young adults, healthy older adults, or subjects with a specific disease, like cardiac problems, asthma or cystic fibrosis. Thus, among the criteria adopted for inclusion or exclusion of studies some characteristics of the study population are generally included, like age range, sex, ethnicity, disease status and so on.

- **Treatment/exposure under study.** The same treatment can have different effects at different doses, or according to route of administration, or in combination with other drugs. In the case of influenza vaccine, for example, inactivated and live-attenuated vaccines were considered separately (Negri *et al.*, 2005).

- **Outcome.** Also the definition of the outcome may be so different across studies that a combination of results would be meaningless. Influenza for example may be clinically defined, serologically confirmed or culture-confirmed (Negri *et al.*, 2005).

# 11.3    Identification of relevant studies

Once it has been made clear which kind of studies is to be included, a search strategy for the identification of the relevant studies must be developed (Lefebvre and Clarke, 2001; Crumley *et al.*, 2005). Identification of studies is generally performed using electronic databases such as Medline (www.ncbi.nlm.nih.gov/pubmed/) and Embase (www.embase.com/home). To search these databases a search strategy including combinations of various relevant keywords is designed.

Previous reviews and the references of identified papers are generally also used in order to identify relevant studies. Hand searching of selected journals is sometimes also performed. If congress abstracts or gray literature (e.g., reports of institutions or doctoral thesis) are also to be included, a search strategy for those too must be defined. Ideally all eligible studies should be included, in order to provide a comprehensive overview of the research question. Failure to identify all (or almost all) eligible studies will decrease the quality of the systematic review.

It is not always easy to determine whether a study meets the inclusion criteria from the title/abstract alone. Thus typically the first sift of the results of electronic databases yields a number of articles for which the full text must be retrieved in order to decide whether to include them or not.

If multiple publications are available for the same study, the most up-to-date one or the one providing the more detailed information may be chosen. In some cases, different publications may present different outcomes.

It is preferable that the decision of whether the study should be included or not is performed independently by two (or more) persons and an additional researcher is involved when differences emerge.

Given the critical importance of study retrieval this must be documented in the report. A flowchart of the selection of publications is often presented.

## 11.4    Statistical analysis

Once the studies have been identified, the statistical strategy originally planned must be revised, according to how many studies are available, their characteristics and what data are available from the individual studies. If the available studies are too different, one may also decide not to perform the meta-analysis. If relatively homogeneous groups of studies can be formed, one may combine studies in each group. As mentioned before, in the meta-analysis on influenza vaccine in children, three different groups were formed according to how the outcome was measured (clinical/serologically-confirmed/culture-confirmed influenza) and these groups were analyzed separately (Negri *et al.*, 2005).

Often, studies are combined also if they differ by some characteristic, and further subgroup analyses are conducted in order to determine whether this characteristic influences the overall result, and explains (part of) the heterogeneity between studies.

The nature of the data (dichotomous or continuous) and the effect measure of interest must be defined.

For *dichotomous outcomes*, the most commonly used effect measures are the risk ratio or relative risk (RR), the odds ratio (OR) and the risk difference (RD) or absolute risk reduction. The OR, under some circumstances, can be considered an estimator of the RR. Thus, if cohort and case-control studies are combined, the RR is defined as the effect measure of interest, and ORs and RRs are sometimes combined. The RR and OR however are different estimators; particularly when the event under study is common they yield different results and these differences must be carefully explored.

For *continuous outcomes* the most used outcomes are the mean difference (MD) and the standardized mean difference (SMD).

For *survival (time to event) outcomes* the most commonly used measure is the hazard ratio (HR), although sometimes survival data are analyzed as dichotomous outcomes. Furthermore, RRs and HRs and ORs are sometimes combined, as estimators of the RR.

The selection of the statistic which summarizes the effect of each study, and that will then be combined in order to obtain a pooled estimate, is an important step. Consistency of effect across studies, ease of interpretation and mathematical properties have been suggested as grounds for the choice. This choice should rely on the understanding of the dynamics of the various models and the evaluation of their consistency as estimators of treatment effects in a specific setting (Deeks, Altman and Bradburn, 2001).

## 11.5    Extraction of study-specific information

Once the studies have been identified and retrieved, the data needed to perform the meta-analysis must be extracted from the publications. This may include information on the study design, the study population, number of subjects in categories of exposure/outcome, statistical methods and so on. Clearly, the data extracted depend on the chosen measure of effect.

All characteristics that will then be used to perform analyses of subgroups of studies, as well as indicators of study quality and other variables that may be important to describe the study (e.g., location, response rate) are also recorded.

The extraction of data from the individual studies is another important step, where often unexpected problems arise. Errors in published articles are quite common, and sometimes a study that meets the inclusion criteria must be excluded because the data in the tables are inconsistent.

It is preferable that two or more researchers extract the data and judge the quality of the study independently, in order to improve the quality of this process.

In general a table presenting the main features of each included study is provided. Sometimes, features of excluded studies are also presented, together with the reason for exclusion (e.g., non-randomized study, no control group)

Not always is all the information needed to perform the meta-analysis available in a published study. In this case the needed information may be requested directly from the authors. If this is not possible, alternative methods may be used.

The two measures needed to combine studies are the study-specific estimate of the effect and its standard error $s_i$, or the data to compute these.

If $s_i$ is not provided, it can be estimated from the confidence interval (CI).

For example, from the RR (or OR) and 95% CI the $s_i$ of the log(RR) can be computed according to the formula:

$$s_i = \frac{\log CI_{up} - \log CI_{lo}}{3.92}$$

where $CI_{up}$ and $CI_{lo}$ are the upper and lower confidence limits.

If only the p-value is provided, then

$$s_i = \frac{\log RR}{Z_p}$$

is considered, where $Z_p$ is the value of the Gaussian distribution that corresponds to the given p-value.

Corresponding formulas can be derived for other estimators.

Methods for imputation of missing standard errors have also been suggested (Furukawa *et al.*, 2006; Ma *et al.*, 2008).

## 11.6   Outcome measures

### 11.6.1   Binary outcome measures

For the standard $2 \times 2$ table in study $i$,

|              | Event |       |
| ------------ | :---: | :---: |
| Group        |  Yes  |  No   |
| Experimental | $a_i$ | $b_i$ |
| Control      | $c_i$ | $d_i$ |

let $N_i = a_i + b_i + c_i + d_i$.

Then the OR, RR and RD and their standard errors are computed as follows:

$$OR_i = \frac{a_i d_i}{b_i c_i}; \quad SE\left[\ln\left(OR_i\right)\right] = \sqrt{\frac{1}{a_i} + \frac{1}{b_i} + \frac{1}{c_i} + \frac{1}{d_i}}$$

$$RR_i = \frac{\dfrac{a_i}{(a_i + b_i)}}{\dfrac{c_i}{(c_i + d_i)}}; \quad SE\left[\ln\left(RR_i\right)\right] = \sqrt{\frac{1}{a_i} + \frac{1}{c_i} + \frac{1}{a_i + b_i} + \frac{1}{c_i + d_i}}$$

$$RD_i = \frac{a_i}{(a_i + b_i)} - \frac{c_i}{(c_i + d_i)}; \quad SE\left(RD_i\right) = \sqrt{\frac{a_i b_i}{(a_i + b_i)^3} + \frac{c_i d_i}{(c_i + d_i)^3}}$$

The *Peto OR* (Yusuf *et al.*, 1985) is based on the differences between observed and expected numbers of events (O-E).

It is defined as follows:

$$OR_{Peto,i} = \exp\left(\frac{O_i - E_i}{V_i}\right),$$

where

$$O_i = a_i; \quad E_i = \frac{(a_i + b_i)(a_i + c_i)}{N_i}$$

are the observed and expected numbers of events in study $i$, respectively, and

$$V_i = \frac{(a_i + b_i)(c_i + d_i)(a_i + c_i)(b_i + d_i)}{N_i^2(N_i - 1)}$$

is the hypergeometric variance of $a_i$.

The standard error is given by

$$SE\left[\ln\left(OR_{Peto,i}\right)\right] = \sqrt{\frac{1}{V_i}}.$$

## 11.6.2    Continuous outcome measures

For each study, results can be summarized in the following table:

| Group | Mean response | Standard deviation | Group size |
|---|---|---|---|
| Experimental | $m_{1i}$ | $s_{1i}$ | $n_{1i}$ |
| Control | $m_{2i}$ | $s_{2i}$ | $n_{2i}$ |

Let $N_i = n_{1i} + n_{2i}$ and

$$s_i = \sqrt{\frac{(n_{1i} - 1)s_{1i}^2 + (n_{2i} - 1)s_{2i}^2}{N_i - 2}},$$

then the *mean difference* (MD) is given by

$$MD_i = m_{1i} - m_{2i}; \quad SE\,(MD_i) = \sqrt{\frac{s_{1i}^2}{n_{1i}} + \frac{s_{2i}^2}{n_{2i}}}.$$

There are several forms for the weighted mean difference (WMD).One is Cohen's *d*, which is the ratio of the difference of the means in the two groups to the pooled standard deviation:

$$d_i = \frac{m_{1i} - m_{2i}}{s_i}$$

and

$$SE\,(d_i) = \sqrt{\frac{N_i}{n_{1i}n_{2i}} + \frac{d_i^2}{2(N_i - 2)}}.$$

Other forms for the WMD corrected for small sample bias can be found in Deeks, Altman and Bradburn (2001).

## 11.7  Estimation of the pooled effect

In general, the summary estimate is a weighted average of the estimates in the single studies (Deeks, Altman and Bradburn, 2001).

There are two different models to estimate the pooled effect: *fixed-effect models and random-effect models.*

### 11.7.1  Fixed-effect models

In the *fixed-effect model* it is assumed that all studies measure the same effect. The estimate $\gamma_i$ of study *i* is a realization of a normal distribution with mean $\theta$, which is the same for each *i*;

$$\gamma_i \approx N\left(\theta, s_i^2\right).$$

Thus, all studies derive from the same homogeneous population. The pooled estimate $\hat{\theta}$ is a weighted average of the effects $\gamma_i$ of the single studies.

$$\hat{\theta} = \frac{\sum w_i \gamma_i}{\sum w_i}.$$

If the $w_i$ are all 1, then $\hat{\theta}$ is simply the mean of the $\gamma_i$.
The variance of $\hat{\theta}$ is given by

$$Var(\hat{\theta}) = \frac{\sum w_i var(\gamma_i)}{\sum w_i}.$$

When dealing with ratio measures (OR, RR, HR), the $\gamma_i$ are the natural logarithms of the measure and $\ln(\hat{\theta})$ substitutes $\hat{\theta}$ in the left-hand side of the previous equation.

A test of heterogeneity between studies is given by:

$$Q = \sum w_i (\gamma_i - \hat{\theta})^2$$

which, under the null hypothesis of no difference across studies ($H_0 : \theta_1 = \theta_2 = \cdots = \theta_k$) follows a $\chi^2$ distribution with $k - 1$ degrees of freedom, where $k$ is the number of studies.

The choice of the weights determines the influence of each single study on the summary estimate. There are several ways to choose the weights. In the following the more often used ones are presented.

### 11.7.1.1   Inverse variance method

A general fixed-effects method to combine the measures from the single studies is the inverse variance method in which the weight of each study is the inverse of the variance $s_i^2$ of the estimate (or of its natural logarithm). Thus, the larger the study the greater its weight is. This method can be used for many types of outcome measures, and it is the (fixed-effects) method usually used for continuous outcome measures; while for binary outcomes the Mantel–Hanszel and Peto methods are preferred.

Thus $w_i = \frac{1}{s_i^2}$ and

$$\hat{\theta} = \frac{\sum \dfrac{\gamma_i}{s_i^2}}{\sum \dfrac{1}{s_i^2}},$$

and the variance is:

$$Var(\hat{\theta}) = Var\left(\frac{\sum \dfrac{\gamma_i}{s_i^2}}{\sum \dfrac{1}{s_i^2}}\right) = \frac{1}{\sum \dfrac{1}{s_i^2}}.$$

### 11.7.1.2   Mantel–Haenszel method

A fixed-effects method often used for binary outcomes is the Mantel–Haenszel method (Mantel and Haenszel, 1959; Robins, Breslow and Greenland, 1986; Deeks, Altman and Bradburn, 2001), where the weights used vary according to the chosen measure of effect (OR, RR, RD). This method has been shown to perform better than the inverse variance method when data are sparse.

The summary statistic is

$$\hat{\theta}_{MH} = \frac{\sum (w_i \gamma_i)}{\sum w_i}.$$

The Mantel–Haenszel pooled estimate differs depending on whether we are pooling ORs, RRs or RDs.

If $\gamma_i = OR_i$ ($\forall i$) then $w_i = \dfrac{b_i c_i}{N_i}$ and

$$SE\left[\ln\left(OR_{MH}\right)\right] = \sqrt{\frac{1}{2}\left(\frac{E}{R^2} + \frac{F+G}{R \times S} + \frac{H}{S^2}\right)}$$

where

$$R = \sum \frac{a_i d_i}{N_i}; \quad S = \sum \frac{b_i c_i}{N_i};$$

$$E = \sum \frac{(a_i + d_i)a_i d_i}{N_i^2}; \quad F = \sum \frac{(a_i + d_i)b_i c_i}{N_i^2};$$

$$G = \sum \frac{(b_i + c_i)a_i d_i}{N_i^2}; \quad H = \sum \frac{(b_i + c_i)b_i c_i}{N_i^2}.$$

If $\gamma_i = RR_i$ then $w_i = \dfrac{c_i(a_i + b_i)}{N_i}$ and

$$SE\left[\ln\left(RR_{MH}\right)\right] = \sqrt{\frac{P}{R \times S}},$$

where

$$P = \sum \frac{((a_i + b_i)(c_i + d_i)(a_i + c_i)) - a_i c_i N_i}{N_i^2};$$

$$R = \sum \frac{a_i(c_i + d_i)}{N_i}; \quad S = \sum \frac{c_i(a_i + b_i)}{N_i}.$$

If $\gamma_i = RD_i$ then $w_i = \dfrac{(a_i + b_i)\,(c_i + d_i)}{N_i}$ and

$$SE\,(RD_i) = \sqrt{\frac{J}{K^2}},$$

where

$$J = \sum \frac{a_i b_i(c_i + d_i)^3 + c_i d_i(a_i + b_i)^3}{(a_i + b_i)(c_i + d_i)N_i^2}; \quad K = \sum \frac{(a_i + b_i)(c_i + d_i)}{N_i}.$$

### 11.7.1.3   Peto method or one-step method

The summary OR is given by (Yusuf *et al.*, 1985; Deeks, Altman and Bradburn, 2001):

$$OR_{Peto} = \exp\left(\frac{\sum V_i \ln\left(OR_{Peto,i}\right)}{\sum V_i}\right)$$

and

$$SE\left[\ln\left(OR_{Peto}\right)\right] = \frac{1}{\sqrt{\sum V_i}}.$$

Thus, the summary $\ln(OR_{Peto})$ is given by the sum of the (O-E) across studies, divided by the sum of their variances. This method makes it very easy to compute summary estimates across subgroups of studies, once the observed and expected numbers and $V_i$ are provided for each study.

The Peto method has the advantage that it works even when there are no events in one group (without need of continuity correction), but it has been shown to be biased when the treatment effect is strong, and when data are unbalanced (Greenland and Salvan, 1990).

## 11.7.2 Random-effects models

In *random-effect models* it is assumed that studies do not measure the same parameter. It is assumed that the estimate in each study derives from a normal population:

$$\gamma_i \approx N(\vartheta_i, s_i^2)$$

(note that in this case $\vartheta_i$ is not the same for all studies)

Moreover, the parameters $\vartheta_i$ from different studies also derive from a normal distribution:

$$\vartheta_i \approx N(\theta, \tau^2).$$

The random-effects model thus takes into account variance between, as well as within, the individual studies.

The random-effects method proposed by DerSimonian and Laird (DL) (DerSimonian and Laird, 1986) is the simplest and most widely used. It is similar to the inverse variance method:

$$\hat{\theta}_{DL} = \frac{\sum w_i^* \gamma_i}{\sum w_i^*},$$

where

$$w_i^* = \frac{1}{s_i^2 + \tau_{DL}^2}$$

and

$$Var(\hat{\theta}_{DL}) = \frac{1}{\sum w_i^*};$$

$\tau_{DL}^2$ is computed from the Q-statistics for heterogeneity:

$$\tau_{DL}^2 = Max\left(\frac{Q - (k - 1)}{\sum w_i - \frac{\sum w_i^2}{\sum w_i}}, 0\right),$$

where the $w_i$ are the inverse variance weights $\frac{1}{s_i^2}$.

If $Q < (k-1)$, then $\tau_{DL}^2$ is set to 0, and the DL method coincides with the fixed-effects inverse variance method. Other more general random-effects methods have also been proposed (DerSimonian and Kacker, 2007).

The *confidence intervals* for the pooled estimates, in all cases, can be computed using the formula

$$\hat{\theta} \pm Z_{\frac{\alpha}{2}} \sqrt{Var(\hat{\theta})}.$$

In the case of rate ratios, $\hat{\theta}$ is the natural logarithm of the OR or RR.

## 11.7.3    Random-effects vs. fixed-effects models

In fixed-effects models it is assumed that the sample error is the only variation between studies, and the studies all measure the same effect, while in random-effects models the studies measure different effects. However, the further assumption is made that the studies are a random sample of a hypothetical distribution of studies. Both assumptions have been criticized, since populations in the various studies have different characteristics, and it is unreasonable to think that the treatment effect may be the same across studies, On the other hand, it is sometimes unreasonable to assume that the available studies are a sample of a hypothetical distribution of possible studies.

Basically, the fixed-effects and random-effects models differ according to the relative weight that they give to large studies as compared to small ones. In fixed-effects models, large studies carry considerably more weight than small studies. In the case where several small studies and one or a few very large studies are available, the influence of the large studies on the pooled estimate may be overwhelming. Random-effects models give comparatively more weight to small studies. When heterogeneity between studies is small, then large studies have considerably more weight than small ones. However, if heterogeneity between studies is large, $\tau_{DL}^2$ will be large as compared to individual study variances, and the weights $\frac{1}{s_i^2 + \tau_{DL}^2}$ will tend to be dominated by it, and therefore become very similar.

Also when using random-effects models one must not fall into the error of thinking that even very heterogeneous studies can be pooled, since random-effects models 'take heterogeneity into account'. Although random-effects models yield a larger variance of the pooled estimate, and hence wider confidence intervals, they are not always conservative, compared to fixed-effects models (Poole and Greenland, 1999). In general, in the presence of considerable heterogeneity the appropriateness of pooling results across studies must be questioned (Poole and Greenland, 1999; Al Khalaf, Thalib and Doi, 2011). On the other hand, there may be good reasons to pool data also under heterogeneity (Peto, 1987).

It has been pointed out that the interpretation of results under random-effects models should be different, and prediction intervals should be computed, which provide the predicted range for the true treatment effect in individual study settings (Riley, Higgins and Deeks, 2011).

If the number of available studies is small, it may not be possible to obtain an accurate estimate of the between-studies variance, which is used by random-effects models to compute the pooled estimate (Borenstein *et al.*, 2002).

## 11.8   Exploring heterogeneity

Heterogeneity can be quantified using the Q-statistic presented before, and comparing it to a $\chi^2$ distribution with $k-1$ degrees of freedom. The power of this test is low when a small number of studies is available.

Another statistic derived from the Q-statistic that has been proposed (Higgins and Thompson, 2002; Higgins *et al.*, 2003) is

$$I^2 = 100\% \times Max \left( \frac{Q - (k-1)}{Q}, 0 \right).$$

$I^2$ ranges from 0 to 100%, and describes the percentage of total variation across studies that is due to heterogeneity rather than chance.

Besides quantifying heterogeneity, an important aspect of meta-analysis is investigating its sources (Glasziou and Sanders, 2002). These can be artifactual or real. Artifactual heterogeneity can arise, for example, when the wrong effect measure has been chosen, or if studies with poorer design (e.g., not blinded) provide stronger effects, or if the outcome has been measured in different ways.

Often meta-analysis has been criticized because, in the case of heterogeneous studies, deriving a summary estimate implies mixing 'apples with oranges'. It has however also been pointed out that exploring real heterogeneity improves our understanding of the effect of a treatment, by identifying groups of patients who will benefit most from the treatment, and avoiding using the same treatment on patients that do not benefit from it.

A way of exploring heterogeneity is to form subgroups of studies (e.g., randomized trials *versus* observational studies, blinded *versus* open-label studies, studies conducted in America *versus* Europe *versus* Asia) and compare the within- and between-studies variances. When data are available, even subgroups of patients within the same studies (e.g., men *versus* women, or, more severe *versus* less severe cases) can be compared. The more the groups appear homogeneous within, and heterogeneity is mostly between groups, the more the grouping variable explains heterogeneity.

Let

$$Q_T = \sum w_i (\gamma_i - \hat{\theta})^2$$

be the heterogeneity between all $k$ studies.

If we divide these studies into two groups, $G_1$ and $G_2$ respectively, of $k_1$ and $k_2$ studies, with $k_1 + k_2 = k$, we can compute the summary estimates $\theta_{G_1}$ and $\theta_{G_2}$ using only the studies in $G_1$ and $G_2$, respectively. Then, again under the null hypothesis of no difference across studies,

$$Q_{G_1} = \sum w_i (\gamma_i - \hat{\theta}_{G_1})^2; \ i \in G_1; \quad Q_{G_2} = \sum w_i (\gamma_i - \hat{\theta}_{G_2})^2; \ i \in G_2$$

follow the $\chi^2$ distribution with $k_1 - 1$ and $k_2 - 1$ degrees of freedom, respectively.

They give a measure of the heterogeneity within groups.

Then $Q_B = Q_T - (Q_{G_1} + Q_{G_2})$ follows the $\chi^2$ distribution with one degree of freedom, and gives a measure of heterogeneity between groups.

This can easily be extended to the case in which more than two groups are formed.

A more sophisticated tool for exploring heterogeneity is *meta-regression* (van Houwelingen *et al.*, 2002; Baker *et al.*, 2009). Its aim is to investigate whether a linear relationship exists between the outcome measure and one or more covariates.

A linear model is fitted where the experimental units are the studies included in the meta-analysis, the dependent variable is the effect size, and the independent variables are study characteristics (e.g., mean age of participants). Weights are generally used, and they can derive from fixed-effect models (e.g., inverse variance weights), or from random-effects models (the DerSimonian and Laird weights).

## 11.9 Other statistical issues

*Influence analysis* is also often performed, by excluding each study in turn (or a group of studies with certain characteristics) and evaluating the change in the summary estimate. This allows evaluation of how influential a study/group of studies is on the overall effect.

Models for performing *dose-response* analysis have also been developed when effect estimates for different levels of exposure or treatment are provided for the included studies. A simple approach is to estimate the linear change in the effect measure (or its natural logarithm in the case of ORs or RRs) per unit of exposure, and to combine these estimates across studies. Given that, in a study, effect estimates at different levels of exposure are often referred to the same baseline level, this implies pooling correlated estimates to compute regression slopes. Greenland and Longnecker (1992) proposed a method that accounts for the correlations but requires only the summary estimates and marginal data from the studies. This method, based on generalized least square regression, estimates the covariance matrix between estimates from the same study and also allows estimation of nonlinear trend components. Methods based on random-effects models have also been proposed (Rota *et al.*, 2010).

*Bayesian methods* for meta-analysis have also been developed (Sutton and Abrams, 2001). Most applications in meta-analysis used non-informative or empirical Bayesian (EB) methods, which estimate the hyper-parameters of the prior distribution from the data. Informative or fully Bayesian (FB) methods use external evidence/subjective beliefs to estimate prior distributions for the model parameters, and have more computational complexities. Recently, however, the development of simulation-based methods (Markov chain Monte Carlo) has rendered the application of FB methods easier, further promoted by the development of the computer software WinBUGS (www.mrc-bsu.cam.ac.uk/bugs/winbugs/contents.shtml). External information can, for example, be derived from the results of a prior meta-analysis or by eliciting the opinion of a group of experts. As an example, Deandrea and colleagues performed a meta-analysis of risk factors for falls in older people, incorporating opinions obtained from geriatricians and general practitioners using an *ad hoc* developed questionnaire (Deandrea, Negri and Ruggeri, 2012).

## 11.10 Forest plots

Graphs are an important tool for presenting results from individual studies and pooled estimates, investigating heterogeneity and publication bias, performing model diagnostics and so on (Anzures-Cabrera and Higgins, 2010).

The *forest plot* presents, in a single graph, results from individual studies as well as the pooled estimate (if computed). In this plot the effect estimate for each study is presented (Anzures-Cabrera and Higgins, 2010); each one is represented by a square, the area of which is proportional to the weight assigned to the corresponding study in the pooled estimate. Thus studies with a larger weight tend to attract the reader's attention. A line through the square and parallel to the axis providing the effect measure scale represents the confidence interval. The pooled effect estimate may also be provided, generally by a diamond centered on the point estimate and whose vertices represent the confidence interval. Studies can be subdivided in subgroups, and pooled estimates for these subgroups can also be provided. Figure 11.1 provides an example of a forest plot evaluating the effect of an active treatment in two subgroups of studies and overall. For ratio measures a logarithmic scale is sometimes used.

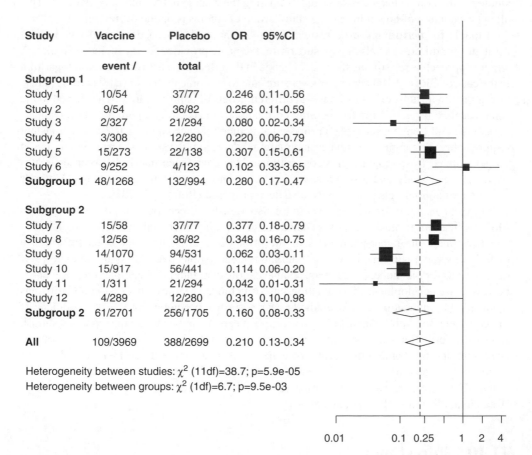

| Study | Vaccine | Placebo | OR | 95%CI |
|---|---|---|---|---|
| | event / | total | | |
| **Subgroup 1** | | | | |
| Study 1 | 10/54 | 37/77 | 0.246 | 0.11-0.56 |
| Study 2 | 9/54 | 36/82 | 0.256 | 0.11-0.59 |
| Study 3 | 2/327 | 21/294 | 0.080 | 0.02-0.34 |
| Study 4 | 3/308 | 12/280 | 0.220 | 0.06-0.79 |
| Study 5 | 15/273 | 22/138 | 0.307 | 0.15-0.61 |
| Study 6 | 9/252 | 4/123 | 0.102 | 0.33-3.65 |
| **Subgroup 1** | 48/1268 | 132/994 | 0.280 | 0.17-0.47 |
| | | | | |
| **Subgroup 2** | | | | |
| Study 7 | 15/58 | 37/77 | 0.377 | 0.18-0.79 |
| Study 8 | 12/56 | 36/82 | 0.348 | 0.16-0.75 |
| Study 9 | 14/1070 | 94/531 | 0.062 | 0.03-0.11 |
| Study 10 | 15/917 | 56/441 | 0.114 | 0.06-0.20 |
| Study 11 | 1/311 | 21/294 | 0.042 | 0.01-0.31 |
| Study 12 | 4/289 | 12/280 | 0.313 | 0.10-0.98 |
| **Subgroup 2** | 61/2701 | 256/1705 | 0.160 | 0.08-0.33 |
| | | | | |
| **All** | 109/3969 | 388/2699 | 0.210 | 0.13-0.34 |

Heterogeneity between studies: $\chi^2$ (11df)=38.7; p=5.9e-05
Heterogeneity between groups: $\chi^2$ (1df)=6.7; p=9.5e-03

0.01        0.1  0.25        1  2  4

Odds ratio

**Figure 11.1** Example of a forest plot evaluating the effect of a vaccine in two subgroups of studies, and overall.

## 11.11   Publication and other biases

If the studies included in a systematic review are prone to bias, this will carry forward to the review as well. The meta-analysis of observational studies has been particularly criticized, since these types of studies are more prone to bias than controlled trials. Therefore, particular attention should be devoted to exploring possible sources of bias in the individual studies, and to evaluating, whenever possible, their effect on the pooled estimate.

Besides the distortions inherent in the individual studies included, causes of bias specifically deriving from the meta-analysis *per se* must also be considered (Sterne, Egger and Smith, 2001). Among these, publication bias is the one more often discussed (Thornton and Lee, 2000). There are several indications that studies that have a statistically significant result are more likely to be published than negative studies; they are more likely to be published in English (language bias), to undergo repeated publications and to be cited by other authors. Therefore, they are also easier to be identified and included in a meta-analysis. Therefore, in a systematic review, efforts must be devoted to ensure the retrieval of (possibly) all relevant studies. The inclusion of studies published in languages other than English, of abstracts and of gray literature (e.g., doctoral theses) has been recommended, although critics have pointed out that these study presentations are generally of lower quality than published studies that have undergone peer review. On the other hand, only if these unpublished studies have been retrieved can their quality and influence on the overall estimate be evaluated, and they can be excluded if deemed necessary (Cook *et al.*, 1993). Results from published and unpublished studies can be compared, in order to investigate publication bias.

Graphical methods and statistical tests for investigating publication bias have been developed (Sterne, Egger and Smith, 2001). They rely on the fact that large trials are more likely to be published, even when negative, than small trials. However, even the quality standards of large trials, which entail considerable investment, are generally (albeit not always) better.

A simple graphical method to investigate the 'small studies effect' is the *funnel plot* (see Figure 11.2 for an example). This is a scatter plot that plots the effect size of a study against

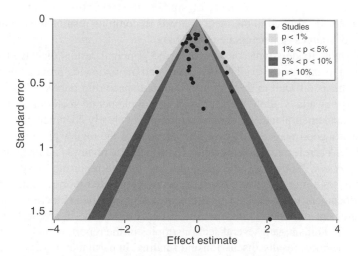

**Figure 11.2**   Example of a funnel plot produced with Stata.

some measure of its size or precision (often the standard error of the effect estimate). Small studies should be more scattered than larger ones. If the differences between effect estimates are due to random variation alone, the plot should resemble an inverted funnel, and studies should be disposed symmetrically around the line representing the fixed-effect summary estimate. Contour lines showing levels of statistical significance (e.g., <0.01, <0.05, <0.1) are often added to funnel plots. If publication bias is an issue, the plot should be asymmetrical and non-significant studies should be missing. An asymmetrical plot where, however, the studies that appear lacking are in the areas of statistical significance, points to the influence of some other factors, rather than publication bias (Sterne et al., 2011).

Statistical tests have also been developed in order to investigate the association between study precision and effect size (Sterne, Egger and Smith, 2001). The two more commonly used ones are a rank correlation test between the (standardized) effect size and its variance (Begg and Mazumdar, 1994) and regressing the standardized (log) effect size $\frac{y_i}{s_i}$ against its precision $\frac{1}{s_i}$ (Egger et al., 1997).

Outcome reporting bias has also been recently highlighted (Moher et al., 2009). In the final report, researchers tend to present the most positive outcome(s), and omit the others. A study comparing study protocols with published reports of a cohort of clinical trials found that these were often incomplete, biased and inconsistent with protocols (Chan et al., 2004). An assessment of each important outcome in each study should be performed in the review. Besides individual studies, selective outcome reporting may affect systematic reviews too.

## 11.12    Interpretation of results and report writing

The quantity and quality of the studies included in the systematic review is important in the interpretation of the results. Clearly, if only poor quality studies are available, the systematic review can explore possible bias but cannot substitute strong evidence from original studies.

Furthermore, a critical evaluation of all aspects of the reviewing process must also be undertaken, including the initial formulation of the research question, the implemented search strategy for identification and retrieval of studies, the extraction of data from individual studies, the methods applied in the meta-analysis to combine results, the quantification and investigation of sources of heterogeneity and bias.

Although most readers will consider only the principal results displayed in the report, some will want to explore the available evidence and the reviewing process more in depth by themselves. This is difficult to do within the limited space of a published article. However, many journals nowadays allow the inclusion of supplemental material on their websites. Provision of supplemental tables and other material that clearly document the various aspects of the review is a good way to guarantee transparency of the review process.

The PRISMA (preferred reporting items for systematic reviews and meta-analyses) statement (Moher et al., 2009) is an updated guideline for the reporting of systematic reviews and meta-analyses aiming to ensure transparent and complete reporting. An explanation and elaboration document to the PRISMA statement is also provided (Liberati et al., 2009). The PRISMA statement provides a checklist of 27 items to include in a report of a systematic review. These 27 items regard several sections/topics of the report; namely the title, abstract, introduction, methods, results, discussion and funding. In particular, in the discussion session it is suggested, besides the discussion of potential biases at both the individual study and the review level, to consider the relevance of the results for key groups (e.g., healthcare providers, users, policy makers), as well as the implications for future research.

## 11.13    Summary

The term meta-analysis refers to the statistical methods used in a systematic review. Statistical issues arise in practically all the steps of a systematic review, including the formulation of the research question, the definition of eligibility criteria for study inclusion, the definition of a search strategy, the choice of the outcome measure, data extraction from the individual studies, the choice of whether to combine and, in that case, how to combine results from included studies, the quantification and investigation of sources of heterogeneity and the presentation and interpretation of results.

The objective of a meta-analysis should not merely be the computing of a combined estimate. Investigating the quality of the included studies, and hence their adequacy to provide information on the investigated issue, the consistency of results across studies and the evidence of publication or other types of bias are fundamental parts of the meta-analytic process.

More important than the choice between fixed-effect or random-effect models, or obtaining p-values of heterogeneity tests, a careful examination of the data at hand and a clear understanding of the strengths and pitfalls of the statistical analysis are essential in order to interpret results in a meaningful way.

## References

Al Khalaf, M.M., Thalib, L. and Doi, S.A. (2011) Combining heterogenous [sic] studies using the random-effects model is a mistake and leads to inconclusive meta-analyses. *J Clin Epidemiol*, **64**, 119–123.

Anzures-Cabrera, J. and Higgins, J.P.T. (2010) Graphical displays for meta-analysis: an overview with suggestions for practice. *Res Synth Meth*, **1**, 66–80.

Baker, W.L., White, C.M., Cappelleri, J.C. *et al.* (2009) Understanding heterogeneity in meta-analysis: the role of meta-regression. *Int J Clin Pract*, **63**, 1426–1434.

Begg, C.B. and Mazumdar, M. (1994) Operating characteristics of a rank correlation test for publication bias. *Biometrics*, **50**, 1088–1101.

Borenstein, M., Hedges, L.V., Higgins, J.P.T. and Rothstein, H.R. (2002) A basic introduction to fixed-effect and random-effects models for meta-analysis. *Res Synth Meth*, **1**, 97–111.

Chan, A.W., Hrobjartsson, A., Haahr, M.T. *et al.* (2004) Empirical evidence for selective reporting of outcomes in randomized trials: comparison of protocols to published articles. *JAMA*, **291**, 2457–2465.

Cook, D.J., Guyatt, G.H., Ryan, G. *et al.* (1993) Should unpublished data be included in meta-analyses? Current convictions and controversies. *JAMA*, **269**, 2749–2753.

Crumley, E.T., Wiebe, N., Cramer, K. *et al.* (2005) Which resources should be used to identify RCT/CCTs for systematic reviews: a systematic review. *BMC Med Res Methodol*, **5**, 24.

Deandrea, S., Negri, E. and Ruggeri, F. (2012) Integrating clinicians' opinions in the Bayesian meta-analysis of observational studies: the case of risk factors for falls in community-dwelling older people. *Submitted*.

Deeks, J.J., Altman, D.G. and Bradburn, M.J. (2001) Statistical methods for examining heterogeneity and combining results from several studies in meta-analysis, in *Systematic Reviews in Health Care: Meta-Analysis in Context*, 2nd edn (eds M. Egger, G. Davey Smith and D. Altman), BMJ Publishing Group, London, pp. 285–312.

DerSimonian, R. and Kacker, R. (2007) Random-effects model for meta-analysis of clinical trials: an update. *Contemp Clin Trials*, **28**, 105–114.

DerSimonian, R. and Laird, N. (1986) Meta-analysis in clinical trials. *Control Clin Trials*, **7**, 177–188.

Dixon-Woods, M., Agarwal, S., Jones, D. *et al.* (2005) Synthesising qualitative and quantitative evidence: a review of possible methods. *J Health Serv Res Policy*, **10**, 45–53.

Egger, M., Davey Smith, G., Schneider, M. and Minder, C. (1997) Bias in meta-analysis detected by a simple, graphical test. *BMJ*, **315**, 629–634.

Egger, M., Davey Smith, G. and Altman, D. (eds) (2001) *Systematic Reviews in Health Care: Meta-Analysis in Context*, 2nd edn, BMJ Publishing Group, London.

Furukawa, T.A., Barbui, C., Cipriani, A. *et al.* (2006) Imputing missing standard deviations in meta-analyses can provide accurate results. *J Clin Epidemiol*, **59**, 7–10.

Glasziou, P.P. and Sanders, S.L. (2002) Investigating causes of heterogeneity in systematic reviews. *Stat Med*, **21**, 1503–1511.

Greenland, S. and Longnecker, M.P. (1992) Methods for trend estimation from summarized dose-response data, with applications to meta-analysis. *Am J Epidemiol*, **135**, 1301–1309.

Greenland, S. and Salvan, A. (1990) Bias in the one-step method for pooling study results. *Stat Med*, **9**, 247–252.

Higgins J.P.T. and Green, S. (eds) (2011) Cochrane Handbook for Systematic Reviews of Interventions. Version 5.1.0 [updated March 2011], The Cochrane Collaboration. Available from: www.cochrane-handbook.org (accessed March 4, 2012).

Higgins, J.P. and Thompson, S.G. (2002) Quantifying heterogeneity in a meta-analysis. *Stat Med*, **21**, 1539–1558.

Higgins, J.P., Thompson, S.G., Deeks, J.J. and Altman, D.G. (2003) Measuring inconsistency in meta-analyses. *BMJ*, **327**, 557–560.

Lefebvre, C. and Clarke, M.J. (2001) Identifying randomised trials, in *Systematic Reviews in Health Care: Meta-Analysis in Context*, 2nd edn (eds M. Egger, G. Davey Smith and D. Altman), BMJ Publishing Group, London.

Liberati, A., Altman, D.G., Tetzlaff, J. *et al.* (2009) The PRISMA statement for reporting systematic reviews and meta-analyses of studies that evaluate healthcare interventions: explanation and elaboration. *BMJ*, **339**, b2700.

Ma, J., Liu, W., Hunter, A. and Zhang, W. (2008) Performing meta-analysis with incomplete statistical information in clinical trials. *BMC Med Res Methodol*, **8**, 56.

Mantel, N. and Haenszel, W. (1959) Statistical aspects of the analysis of data from retrospective studies of disease. *J Natl Cancer Inst*, **22**, 719–748.

Moher, D., Liberati, A., Tetzlaff, J. and Altman, D.G. (2009) Preferred reporting items for systematic reviews and meta-analyses: the PRISMA statement. *BMJ*, **339**, b2535.

Negri, E., Colombo, C., Giordano, L. *et al.* (2005) Influenza vaccine in healthy children: a meta-analysis. *Vaccine*, **23**, 2851–2861.

Normand, S.L. (1999) Meta-analysis: formulating, evaluating, combining, and reporting. *Stat Med*, **18**, 321–359.

Peto, R. (1987) Why do we need systematic overviews of randomized trials? *Stat Med*, **6**, 233–244.

Poole, C. and Greenland, S. (1999) Random-effects meta-analyses are not always conservative. *Am J Epidemiol*, **150**, 469–475.

Riley, R.D., Higgins, J.P. and Deeks, J.J. (2011) Interpretation of random effects meta-analyses. *BMJ*, **342**, d549.

Robins, J., Breslow, N. and Greenland, S. (1986) Estimators of the Mantel-Haenszel variance consistent in both sparse data and large-strata limiting models. *Biometrics*, **42**, 311–323.

Rota, M., Bellocco, R., Scotti, L. *et al.* (2010) Random-effects meta-regression models for studying nonlinear dose-response relationship, with an application to alcohol and esophageal squamous cell carcinoma. *Stat Med*, **29**, 2679–2687.

Sackett, D.L., Rosenberg, W.M., Gray, J.A. *et al.* (1996) Evidence based medicine: what it is and what it isn't. *BMJ*, **312**, 71–72.

Shrier, I., Boivin, J.F., Steele, R.J. *et al.* (2007) Should meta-analyses of interventions include observational studies in addition to randomized controlled trials? A critical examination of underlying principles. *Am J Epidemiol*, **166**, 1203–1209.

Sterne, J.A., Egger, M. and Smith, G.D. (2001) Systematic reviews in health care: investigating and dealing with publication and other biases in meta-analysis. *BMJ*, **323**, 101–105.

Sterne, J.A., Sutton, A.J., Ioannidis, J.P. *et al.* (2011) Recommendations for examining and interpreting funnel plot asymmetry in meta-analyses of randomised controlled trials. *BMJ*, **343**, d4002.

Sutton, A.J. and Abrams, K.R. (2001) Bayesian methods in meta-analysis and evidence synthesis. *Stat Methods Med Res*, **10**, 277–303.

Thornton, A. and Lee, P. (2000) Publication bias in meta-analysis: its causes and consequences. *J Clin Epidemiol*, **53**, 207–216.

van Houwelingen, H.C., Arends, L.R. and Stijnen, T. (2002) Advanced methods in meta-analysis: multivariate approach and meta-regression. *Stat Med*, **21**, 589–624.

Yusuf, S., Peto, R., Lewis, J. *et al.* (1985) Beta blockade during and after myocardial infarction: an overview of the randomized trials. *Prog Cardiovasc Dis*, **27**, 335–371.

# Part Three

# STATISTICAL PROCESS CONTROL IN HEALTHCARE

# 12

# The use of control charts in healthcare

## William H. Woodall[1], Benjamin M. Adams[2] and James C. Benneyan[3]

[1]*Department of Statistics, Virginia Tech, Blacksburg, VA, USA*
[2]*Department of Information Systems, Statistics and Operations Management, University of Alabama, Tuscaloosa, AL, USA*
[3]*Healthcare Systems Engineering Institute, Northeastern University, Boston, MA, USA*

## Synopsis

Statistical process control (SPC) charts are increasingly being used in healthcare to aid in process understanding, assess process stability, and identify changes that indicate either improvement or deterioration in quality. They are used in hospital process-improvement projects, by accrediting bodies and governmental agencies, and for public health surveillance. We provide an overview of common uses of SPC in healthcare, and some guidance on the choice of appropriate charts for various applications. Implementation issues and more advanced SPC and related methods also are discussed.

## 12.1 Introduction

Continuous improvement of healthcare systems requires the measuring and understanding of process variation. It is important to eliminate extraneous process variation wherever possible, while moving well-defined metrics toward their target values. In healthcare, most performance

*Statistical Methods in Healthcare*, First Edition. Edited by Frederick W. Faltin, Ron S. Kenett and Fabrizio Ruggeri.
© 2012 John Wiley & Sons, Ltd. Published 2012 by John Wiley & Sons, Ltd.

metrics are of the lower-the-better or higher-the-better variety. Examples of important variables in healthcare involve lab turnaround times, days from positive mammogram to definitive biopsy, waiting times, patient satisfaction scores, medication errors, emergency service response times, infection rates, mortality rates, numbers of patient falls, post-operative lengths of stay, 'door-to-needle' times, counts of adverse events, and many others. Careful monitoring and study of such variables often can lead to significant improvements in quality. For example, monitoring infection rates, as discussed by Morton *et al.* (2008), can provide insights leading to improved standardized cleaning procedures or the early detection of new outbreaks.

Within this context, statistical process control (SPC) charts are very useful tools for studying important process variables and identifying quality improvements or quality deterioration. A control chart is a chronological time series plot of measurements of an important variable. The statistics plotted can be averages, proportions, rates, or other quantities of interest. In addition to these plotted values, upper and lower reference thresholds called *control limits* are plotted. These limits are calculated using process data and define the natural range of variation within which the plotted points almost always should fall. Any points falling outside of these control limits therefore may indicate that all data were not produced by the same process, either because of a lack of standardization or because a change in the process may have occurred. Such changes could represent either quality improvement or quality deterioration, depending on which control limit is crossed. Control charts are thus quite useful both for monitoring if processes get worse and for testing and verifying improvement ideas.

As an example, consider the time (in hours) required to complete a particular lab procedure. Suppose completion times are collected over time and plotted as shown in Figure 12.1. In this example, the observation at time period 40 falls below the lower control limit, thereby formally signaling a process change. During the time of this study, an improvement project resulted in a new standardized operating procedure implemented at time period 31. This

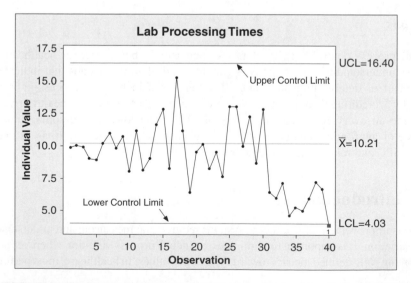

**Figure 12.1** Example of a control chart to verify a process improvement, here in laboratory processing times.

control chart provides statistical evidence that the new procedure did, in fact, change the lab processing times for the better. The amount of improvement (here, reduction) in both the duration average and variation can be quantified from the plotted values that occur after time period 31. New control limits now could be calculated based on these improved values, and the process monitored to ensure these quality gains are maintained.

In process improvement projects such as the above example, the control limits are calculated initially based on a historical set of data. For another example one could consider the proportion of Caesarean section deliveries in a hospital each month for the past three years. Initially, the control limits are used to assess the stability of the process and to identify unusual events (outliers). Once the analyst is confident the data reflect a stable process (points falling within the control limits and showing no clearly non-random patterns), the parameters of the statistical model used to determine the control limits are estimated. These control limits then are used for on-going monitoring as new data are collected and plotted. The retrospective analysis of historical data is referred to as Phase I; whereas the prospective monitoring of future data is referred to as Phase II. Essentially one checks whether the process historically was stable and consistent ('in statistical control' in SPC terminology) in Phase I and, if so, one checks whether the process continues to behave consistently or whether any process changes are evident ('out of control' in SPC terminology) in Phase II.

Analysts have many types of control charts at their disposal. An appropriate choice of control charts depends on the type of data being analyzed, the behavior of the data, and the assumed underlying probability distribution used for modeling. Appropriate chart and sample size selection often is difficult for practitioners due to the subtleties involved, but the correct choice is essential for meaningful results to be obtained. Since computer software is typically used for control chart generation, most calculations are not discussed in detail in this chapter. Many software options exist, a common choice being MINITAB (www.MINITAB.com). Version 16 of MINITAB also includes tutorials for the proper selection of control chart methods.

Readers can find detailed information on control charting assumptions, formulae, and implementation (but with an engineering focus) in Montgomery (2008). Several more practitioner-focused books cover SPC for healthcare applications along with detailed case studies; see, for example, Hart and Hart (2002) and Carey (2003), with a comparison and discussion of these two books given by Woodall (2004). Advice on the selection, design, and performance of control charts in healthcare applications was given by Benneyan (1998a, 1998b, 2006); Benneyan, Lloyd, and Plsek (2003); and Mohammed, Worthington, and Woodall (2008). Winkel and Zhang (2007) covered some more advanced control charting methods used in healthcare, as well as the basic control charting methods. Examples of healthcare process improvement projects involving SPC were reviewed by Thor *et al.* (2007).

## 12.2   Selection of a control chart

### 12.2.1   Basic Shewhart-type charts

The choice of an appropriate control chart depends on the type of data to be plotted. The most common types of data therefore need to be understood in order to identify the most appropriate control chart. All data can be classified as either continuous (variable) or discrete (attribute). Numerical measurements that can assume any values over some defined range are referred to as continuous, or variables, data. Examples include patient waiting times, times between adverse events, and blood pressure measurements. Even though these variables are always rounded in practice, in theory an infinite number of values between any two possible values also are possible, and thus such data are usually treated as continuous variables. If several samples are collected during each time period; for example, 20 emergency department waiting times for each day for a month, then an $\bar{X}$ and $S$ chart combination may be required. The statistic $\bar{X}$ (pronounced 'X-bar') represents the sample mean and $S$ represents the sample standard deviation. The $\bar{X}$ chart is used to monitor the mean of a process whereas the $S$ chart monitors process variation or inconsistency. An example of an $\bar{X}$ chart is given in Chapter 15. If only individual continuous measurements are available at each time period, for example, systolic blood pressure readings for a patient taken once a day for a month, then use of an $X$ chart ('individuals') typically is recommended. This type of chart is also illustrated in Chapter 15.

As discussed further in Chapter 13, quantitative variables data contain much more information than 'attribute' data, which are based on counts or rates of a particular event of interest. Thus it is not advisable to convert quantitative data into attribute data, such as for waiting times recording only whether or not each time met a given standard. This unfortunately was done in several published case studies on the use of Six Sigma in healthcare, with an unnecessary resulting loss of information and an associated loss in the ability to detect important process changes. See Chapter 13 for further discussion of this practice.

Continuous variables are usually modeled with probability distributions such as the normal, lognormal distribution, or exponential distribution. These probability distributions form the basis for mathematically establishing valid control limits. The $\bar{X}$, $S$, and $X$ control charts are most appropriate for normally distributed data, which are symmetric and bell-shaped when plotted on a histogram. If the data are skewed, such as for lognormal or exponential distributions, then the usual $\bar{X}$ or $X$ chart may not perform well. From a practical perspective, this is more important if a small sample size is used to calculate the average at each time period. In such cases, exact limits can be computed from knowledge of the appropriate probability distribution, which usually requires a skilled analyst. More simply, an appropriate normalizing transformation can be used and the transformed data then simply used with a conventional $\bar{X}$ or $X$ chart. For example, for lognormal data taking the logarithm of all measurements transforms them to being normally distributed, whereas raising exponential data to the power 0.2777 is one of several normalizing transformations. An example where this latter transformation was used is given in Chapter 15. One must be careful with these Transformations, however, since recent research shows that they can result in a loss of power to detect worsening quality.

In contrast to continuous data, attribute data most often involve counts (e.g., the number of falls per day), proportions (e.g., the proportion of patients receiving the correct antibiotic), or rates (e.g., the number of falls per 1000 patient-days). The Poisson distribution is typically an underlying assumption in the construction of charts for counts and rates. The corresponding control charts are the $c$-chart (counts) and the $u$-chart (rates), respectively. Generally the use of rates is more informative and conventional than counts, especially when the opportunity for adverse events varies over time. Examples include monthly falls per 1000 patient-days or catheter infections per 1000 device-use-days, where the number of patients at risk or device-use-days vary over time. A second type of attribute data is the proportion or percentage of a fixed number of cases for which an outcome of interest occurs. An example is the percentage of similar surgeries that result in a post-operative infection. In such cases, the binomial probability distribution is usually assumed to be appropriate and $p$-charts can be used.

In some cases the outcome of interest is known for each individual patient; for example, whether or not each surgical patient developed a particular type of infection. Each case then is a Bernoulli random variable, or equivalently a binomial variable with a sample size of one. As an alternative to the $p$-chart, one can plot the total number of patients until the infection occurs, with an assumed underlying geometric distribution. This is referred to as a $g$-chart by Benneyan (2001), who explored their detection performance and variations at length. Although charts based on Bernoulli and geometric data are very useful in healthcare applications, they are rarely included in standard statistical software. An exception is the Electronic Infection Control Assessment Technology (eICAT) software package, with information available at www.eicat.com.au/. Szarka and Woodall (2011) provided a detailed review of charts for monitoring Bernoulli processes.

Many sources exist to which the reader can turn for additional information on the selection of an appropriate control chart. We recommend Adams (2007), Montgomery (2008), Benneyan (2008), Lee and McGreevey (2002), and Winkel and Zhang (2007), in particular.

The charts discussed thus far in this chapter are referred to as Shewhart-type control charts, after Walter Shewhart, the inventor of the control chart. The estimated control limits usually are placed at plus and minus three standard deviations of the plotted statistic above and below a center line, which is placed at the estimated mean of the statistic. Three-sigma limits are used so that it is unlikely that a plotted point would fall outside the control limits if the process remains stable. Importantly, one should not overreact to each random movement in a plot of a statistic over time since this leads to wasted time and resources. One should seek to react to only true process changes. Control charts help separate such natural random process variation, referred to as 'common cause variation', from unusual variation caused by influences on the process to which some action is required. These influences are referred to as 'assignable causes' in the SPC literature.

## 12.2.2   Use of CUSUM and EWMA charts

An important distinction between Shewhart and some other types of control charts is that in the Shewhart charts the decision of whether the process is stable is made based on only the most recent information, unless supplementary rules are used, such as signaling if eight consecutive plotted values are all on the same side of the centerline or if two out of three consecutive values are beyond the same two-sigma limit. Runs rules can increase the ability of the chart to detect sustained process shifts, but can also increase the number of false alarms. Common supplementary rules are discussed in several of our recommended references. In particular, we recommend the discussion in Montgomery (2008). In contrast, cumulative sum (CUSUM) and exponentially weighted moving average (EWMA) charts are based (in different ways) on past data. While a bit more advanced to use and interpret, CUSUM and EWMA charts can detect small and moderately sized sustained changes in quality on average much more quickly than Shewhart charts, although they tend to be poorer at detecting one-time or short-term spikes.

Details of the construction of EWMA charts are given in Chapter 15 along with an example. To illustrate the construction of a CUSUM chart, suppose we wish to monitor the mean of a normally distributed random variable $X$ with individual and independent observations, $X_1, X_2, X_3, \ldots$ observed over time. We assume that these measurements have been standardized by subtracting the in-control mean and dividing by the standard deviation in order to have unit variance and in-control mean of zero. If the smallest shift in the mean in either direction that we want to detect quickly is $\delta$ standard deviations in size, then the following two sets of cumulative sum statistics, $X_t^+$ and $X_t^-$, are plotted over time:

$$X_t^+ = \max(0, X_{t-1}^+ + X_t - \delta/2),$$

and

$$X_t^- = \min(0, X_{t-1}^- + X_t + \delta/2), \quad t = 1, 2, 3, \ldots,$$

(12.1)

where $X_0^+ = X_0^- = 0$ and the index $t$ indicates the time period. The upper part of the CUSUM chart is designed to detect increases in the mean, and the lower part is designed to detect decreases in the mean. An out-of-control signal is given as soon as $X_t^+ > h_1$ or $X_t^- < h_2$, where the values of the thresholds $h_1 > 0$ and $h_2 < 0$ are selected to ensure a reasonably long average time between false alarms. Frequently the values $\delta = 1$ and $h_1 = -h_2 = 4$ or $h_1 = -h_2 = 5$ are used.

A simulated example of a CUSUM chart is shown in Figure 12.2. The chart was constructed with $\delta = 1$ and $h_1 = -h_2 = 4$. The first 100 observations all come from the same process, standard normal variables; while for the last 15 observations the mean increased by one standard deviation. The upper CUSUM chart signaled an increase in the mean at time 103.

Figure 12.3 shows the raw data in the simulation used to obtain Figure 12.2. Note that the increase in the mean is not nearly as evident visually in this plot, but it is very clear in the CUSUM plot of Figure 12.2. An $X$ chart with three-sigma limits would generate only a very slight signal at time 106. This example illustrates the value of CUSUM charts for better detection of subtle changes by incorporating more information in the plotted statistics.

EWMA and CUSUM charts have been developed for other types of data as well, including binomial, Poisson, and geometric random variables. Cumulative sum methods also have been used in healthcare to subjectively fit learning curves. See, for example, Young, Miller, and Azarow (2005) or Winkel and Zhang (2007, Ch. 8). This application is not a part of

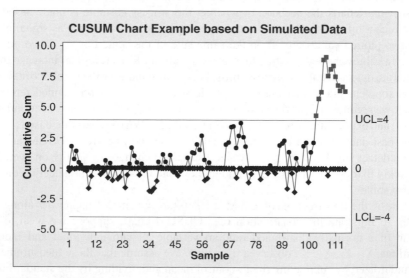

**Figure 12.2**   A CUSUM chart for normally distributed data with $\delta = 1$ and $h_1 = h_2 = 4$.

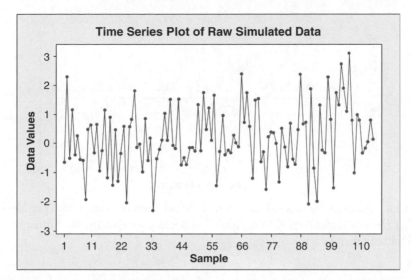

**Figure 12.3**    Simulated normally distributed observations with mean shift at sample 100.

traditional SPC, however, and should not be confused with the use of CUSUM charts for process monitoring. An important method closely related to cumulative sum charts is a sequential probability ratio test (SPRT), which is also based on a very similar likelihood ratio mathematical justification.

## 12.2.3    Risk-adjusted monitoring

In many healthcare applications the concept of acuity or risk adjustment is important, such as when the analysis includes comparisons of different physicians or hospitals with varying patient mix. Risk factors such as age, weight, gender, co-morbidities, fitness, and others affect the probability of a particular outcome occurring (such as the presence of diabetes or hypertension). Relevant risk factors vary depending on the outcome being evaluated or monitored. A considerable amount of effort has gone into developing risk-adjustment models over the past several decades. See, for example, Iezzoni (2003). Even though these models are not perfect, comparisons of some healthcare performance metrics are not meaningful without them. Reviews of risk-adjusted monitoring were provided by Grigg and Farewell (2004) and Woodall (2006), but a considerable amount of work has been done on this topic in the last five years.

Two basic types of risk adjustment occur in practice, with a patient either being placed into one of several risk categories (e.g., very low, low, medium, high, very high) or with a risk probability being assigned to each patient. The latter is often done through a logistic regression model, as described in detail in Chapter 15. If, for example, 30-day mortality rates following surgery are of interest, then a predicted mortality rate is obtained for each patient. The Bernoulli outcomes and the predicted mortality rates can be used as input into the risk-adjusted CUSUM charts of Steiner *et al.* (2000). These charts have been used in a number of applications, including monitoring cardiac surgery results. Taseli and Benneyan (2008) developed similar types of risk-adjusted SPRTs and investigated their

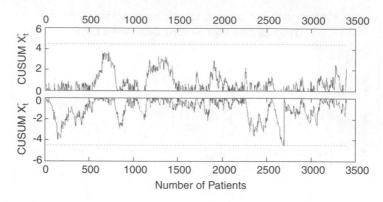

**Figure 12.4**  An example of a risk-adjusted CUSUM chart (reprinted with permission from *Journal of Quality Technology* ©2006 American Society for Quality. No further distribution allowed without permission.).

detection performance. As another example, Axelrod *et al.* (2006) discussed the use of a Poisson hazards-based risk-adjusted CUSUM chart in monitoring the performance of organ transplant centers.

An example of a risk-adjusted CUSUM chart used to monitor cardiac surgery is shown in Figure 12.4. The upper part of the CUSUM chart was designed to detect deterioration in quality, while the lower part was designed to detect improvements in performance. A signal is given when either control limit is crossed. If a patient dies within 30 days of surgery, both CUSUM statistics increase by specified amounts. If the patient lives, the CUSUM statistics decrease by specified amounts. As with the CUSUM chart defined for normally distributed data given in equation (12.1), neither CUSUM statistic is allowed to pass the reflecting barrier at zero. The amount that each CUSUM statistic increases or decreases for an individual patient depends on the predicted mortality rate for the patient and the smallest increase and decrease in the odds of mortality one is interested in detecting quickly.

In the above example, the Parsonnet scoring system was used in the risk-adjustment approach. If $p_t$ is used to represent the predicted 30-day mortality rate for the $t$th patient, then the regression model used was

$$\text{logit}(p_t) = -3.68 + 0.07 X_t,$$

where $X_t$ is the Parsonnet score for the $t$th patient. The Parsonnet score is based on the gender, age, and obesity level of the patients, as well as the presence or absence of health characteristics such as hypertension. (See Parsonnet, Dean, and Bernstein, 1989.) The chart was set up to detect a process deterioration corresponding to a doubling of the odds ratio corresponding to mortality and a process improvement corresponding to a halving of the odds ratio. An improvement in quality was detected around the 2700th patient, as seen by the plotted data reaching the lower limit, and the two CUSUM chart statistics then were reset to zero before monitoring was continued.

The risk-adjusted CUSUM chart of Steiner *et al.* (2000) is a generalization of the Bernoulli CUSUM chart of Reynolds and Stoumbos (1999). Under the Reynolds and Stoumbos (1999) and Leandro *et al.* (2005) framework there is a constant probability $p_0$ of an adverse event occurring when the process is stable, and detecting a sustained shift to an out-of-control value $p_1$ is of primary interest. Ismail, Pettitt, and Webster (2003) and others recommended a scan method in this situation that signals as soon as the number of adverse events in the last $m$ Bernoulli trials exceeds a specified value. Joner, Woodall, and Reynolds (2008) showed, however, that the Bernoulli CUSUM chart was more effective.

Sometimes a variable life adjusted display (VLAD) is used instead of plotting a risk-adjusted CUSUM chart. In the case of monitoring mortality rates, this chart would be a plot over time of the sum of the predicted number of deaths minus the observed number of deaths. The vertical axis is frequently labeled 'statistical lives saved' and the horizontal axis is the number of patients. A related risk-adjusted metric often used in practice is a ratio of the observed over expected number of outcomes, or the O/E ratio. If the VLAD shows an increasing trend (or if O/E < 1), then performance is better than indicated by whatever risk-adjustment model is used. A decreasing trend (or O/E > 1) conversely indicates performance poorer than would be expected by the model. The risk-adjusted CUSUM method also can be used in the background to signal when performance seems to reflect more than simply random variation, as recommended by Sherlaw-Johnson (2005). The book produced by the Clinical Practice Improvement Centre (2008) explains in detail the use of VLADs in the monitoring of healthcare outcomes in Queensland, Australia.

## 12.3   Implementation Issues

### 12.3.1   Overall process improvement system

The use of control charts is most beneficial as a component within an overall well-structured quality improvement program. We support the use of the Six Sigma process design strategy and its Define-Measure-Analyze-Improve-Control (DMAIC) process improvement strategy. The history and principles of Six Sigma were reviewed by Montgomery and Woodall (2008). There are quite a few books available on the use of Six Sigma in healthcare applications; for example Bisgaard (2009) and Trusko *et al.* (2007). In addition, Chapter 14 is devoted to this topic.

Most hospitals in the United States are accredited and evaluated by the Joint Commission (formerly the Joint Commission on Accreditation of Healthcare Organizations, or JCAHO), which evaluates each hospital's compliance with federal regulations, including their internal processes aimed at continuously improving patient outcomes. The Joint Commission is a private, not-for-profit organization that operates accreditation programs for a fee to subscriber hospitals and other healthcare organizations. Over 17 000 healthcare organizations and programs are inspected for accreditation on a three-year cycle, with periodic unannounced inspections. A few smaller accrediting organizations also exist, most notably the European DNV organization that began accrediting US hospitals in 2008. Accreditation by one of these organizations is required by many states as a condition of licensure and Medicaid reimbursement. In 2009 the Joint Commission Center for Transforming Healthcare (www.centerfortransforminghealthcare.org/) was established to help solve critical healthcare safety and quality problems. The use of Lean and Six Sigma methods is said to be an important component of this center's efforts. In our view a greater focus on process improvement is necessary.

### 12.3.2   Sampling issues

The benefits of control charting can be compromised if the quality of collected data is poor. Ensuring that variables are carefully defined and that the measurement system is accurate are key components of the Six Sigma approach. The sampling approach used by the National Surgical Quality Improvement Program, described by Ko (2009) is exemplary. With any improvement project, one must carefully consider what data to collect, with the purpose of the project driving data-collection decisions. In order to characterize emergency department waiting times, for example, one must decide how often to collect data and how large each sample should be. If the variation within the day is to be understood, then samples would need to be taken frequently, say every hour. If only the longest waiting times for each day are of interest then sampling could be restricted to known peak periods of emergency department admissions.

Biased sampling should be avoided whenever possible. As an example, healthcare data collected for insurance purposes in the USA can produce bias if there is any 'upcoding' to justify higher payments. Generally the choice of what variables to measure and how often to collect data is decided to ensure that important magnitudes of changes in quality levels can be detected in a reasonable amount of time for that particular application. When possible, samples also are collected in such a way that process changes are most likely to occur between (rather than within) samples, in order to maximize detection power. This practice often is referred to as 'rational subgrouping' in the industrial SPC literature, and is particularly important when computing control limits in the Phase I use of SPC described earlier.

### 12.3.3   Violations of assumptions

All control charts are most effective under their specified statistical assumptions. As discussed in Chapter 15, a standard assumption is that all data collected over time are independent. This means, for example, that there is not a tendency for large values to follow other large values and for small values to follow other small values; that is, there is no positive autocorrelation. With positive autocorrelation some types of charts, such as the $X$ chart with limits based on the moving ranges, will produce a large number of false alarms.

Checking for autocorrelation and selecting an appropriate control chart is important for understanding the behavior of a process over time. If autocorrelation or systematic seasonal variation, such as a day-of-the-week effect, exists but in the particular setting is considered 'unnatural' variation, then it should be removed or reduced if possible. If this is not possible or if the autocorrelation is considered part of the natural process, such as with a daily bed census, then Phase II monitoring becomes more complicated and special-purpose control charts should be used. Winkel and Zhang (2007, Ch. 4) and Montgomery (2008) discussed the use of control charting with autocorrelated data. One commonly recommended approach is to use a time series model to predict one time period ahead and to then plot the one-step-ahead forecast errors on a control chart. If the correct time series model is fitted then these forecast errors, sometimes referred to as residuals, are independent random variables.

Numerous other ways exist by which distributional assumptions can be violated. As one of several examples, some count data may exhibit more variability than they would under a Poisson model. This is referred to as overdispersion, and another probability model such as a negative binomial distribution should be used. In other applications where there are more zeros in count data than expected under the Poisson model, a zero-inflated Poisson distribution could be used. Within most Six Sigma programs there usually is an individual available who is designated as a 'Master Black Belt' who can provide expert guidance when such statistical complications arise.

### 12.3.4    Measures of control chart performance

If basic chart selection and sample size guidelines are followed and all assumptions are reasonable, then control charts will perform well. SPC researchers use several metrics to investigate detection performance and develop sample size guidelines. The most common performance metric is the average run length (ARL), which is the average number of plotted points until the control chart generates an out-of-control signal. Control limit formulae are set so that the in-control ARL, $ARL_0$, is sufficiently large. For example, the ARL for an $\bar{X}$ chart with 3-standard-deviation control limits is roughly 370 plotted points. This is the average number of plotted values between false alarms. Conversely, low ARL values are desirable to quickly detect true sustained process shifts. When samples are collected periodically, if there are $m$ cases between samples and samples are of size $n$, then a related important metric is the average number of items (ANI) until a signal, where here $ANI = ARL \times (n + m)$. For charts such as the $g$-chart, the number of cases between plotted points varies, so the average number of (Bernoulli) observations until a signal (ANOS) is used, where here ANOS equals the ARL divided by the probability that the event being monitored occurs in one of the Bernoulli trials.

   As an alternative to 3-sigma control limits, Shewhart-type chart limits often are computed so that the false-alarm probability per sample is a specified value $\alpha$, such as 0.001, for example. If the in-control parameters of the process are assumed to be known, then $ARL_0 = 1/\alpha$. As mentioned earlier, conventional three-standard-deviation control limits most often are used with Shewhart-type charts, which for normally distributed continuous data results in $\alpha = 0.0027$. For charts based on attribute data the discrete nature of the underlying distributions usually makes it impossible to obtain a false-alarm rate of exactly any given value of $\alpha$, and the limits are set to obtain as close a value as possible. For EWMA, CUSUM, and other more advanced charts, computing the ARL or any of the other performance measures is more complicated; so the practitioner needs to rely on published values.

   If outbreaks or problems to be detected with control charts are temporary, not sustained over time, then the usual metrics for evaluating control chart performance are not valid. For discussion of this situation and additional metrics, such as power and the probability of successful detection, the reader is referred to Fraker, Woodall, and Mousavi (2008).

## 12.4    Certification and governmental oversight applications

Control charts are increasingly being used by certification bodies and governmental agencies in order to assess hospital performance. The Joint Commission's ORYX® initiative, for example, integrates outcomes and other performance measurement data into its accreditation process. These performance data are analyzed with control charts and 'target analysis'. The control chart analysis is used to assess stability of processes; whereas target analysis, introduced in 2009, is used to assess the performance of the healthcare provider relative to relevant standards. A process can be stable and in 'statistical control', but still with overall poor performance compared to other providers, so both types of analyses are required. This distinction is similar conceptually to the dual use in manufacturing of control charts to assess stability, and process capability analysis to assess compliance to specifications. Lee and McGreevey (2002) reviewed the control charting approaches used by ORYX.

The healthcare regulator in England is the Care Quality Commission. Spiegelhalter *et al.* (2012) described this commission's methods for rating, screening, and surveillance of healthcare providers. The surveillance methods used are somewhat complicated and not straightforward applications of standard control charts. First, each of the many input data streams are standardized to be approximately normally distributed with a mean of zero and a standard deviation of one. After some accounting for variance components and using some robust estimation, $p$-values are calculated based on CUSUM charts, and false discovery rate (FDR) methods are used to identify the providers with the most outlying performance. The $p$-values are the probabilities of obtaining CUSUM values as large as the ones obtained given that the process is stable at the overall average. Roughly 200 000 CUSUM charts are used as part of this surveillance system, which produces about 30 alerts per quarter. More information about these methods can be obtained from Healthcare Commission (2009).

## 12.5    Comparing the performance of healthcare providers

Although not a control chart, there is another type of increasingly common charting activity but that should be used with some caution. When comparing the rates of adverse events among a number of healthcare providers, perhaps risk-adjusted, it is becoming more common to order the providers from the one with the lowest rate to the one with the highest rate. Confidence intervals then are used to identify any providers with significantly different performance, in a statistical sense, from the average overall rate. This type of plot, sometimes called a league table, can easily be misinterpreted since much of the ordering reflects only random variation. Being located at the 25th percentile is not necessarily different, in the sense of statistical significance, from being at the 75th percentile. It is a misuse of statistics, however, to place undue importance on the numerical ordering of providers since much of the variation is random. The ordering will vary considerably from one reporting period to another.

These types of charts are used, for example, in the semiannual reports provided to participating sites by the National Surgical Quality Improvement Program (NSQIP). For further details and examples, a sample NSQIP report is available at acsnsqip.org/main/resources_semi_annual_report.pdf. Also note that risk-adjustment models are contained in this report for a large number of surgical outcomes.

As a better approach, funnel plots (Spiegelhalter, 2005a, 2005b) are more informative than league tables. In a funnel plot the rate of interest is plotted on the $Y$-axis and the number of patients treated is plotted on the $X$-axis. Confidence interval bands drawn on the plot take a funnel shape as illustrated in Figure 12.5. Providers corresponding to points outside the confidence bands are outliers with performance that may be statistically different from the overall average performance. In this case, two of the hospitals have statistically significant MRSA rates below the lower confidence band. Study of these hospitals' procedures and processes could lead to understanding ways to also lower rates at other hospitals.

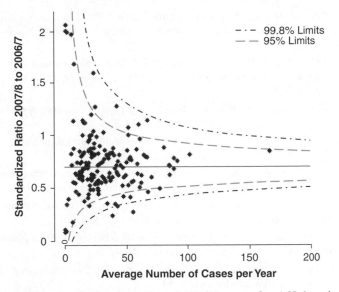

**Figure 12.5**   An example of a funnel plot of MRSA rates for 168 hospitals in the UK. Reproduced by permission of John Wiley & Sons, Ltd.

## 12.6   Summary

Process monitoring with control charts is an important component within an overall process evaluation and improvement framework in healthcare. Control charting methods, frequently as part of Six Sigma initiatives, are being used increasingly in healthcare, but greater use of these and other quality improvement methods is needed. Training in the use of control charting methods is best accomplished within an overall process improvement context, such as Six Sigma, Lean, or Lean Six Sigma.

In addition to standard control charting methods used in other industries, special-purpose charts for risk-adjusted and rare event data are particularly useful. Funnel plots are also a very useful, and relatively new, tool for evaluating the relative performance of a number of healthcare providers with respect to some outcome measure. These plots contain more information than league tables and are less prone to misinterpretation.

## Acknowledgements

Professor Woodall's work was supported in part by NSF Grant CMMI-0927323.

## References

Adams, B.M. (2007) Selection of control charts. *Encyclopedia of Statistics in Quality and Reliability*, **1**, 432–438.

Axelrod, D.A., Guidinger, M.K., Metzger, R.A. *et al.* (2006) Transplant center quality assessment using a continuously updatable, risk-adjusted technique (CUSUM). *American Journal of Transplantation*, **6**, 313–323.

Benneyan, J.C. (1998a) Statistical quality control methods in infection control and hospital epidemiology, Part 1: introduction and basic theory. *Infection Control and Hospital Epidemiology*, **19**, 194–214.

Benneyan, J.C. (1998b) Statistical quality control methods in infection control and hospital epidemiology, Part 2: chart use, statistical properties, and research issues. *Infection Control and Hospital Epidemiology*, **19**, 265–277.

Benneyan, J.C. (2001) Performance of number-between g-type statistical control charts for monitoring adverse events. *Health Care Management Science*, **4**, 319–336.

Benneyan, J.C. (2006) Discussion of 'Use of control charts in health-care and public-health surveillance' by W. H. Woodall. Journal of Quality Technology, **38**, 113–123.

Benneyan, J.C. (2008) The design, selection, and performance of statistical control charts for healthcare process improvement. *International Journal of Six Sigma and Competitive Advantage*, **4**, 209–239.

Benneyan, J.C., Lloyd, R.C., and Plsek, P.E. (2003) Statistical process control as a tool for research and healthcare improvement. *Quality & Safety in Health Care*, **12**, 458–464.

Bisgaard, S. (ed.) (2009) *Solutions to the Healthcare Quality Crisis: Cases and Examples of Lean Six Sigma in Healthcare*, ASQ Quality Press, Milwaukee, WI.

Carey, R.G. (2003) *Improving Healthcare with Control Charts: Basic and Advanced SPC Methods and Case Studies*, ASQ Quality Press, Milwaukee, WI.

Clinical Practice Improvement Centre (2008) *VLADs for Dummies*, John Wiley & Sons Australia Ltd, Milton, Queensland (request for a free copy can be sent to vlad_queries@health.qld.gov.au).

Fraker, S.E., Woodall, W.H., and Mousavi, S. (2008) Performance metrics for surveillance schemes. *Quality Engineering*, **20**, 451–464.

Grigg, O. and Farewell, V. (2004) An overview of risk-adjusted charts. *Journal of the Royal Statistical Society – Series A*, **167**, 523–539.

Hart, M.K. and Hart, R.F. (2002) *Statistical Process Control for Health Care*, Duxbury, Pacific Grove, CA.

Healthcare Commission (2009) Following up mortality 'outliers': a review of the programme for taking action where data suggest there may be serious concerns about the safety of patients. http://archive.cqc.org.uk/_db/_documents/Following_up_mortality_outliers_200906054425.pdf (accessed April 5, 2012).

Iezzoni, L. (ed.) (2003) *Risk Adjustment for Measuring Health Care Outcomes*, 3rd edn, Health Administration Press, Chicago, IL.

Ismail, N.A., Pettitt, A.N., and Webster, R.A. (2003) 'Online' monitoring and retrospective analysis of hospital outcomes based on a scan statistic. *Statistics in Medicine*, **22**, 2861–2876.

Joner, M.D. Jr., Woodall, W.H., and Reynolds, M.R. Jr. (2008) Detecting a rate increase using a Bernoulli scan statistic. *Statistics in Medicine*, **27**, 2555–2575.

Ko, C.Y. (2009) Measuring and improving surgical quality. Patient Safety and Quality Healthcare, **6**(6), 36–41.

Leandro, G., Rolando, N., Gallus, G., Rolles, K., and Burroughs, A.K. (2005) Monitoring surgical and medical outcomes: the Bernoulli cumulative SUM Chart. A novel application to assess clinical interventions. *Postgraduate Medical Journal*, **81**, 647–652.

Lee, K. and McGreevey, C. (2002) Using control charts to assess performance measurement data. *Journal on Quality Improvement*, **28**, 90–101.

Mohammed, M.A., Worthington, P., and Woodall, W.H. (2008) Plotting basic control charts: tutorial notes for healthcare practitioners. *Quality and Safety in Health Care*, **17**, 137–145.

Montgomery, D.C. (2008) *Introduction to Statistical Quality Control*, 6th edn, John Wiley & Sons, Inc., Hoboken, NJ.

Montgomery, D.C. and Woodall, W.H. (2008) An overview of Six Sigma. *International Statistical Review*, **76**, 329–346.

Morton, A.P., Clements, A.C.A., Doidge, S.R. *et al.* (2008) Surveillance of healthcare-acquired infections in Queensland, Australia: data and lessons from the first 5 years. *Infection Control and Hospital Epidemiology*, **29**, 695–701.

Parsonnet, V., Dean, D., and Bernstein, A.D. (1989) A method of uniform stratification of risks for evaluating the results of surgery in acquired adult heart disease. *Circulation*, **779** (Supplement 1), 1–12.

Reynolds, M.R. Jr. and Stoumbos, Z.G. (1999) A CUSUM chart for monitoring a proportion when inspecting continuously. *Journal of Quality Technology*, **31**, 87–108.

Sherlaw-Johnson, C. (2005) A method for detecting runs of good and bad clinical outcomes on variable life-adjusted display (VLAD) charts. *Health Care Management Science*, **8**, 61–65.

Spiegelhalter, D.J. (2005a) Funnel plots for comparing institutional performance. *Statistics in Medicine*, **24**, 1185–1202.

Spiegelhalter, D.J. (2005b) Handling over-dispersion of performance indicators. *Quality and Safety in Healthcare*, **14**, 347–351.

Spiegelhalter, D., Sherlaw-Johnson, C., Bardsley, M. *et al.* (2012) Statistical methods for healthcare regulation: rating, screening and surveillance (with discussion). *Journal of the Royal Statistical Society – Series A*, **175**(1), 1–47.

Steiner, S.H., Cook, R.J., Farewell, V.T., and Treasure, T. (2000) Monitoring surgical performance using risk-adjusted cumulative sum charts. *Biostatistics*, **1**, 441–452.

Szarka, J.L. III and Woodall, W.H. (2011) A review and perspective on surveillance of high quality Bernoulli processes. *Quality and Reliability Engineering International*, **27**(6), 735–752.

Taseli, A. and Benneyan, J.C. (2008) Cumulative sum charts for heterogeneous dichotomous events. Industrial Engineering Research Conference Proceedings, pp. 1754–1759.

Thor, J., Lundberg, J., Ask, J. *et al.* (2007) Application of statistical process control in healthcare improvement: systematic review. *Quality and Safety in Health Care*, **16**, 387–399.

Trusko, B.E., Pexton, C., Harrington, J., and Gupta, P. (2007) *Improving Healthcare Quality and Cost with Six Sigma*, FT Press.

Winkel, P. and Zhang, N.F. (2007) *Statistical Development of Quality in Medicine*, John Wiley & Sons, Inc., Hoboken, NJ.

Woodall, W.H. (2004) Review of *Improving Healthcare with Control Charts* by Raymond G. Carey. *Journal of Quality Technology*, **36**, 336–338.

Woodall, W.H. (2006) Use of control charts in health-care and public-health surveillance (with discussion). *Journal of Quality Technology*, **38**, 89–104.

Young, A., Miller, J.P., and Azarow, K. (2005) Establishing learning curves for surgical residents using cumulative summation (CUSUM) analysis. *Current Surgery*, **62**, 330–334.

# 13

# Common challenges and pitfalls using SPC in healthcare

## Victoria Jordan[1] and James C. Benneyan[2]

[1] *Office of Performance Improvement, University of Texas, MD Anderson Cancer Center, Houston, TX, USA*
[2] *Healthcare Systems Engineering Institute, Northeastern University, Boston, MA, USA*

## Synopsis

Effectiveness of the growing use of statistical process control (SPC) methods in healthcare has been limited by a number of technical and non-technical factors. This chapter addresses the impediments which have given rise to this situation, ranging from cultural factors and conceptual framework, to issues of data availability and misuse of otherwise appropriate statistical techniques. A variety of examples are presented throughout to compare the efficacy of alternative approaches, and to illustrate how prudent method choices can positively impact opportunities for improvement of patient care.

## 13.1 Introduction

Statistical process control (SPC) charts have been used successfully in manufacturing since the 1920s, but only recently have gained general recognition as useful tools within healthcare. A number of publications (Benneyan, 1998; Mohammed, Worthington and Woodall, 2008) and Chapters 8, 12 and 15 of this book illustrate how control charts can help differentiate between common and special causes of healthcare variation in important clinical and

*Statistical Methods in Healthcare*, First Edition. Edited by Frederick W. Faltin, Ron S. Kenett and Fabrizio Ruggeri.
© 2012 John Wiley & Sons, Ltd. Published 2012 by John Wiley & Sons, Ltd.

non-clinical applications. Several challenges and implementation errors, however, often limit the potential and effectiveness of SPC for improving such processes.

This chapter discusses issues most commonly seen in practice, most of which fall into three general categories: cultural, implementation, and statistical. The net result can be either (1) decreased ability to detect meaningful process changes or (2) dramatic increases in false signals when no special causes actually exist, or both. Additional information on the use of control charts in healthcare can be found in Benneyan (1999, 2008) and in Chapters 8, 12 and 15.

## 13.2    Assuring control chart performance

Since almost all of these issues in some way relate to the ability of a control chart to detect if a process is stable – the fundamental purpose of SPC – we first discuss the important topic of chart performance. The selection and design of an appropriate control chart is discussed below. Two of the most important charts, however, are discussed much less frequently in practitioner literature yet are critical to understand. These charts plot what are called OC (operating characteristic) or ARL (average run length) curves that describe the ability of a control chart to perform as desired – concepts related to type I and type II statistical errors (i.e. specificity and sensitivity). These properties can be affected quite significantly by the type and accuracy of data collected, the type of chart selected, the manner in which control limits are calculated and other decisions. The mathematical relationships between OC, ARL and related performance metrics are discussed in Chapter 12, and computations are provided by Benneyan (2001, 2008) and Montgomery (2009).

Examples of four OC curves are shown in Figure 13.1 that correspond to four control chart options for monitoring the rate of ventilator-associated pneumonia (VAP). For these OC curves, the control chart was established with a stable process with an average VAP = 0.0010. The x-axis indicates the average VAP following a change in the process, and the y-axis indicates the probability of no signal (i.e. the probability that the chart does not signal

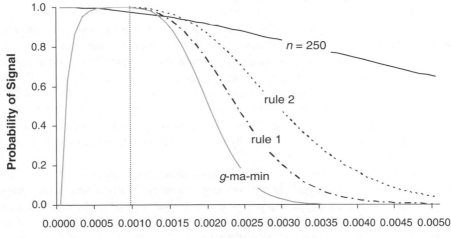

**Figure 13.1**   Example of OC curves.

an out-of-control condition even though the process average has changed.) The amount of change ($\delta$) often is expressed either as a percentage of the baseline or as a multiple of the process standard deviation, although other formats exist. As a general guideline, the time until an out-of-control signal should be long when the process has not changed ($\delta = 0$), shorter when the process has changed, and very short for large changes. Thus graphically a tall and narrow OC curve generally is better than a short and wide one.

In the illustrated case, the wider three curves correspond to $p$ type of control charts using three different subgroup size rules, discussed later in this chapter. The narrowest OC curve (i.e. the best) describes the performance of a $g$ type of control chart, which in this case exhibits the best choice in terms of statistical performance (and more specifically in terms of the probability that the next plotted point detects the rate increase). To illustrate, if the VAP rate roughly doubles from 0.0010 to 0.0020, the worst $p$ chart will detect this increase on the next subgroup with probability roughly 0.05 (for an ARL of ~20 subgroups), whereas the $g$ chart will detect it roughly with probability 0.50 (or an ARL of ~2 subgroups).

## 13.3   Cultural challenges

### 13.3.1   Philosophical and statistical literacy

Aside from the more technical issues discussed below, several cultural and conceptual barriers exist to maximizing the value of SPC to help improve healthcare processes. The three primary goals of statistical quality control and control charts in any industry are to attain a stable process, monitor that process for changes, and improve the process so that it performs with acceptable capability relative to needs (Juran and Gryna, 1988). Overall, the objective is to achieve and then maintain an acceptable state of statistical control (consistency) that then will allow one to monitor for special or assignable cause variation. This objective and the deliberate methodical approach it requires, however, can be at odds with current cultural trends in healthcare, especially as they relate to standardization, physician autonomy and simplified process improvement methods.

As a fundamental concept, statistical stability is synonymous with standardized processes in which the same basic steps are followed in a consistent manner by everyone involved in the process. This notion – standardization – is both a hard-sought goal in healthcare and a frequent point of contention. In many circles standardization is rejected as a loss of physician autonomy and expertise, 'cookbook medicine', and contrary to the 'art of medicine'. Recent experiences, especially with respect to patient safety, however have shown that standardized processes can result in safer (and more consistent) care. The World Health Organization (WHO) surgical checklist (Gawande, 2009), for example, provides a standardized list of surgery preparation steps that in an eight-city pilot reduced non-fatal complications by 36% and deaths by 47%.

As indicated throughout the discussions in this chapter, the correct use of control charts at times requires a deliberate and careful approach – whereas in many healthcare settings a sense of urgency exists to spread improvement widely and with broad brush strokes rather than methodically and precisely. The current state of healthcare and existence of many improvement opportunities often tempts organizations to work on 'everything', and, with SPC, translating to constructing control charts on nearly every data element possibly available. This typically has led organizations in other industries to create charts for charts' sake and to lose sight of the real objective. Like any tool, left unused in any deep meaningful way to improve processes eventually control charts are perceived as not helpful. A better path instead can be to strategically focus one's use of SPC and other improvement methods on a manageable number of key process indicators and pervasive problems.

While software packages definitely can be a tremendous help for calculating and displaying charts with very little effort, they also make it easier for users to skip the important first phase of using SPC (discussed below), which is a highly people-based activity, and to miss opportunities to identify and eliminate assignable causes. More generally, it becomes very easy to simply click-and-point and believe the correct SPC chart is being used and is being used correctly. Two of the more common consequences are using the wrong chart or recalculating the limits with every data new point that is added, both of which can reduce the ability to detect small, gradual process changes.

Even with the use of software, a certain amount of statistical literacy is important to maximize the effectiveness of control charts. Key issues include understanding that almost everything naturally exhibits variation and therefore that one should expect roughly half of all results to be above (or below) average. More deeply, the distinctions between different types of discrete and continuous data, key assumptions under which common probability distributions apply, and concepts of statistical versus practical significance all are important. Often one also encounters rare events, risk-adjusted, stratified, surrogate, naturally cyclic, correlated and under-reported data, each of which needs treatment and consideration in some way beyond the scope of this chapter and beyond the level at which most healthcare quality improvement specialists are trained.

## 13.3.2   Acceptable quality levels

A large part of the motivation for using SPC in other industries is to reduce variability and defects to near-zero. While zero-defect cultures exist in many manufacturing companies, the same obsession is not as widespread in healthcare. For example, the 'Six Sigma' focus initiated by Motorola in 1981 was designed to reduce variability to the point where processes produce less than 3.4 failures per million opportunities. This focus originally came from the concept that if variability could be reduced to the point where (in the bilateral specifications and normal distribution case) the mean plus or minus six standard deviations ($\mu \pm 6\sigma$) of the random variable of interest is centered within specification limits, then there would be less than two defective parts per billion produced (or 3.4 defects per million after allowing for the mean to be $1.5\sigma$ off target).

Over the past 30 years, this specific statistical definition has evolved into a more general management metaphor for aggressively reducing defects, however defined, to successively lower levels through continuous improvement. Related terminology has developed that generally describes defect rates in terms of single digit occurrences per $10^n$ opportunities (e.g. $10^{-2}$, $10^{-3}$ and $10^{-4}$ quality levels, meaning a few failures per 100, 1000 and 10 000 opportunities). One such common metric is Defects per Million Opportunities, or DPMO. As organizations reduced variability toward any of these levels, control charts were important tools for differentiating between common (natural) and special (assignable) causes of variation that could be identified and acted upon in different manners to reduce variation.

However, existing and culturally acceptable 'defect' levels in healthcare are both relatively high in comparison. According to the WHO, for example, adherence of healthcare workers to recommended hand hygiene procedures is dismally low and highly variable, ranging from

**Table 13.1**  Comparison of healthcare defect rates versus Six Sigma processes.

| Metric | Compliance or defect-free rate (%) | Equivalent sigma level | DPMO |
|---|---|---|---|
| Medication errors | 99.4 | 4.01 | 6000 |
| Antibiotic one-hour before surgery | 91 | 2.84 | 90 000 |
| Deep vein thrombosis blood clotting prevention | 88 | 2.68 | 120 000 |
| Hospital readmissions | 75.7 | 2.20 | 243 000 |
| Hand hygiene | 38.7 | 1.21 | 613 000 |
| Evidence-based care compliance | 33.3–87.2 | 1.07–2.64 | 128 000–667 000 |
| Six Sigma process | 99.99966 | 6.0 | 3.4 |

5 to 89% with an overall average of 38.7% (WHO, 2009). Centers for Medicare and Medicaid Services (CMS) 'core measures' publically reported by most hospitals include process metrics that also are at unacceptable quality levels. For example, in 2010 only 91% of surgery patients were given antibiotics at the right time to prevent infection (within one hour before surgery), and only 88% were given appropriate treatment to prevent blood clots after certain types of surgeries (Hospital Compare, 2010), both at the $\sim 10^{-2}$ or roughly 2.8-sigma quality level. Table 13.1 summarizes sigma levels for several other common healthcare metrics.

## 13.4    Implementation challenges

### 13.4.1    Data availability and accuracy

SPC or any statistical method, of course, works best with accurate data. Access to the types of healthcare process and clinical data that are useful for process improvement, however, often lags behind other industries. In the United States, recent efforts to improve access to medical records, such as the Meaningful Use Act (2009), is increasing availability of medical history information, but less improvement has occurred with respect to process and defect causal data. Many healthcare organizations have started automating clinical performance metrics, although significant challenges still exist for aggregating information across patients without tedious manual chart abstraction. Examples include computing National Quality Forum metrics such as the percentage of patients with coronary artery disease who were prescribed antiplatelet therapy (American College of Cardiology et al., 2005) and the number of eligible patients who received venous thromboembolism prophylaxis within a specified time window (The Joint Commission, 2009).

Sometimes when manual data collection remains tedious, creative surrogate measures can be used (such as monitoring soap and towel consumption instead of hand washing compliance via direct observation). In contrast, at times poor data availability is used as an excuse for not conducting important analyses. Even data that are available often can contain an unknown amount of error, compromising the statistical value and cultural buy-in associated with results.

Examples include undetected or under-reported nosocomial infections, medication errors, patient falls and near-misses. Under-reporting is known to reduce the ability of a $p$ chart to detect changes, potentially as much as doubling the ARL time until detection (Benneyan, 1997). Very little methodological work, however, has been conducted in healthcare quality control to understand the degree and corresponding implications of measurement error, as would be conventional practice in manufacturing industries.

## 13.4.2    Rational subgroups

An important sampling concept in statistical quality control is the value of defining rational subgroups, which are based on the assumption that all data within a subgroup to the greatest extent possible are in-control and subject to only natural variation. These data are collected in such a manner that any process changes and special cause variation, conversely, for the most part are likely to occur between subgroups; that is, a rational subgroup is 'a sample in which all of the items are produced under conditions in which only random effects are responsible for the observed variation' (Nelson, 1988). In practice, of course, this theoretic concept can be easier to implement in some settings than in others.

In manufacturing, rational subgroups often are created by sampling consecutive pieces over a short time period and then waiting a period of time before collecting another such subgroup. In healthcare, the registration durations for the first five patients each hour is a good example of a rational subgroup, although in other settings they can be difficult to form in this manner (for example, if using historical data collected for other purposes). While some authors (erroneously) state that rational subgroups are absolute necessities, the greater extent to which they can be implemented, the greater the ability a control chart has to detect process changes. In some cases, in fact, it can be better to sample fewer data that form rational subgroups than to use all available data, in order to avoid misplaced control limits and negative impacts on detection run lengths. Care also should be taken not to combine data across different processes (e.g. different shifts) or populations (e.g. types of procedures), for the same reasons.

## 13.4.3    Specification threshold approaches

Due to a combination of convenience, reporting simplification, and a lack of automatically available data, many common performance metrics are based on dichotomous (yes/no) compliance to thresholds (e.g. antibiotics within/not within 60 minutes, thrombolytic within/not within three hours, door-to-balloon within/not within 90 minutes), rather than based on the raw data themselves (e.g. average and standard deviation of the timing of these same events). Other common performance measures often are measured by the number or rate of occurrences (pressure ulcers, falls, infections) and compliance to standards (hand-washing, use of surgical checklist, checking identification). Consequently, in healthcare, currently attribute ($p$, $np$, $c$, $u$) control charts are used much more frequently than variables ($Xbar$, $R$, $S$) control charts.

While there is nothing mathematically wrong with these charts, *per se*, the consequence of treating continuous data as discrete is to unnecessarily cause longer detection times; that is, a loss of statistical power. Figure 13.2 illustrates this consequence generally, where $\varepsilon$ is the distance of the in-control process mean from the specification (e.g. acceptable maximum time) and $\delta$ is the magnitude of a process change, both in standard deviation units. For

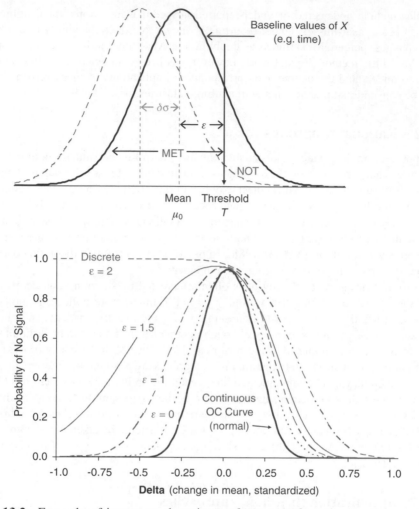

**Figure 13.2**   Example of impact on detection performance of treating continuous data as discrete data.

example, a common performance specification for heart attack patients is reperfusion within 90 minutes of arrival to the emergency department ('door-to-balloon' time). Typically the fraction of patients for whom this level of care was met is monitored over time (such as on a $p$ chart), rather than the actual door-to-balloon times themselves (such as on $Xbar$ and $S$ charts).

Using the actual times would still allow one to compare compliance with the standard, but also would provide more information on process performance and greater sensitivity with no specificity loss. In this case, suppose the mean and standard deviation of door-to-balloon times are 70 and 20 minutes respectively (so $\varepsilon = 1.0$) and that, due to some assignable cause(s), the mean increases to 75 minutes (so $\delta = 0.25$). An $XmR$ chart would detect this shift roughly with probability 0.60 (or an ARL of $1/0.60 \approx 1.67$), whereas the ARL for a $p$ chart would be roughly $1/0.20 = 5$, nearly triple.

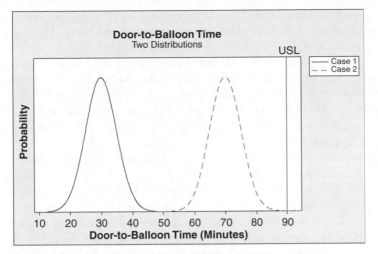

**Figure 13.3**   Illustration of compliance to standards versus quest for quality. USL = upper specification limit.

More simply, this also is a good example of the fallacy of 'management by averages'. In both the in-control and out-of-control cases the mean door-to-balloon time met the 90 minute standard. But in a post-shift case where $\mu = 75$ minutes, approximately 23% of all patients will have a door-to-balloon time longer than the specification standard. Even in the pre-shift case roughly 16% of patients will exceed the 90 minute threshold. Manufacturing firms learned in the 1970s that similarly focusing on all cases meeting specifications was a misleading mindset, as illustrated in the Ford Batavia, Ohio example (Montgomery, 2009). For example, an in-control emergency department process for which door-to-balloon times have an average of 70 minutes with a standard deviation of 5 minutes would arguably not be as good as one with a mean of 30 minutes and the same standard deviation, even though both meet the standard for nearly all patients (see Figure 13.3).

## 13.4.4   Establishing versus maintaining stability

Regardless of data type and integrity, control charts are useful for helping establish control, test the impact of interventions and detect unexpected events. These uses of control charts often are described as being conducted in two sequential phases: first testing for stability and then monitoring for instability. Awareness of the distinction between these two phases, the importance of establishing a state of statistical control, and the relation of this concept to standardized work tends to be lower than in other industries.

In the first phase, often called Phase I, the control limits commonly are calculated from historical data (or less commonly from standards), and any assignable causes or occurrences of irregular variation are identified and eliminated from the process. After this activity is completed, the control chart should exhibit a state of statistical control, with only natural common variability present. The control limits then may be recomputed, to now define the stable process, and used in the second phase to monitor and identify process improvement or deterioration.

It is important to underscore that when first starting to work on many applications, healthcare or otherwise, processes often are not stable and consistent. The analyst therefore should not expect a 'textbook' example for which all data immediately fall between control limits, or for which just one simple assignable cause needs to be removed to magically and quickly reach a state of statistical control. In practice, more often this Phase I 'identify-remove-recompute' activity is an iterative process of calculating control limits, identifying and addressing out-of-control conditions, removing data associated with those assignable causes (that have been addressed), and re-calculating control limits – repeating this process many times until a state of statistical control is established.

As assignable causes of variability are identified and addressed (eliminated if undesirable, standardized if favorable), the process gradually becomes more consistent and predictable. This often is best done by using 'Lean', 'Six Sigma' and other process improvement tools to standardize processes and eliminate unnecessary variation. This activity alone sometimes can take many months, and the analyst or process improvement team should not be discouraged. Eventually achieving a state of control is a major milestone and a good deal of the value of using SPC. Only at that point can it be said that a consistent standard process exists. When Phase I is ignored, opportunities to reduce and control variability can be missed. Achieving an in-control process also is important for comparing performance to standards or benchmarks, since an implicit assumption is that the sampled data represent the overall process (which would not be the case if the process is not in control).

Once a stable process is achieved, one can move to Phase II to monitor the process prospectively using new control limits that now define the expected process variability. This is the more well-known use of control charts, such as to detect an unexpected process change or to verify whether an intentional intervention (such as a change to the work flow or new equipment) has a desired effect. Examples of this more passive phase can be found in numerous publications; so these points are not repeated here. The control limits, however, should not be revised in Phase II without evidence of a changed process. The impact of improvement interventions first should be determined by assessing where points fall on the current control chart and recalculating the limits only if (1) a change has occurred that is expected to be maintained and (2) this change has significantly (statistically) modified the average or variability of the process, usually as evidenced by a now out-of-control condition.

Figure 13.4, for example, illustrates a control chart constructed by a process improvement team working to reduce time to transfer patients from an emergency department to a medical intensive care unit. The team made a change to the process and computed separate control limits for the time periods before and after this change (Figure 13.4a). Note however (Figure 13.4b) that the process was stable (in-control) over the entire time period and exhibits no significant before–after differences. The conclusion instead should be that the tested change did not impact transfer time and that the new control limits should not be revised.

# 13.5    Technical challenges

## 13.5.1    Common errors

By far the four most common mistakes when using basic SPC are (1) selecting an inappropriate control chart, (2) using an inappropriate subgroup size, (3) rampant misuse of 'individuals'

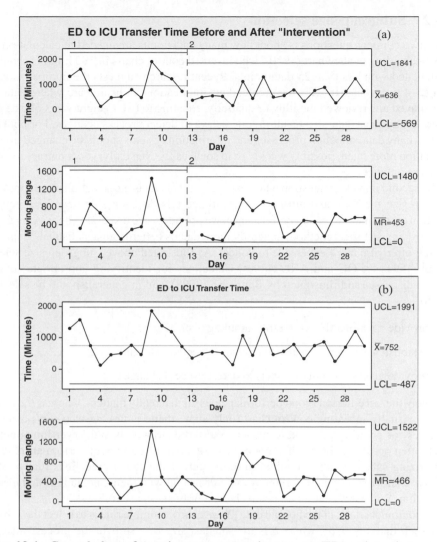

**Figure 13.4** Control charts for patient emergency department (ED) to intensive care unit (ICU) transfer times (a) erroneously suggesting improvement occurred and (b) showing that the tested process change did not impact patient transfer time. UCL = upper control limit; LCL = lower control limit.

*XmR* charts, and (4) failing to verify that statistical assumptions for a given chart are reasonably met. Guidance for selecting a correct chart for given applications has been well-discussed elsewhere (Benneyan, Lloyd and Plsek, 2003; Benneyan, 2008), so we do not discuss this subject at length here. Selecting an appropriate subgroup size and checking assumptions, however, are important practical (and performance) questions that are not discussed much in practitioner-focused literature. Unfortunately *XmR* charts also are encouraged far too much in such publications, in our opinion, from the perspective of performance.

## 13.5.2    Subgroup size selection

One of two common questions is about how many data points are needed to calculate control limits. According to Shewhart (1980), who invented control charts in 1924, limits should not be calculated with less than 25 data points. Recent research suggests the number should be much (2–4 times) higher. This has tremendous implications in healthcare where data often are displayed and reviewed monthly or quarterly, equating to two to eight years of data being required. Infrequent data also result in long delays to detect process changes. For both these reasons, many data collection processes and information systems should be changed to collect information more often, possibly weekly or in some cases even daily, very contrary to current healthcare practices.

The second important question when using control charts is the selection of an appropriate subgroup size for *Xbar* and attribute charts. Since this decision significantly affects data collection costs, time, effort and performance, we provide some discussion here. As is the case for almost any statistical method, generally more data is better from a statistical perspective, although often also more expensive to collect. As illustrated above, subgroup size selection directly affects the OC and ARL curves. Guidelines for identifying appropriate subgroup sizes are discussed and illustrated by Benneyan (2008), and in general should be selected in order to:

- provide a reasonably symmetric sampling distribution;

- establish a non-zero (greater than zero) lower control limit (LCL);

- provide good sensitivity (power) to detect process changes.

Ultimately the last criterion (good performance) is all that really matters, whereas the first two ensure a visually appealing control chart (only an aesthetic issue) but also serve as general surrogates for ensuring good performance. Skewed distributions and lower limits below 0 (which often occur together), while not bad *per se*, often result in poor performance. A table summarizing subgroup sizes required to meet each of the above guidelines for *np*, *p*, *c*, *u* and *Xbar* charts can be found in Benneyan (2008) along with their calculations and theoretic justification. Without repeating all details here, a brief summary follows.

For continuous data, in the normal case (*Xbar* chart), a simple rule is to select the subgroup size $n$ such that $n \geq 9/\delta^2$, where $\delta$ is the smallest size of a shift in the process mean that would be important to detect on average in two plotted points (e.g. two months, quarters). The shift size is stated in standard-deviation units. For example if the mean time to deliver treatment to an emergency department patient was 80 minutes with a standard deviation of 20 minutes, and it were felt important to quickly detect an increase to 90 minutes (i.e. a change in the mean by half a standard deviation), then the minimum subgroup size should be $n = 9/(0.5)^2 = 36$ patients per subgroup. Note that detecting an increase to 100 minutes (i.e. a one-standard-deviation shift) would require only $n = 9/(1)^2 = 9$ patients per subgroup. This example illustrates the general result that larger subgroup sizes are required to detect smaller process changes equally fast.

For discrete data, the standard attribute charts (*p*, *np*, *c*, *u*) all tend to perform reasonably well when their parameters are such that the underlying binomial or Poisson distributions are reasonably approximated by normal distributions. This occurs when the subgroup sizes are sufficiently large relative to the adverse event (AE) rate being studied. In the binomial case (*np* and *p* charts), the subgroup size should be selected so that the centerline $\geq 5$ or

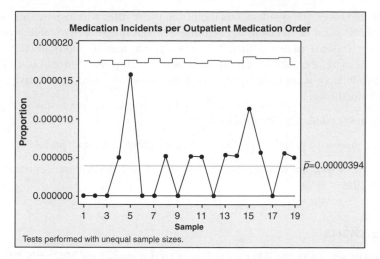

**Figure 13.5**  Example of *p* chart for which subgroup sizes are not large enough for a normal approximation to apply.

equivalently $n \geq 5/p$, where $p$ denotes the AE rate for the particular application. In practice this often is estimated from past data and denoted in SPC by $\bar{p}$. In the Poisson case (*c* and *u* charts), the corresponding rule is that the centerline $\geq 5$ or equivalently $n \geq 5/\lambda$, where $\lambda$ is the average number of occurrences per some unit (e.g. number of falls per 1000 patient-days) and is estimated in SPC by $\bar{c}$. In both cases note that lower AE rates require larger subgroup sizes (ironically, better processes require more data).

If these guidelines are not met, often the LCL will be negative, which motivates the first rule of thumb. Since points cannot fall below zero, the LCL also loses any ability to signal improvements. Figure 13.5 illustrates medication incidents that do not satisfy the above rules and produce negative lower limits (here, and by convention, rounded up to 0).

In this example, $n$ is the number of medication orders per month (on average about 200 000 in this data) and $\bar{p}$ is the proportion of those that resulted in an incident. Since $\bar{p} = 0.00000394$ and $n\bar{p} \approx 0.74$ (using the average subgroup size), the control chart will not be very powerful at detecting process changes. In this example, in order to satisfy the sample-size guideline, $n$ would have to be approximately 1 200 000. In healthcare, if all data are readily available, sample size often is the total number of patients seen and thus cannot be increased within a time frame. One option is to use larger time frames (e.g. sample every quarter instead of every month), but that makes for slower response. Unlike *Xbar* and *S* charts, with attribute control charts, as the process improves more data is required to indicate a change in the process. This is another reason why, where possible, measuring performance on a continuous scale is preferable.

### 13.5.3  Over-use of supplementary rules

Many authors describe the use of supplementary rules for detecting out-of-control conditions and their value for increasing a chart's performance. In cases where sampling logistics prevent LCL > 0, such rules can make control charts more powerful, especially in cases of limited data. However, the simultaneous use of too many rules will increase the overall false alarm rate to the point of frequently generating a signal for perfectly stable processes. The use of all conventional rules together, for example, can lead to approximately a 5% false alarm rate; meaning one false signal on average every 20 points. Instead use of just a few rules will produce an acceptable balance between sensitivity and specificity, with a good recommendation being:

- one point outside of the control limits;
- eight consecutive points all on the same side of the center line; and
- four out of five consecutive points between 1 and 3 standard deviations from the center line.

### 13.5.4   *g* charts

A second approach when the AE rate is low is to use rare-event SPC methods, such as *g* control charts for the number of cases or time between data. These charts were introduced in healthcare by Benneyan and Kaminsky (1995), and the mathematics and performance can be found in Benneyan (2001). To illustrate, recall that Figure 13.5 contained a *p* chart of the proportion of medication orders that resulted in an incident. Since the number of incidents per month is relatively small, the calculated lower control limit is less than zero. Increasing the inter-subgroup time to quarterly would increase the subgroup size but would also require several years to acquire enough data to demonstrate process stability. Figure 13.6 shows these same data presented on a *g* chart in the context of the number of medications (visits) between

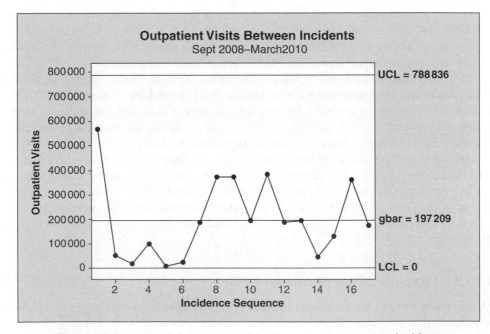

**Figure 13.6**   *g* chart of outpatient visits between adverse event incidents.

events. For this type of chart, a downward trend now indicates an increase in the AE rate (fewer cases between AEs), but otherwise these charts are interpreted the same as any others. While both these charts indicate that the AE rate is stable, if the rate were to change, $g$ charts have the advantage of faster detection (as suggested earlier in Figure 13.1).

### 13.5.5   Misuse of individuals charts

In addition to the standard types of control charts described above ($p$, $np$, $u$, $c$, $Xbar$, $S$), a less powerful chart called an 'individuals' ($XmR$) chart has become more common in healthcare than in other industries. These charts are intended to be used for continuous normally distributed data when plotted individually, rather than aggregated into subgroups. The advantage of using an $Xbar$ chart over an $XmR$ chart is that it is more powerful for detecting process changes faster. That is, power increases as subgroup size increases. $XmR$ charts are becoming routinely recommended as an 'always works' choice even in cases where sufficient data or better chart options exist. In addition to the loss of power, these charts also are much more sensitive to non-normality, since no central limit effects apply, again with consequences on performance. A second common (but inappropriate) practice in healthcare is to use $XmR$ charts for discrete data such as percentages and rates, rather than the more appropriate $p$ and $u$ charts.

A related common error is to apply these charts to aggregated data, such as averages or sums, rather than using the more advisable $Xbar$ or $T$ charts for means or totals. Without going into mathematical details, the consequence of each of these three blunders is to worsen detection performance. Figure 13.7 illustrates an $XmR$ chart applied to length of stay (LOS) data averaged by month. Nonetheless, this chart suggests an out-of-control condition, with a point above the moving range upper confidence limit (UCL) indicating that the variation in the average LOS between June and July of 2007 was unusually high. Note that lost is any knowledge and analysis of the within-month (within-treatment) variability, a fundamental building block in SPC and other statistical methods, with an associated loss in power as

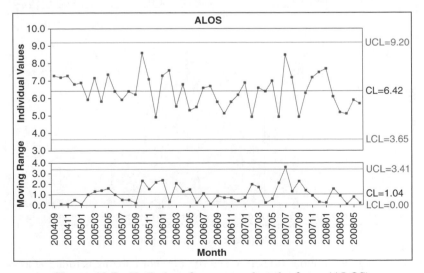

**Figure 13.7**   *XmR* chart for average length of stay (ALOS).

would be expected. Typically, the result is to fail to detect statistical differences in the data or erroneously conclude that an out-of-control process is stable.

### 13.5.6    Distributional assumptions

*XmR* charts assume that the plotted data can be approximated by a normal distribution. Although some authors assert that Chebyshev's theorem allows these charts to be used as a non-parametric tool even if the distribution is non-normal, it is a simple exercise to show that this approach can radically compromise both detection performance and false alarm rates. To illustrate this type of incorrect application of an *XmR* chart, Figure 13.8a plots the duration

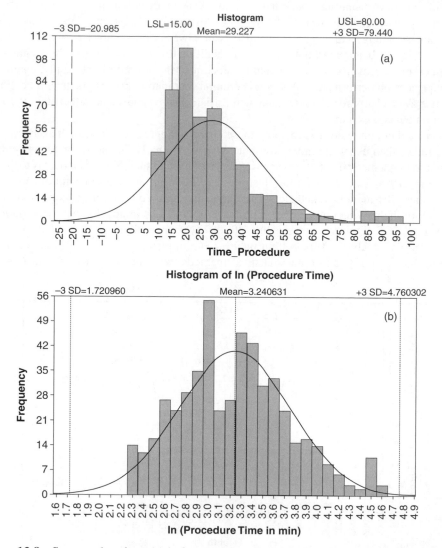

**Figure 13.8**    Surgery durations (a) before and (b) after normalizing natural log transformation. USL = upper specification limit; LSL = lower specification limit.

(in minutes) for a surgical procedure. Note the significant non-normality of these data and the fact that the mean minus three standard deviations (i.e. roughly the LCL) is far below zero. When estimated in the usual manner using moving ranges, the exact control limits are shown in Figure 13.9a. Many points fall above the upper control limits of both the $X$ and $MR$ charts, either because the process truly is out of control or because of natural non-normality. Unfortunately, even an informed analyst has no way of knowing which situation is the case.

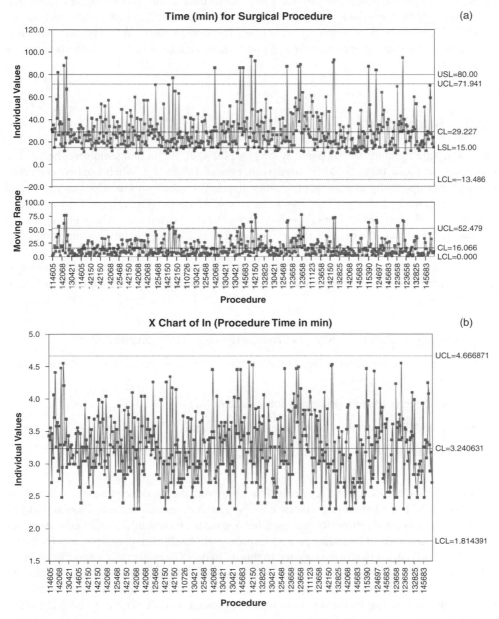

**Figure 13.9**   Individuals chart of (a) original, versus (b) transformed surgery durations.

Figure 13.8b illustrates a histogram of the natural log of each data value, which in this case results in approximate normality. As shown in Figure 13.9b, these transformed data now exhibit a state of statistical control and the correct conclusion therefore is that surgery durations appear consistently random over time, whereas the three to four dozen points above the UCL for the untransformed data appear all to be false alarms. The opposite conclusion (i.e. significant process instability) just as likely may have resulted after transformation.

Similarly, naively applying *XmR* charts to number-between and time-between data, increasingly frequent and very poor advice, can produce false alarm rates of roughly 1.8%; that is, one false signal every ARL = 55 plotted points (versus a more acceptable and conventional $\alpha = 0.0027$, with one false alarm every ARL = 370 plotted points). While beyond the scope here, a related disturbing theoretic error is poorly advised transformation methods for these types of data.

## 13.6   Summary

Statistical quality control charts are a very useful tool for helping improve healthcare processes, and one that should be used with greater frequency. When applied correctly, tremendous opportunity exists to apply industrial quality control tools to help standardize and improve healthcare delivery across all six Institute of Medicine dimensions of care – safety, timeliness, efficiency, effectiveness, equity and patient-centeredness. Although seemingly simple on the surface, however, a fair amount of statistical theory is involved in using them correctly and for greatest impact.

This chapter discussed several implementation challenges, conceptual misunderstandings, and common pitfalls in using control charts in healthcare settings. The most common of these include:

- selecting an inappropriate type of chart, subgroup size or sampling interval;
- conceptual misunderstandings of the meaning of process stability and its relationship to standardized processes;
- lack of access to appropriate and accurate data;
- skipping the important 'Phase I' use of control charts;
- poorly advised over-simplified charts, calculations and transformations.

The contribution of SPC can be accelerated by improving the knowledge base within healthcare about SPC and by removing common misunderstandings and barriers discussed in this chapter. This has implications for the need for a greater amount of *accurate* education developed and delivered to front-line process improvement healthcare personnel, and for better education materials and software targeted to this audience. Currently only a handful of either exist, and fewer still are error free. Some well-meaning methods currently being taught and implemented in software in fact may be slowing down healthcare improvement. Train-the-trainer programs are somewhat at fault as well. As Einstein said, 'Everything should be made as simple as possible, but not simpler.'

# References

American College of Cardiology, American Heart Association and Physician Consortium for Performance Improvement (2005) Clinical Performance Measures: Chronic Stable Coronary Artery Disease. Tools Developed by Physicians for Physicians, American Medical Association.

Benneyan, J.C. (1997) Approaches to Quality in the Presence of Inspection Error. Doctoral dissertation, University of Massachusetts-Amherst.

Benneyan, J.C. (1998) Use and interpretation of statistical quality control charts. *International Journal for Quality in Health Care*, **10**(1), 69–73.

Benneyan, J.C. (1999) Some control chart caveats. *Infection Control and Hospital Epidemiology*, **20**(8), 526–527.

Benneyan, J.C. (2001) Performance of number-between g-type statistical control charts for monitoring adverse events. *Health Care Management Science*, **4**, 319–336.

Benneyan, J.C. (2008) Design, use, and performance of statistical process control charts for clinical process improvement. *International Journal of Six Sigma*, **4**(3), 219–239.

Benneyan, J.C. and Kaminsky, F.C. (1995) Successfully applying SPC to improve health care. *American Society for Quality Control Annual Quality Congress Transactions*, **49**, 578–586.

Benneyan, J.C., Lloyd, R.C. and Plsek, P.E. (2003) Statistical process control as a tool for research and healthcare improvement. *Quality Safety Health Care*, **12**, 458–464.

Gawande, A. (2009) *The Checklist Manifesto – How to Get Things Right*, Henry Holt and Company, New York.

Hospital Compare (2010) http://www.hospitalcompare.hhs.gov/Hospital/Search/compareHospitals.asp, US Department of Health and Human Services (accessed March 18, 2010).

The Joint Commission (2009) Venous Thromboembolism (VTE) Core Measure Set. VTE-1: Venous Thromboembolism Prophylaxis. Available at: www.jointcommission.org/venous_thromboembolism/ (accessed April 11, 2012).

Juran, J.M. and Gryna, F. (1988) *Juran's Quality Control Handbook*, 4th edn, McGraw-Hill, New York.

Meaningful Use Act (2009) Medicare and Medicaid Programs, Electronic Health Record Incentive Program, part of the American Recovery and Reinvestment Act of 2009, ARRA, Pub. L. 111-5, published by Health and Human Services, Centers for Medicare and Medicaid Services.

Mohammed, M.A., Worthington, P. and Woodall, W.H. (2008) Plotting basic control charts: tutorial notes for healthcare practitioners. *Quality Safety Health Care*, **17**, 137–145.

Montgomery, D.C. (2009) *Introduction to Statistical Quality Control*, 6th edn, John Wiley & Sons, Inc., New York.

Nelson, L.S. (1988) Control charts: rational subgroups and effective applications. *Journal of Quality Technology*, **20**, 1.

Shewhart, W.A. (1980) *Economic Control of Quality of Manufactured Product*, American Society for Quality Control, Milwaukee, WI.

WHO (2009) *WHO Guidelines on Hand Hygiene in Health Care: a Summary – First Global Patient Safety Challenge – Clean Care is Safer Care*, WHO/IER/PSP/2009.07, World Health Organization, Geneva.

# 14

# Six Sigma in healthcare

**Shirley Y. Coleman**
*Industrial Statistics Research Unit, Newcastle University,*
*Newcastle upon Tyne, UK*

## Synopsis

Spurred on by hopes of similar gains to those found in the manufacturing sector and enthusiasm for the methodology, Six Sigma has spread from manufacturing and process industries into the service sector, finance, research, public service, education and healthcare. Healthcare, however, is one of the most important application areas, partly because of the enormous size of the healthcare sector, but also because of the intrinsic value and importance of healthcare to everyone's well being; and because of the inherent complexity and inter-dependence of the many activities associated with it. Healthcare is different to other sectors. Patients are sick and in danger of becoming sicker. They are extremely variable, and treating their ailments is a complex business involving many departments and many people. Six Sigma is characterised by its DMAIC phases and structured approach to problem-solving. This has the advantage of helping people to work together and makes it easier to document projects and share with other interested parties. A project charter records: the team members, the objectives, the methodology, resources required, the reporting structure and the timescale of the project. Participatory learning is more enjoyable than being a passive receptor and it is much more effective at embedding knowledge and skills. A feature of Six Sigma is an event to celebrate the outcomes and to share the benefits and learning with a wider community. At one time statisticians were in the role of technical advisers; a task came along and the statistician applied their art and presented a solution. There was less attention paid to whether it was the right problem, whether it was a sensible solution, whether the stakeholders understood and could use the solution, whether the solution was robust to change, whether the solution

*Statistical Methods in Healthcare*, First Edition. Edited by Frederick W. Faltin, Ron S. Kenett and Fabrizio Ruggeri.
© 2012 John Wiley & Sons, Ltd. Published 2012 by John Wiley & Sons, Ltd.

was value for money. Six Sigma has helped statisticians to work in a more professional way, raising their professional status and making them more useful partners with other healthcare professionals.

## 14.1 Introduction

Six Sigma was developed as a methodology for improving efficiency and profitability in manufacturing. It combines quality improvement and statistical data analysis in a business-oriented, inclusive methodology. It has grown out of earlier quality initiatives and arguably combines the best parts of them all. Six Sigma is now producing some important results in the healthcare arena in terms of improvement of services, breakthroughs in understanding and communication, and new ways of working of mutual benefit to consumers and providers of healthcare.

Healthcare involves a wide range of services, stakeholders and functions and is characterised by large buildings, multiple wards and beds, car parks, injured and sick people, doctors, nurses, professions allied to medicine, ambulances, mental health patients, paramedics and pharmacists. In other words it is a complicated mix of vested interest, variability and urgency.

Six Sigma has been shown to be widely applicable; examples and case studies can be found in many websites and journals, see for example, www.asq.org/healthcaresixsigma/articles/ssfhc-form.html.

Healthcare workers in all departments are expected continuously to improve the quality, timeliness and cost of their services to the community. Six Sigma appeals to the practical enthusiasm of healthcare workers to get more for their patients and increase the effectiveness of the services they provide. Mukherjee (2008) describes a Six Sigma project to increase take up of pharmacy facility in a hospital. The result is a win, win, win situation in which hospital profits increase, patients receive a better service and staff develop new skills.

Six Sigma is ideally placed to address:

- the delivery of healthcare by integrating patient care and safety improvements

- healthcare efficiencies and efficacy by checking that the right things are being done at the right cost

- an operational approach to evidence-based medicine and risk management.

Staff require skills to manage both the quality and cost of healthcare, and this is facilitated by Six Sigma methodology that is interdisciplinary and project based. Six Sigma projects are circumscribed and well defined. Projects help to ensure the ring-fenced time and effort and freedom from interference so vital to successful outcomes.

Statisticians have provided sound statistical support and analysis to healthcare for many years. Six Sigma, however, takes statistical support one step further as it incorporates the statistical intervention within a sound business methodology consisting of good problem definition up front and solid appraisal and evaluation at the end of the work. Communication skills are given a high profile, as the importance of effective exchange of ideas is well recognised (Caulcutt, 2008).

In this chapter, we will give an overview of Six Sigma, including its historical roots and the way it is currently evolving. We will consider the special features of healthcare and compare the healthcare sector with other sectors also making use of Six Sigma. We will look at each phase of Six Sigma in the context of healthcare. Lean Six Sigma combines the waste and complexity reduction of Lean manufacturing with the statistics, problem-solving and project management aspects of Six Sigma. Lean and Lean Six Sigma have proved accessible to healthcare and this will also be discussed. We will consider barriers to adopting Six Sigma and look at the way forward for Six Sigma in healthcare.

## 14.2    Six Sigma background

In the early 1980s Motorola launched their application of standard statistical analysis to process improvement. Six Sigma was 'released' as a formal methodology in the early 1990s, and Motorola owns the copyright of the term 'Six Sigma'. Six Sigma is a project-based quality improvement methodology in which projects are tackled by focusing on five phases, DMAIC: Define, Measure, Analyse, Improve and Control. A final phase of Transfer may also be included. Six Sigma started in manufacturing but has now spread to other sectors. Each of the phases makes use of various statistical and problem-solving techniques. Six Sigma is more than the sum of its parts. Its success has been credited to advantages such as the adoption of a common nomenclature and cross-departmental team working. Bob Galvin, past chairman of Motorola said 'At Motorola we use statistical methods daily throughout all of our disciplines to synthesize an abundance of data to drive concrete actions... How has the use of statistical methods within Motorola Six Sigma initiative, across disciplines, contributed to our growth? Over the past decade we have reduced in-process defects by over 300 fold, which has resulted in cumulative manufacturing cost savings of over 11 billion dollars' (referred to by Kenett and Zacks, 1998).

Six Sigma was further developed by General Electric in the later 1990s. In 1995 General Electric mandated each employee to adopt Six Sigma methodology, and extensive training was carried out. Jack Welch, as Chief Executive Officer of General Electric said Six Sigma was 'the most important initiative GE has ever undertaken'. In 1998 investments in Six Sigma training and projects reached 45 million US dollars; profits increased by 1.2 billion US dollars.

General Electric's undoubted success in using this Six Sigma methodology and publically attributed large cost savings assured its rapid uptake by many other companies. The list is increasing all the time, but early participants included Bank of America, Caterpillar and Honeywell International (previously known as Allied Signal). The January/February 2007 issue of *iSixSigma Magazine* (www.isixsigma-magazine.com) stated that 'Over the past 20 years, use of Six Sigma, the popular business improvement methodology, has saved Fortune 500 companies an estimated $427 billion.'

The interest in Six Sigma has grown over the years, for example a search for 'Six Sigma' in Google in September 2005 yielded 4 460 000 entries; a search in September 2007 yielded 18 200 000 entries. In June 2010 there were 7 950 000 entries with 10 101 000 for Lean Six Sigma and 46 100 000 for Lean, which shows how Six Sigma has spread out into additional associated methodologies.

Six Sigma builds on the quality improvement philosophies of major figures, such as Walter Shewhart, W. Edwards Deming, Joseph Juran and Kaoru Ishikawa. It draws on the achievements of earlier quality improvement initiatives, such as Total Quality Management (TQM) and the European Foundation for Quality Management (EFQM) Excellence model; see for example Juran (1999); Montgomery and Woodall (2008).

The term 'Six Sigma' has a statistical interpretation: 'sigma' is the term for standard deviation and 'Six Sigma' refers to the aim of having process variation so low that the mean plus and minus six standard deviations fits within the specification limits. Allowing for the process mean to deviate from target by up to 1.5 standard deviations, Six Sigma translates to having no more than 3.4 defects per million;[1] see, for example, Henderson (2006). Six Sigma is a catchy name and initially divided the statistical community. Some statisticians embraced the idea as an excellent opportunity for statisticians and for increasing the respect given to the scientific method. Other statisticians were concerned about the possible misuse of powerful statistical techniques such as design of experiments, statistical process control and multiple regression (Coleman, 2008).

Six Sigma is part of a widespread movement towards valuing the scientific/engineering method for facilitating improvement and innovation. See for example chapters on Six Sigma, Lean Six Sigma and Quality by Design in Ruggeri, Kenett and Faltin (2007). Six Sigma fits in with the PDCA (Plan-Do-Check/Study-Act) cycle described by Deming (1986), as it is usually part of a continual improvement culture.

Spurred on by hopes of similar gains to those found in the manufacturing sector and enthusiasm for the methodology, Six Sigma has spread from manufacturing and process industries into the service sector (see for example Hoerl and Snee, 2005), and from there into all sectors including finance, research, public service, education and healthcare. Healthcare, however, is one of the most important application areas partly because of the enormous size of the healthcare sector, but also because of the intrinsic value and importance of healthcare to everyone's well being; and because of the inherent complexity and inter-dependence of the many activities associated with it.

## 14.3   Development of Six Sigma in healthcare

There is a long history of statistics in healthcare research; for example clinical trials, longitudinal studies, risk analysis (see for example Bradford Hill, 1967). However, statistical analysis of healthcare processes was less common until relatively recently. Economic forecasts and planning were based on models which did not include the actual experience of what happens day to day in a ward or operating theatre.

Statistical measurement in the UK NHS (National Health Service) had a boost with the Patient's Charter in 1991. This led to a mass of ideas for applying management quality improvement methodologies to achieve productivity increases and cost cutting; for example recording snap shots of what everyone was doing at a certain time point and several attempts to apply TQM, including quality circles, to hospitals.

Healthcare is different from other sectors. Patients are sick and in danger of becoming sicker. They are extremely variable, and treating their ailments is a complex business involving many departments and many people. A tangible, practical example of the difficulties is conformance to requirements. In the manufacturing sector, it is expected that employees will conform to rules; however, in the healthcare sector employees are carers who are very aware of their primary responsibility to their patients. For example, it is a requirement for midwives to recommend pregnant women who smoke to attend the smoking cessation service. However,

---

[1] The probability of 3.4 per million is calculated for the variable to be between 7.5 and 4.5 standard deviations of the mean rather than symmetrically six standard deviations either side of the mean.

**Table 14.1**   Healthcare compared to manufacturing.

| Manufacturing | Healthcare |
| --- | --- |
| Large variability in quality of product | Large variability in time taken to carry out 'jobs' |
| Unavailable parts/materials | Staff waiting on information |
| Excessive material/parts handling | Duplication/excessive information transfers |
| Errors *and* waste | Errors *and* waste |
| Frequent re-work, scrapped product | Relapse, recurrence, demise |

the subject of a Six Sigma project was to improve the conformance from 70 to 90%. This was surprising; why isn't there conformance already? In manufacturing, if members of a work cell are told, for example, to check the measurements of a component before fitting, then there would probably be 100% conformance. However, in healthcare, the situation is different. Midwives who deal with smoking pregnant women may well encounter women who have very difficult lives, for example with children in care, drug addiction and deprivation. Trying to give up smoking would be an additional problem for them; therefore the midwives do not send them to anti-smoking classes. Interestingly, there is currently a hot debate in the UK as to whether pregnant women should be automatically given smoke-detecting breath tests. This shows the complicated issues that exist when systems are dealing with human beings in challenging circumstances.

The intellectual capital in a hospital is enormous, and all departments are inter-related. Unlike other sectors, the effect of errors and mistakes can be the actual loss of a fellow human being. Nevertheless, issues which encouraged the development of Six Sigma in manufacturing also affect healthcare. Some of these are given in Table 14.1. The drive towards quality improvement has been unstoppable, however, and the Intelligent Board was an attempt to bring evidence-based decision making into the UK NHS health authorities. It was well received and led to the use of key performance indicators in board-level meetings and a number of useful software packages, for example Dr Foster (www.drfosterintelligence.co.uk/), and now CHKS (Comparative Health Knowledge System; www.chks.co.uk/).

Some of the facts about healthcare are surprising and worrying. According to the UK All-Party Parliamentary Group on Patient Safety, 'Patient safety is rightly a top priority for the NHS and is of increasing concern to the general public. Each year 400,000 avoidable adverse incidents occur in patient care that directly lead to 40,000 deaths. This is costing the NHS £2 billion a year in extended hospital stays alone' (see www.dh.gov.uk/en/ Publicationsandstatistics/Publications/PublicationsPolicyAndGuidance/Browsable/DH_409 7460). Risks to patients of around 20% are common, and there is increasing interest in improving patient safety (Health Foundation, 2010). In fact, many excellent Six Sigma case studies have arisen from the Institute of Healthcare Improvement (www.ihi.org/ihi) in the USA, who instigated an initiative to save 100 000 avoidable deaths after the publication of a report by the Institute of Medicine (1999). They claim to have achieved the target making changes such as: deploying rapid response teams; preventing adverse drug events; preventing infections. Their next aim is to save five million patients from avoidable harm.

Six Sigma is being deployed in healthcare, but it is not necessarily always for the best. Systems thinking and a holistic approach are particularly important. A project which concludes that nurses will be less stressed if patient access is restricted to clearly delineated times of the day will not be similarly welcome to patients' relatives. It is particularly important to establish what the patient wants; that is, to listen to the voice of the customer. One patient may want to have their elective surgery as soon as possible after diagnosis; another may want time to come to terms with the idea. In some ways, healthcare presents an impossible conflict of interest because patients want to have as much attention as possible, doctors and nurses want to have enough time and space to do their job properly without interruption, and healthcare funders want to limit their costs.

As an indication of the interest in quality improvement, all 378 NHS Trusts providing health services in England since April 2010 are required to register with the newly reorganised Care Quality Commission under a new tougher system for regulating standards (Care Quality Commission, 2012). One of the activities is to check that Trusts meet 16 essential standards of quality and safety. The fourth standard – meeting nutritional needs – requires that 'You are supported to have sufficient food and drink and a choice of food and drink to meet your diverse needs.' Hospital catering is an area that can benefit from the application of Six Sigma. The enormous amount of food waste in hospitals is well documented (Department of Health, 2005) and attempts have been made to improve the situation. The complexities are enormous, however, with waste arising from many sources: for example patients feeling ill and changing their mind about eating; poor timing resulting in unattractive meals. There are many barriers to reducing problems such as food waste, including reluctance to share information, fear of reduction of benefit to patients by tampering with a system that currently works. Nevertheless, when the complexities of healthcare are acknowledged and there is allowance for dealing with people instead of objects, Six Sigma has had some excellent successes. Interesting case studies can be found at www.isixsigma.com, the NHS Institute for Innovation and Improvement (www.institute.nhs.uk), the American Society for Quality Healthcare Division (www.asq.org) and elsewhere.

Healthcare funding differs enormously from country to country, and this has a profound impact on the way it is run. Healthcare stakeholders are also characterised by different roles:

- clinicians want to make people well

- management want to make the provision cost effective.

Nevertheless, all healthcare organisations and stakeholders have a joint interest in providing a service which is

- timely

- safe

- fair.

Consequently, most successful Six Sigma projects are collaborative.

Some in healthcare dislike the assumption that they have much to learn from manufacturing; they want manufacturing to learn from them. This is a positive sign and suggests that ownership is leading to a new stage in Six Sigma in healthcare.

## 14.4    The phases and tools of Six Sigma

*Tools of Six Sigma:* Six Sigma includes problem definition, problem analysis, team working, statistical analysis, data presentation and evaluation. The syllabus (or Body of Knowledge) used by the American Society for Quality for certification is available at www.asq.org/certification/six-sigma/bok.html.

A wide range of tools are relevant. There are many free internet resources describing the tools; for example the world class manufacturing site http://wcm.nu. Some of the most popular tools are the graphical tools including Ishikawa's seven quality improvement tools.

*Ishikawa quality improvement tools:*

- flow charts

- data collection forms

- histograms

- scatterplots

- Pareto charts

- run/control charts

- cause and effect diagrams.

In addition there are other excellent graphical tools; for example the location plots which were instrumental in identifying the source of a cholera outbreak in London in1854 (see for example Magnello, 2009). More recently, websites such as www.gapminder.org have vivid graphical representations of data showing patterns and correlations hitherto unrecognised.

The international standard ISO9004 (ISO, 1993) describes the so-called modern improvement tools which are also part of Six Sigma; for example affinity and tree diagrams. The NHS Institute for Innovation and Improvement gives detailed guidance on how to use tools, for example Force Field Analysis, which is at www.institute.nhs.uk/quality_and_service_improvement_tools/quality_and_service_improvement_tools/force_field_analysis.html.

## 14.5    DMAIC overview

Six Sigma is characterised by its phased and structured approach to problem-solving. This has the advantage of helping people to work together and for the work to be thorough. It also makes it easier to document projects and share with other interested parties.

### 14.5.1    Define

The first phase is arguably the most important and certainly tends to absorb people the most. In fact it is often difficult to move people on to the subsequent phases. This phase captures the imagination and helps clarify the problem as well as focusing everyone's attention on the project. The Define phase helps to avoid starting on projects which cannot be completed, as it ensures that issues of resources, time scale and purpose are thoroughly explored before the project actually starts. One of the Define phase features is to specify SMART objectives.

These are Specific, Measureable, Achievable, Realistic and Timely. The SMART objectives help to formulate the business case for the project. It should be checked that the objectives are in line with the strategic objectives of the institution. The project scope should not be too large. Each project should aim to be completed in about six months. Deliverables should be outlined and agreed in principle. As part of the project definition, the current baseline is stated.

*Some tools of the Define phase:*

- problem analysis methods, for example Kepner-Tregoe;

- team building, Six hats of Edward de Bono;

- TRIZ theory of inventive problem-solving;

- BS 7850 I and II (ISO 9004-4:1993) Total Quality Management tools;

- value stream mapping;

- process cycle efficiency;

- FMEA (failure mode and effect analysis) and QFD (quality function deployment).

*Example*

Day surgery waiting times at South Tyneside District Hospital were slashed from nine months to three weeks as a result of a business improvement technique called Process Improvement for Strategic Objectives (PISO) developed by the University of Sunderland. PISO uses data flow diagrams to allow managers to see how their strategic objectives can be achieved. The process can be taught to anyone with a basic understanding of business in only a few hours and provides a means of solving organisational problems that can make working life so frustrating. The results for the hospital were outstanding, and a new Day Surgery Direct service was successfully trialled on patients with groin hernias. As well as dramatically reducing waiting times, quality improvements have also been made. For instance, a sick note is provided at discharge to cover the whole period that the patient will need off work. Ms Tann, head of the Trust's performance management, said: 'The approach used in PISO is potentially transferable to other elective procedures and will assist the Trust in achieving its aim of becoming a "no waiting" Trust. We are currently reviewing our pre-operative assessment service using PISO.'

www.medicalnewstoday.com/articles/35877.php

## 14.5.2  Measure

The Measure phase focuses attention on all aspects of evaluation. Measurements should represent the problem at hand and also be reliable, precise and repeatable and have sufficient information content to be analysable effectively. Measuring effectiveness of interventions is one of the most sought-after skills.

*The activities in this phase include:*

- identify key metrics

- measurement system analysis

- assess 'current cost' of problem

- data collection, surveys and questionnaires

- operational definitions

- qualitative data analysis, for example diaries, observation

- Statistical Process Control (SPC).

*Typical clinical measures, process and outcomes include:*

- lab turnaround time

- days from positive mammogram to definitive biopsy

- patient satisfaction scores

- medication error counts

- emergency service response times

- infection rates

- mortality rates

- number of patient falls

- post-operative length of stay

- 'door-to-needle' time.

Charting is a familiar concept in healthcare. However, the way charts are used, for example a temperature chart, is intrinsically different to an SPC chart. Training in SPC has been ongoing in healthcare for many years. SPC has been well accepted, as implied by the other chapters in this book. The NHS Scotland website www.indicators.scot.nhs.uk/SPC/Main.html provides an SPC tutorial guide and free Excel SPC chart tool. Some excellent healthcare examples of SPC are given in Woodall (2006); Mohammed, Worthington and Woodall (2008); and Henderson *et al.* (2008).
   *Some tools of the Measure phase are:*

- data quality and access

- variation

- summary statistics

- probability distributions

- measurement system analysis

- process capability

- customer surveys.

*Example* Six Sigma promotes holistic problem-solving, emphasising circumspection before jumping into action. Consider the following scenario:

One month, 30% of patients had medication errors. What did the Six Sigma–trained staff do?

1. Panic and double the staff numbers to allow double checks? *No*

2. Check the figures to make sure they were correct? *No*

3. Compare the error rate with previous months? *Yes*

It may well be found that the current rate is not dissimilar from previous months and 30% is not uncommon for medication errors. Recording error is not the problem here, and doubling the staff numbers is not (necessarily) the best option. Improvement requires root cause analysis and fundamental change. Although this is a hypothetical scenario, a Six Sigma project which may have resulted from just such a panic is reported at www.ncbi .nlm.nih.gov/pubmed/15999960.

## 14.5.3   Analyse

This is the most interesting area as it involves root cause analysis. Often there is a lot of data around and this phase involves sifting through it identifying important factors (sometimes called the red Xs) and generally looking for patterns and correlations. Some surprising results can be found. For example, the waiting time for a coronary artery by-pass graft is less the closer to the hospital the patient lives.

The data must be compatible and of good quality. Care must be taken to ensure that metadata – that is, data describing start dates, operational definitions, purpose of collection, timeliness and so on – are available and well understood, otherwise false alarms can occur.

Statistical tools can be used as well as graphical tools. In addition, if there are sufficient data, some of the data mining tools are useful, for example recursive partitioning and cluster analysis, as well as partial least squares and principal components regression.

*Some of the activities involved in this phase are:*

• examine process variation and capability

• analyse data

• identify factors believed to influence the problem.

Data displays are useful in this phase, for example, looking at a typical set of data, visualising data with creative graphics, comparing before and after figures. Unfortunately analysis is often limited because the data are incomplete and unreliable.

*Some tools of the Analyse phase are:*

• looking for causes

• comparative tests, for example *t*-tests

• confidence intervals

• correlation and regression

• analysis of variance

- non-parametric tests
- reliability.

*Example* When patients are discharged from hospital they are invited to press one of two buttons on their way out: one button says that they are satisfied with their treatment, the other says that they are dissatisfied with their treatment. Data are collected from all wards and are analysed to look for factors which give satisfaction; potential explanatory factors are type of ward, day and time of discharge. A decision tree shows which factors are most important for separating satisfied patients from dissatisfied patients. The recursive partition analysis is just the initial analysis and points to further statistical analysis using logistic regression, and presentation via slicing and dicing in pivot tables.

## 14.5.4   Improve

Now that the problem has been well defined, measures and past data have been analysed, the focus moves to how the current situation can be improved.

   *The activities in this phase include:*

- investigate vital factors – determine 'best settings'
- interpret: do changes give desired consequences?
- carry out cost analysis of changes
- designed experiments; some need ethical approval. Table 14.2 shows some possible types of experiment which could be applicable.

It is often thought that determining basic issues like when to discharge patients is impossible because the enormous amount of patient variability makes a large number of trials necessary and this could take a lot of time, and the whole system changes with time, making experiments infeasible. However, large samples are required when the differences being sought are small, as they often are in clinical research. But in healthcare we may be interested in large changes and therefore require fewer trials. For example, is it better to send mental illness patients or elderly

**Table 14.2**   Types of experiment for the Improve phase.

| Type of experiment | Application | Comments |
| --- | --- | --- |
| Kano analysis | Identify features which are expected, which please and which delight | Not all features may be provided |
| Conjoint analysis | Identify important factors by presenting scenarios and asking subjects to consider the factors jointly | Many patients are elderly and unable to cope with complicated questionnaires; easier to ask carers |
| Factorial experiments | Look for best methods, e.g. of training personnel | May take time to set up |

people home quickly after treatment or to keep them in hospital? There is copious information on this, and an experiment could readily be carried out looking for large differences in outcome. The main problem is that it would require a lot of agencies working together, and that is the real drawback.

Another problem with statistical experiments is that large differences are obvious; smaller differences may not be statistically significant and so the opportunities for statistics to make a difference are limited. Similarly, real data are messy and may not adhere to assumptions, and yet non-parametric alternative tests are usually much less powerful than parametric tests, such as $t$-tests and analysis of variance. Data mining may well be the way forward, providing that apparent relationships are checked and confirmed before action is taken.

The major problem with trying to improve a complex system is that changing one part can impact on another. For example, to release beds for new patients, a solution is to send some patients home, but this puts much more work on external agencies and also increases re-admissions to hospital.

*Some tools of the Improve phase are:*

- design of experiments
- robust designs
- risk management
- graphical presentation
- Poka Yoke or fault proofing
- theory of constraints
- Pull and 5S.

## 14.5.5   Control

The most important part of a Six Sigma project is realising the benefits of the project. This involves evaluating the work, giving feedback to stakeholders and trying to ensure that the benefits are maintained.

*Some of the activities of the Control phase are:*

- implement changes
- hold the gains
- review the project
- dashboard creation.

*Some of the tools of the Control phase are:*

- design and implementation of SPC
- different types of charts

- guidelines and control plans

- review meetings

- holding the gains

- visual management.

Peer comparison is a powerful tool in healthcare, but it can be demoralising if it used instead of statistical process control. Organisations can compare themselves to similar groups using funnel charts (Spiegelhalter, 2005). Some organisations are signed up to a system that instigates an enquiry whenever an organisation is outside of the funnel plot control limits. An Excel spreadsheet to construct a funnel plot is given at www.apho.org.uk/resource/view.aspx?RID=47239.

### 14.5.6    Transfer

After all the work of a successful Six Sigma project, the final phase is to look carefully at where the lessons learnt and the methodology developed can be used in other departments to find similar solutions and benefits.

An example of the difference that the Six Sigma approach can make to a project (Toolan and Coleman, 1994) is shown in Table 14.3.

## 14.6    Operational issues of Six Sigma

### 14.6.1    Personnel

Six Sigma requires fundamental training for all personnel. The majority of staff are given an appreciation of Six Sigma combined with a review of the strategic goals of the organisation and of the current initiative. The depth of training for those more actively involved varies. Some prefer to announce the new initiative and try to include all staff at the start; others recommend a more gradual 'crawl-walk-run' process in which projects are addressed using Six Sigma methodology and the good results inspire others to join in (Arthur, 2005).

The most familiar name for Six Sigma personnel is 'black belt'. Such martial arts names, however, are not popular with healthcare workers, who see themselves more in a saving and caring role than in attacking and defending. Some companies have used more corporately associated names, such as 'high-performance action team', and some avoid the names as they don't want to be associated with yet another fad. However, regardless of the actual names, the roles of the different personnel still stand. Typically the roles are the following.

- **Black Belts (BBs)** are trained in all Six Sigma methods and manage the process improvement, leading projects and training other staff.

- **Green Belts (GBs)** help gather data and keep the process going, sometimes they also lead projects.

- **Yellow Belts (YBs)** are briefed in Six Sigma methodology and support the green and black belts; yellow belts can be drawn from higher management, operational, technical or administrative roles.

**Table 14.3** Example: music therapy.

| Six Sigma phase | Pre-Six Sigma version | Post-Six Sigma version |
|---|---|---|
| Define project | Use music to provide therapy for patients with learning disabilities. | Provide evidence of benefit of music therapy for patients with a range of learning disabilities. |
| Measure | Three observers score video recording of the patients' engagement every minute for five weekly, 30-minute sessions. | Calculate cost of music therapy and benchmark with other therapies. Establish baseline engagement. Three observers score the patients' engagement every minute for five weekly, 30 minute sessions. Check measurement reliability. |
| Analyse | Conduct literature review. Study the engagement over time. | Conduct literature review. Plot the engagement over time, compare changes between and within patients. Include input from music therapist. |
| Improve | Hope to show increase in engagement, thereby justifying cost of music therapist. | Experiment with time, location, timing, type of music and instruments. |
| Control | | Recommend best practice and maintain. Periodically review patients' engagement. Assess cost benefit of music therapy and decide salary for therapist. |
| Transfer | | Consider using above methodology to assess effectiveness of other interventions, e.g. art therapy. |

- **Master Black Belts (MBBs)** have extensive experience including time as a black belt, act as mentors to others and help in certification; they have shown competence in the deeper aspects of Six Sigma methodology.

- **Champions** smooth the path to make projects happen; champions are usually in higher management.

Black belts spend the majority of their time on Six Sigma projects, but are usually expected to move on from the role after about two years (Hoerl, 2001). The job prospects for black belts are very good, making the training highly sought after. This gives issues in terms of how to keep good staff.

In the healthcare arena, great attention is quite rightly given to choosing the right people to train in Six Sigma. Amongst other requirements, people need to have a thirst for new ideas; good communication skills; interest in the scientific problem-solving method; be at a suitable point in their healthcare careers; be willing and able to challenge and to present the results of their work. Putting findings into action will require determination and ability to manage change.

The numbers of Six Sigma black, green and yellow belts is often discussed. They vary considerably from organisation to organisation and there is no fixed ratio.

## 14.6.2    Project selection

Six Sigma training is practically orientated and is best carried out around a relevant project that the tools and techniques can be related to. Certification usually involves the successful completion of one or more projects. Projects are usually expected to be completed in about six months and to have a quantifiable benefit.

Project selection can be facilitated in a number of ways, but what is most important is that the projects are chosen before the training is carried out and that the choice of project is acknowledged to be as important as the choice of personnel.

The matrix method helps to formulate ideas and also to justify the eventual choice. Each potential project is assessed in terms of relevant criteria such as impact on customer satisfaction, required investment, ability to implement and so on. Each potential project can then be scored and a prioritisation be made.

Some possible areas for projects in healthcare are:

- patient satisfaction level

- reduction in medical errors

- documentation errors

- speed and accuracy in admission of patients

- insurance claim processing accuracy and time

- bed availability

- billing accuracy

- care co-ordination

- supply chain of medicines, equipments and instruments

- laboratory results accuracy level

- quick emergency room treatment

- surgery planning *and* scheduling

- reduction in customer waiting time

- increase in patient safety level.

Having selected the project, the next important step is to complete a project charter. This records: the project title, the team members, the objectives, the methodology, resources required, the reporting structure and the timescale of the project.

### 14.6.3   Training

Participatory learning is more enjoyable than being a passive receptor, and it is much more effective at embedding knowledge and skills. Adults as well as children like to have the opportunity to interact with the learning process. Practicals and games are a vital part of Six Sigma training, and some excellent ideas are available; see for example Chen and Roth (2005). The following is a very effective 50-second practical that thoroughly imparts an appreciation of how difficult it is to ask people to adopt new methods of working: ask the class to write their name on a sheet of paper; ask them to observe how they feel about the task and how they feel generally; now ask them to write their name with the opposite hand; ask them to compare how they feel now as compared to before. It is quite surprising how a simple task can change your feeling from confident and in control to feeling inadequate and unsure.

Much has been written about the syllabus of Six Sigma training. Although the name is copyrighted by Motorola, there are many versions of the knowledge base expected of Six Sigma personnel. A wide range of tools is cited by GE in their toolbox. The variation in syllabus is naturally linked in with certification issues. In applying for Six Sigma jobs, it is usually sufficient to state where Six Sigma training was carried out and to give examples of projects completed, in addition to supplying references.

*Typical black belt programme:*

- project work

- 20 days of core training (DMAIC)

- 2 extra Define days (complete project charter)

- Kaizen workshops (6 days)

- review days.

*Typical green belt programme:*

- project work

- 10 days of core training (DMAIC)

- 1 extra Define day (complete project charter)

- Kaizen workshops (6 days)

- review days.

### 14.6.4   Kaizen workshops

Sometimes the effort involved in a six-month project seems large and unappealing at the start of a programme. To encourage team motivation and to try to make quick progress, smaller sub-projects are tackled in Kaizen workshops. Typical sub-projects may be to reduce time taken for a process or to reduce waste; see for example Kaizen in Ruggeri, Kenett and Faltin (2007).

The Six Sigma Kaizen model has been adapted from its manufacturing origin for the healthcare environment in the following ways:

- shorter duration than a traditional manufacturing Kaizen

- recognition that process changes potentially affect patient care

- recognition that multiple stakeholder sign-offs may be required.

Solutions are identified, but it may not be possible to trial them during the event. Kaizen team members are expected, however, to maintain project momentum and implement solutions as soon as possible. An example of a successful four-day Kaizen event in an emergency department is given in www.gehealthcare.com/usen/ultrasound/genimg/docs/GEHCKaizenCaseStudy.pdf.

### 14.6.5    Organisation of training

A typical Six Sigma programme takes at least a year to complete. The following case study illustrates the process.

**Case study: Teaching Primary Care Trust**

A Six Sigma implementation programme delivered by an external provider allowed a Teaching Primary Care Trust to improve patient care pathways and reduce expenditure. The programme demonstrated the absolute transferability of this approach from industrial to public sector service settings. Members of staff from a wide range of areas and levels within the trust undertook the programme, from community nursing staff to the director of corporate management.

*Three-phase approach:*

1. preparation

2. learning transfer

3. evaluation and forward planning.

**Phase 1: preparation (three months)**
The preparation of the Trust aimed to ensure that the investment in the programme yielded proper returns. The components were:

- candidate selection and preparation

- selection of Six Sigma projects

- management training.

**Phase 2: learning transfer (six months)**
The core learning programme for black, green and yellow belts was divided into five major sections:

- Define

- Measure

- Analyse

- Improve

- Control.

Each section of training was separated by a suitable time period to allow essential project work to take place.

**Phase 3: evaluation and forward planning (three months)**
This phase offered a review of all aspects of phases 1 and 2. Projects were reported and financially evaluated and there was black belt, green belt and yellow belt accreditation.

The Six Sigma approach suited the staff culture and had the following features:

- team working ethic
- strong focus on patient impact projects
- projects tied in with strategic objectives
- strong focus on costs
- the correct application of statistical and problem-solving tools
- the structured approach to projects.

*Projects included:*

- reducing the expenditure on tertiary contracts
- reducing the number of delayed discharges in community hospitals
- reducing average waiting times to receive drug treatment
- optimising access times to primary care services.

Due to the team and project-based nature of Six Sigma, it is very important to have an event to celebrate the outcomes and to share the benefits and learning with a wider community. Accordingly a celebration day was organised at the end of the programme. The event was well publicised and was well attended. Teams were encouraged to prepare posters showing their work, and colleagues and stakeholders were invited to join the teams for the day.

# 14.7    The way forward for Six Sigma in healthcare

## 14.7.1    Variations

Six Sigma has evolved as its range of applications has increased, and there are notable adaptations.

The pharmaceutical industries, in particular, spend a lot of time in new product design. Design for Six Sigma (DFSS) and Quality by Design (QbD) focus on designing new products and processes; see for example Ruggeri, Kenett and Faltin (2007); DMADV (Define, Measure, Analyse, Design, Verify) is also specially focused on innovation (Stevenson and Kashef, 2008).

In response to a determination to improve the environmental impact of products and services, Green Six Sigma is environmentally focused and emphasises green issues; the inaugural Green Six Sigma Conference took place in 2009 in Chicago.

Six Sigma for research differs in the control phase, as research results are usually fed into the process and are part of an overall drive for change (Coleman *et al.*, 2008).

One criticism of Six Sigma is a perceived overdependence on statistical analysis. Visual Six Sigma seeks to rectify this by shifting the focus to letting the data speak for itself. The Visual Six Sigma roadmap is:

- uncover relationships
- model relationships
- revise knowledge.

Visual Six Sigma uses data visualisation and exploratory data analysis, reserving statistical analysis for when the conclusions are not obvious (Cox *et al.*, 2010).

## 14.7.2   Six Sigma and the complementary methodology of Lean Six Sigma

*Six Sigma:*

- is logical, data driven, well established
- aims to reduce variation in order to deliver high-quality services
- aims to eliminate errors/defects
- uses a powerful set of statistical *and* quality tools within an effective framework for problem-solving
- visual Six Sigma goes from data to decision – uncover and model relationships, revise knowledge.

*Lean:*

- aims to maximise service/process speed
- uses tools to analyse flow *and* delay times in a process
- distinguishes between 'value-added' and 'non-value-added' work and aims to eliminate the root causes of 'non-value-added' activities.

*Lean Six Sigma:*

- combines 'just speed' (Lean) and 'just quality' (Six Sigma)
- acknowledges the importance of measurement and statistics as well as process flow and value adding.

Healthcare workers, like many others, are 'right brain' thinkers, and some do not enjoy the statistical elements of Six Sigma. Some institutions have responded to the dislike of statistics by reducing the statistical content of the Six Sigma programme; others have moved to Lean Six Sigma or to Lean. Statistical Process Control, however, is more readily accepted in healthcare and has been adopted by generations of staff, with continual waves of interest and sustained wide use.

## 14.7.3   Implementation issues

Announcing a Six Sigma initiative in a healthcare organisation is the first step; the second is to carry out training; the third is to embed the methodology and develop it within the organisation. There are many reasons why this last step can fail. Healthcare is vulnerable to continual re-organisation which is naturally disruptive; staff are overworked and find that they do not have the promised 'protected' time to carry out their Six Sigma projects; staff may not be confident that Six Sigma has any benefit. These problems are shared with other sectors.

There may also be situations where problem solutions are just too difficult to implement. A series of programmes for British television (BBC) explored the difficulties of implementing quality improvement in hospitals and made very entertaining, if frustrating viewing. There were lots of problems with lack of authority and poor communication (Robinson, 2006).

There is a fundamental dislike of treating patients as numbers by the staff most concerned with caring for them. Management should be in a better position to be more dispassionate, but have to tread very carefully to take the hearts and minds of the rest of the team with them. Some decisions are very difficult to make; for example, a project showed that a particular local hospital should close, but this meant moving a small number of resident patients. There was enormous public opinion against closure and so the hospital was left running, even though the potential cost savings of closing it were translated into the large number of extra hip replacements that could have been carried out. In the end the upset to the residents was considered more important.

Six Sigma projects have been carried out to streamline decision making, for example in pre-operative checks, day surgery and fast-tracking. Although this may help cut costs for the majority it can lead to duplication of checks and frustration for a minority of patients.

Examples of patient intransigence to change include the desire to be treated near to home or at the healthcare provider traditionally linked to their area, even if this service is less comprehensive or more expensive or has a longer waiting list. Strong personal connections between doctors can affect their referral pattern and encourage them to refer to each other or in a particular direction for the benefit of the patient, but leaving some provision underused. There may be similar problems with the drugs prescribed: the doctor chooses on the basis of clinical need but can be influenced unduly by historical allegiance. The responsibility has to stop with someone, and that person, usually the doctor, has in return the privilege of some free choice made on grounds other than cost.

Six Sigma training is taken up less by doctors, with the typical mix being managers, nurses and support staff. This can lead to divisions within units and misunderstanding. One possible solution is for the traditional teaching of statistics to medical students to include Six Sigma topics, especially SPC. Six Sigma should be recognised in postgraduate medical education.

Awards and recognition play an important role in encouraging implementation. For example:

> Recognising and rewarding 40 of the best-performing acute trusts across the UK, the CHKS 40 Top Awards are based on the evaluation of 21 indicators of clinical effectiveness, health outcomes, efficiency, patient experience and quality of care.

Revised annually to take account of newly available performance information, this year's indicators include:

- risk-adjusted mortality
- risk-adjusted length of stay
- rate of emergency readmission to hospital – 28 days
- rate of emergency readmission to hospital following treatment for a fractured hip
- day case rate for target procedures (case-mix adjusted)
- day case conversion rate (case-mix adjusted)
- overall data quality
- rate of emergency readmission to hospital following AMI (acute myocardial infarction) within 28 days
- rate of emergency readmission to hospital within 14 days – COPD (chronic obstructive pulmonary disease)
- percentage of elective in-patients admitted on day of procedure
- pre-op length of stay for fractured neck of femur
- pre-op length of stay for elective surgery
- percentage of elective in-patient admission with no procedure
- reported MRSA bacteraemia rate
- reported *C. difficile* rate for patients aged 65 and over
- procedure not carried out – hospital decision
- in-patient survey
- Accident and Emergency survey
- patient misadventures
- obstetrics complications for delivery spells
- outpatient DNA (Did Not Attends) – first attendance.

http://tophospitals.chks.co.uk/index.php?id=803

## 14.7.4   Implications of Six Sigma for statisticians

At one time statisticians were in the role of technical advisers; a task came along and the statistician applied their art and presented a solution. There was less attention paid to whether it was the right problem, whether it was a sensible solution, whether the stakeholders understood and could use the solution, whether the solution was robust to change, whether the solution was value for money. Six Sigma has helped statisticians to work in a more professional way, raising their professional status and making them a more useful partner with other healthcare professionals.

Six Sigma has led to widespread application of statistical methods by people with no formal training in statistics. However, the democratisation of statistics also has a worrying side. Shallow knowledge can lead to fundamental mistakes, such as having too small a number of yes/no responses as the output of a designed experiment; naïve use of normal approximations to low-occurrence data in SPC; wrongly positioned control limits resulting in too few or too many action signals; or poorly chosen settings for factor levels leading to one factor dominating a designed experiment.

Some potential statisticians may be disappointed with their first taste of statistics because of the basic level at which it is taught and applied in Six Sigma. Hopefully the increasing number of successful applications of Six Sigma will lead to continued interest and more healthcare professionals will develop their statistical skills and use Six Sigma to address the many challenges encountered in healthcare.

## 14.8   Summary

The chapter reviewed the background to the revolutionary Six Sigma approach to process improvement and the gradual increase in its influence from the manufacturing to other sectors including healthcare. It was shown how special features of healthcare, such as the independence of multiple stakeholders, the fundamental importance of each patient and the potential conflicts of satisfying funders, employees and users, make adaptation to healthcare an interesting and complex exercise. Each of the Define, Measure, Analyse, Improve, Control and Transfer phases was described with examples of their use in the healthcare scenario. Typical Six Sigma roles, activities and time scales both for training and for projects were reviewed, and also implementation issues, such as careful management of change and attention to potential knock-on effects in other departments. Finally, the opportunities and challenges for statisticians are considered, as Six Sigma is increasingly embraced by healthcare.

## References

Arthur, J. (2005) Seduce them with success. *Quality Progress*, **38**(9), 35–40.

Bradford Hill, A. (1967) *Principles of Medical Statistics*, 8th edn, The Lancet Ltd.

Care Quality Commission (2012) Government standards, www.cqc.org.uk/public/what-are-standards/government-standards (accessed 5 April 2012).

Caulcutt, R. (2008) Black belt types, in *Statistical Practice in Business and Industry* (eds S. Coleman, T. Greenfield, D. Stewardson and D. Montgomery), John Wiley & Sons, Ltd, pp. 34–41.

Chen, C. and Roth, H. (2005) *The Big Book of Six Sigma Training Games*, McGraw-Hill.

Coleman, S.Y. (2008) Six Sigma – an opportunity for statistics and statisticians. *Significance*, **5**(2), 94–96.

Coleman, S.Y., Fouweather, T., Henning, H. and Uygun, O. (2008) *Six Sigma Green Belt training for Researchers*. 4th Virtual International Conference 'Innovative Production Machines and Systems', IPROMS 2008, Cardiff, UK, July 1st–14th, 2008.

Cox, I., Gaudard, M.A., Ramsey, P.J., Stephens M.L. and Wright, L.T. (2010) *Visual Six Sigma – Making Data Analysis Lean*, John Wiley & Sons, Inc.

Deming, W.E. (1986) *Out of the Crisis*, MIT Press. ISBN 0-911379-01-0. OCLC 13126265.

Department of Health (2005) Managing food waste in the NHS, www.hospitalcaterers.org/documents/foodwst.pdf (accessed 28 June 2010)

Health Foundation (2010) Evidence in Brief: How safe are clinical systems? www.health.org.uk/publications/evidence-in-brief-how-safe-are-clinical-systems/ (accessed 5 April 2012).

Henderson, G.R. (2006) *Six Sigma Quality Improvement with Minitab*, John Wiley & Sons, Ltd.

Henderson, G.R., Mead, G.E., van Dijke, M.L. *et al.* (2008) Use of statistical process control charts in stroke medicine to determine if clinical evidence and changes in service delivery were associated with improvements in the quality of care. *Quality and Safety in Health Care*, **17**, 301–306.

Hoerl, R.W. (2001) Six Sigma black belts: what do they need to know? *Journal of Quality Technology*, **33**(4), 391–406.

Hoerl, R.W. and Snee, R. (2005) *Six Sigma beyond the Factory Floor: Deployment Strategies for Financial Services, Health care and the Rest of the Real Economy*, Prentice Hall.

Institute of Medicine (1999) *To Err is Human: Building a Safer Health System*, The National Academies Press. www.saynotocaps.org/reports/To%20Err%20Is%20Human%20Building%20a %20Safer%20Health%20System.htm.

ISO (1993) ISO 9004-4:1993 *Total Quality Management. Guidelines for Quality Improvement*, International Organization for Standardization, Geneva.

Juran, J. (1999) *Quality Handbook*, 5th edn, McGraw-Hill.

Kenett, R. and Zacks, S. (1998) *Modern Industrial Statistics: Design and Control of Quality and Reliability*, 2nd edn, Chinese edition 2004, Duxbury Press, San Francisco.

Magnello, E. (2009) Eminent Victorians and early statistical societies. *Significance*, **6**(2), 86–88.

Mohammed, M.A., Worthington, P. and Woodall, W.H. (2008) Plotting basic control charts: tutorial notes for health care practitioners. *Quality and Safety in Health Care*, **17**, 137–145.

Montgomery, D.C. and Woodall, W.H. (2008) An overview of Six Sigma. *International Statistical Review*, **76**(3), 329–346.

Mukherjee, S. (2008) A dose of DMAIC. *Quality Progress*, **8**, 44–51.

Robinson, G. (2006) BBC/OU programme 'Can Gerry Robinson fix the NHS?', www.open.edu/ openlearn/whats-on/ou-on-the-bbc-can-gerry-robinson-fix-the-nhs-interview-gerry-robinson    (accessed 5 April 2012).

Ruggeri, F., Kenett, R.S. and Faltin, F.W. (eds) (2007) *Encyclopaedia of Statistics in Quality and Reliability*, John Wiley & Sons, Ltd.

Spiegelhalter, D.J. (2005) Funnel plots for comparing institutional performance. *Statistics in Medicine*, **24**, 1185–1202.

Stevenson, J.R. and Kashef, A.E. (2008) Newer, better, faster. *Quality Progress*, **9**, 34–39.

Toolan, P.G. and Coleman, S.Y. (1994) Music therapy, a description of process: engagement and avoidance in five people with learning disability. *Journal of Intellectual Disability Research*, **38**, 433–444.

Woodall, W.H. (2006) The use of control charts in health-care and public-health surveillance. *Journal of Quality Technology*, **38**(2), 89–104

# 15

# Statistical process control in clinical medicine

## Per Winkel[1] and Nien Fan Zhang[2]

[1]*The Copenhagen Trial Unit, Centre for Clinical Intervention Research, Rigshospitalet, Copenhagen University Hospital, Copenhagen, Denmark*
[2]*Statistical Engineering Division, National Institute of Standards and Technology, Gaithersburg, MD, USA*

## Synopsis

A control chart may be used to characterize a clinical process and subsequently to monitor it. The chart generally depicts a center line indicating the targeted outcome of the process, an upper and a lower control limit, and the values of a measurable quantity characterizing the process, for example the fraction of medication errors occurring per month. When the results of the process are stable, the quality of the process may be assessed, for instance by estimating the fraction of results that do not have an acceptable quality.

Examples include the monitoring of the daily average of patient waiting times at an outpatient clinic and the monitoring of the period elapsed between consecutive *Clostridium difficile* infections.

The process of interest may also be confined to a single patient, for example the process necessary to regulate the patient's blood pressure. Two examples are presented here: the monitoring of the blood pressure of patients treated for hypertension and the monitoring of peak expiratory flow rate in a patient treated for asthma.

The initial data for a control chart should be checked for autocorrelation, in particular if they are obtained from a single patient. Positive autocorrelation may cause the control limits to be too narrow, resulting in too many false alarms.

*Statistical Methods in Healthcare*, First Edition. Edited by Frederick W. Faltin, Ron S. Kenett and Fabrizio Ruggeri.
© 2012 John Wiley & Sons, Ltd. Published 2012 by John Wiley & Sons, Ltd.

The outcome results from several healthcare providers (e.g., hospital departments) may be compared if the patients are assigned at random to the providers. If observational data are used instead, risk-adjustment is necessary in order to adjust for variation between the patients in terms of severity of disease, co-morbidities, age, sex, and so on. A potential problem is that important risk factors may not be known or measured. Using simulation we illustrate how an unknown or unmeasured risk factor may bias the comparison of the quality of care between two healthcare providers if observational data are used.

## 15.1    Introduction

The quality of a clinical process may be assessed provided it is in a state of statistical control; that is, stable. Control chart techniques originally developed for industrial process control [1] may be applied to characterize and monitor the quality of a clinical process [2, 3, 4, 5]. However, if the quantity characterizing the quality of the process is an outcome measure, for example mortality following a coronary artery bypass graft operation, its value depends not only on the quality of the clinical process, but also on risk factors – severity of the patient's disease, co-morbidity, age, sex, and so on. Various risk-adjusted control charts may then be used [6]. This important and rather difficult area is covered in another chapter in this book to which the reader is referred (Chapter 12).

Outcomes from several healthcare providers (physicians, hospital departments, etc.) may be compared if the patients are assigned at random to the providers. Usually (but not always [7]) this is not possible for practical and/or economical reasons. Then, one has to use observational data. The influence of patient case-mix differences between the providers, therefore, has to be adjusted for, prior to the comparison [8]. This is usually achieved by regressing the provider category and important risk factors on the outcome. Other approaches are also possible [8, 9, 10]. We will only touch on the problem of risk-adjustment in this chapter, playing the devil's advocate by showing a simulated example demonstrating the potential perils of using this approach. Risk-adjustment is covered more fully in Chapter 12 of this book.

In Section 15.2 we will present overviews of the various statistical techniques used in this chapter (the reader may want to proceed to Section 15.3 and then refer back to Section 15.2 as needed). We then demonstrate the construction and subsequent use of two types of control charts, the Shewhart chart [2] and the exponentially weighted moving average (EWMA) chart [2] by way of examples. We then present examples where control charts are used for patient monitoring (e.g., the monitoring of blood pressure), and finally illustrate and discuss the perils of risk-adjustment, as mentioned above.

## 15.2    Methods

### 15.2.1    Control charts

#### 15.2.1.1    The Shewhart chart

A Shewhart control chart is one relatively simple type of chart that can be used to characterize a clinical process and subsequently monitor it [2]. The chart depicts the values of a measurable quantity describing the quality of the process over time. Examples of the types of quantities that might be monitored include the fraction of patients dying per month during a specified surgical procedure, the weekly mean of patients' waiting times until seen by a physician, and the cost per patient treated for a hip fracture, and so on.

If a clinical process is in statistical control, the results will follow some type of probability distribution, for example a Gaussian distribution, that characterizes the typical value and the random variation of the process. Usually, the mean of this distribution ($\mu$) and its standard deviation ($\sigma$) define the state of the process.

The Shewhart control chart is constructed using 20 to 30 samples obtained while the process is in statistical control. It is furnished with a center line (the grand mean of the samples), upper and lower control limits (the grand mean plus, and respectively minus, three times the *sample* standard deviation), and a time axis. The control limits are constructed so that, as a rule, the sample means of the observed values will be located within the control limits when the process is in statistical control. If a sample mean value falls outside the control limits, the added variation that pushed it outside the limits should have an assignable cause (with high probability), and a search for this cause is initiated.

### 15.2.1.2   The exponentially weighted moving average (EWMA) chart

The EWMA chart is a slightly more complicated control chart that was introduced by Roberts (1959) [2, 11]. The quantity monitored is the cumulative sum of the weighted values of the current and all previous observations. The largest weight, $\lambda(0 < \lambda \leq 1)$, is assigned to the current observation. The weights of the previous observations then decrease exponentially relative to the parameter $\lambda$. Thus, the older an observation is, the smaller weight it is assigned. The mathematical details of the EWMA chart are given in Appendix 15.A.1.

## 15.2.2   Measuring the quality of a process

Assume that the results of a clinical process in statistical control follow a Gaussian distribution with mean $\mu$ and standard deviation $\sigma$, which are known. Let the upper specification limit (USL) be a value separating acceptable results from unacceptable results that are larger than this value. Then, $C_{pu} = (\text{USL} - \mu)/(3\sigma)$ is a measure of the quality of the process. If $C_{pu} = 1.00$, then 0.135% of the values of the process are expected to exceed the USL, and if $C_{pu} > 1.00$, then fewer than 0.135% are expected to exceed the USL, provided the true values of $\mu$ and $\sigma$ are known. According to industrial standards, $C_{pu} \geq 1.66$ is an acceptable quality. If the values of the parameters $\mu$ and $\sigma$ are not known and must be estimated using data, the number of observations should be 100 or more [12]. In that case, the estimate of $C_{pu}$ is calculated by $(\text{USL} - \hat{\mu})/(3\hat{\sigma})$, where $\hat{\mu}$ and $\hat{\sigma}$ are the estimates of $\mu$ and $\sigma$, respectively.

## 15.2.3   Logistic regression

If two or more patient categories are compared and the outcome of interest is an event such as the death of a patient, it is customary to compare the odds of the event occurring between the categories. The odds of an event are defined as $p/(1 - p)$: the probability ($p$) that the event occurs divided by the probability $(1 - p)$ that it does not occur. If patient categories (say two) are compared, one of them is assigned to be the reference category, and the ratio of the odds of the other category to the reference category is calculated. If the ratio is 1, the odds of the two categories do not differ. If it is larger than 1, the odds of the other category are larger than those of the reference category, and so on.

In addition to the influence of the patient category on the odds ratio, the simultaneous influence of other covariates such as age, sex, blood pressure, and so on, may be of interest to study. Such relationships are usually studied using linear regression. However, if the observed odds are used as the dependent variable, the typical assumptions underlying linear regression will not be fulfilled [2]. This shortcoming may be remedied by performing a linear regression on the logarithm of the observed odds (referred to as logistic regression). The resulting regression coefficients may then be converted back to the odds scale by transforming them using the inverse of the logarithm; that is, the exponential transformation. The resulting transformed value of each covariate's coefficient gives the change in the odds obtained when the covariate changes by one unit while the other covariates remain fixed (e.g., the change in odds when the patient gets one year older, in the case that the covariate is age and the unit is year). Choosing an indicator of healthcare provider and risk factors as covariates, the impact of healthcare provider choice may be studied while compensating for the effect of risk factors (mathematical details are given in Appendix 15.A.2).

### 15.2.4    Autocorrelation of process measurements

A series of measurements obtained from a process during some period and ordered in time is a 'time series', which can be viewed as the values taken on by a sequence of random variables ordered in time. The sequence is *stationary* if it is in a state of 'statistical equilibrium'. This implies that the basic behavior of the time series does not change in time. In particular, the mean and variance are stable. The process corresponding to a stationary sequence of random variables is referred to as a *stationary process*.

Autocorrelation refers to internal correlation between paired observations in a time series. To examine the dependency between values in a stationary time series, the correlation coefficient between values that are a specified number of time units ($\tau$) away from each other is used and called autocorrelation of lag $\tau$.

Intuitively, it makes sense to use the autocorrelation as a measure of the dependency between variables which are a specific number of time units apart, as may be understood from the following reasoning: we define high values as values that are higher than the mean, and low ones as values lower than the mean. If $X_i$ and $X_j$ are positively related, their values tend to be either both high or both low. In either case, the corresponding autocorrelation will be positive. If they are negatively related, a high $X_i$ value tends to be accompanied by a low $X_j$ and vice versa. In either of these cases, the corresponding autocorrelation will be negative. The mathematical details of autocorrelation are given in Appendix 15.A.3.

In biology, random biological variation, for example the random burst in the secretion of some substance that influences the blood pressure, may have a sustained effect, so that several consecutive measurements are all influenced by the same random phenomenon. When the sampling interval is short, autocorrelation, especially positive autocorrelation, of the data may be of concern [13, 14].

### 15.2.5    Simulation

Assume, for example, that we have two types of patients. The probability that a type-1 patient dies during a specified and properly administered surgical procedure is 10%, and the probability that a type-2 patient dies is 30%. If these probabilities are constant over time, the quality of the surgical procedure is stable. To study the properties of procedures like these without actually needing to perform surgery, the behavior of such a process over time may be simulated. Assume we wanted to simulate the outcome of 1000 consecutive type-1 patients subjected to the surgical procedure. Performing 1000 independent experiments each simulating the outcome of one consecutive patient does this. Each experiment may be viewed as a random draw, with replacement, of one ball from an urn, containing 10% red balls and 90% white balls. Thus, the probability of drawing a red ball is 10%, simulating the 10% probability of death during operation. If we wanted to simulate the outcome when a mixture of type-1 and type-2 patients were operated on, we would use two urns: one for type-1 patients containing 10% red balls and another for type-2 patients containing 30% red balls. Instead of physically drawing balls from urns, however, the experiments are typically done virtually, using a computer with standard statistical software for generating random numbers from different types of probability distributions.

## 15.3 Clinical applications

To set the scene, this section starts with a brief review of the measures and indicators of the quality of healthcare. Then we present an example detailing the various phases involved in constructing a control chart. We proceed by demonstrating the usefulness of combining two types of control charts; one that is sensitive to abrupt transient changes in the process monitored (the Shewhart $X$ chart) and one that is sensitive to smaller sustained changes (the EWMA chart). Then we present some examples where control charts have been used to monitor the patient as his/her own control.

### 15.3.1 Measures and indicators of quality of healthcare

The quality of care can be evaluated on the basis of structure, process, and outcome. Structural data are the characteristics of physicians and hospitals. They could include a physician's specialty, the ownership of a hospital, availability of equipment, staffing levels, and so on. Process data are the components of the encounter between a healthcare professional and a patient; for instance the medication administered. A clinical process measure assesses performance based on adherence to established clinical standards. Throughput process measures are based on management data. They include such measures as waiting lists, ambulance response times, delays in emergency departments, and so on. Result data include outcome data and costs incurred by producing a specified healthcare output. Outcome data refer to the patient's subsequent health status (e.g., improvement in mobility). They include observed outcomes – for example death, morbidity – and patient perceived outcomes such as satisfaction and quality of life.

Many of the characteristics assessed in the analysis of healthcare quality are properties of larger clinical and organizational systems in which individuals work. Safety, patient satisfaction, surgical outcomes, infection rates, and so on are all linked to systems of information, architecture, scheduling, resource allocation, and so on. Therefore, organizational quality measurement systems are more powerful in improving care than individually focused measurement systems. For instance, differences in structural factors (e.g., availability of equipment and staffing levels) are correlated with outcome [15]. Several institutional management processes have been found to be associated with improved outcomes in intensive care units [16].

It is important to make a distinction between a measure of quality and an indicator of quality. An example of a quality measure would be a clinical process measure based on agreed criteria supported by evidence or logic. For instance avoiding delay in the use of antibiotics in pneumonia. A quality indicator would, for example, be the death of a patient during a surgical procedure, because the outcome is not only influenced by the quality of care but also by other factors, for example severity of disease, co-morbidity, and the patient's socio-economic status.

In the design of control charts depicting result indicators, risk-adjustment is mandatory for the reasons mentioned above. From a statistical point of view, therefore, it makes sense to distinguish non-risk-adjusted control charts, used for quality measures, from risk-adjusted control charts that require special and rather difficult techniques. In this chapter we will focus on examples from applications where risk-adjustment is not needed.

## 15.3.2    Applications of control charts

In the first example we demonstrate how to build and use a control chart. The second example illustrates the combined use of the Shewhart and the EWMA chart, and the last two examples illustrate the use of control charts for patient monitoring purposes.

### 15.3.2.1    The construction and use of a control chart (patient waiting times)

**15.3.2.1.1    Problem**    At an outpatient clinic the management was notified that the upper specification limit for a patient's waiting time from arrival until blood sampling and/or electrocardiogram (ECG) recording begins is 30 min.

**15.3.2.1.2    Design of experiment**    The management decided firstly to monitor the average waiting time of daily random samples, each including 30 outpatients. Sampling took place on each weekday for four weeks. The employees at the outpatient clinic were not aware of this investigation. The waiting time from arrival until seen by a technologist was recorded for each patient.

**15.3.2.1.3    Analysis of data**    The mean and standard deviation of each sample was calculated. The grand mean ($\hat{\mu} = 15.93$ minutes) estimates the process mean. An unbiased estimate of the process standard deviation ($\hat{\sigma}$) is calculated by dividing the average of the sample standard deviations by a factor removing the bias [2, Equ. 2.19 on p. 47]. Dividing this estimate by $\sqrt{30}$ (here the sample size is 30), one obtains an estimate of the standard deviation of each sample mean.

Figure 15.1 shows the $\bar{X}$ chart with the control limits equal to the grand mean $\pm 3$ sample standard deviations. The observed sample means are depicted on the chart. Three of the values (sample numbers 5, 10, and 15, all sampled on a Friday) are located above the upper control limit (UCL). Therefore, in all likelihood the process is not in statistical control. When

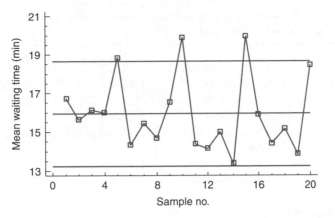

**Figure 15.1**   Mean of waiting time in minutes of patients received at an outpatient clinic on weekdays.

these values were removed and a new chart calculated using the remaining values (chart not shown), the value corresponding to the fourth Friday (sample no. 20) lay above the UCL.

It turned out that on Fridays the patient mix differed from the other weekdays in that an unusually large number of patients from the cardiology department were scheduled for ECG recordings in addition to blood specimen collection. These patients required more time than patients not scheduled for ECG recordings, and a retrospective analysis revealed that overtime was much more usual on Fridays than on any other weekday.

Figure 15.2 shows the control chart based on the remaining values. The points marked as crosses correspond to the Fridays. Now, the process seems to be in control. The management reorganized the technologist shifts and staffing. New data were collected for a three-week period and a new control chart made using these data. This chart was similar to that shown in

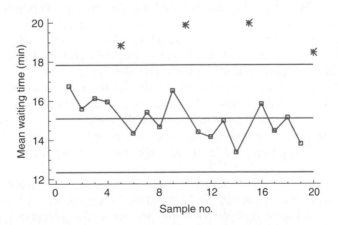

**Figure 15.2**   Mean of waiting time in minutes of patients received at an outpatient clinic on weekdays. The crosses represent mean values recorded on Fridays. They were not used when the control chart was calculated.

**Table 15.1** Procedure for investigating outlying values of daily mean waiting times (start at step 0 and proceed from left to right).

| Step | Actions | Questions and routing in table | |
|------|---------|-------------------------------|---|
| 0 | Control data and data-processing. | Data error? | If yes go to Step 4. If no go to Step 1. |
| 1 | Compute production in number of venipuncture equivalents. Control staffing of ambulatory. | Production or staffing changed? | If yes go to Step 4. If no go to Step 2. |
| 2 | Define productivity as venipunctures/technologist hour. Compute: (1) average productivity, (2) average productivity for each 30 min period, (3) average productivity for each technologist, (4) average productivity for each technologist in each 30 min period. Identify significantly outlying values. | Go to step 3. | |
| 3 | Interview manager of ambulatory and technologists. | Go to step 4. | |
| 4 | Write report and stop. | | |

Figure 15.2, without the out-of-control values on Fridays. The estimated process mean and standard deviation (of the distribution of the waiting times, not the mean waiting times) were 15.72 and 4.85 minutes, respectively.

To implement the system of control charting after determining the process mean and the control limits, the management purchased a system for automatic recording of waiting times. The ID of a technologist servicing a given patient was already automatically captured by the current clinical data-processing system. They also designed a protocol (see Table 15.1) to be followed if daily mean values outside control limits were found.

The initial $C_{pu}$ calculated to assess the quality of the process was $(30.00 - 15.72)/(3 \cdot 4.85) = 0.98$, based on 16 samples of a sample size of 30. This is a questionable quality according to industrial standards. The management, therefore, (1) reorganized and upgraded the staffing, (2) collected new data, (3) computed new control limits, and (4) calculated $C_{pu}$ to see if the state of the process had improved sufficiently. They repeated this cycle until the quality was acceptable.

Using the resulting control chart, they subsequently monitored the quality of the process by plotting the daily mean values on the chart and used the procedure in Table 15.1 to track assignable causes of excess variation. Once the process is of an acceptable quality and the data capture is fully automated, it is of course also possible to construct daily $X$ charts to monitor the waiting times of the individual patients to obtain a more detailed picture of the process. However, the distribution of such waiting times may not be Gaussian, so either a transformation of the process variable or another type of control chart may be required.

### 15.3.2.2    Combined use of the Shewhart and EWMA chart (monitoring the occurrence of *Clostridium difficile* infections)

The risk of infection would seem to be naturally estimated by the relative frequency of infections; that is, the number of patients who have acquired an infection during a specified period divided by the number of patients who have been exposed to the risk of getting an infection during that period. When one is monitoring the relative frequency of infections, rather large patient samples are usually required to ensure that each patient sample contains a few infected patients. This implies that the main significance of the samples is only a matter of history since it will usually be too late to take any action when a sufficiently large sample of patients has finally been collected.

Therefore, recording the period between consecutive infections is often used instead. If the number of patients exposed to the risk of being infected is constant over time, the period between infections will decrease as the relative frequency of infections increases, and vice versa. For a review of the use of statistical quality control methods in infection and hospital epidemiology the reader is referred to [17, 18].

The data used in the present example were read from a figure in a study [19] of the relation between the number of days elapsed between consecutively registered *Clostridium difficile* infections and the sequence number of the infections. In this case we need to use a Shewhart chart for continuous data where the sample size is only 1 (the specific calculations necessary to construct an $X$ chart may be found in [2, p. 56]). Because the observations to be charted are not averages in this case, the assumption that they follow a Gaussian distribution, therefore, may very well be violated. It turns out that the present data follow an exponential distribution. To arrive at a Gaussian distribution from an exponential one, it is recommended [1] to use the transformation $Y = X^{0.2777}$, where $X$ is the original variable and $Y$ the transformed one. We will use this approach.

Table 15.2 shows the sequential number of each infection (column 1) and the number of days elapsed between this and the subsequent infection (column 2). The corresponding value obtained using the above transformation is also shown (column 3).

Figure 15.3 shows the data depicted on a combined $X$-EWMA chart. The period between the 11th and the 12th infection exceeds the UCL of the $X$ chart. The most likely explanation is that the laboratory had some problems with the *Clostridium difficile* assay so that the presence of *C. difficile* was sometimes overlooked. This large increase in the period length was not picked up by the EWMA chart.

By contrast the EWMA detects a small decrease in the mean value that was not picked up by the $X$ chart. This illustrates how the two charts supplement each other. Large, but transient changes in the mean value are missed by the EWMA chart, but picked up by the $X$ chart. Small but persistent changes in the mean value are picked up by the EWMA chart, but may go unnoticed for a long period if the $X$ chart is used alone.

### 15.3.2.3    Using control charts for patient monitoring

Control charts may also be used to monitor a single patient. Tennant *et al.*, reviewed the literature and searched for the application of control charts to monitor variation in clinically relevant markers of disease or risk factors for disease at an individual patient level [20]. The reader is referred to this work for a more comprehensive discussion of the potentials and limitations in using control charts for patient monitoring. Despite their potential

**Table 15.2**   The number of days between registered *Clostridium difficile* infections.

| Infection no. | Number of days elapsed between present and subsequent infection ($X$) | $X^{0.2777}$ ($Y$) |
|---|---|---|
| 1 | 30 | 2.572 |
| 2 | 18 | 2.231 |
| 3 | 31 | 2.595 |
| 4 | 129 | 3.856 |
| 5 | 102 | 3.612 |
| 6 | 18 | 2.231 |
| 7 | 8 | 1.782 |
| 8 | 6 | 1.645 |
| 9 | 19 | 2.265 |
| 10 | 169 | 4.156 |
| 11 | 283 | 4.796 |
| 12 | 99 | 3.583 |
| 13 | 75 | 3.317 |
| 14 | 4 | 1.470 |
| 15 | 3 | 1.357 |
| 16 | 2 | 1.212 |
| 17 | 3 | 1.357 |
| 18 | 4 | 1.470 |
| 19 | 5 | 1.564 |
| 20 | 1 | 1.000 |
| 21 | 1 | 1.000 |
| 22 | 14 | 2.081 |
| 23 | 8 | 1.782 |
| 24 | 9 | 1.841 |

and ease of use, dissemination and uptake of these applications appear to have been less widespread [20, 21]. Here we will only present a few anecdotal examples for illustrative purposes.

During a stable period, measurements (e.g., of blood pressure) are used to develop a control chart characterizing a given patient. The chart is subsequently used to check that the patient remains stable. Data of this type may be autocorrelated, especially if the frequency of observation is high, causing the performance of the control chart to deteriorate. Thus it is important to check if autocorrelation is present in the data. In the following we will present two examples of this type of application.

**15.3.2.3.1   Monitoring a patient with asthma**   A patient suffering from asthma made daily measurements of her peak expiratory flow rate (PEFR) in l/min, in the morning, prior to bronchodilator treatment. The data used in this example have been extracted from a paper by Boggs *et al.* [22] and modified slightly. The results of the first 19 measurements (see Table 15.3) were used to calculate an $X$ chart.

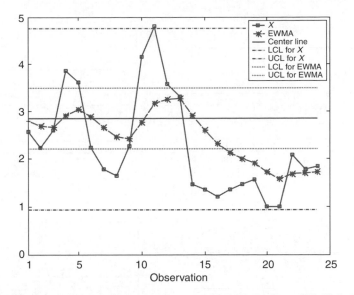

**Figure 15.3**  The time in days ($X$) between consecutive *Clostridium difficile* infections transformed using the transformation $Y = X^{0.2777}$ and then depicted on an $X$ chart. The initial six transformed values were used to calculate the $X$ chart. Superimposed on this chart is the corresponding exponentially weighted moving average (EWMA) chart with $\lambda = 0.20$ and $L = 3.00$. UCL is the upper control limit and LCL is the lower control limit.

**Table 15.3**  Peak expiratory flow rate in l/minute (PEFR) measured daily in the morning in the same patient suffering from asthma.

| Day no. | PEFR before change of treatment | Day no. | PEFR after change of treatment |
|---|---|---|---|
| 1 | 121 | 1 | 310 |
| 2 | 140 | 2 | 307 |
| 3 | 99 | 3 | 325 |
| 4 | 150 | 4 | 346 |
| 5 | 268 | 5 | 380 |
| 6 | 150 | 6 | 312 |
| 7 | 100 | 7 | 384 |
| 8 | 122 | 8 | 376 |
| 9 | 152 | 9 | 354 |
| 10 | 315 | 10 | 370 |
| 11 | 321 | 11 | 365 |
| 12 | 275 | 12 | 325 |
| 13 | 367 | 13 | 368 |
| 14 | 200 | 14 | 350 |
| 15 | 138 | | |
| 16 | 175 | | |
| 17 | 150 | | |
| 18 | 150 | | |
| 19 | 180 | | |

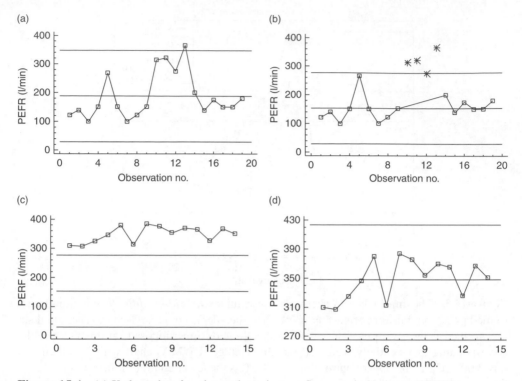

**Figure 15.4** (a) $X$ chart showing the peak expiratory flow rate in l/minute (PEFR) measured daily in the same patient suffering from asthma. (b) $X$ chart showing PEFR measured daily in the same patient. The chart was calculated using the values shown in figure (a) following exclusion of values numbered 10, 11, 12, and 13, depicted as crosses. (c) $X$ chart showing PEFR measured daily in the same patient. The $X$ chart was calculated using values measured in the same patient, prior to a change in therapy (see part (b)). The 14 PEFR values depicted on the $X$ chart were measured after the treatment had been changed and starting two weeks after the change had been initiated. (d) $X$ chart calculated from the PEFR values depicted in (c). These values are depicted on the $X$ chart.

If the values of the $X$ chart appear to be randomly distributed and are all within the control limits, the patient's PEFR is stable. This is good if the patient is stable at a level that is clinically acceptable. However, special causes may disturb a given balance, no matter whether the latter is clinically satisfying or not, and cause additional variation. These causes may be a sudden change in the patient's exposure to allergens, a change in unspecific irritation, or the appearance of infections.

Figure 15.4a shows the $X$ chart calculated using the first 19 values, which are also depicted on the chart. Value number 13 lies above the UCL, and three out of four consecutive values (numbers 10, 11, 12, and 13) lie above the outer upper warning limit (294 l/min).

However, the series is significantly autocorrelated.

As the statistical test for autocorrelation assumes that the mean of the process is stable, a search for assignable causes of variation should be undertaken before one accepts auto-correlation as the explanation. As it turned out, during the period when the four values had been measured the patient had lived with her aunt. Here the patient was no longer exposed to a dog, tobacco smoke, or mittens. Therefore, the values numbered 10, 11, 12, and 13 were deleted, and a revised control chart was calculated, using the remaining values.

The purpose of this was to see if the patient's condition was stable when she was staying at her home, and if so, to learn what the nature of her condition would then be. The mean value of the remaining 15 values was 153.00 l/min, and the standard deviation was 41.22 l/min. The $X$ chart has UCL $= 153.00 + 3 \cdot 41.22 = 276.66$ l/min, center line $= 153.00$ l/min, and LCL $= 153.00 - 3 \cdot 41.22 = 29.34$ l/min.

Figure 15.4b shows the $X$ chart with the values entered. Now, the patient's condition appears to be stable. However, it is clinically unsatisfactory since the PEFR is so low and just a few negative external influences could cause the patient to develop an asthma attack. Therefore, the treatment schedule was altered, taking advantage of the experiences gained from the patient's stay at her aunt's house.

Figure 15.4c shows 14 daily values measured after the patient had been subjected to the new treatment for some time. The values have been entered on the original $X$ chart shown in Figure 15.4b. Since all values lie above the UCL, it is quite clear that the change of treatment (changing the system) has brought the patient out of her previous stable, but clinically unsatisfying condition. The question, now, is if the patient's new condition is stable. Figure 15.4d shows the $X$ chart, calculated using the last 14 values that are depicted on the chart. Since they all lie within the control limits and are randomly scattered, it appears that the patient's new and improved condition is stable. It may be added that the series is not autocorrelated.

### 15.3.2.3.2    Monitoring patients treated for hypertension

*Example 1*    This example shows retrospective data obtained from a male patient treated for hypertension.

Figure 15.5a shows a control chart with 133 measurements of systolic blood pressure (BP) in mm Hg depicted on the chart. The chart is based on the first 29 measurements obtained when the patient did not receive any medication. They were not autocorrelated. We note that the process was in statistical control when the control chart was made, since all 29 points are within the control limits.

The 133 measurements were made between January 11, 2005 and September 19, 2007. The first 98 observations were measured every five to six days from January 11, 2005 to July 26, 2006. The last 31 measurements (nos. 103 through 133) were made one year subsequent to this period from July 26, 2007 to September 19, 2007 with one to two days' interval between measurements. Observations no. 99 through 102 are scattered at random between the two periods.

Starting between observation no. 29 and no. 30, the patient received 25 mg of Tenormin® (atenolol) daily. This dosage was increased to 37.5 mg between observation no. 67 and no. 68 due to the up-going trend, and maintained at that level throughout the rest of the period. Since a number of values between observation no. 30 and no. 55 are below the lower control limit then it may not be unreasonable to assume that overall the medication did have an effect, at least initially.

We now construct an EWMA control chart (Figure 15.5b) based on the first 33 measurements made after the high doses had been initiated (nos. 68 through 100) and depict the 133 measurements on this chart.

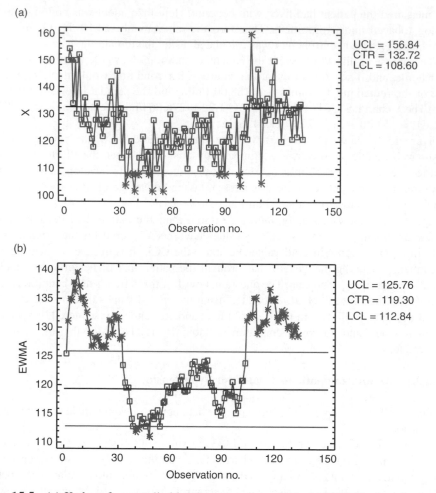

**Figure 15.5** (a) *X* chart for systolic blood pressure (mm Hg). (b) EWMA chart for systolic blood pressure (mm Hg). CTR stands for center line, and LCL, UCL for lower and upper control limits.

The process was in statistical control while the control chart was made since all points between no. 68 and no. 100 are within the control limits and there was no autocorrelation. However, one year later (observation no. 103 and on) the systolic BP is clearly out of control.

The mean BP shows a similar pattern. However, the diastolic BP, once stabilized following the increase of the doses to 37.5 mg, remained in statistical control throughout the period. So it is the systolic BP that is unstable. In this case it appears that, using a control chart, the doses might have been changed at an earlier date.

***Example 2*** This example includes the analysis of prospective blood pressure and body weight measurements made in a hypertensive male on 5 mg of Norvasc® (amlodipine), 50 mg of metoprolol, and 5 mg of ramipril, combined with 25 mg of chlorothiazide daily.

First 30 consecutive daily measurements were made. Then the subject began enjoying daily walks for 30 to 45 minutes and abstained from alcoholic drinks except at dinner, where he enjoyed one to two glasses of vintage red wine. After one month the daily measurements were resumed for 35 days. Control charts of body weight, systolic BP, diastolic BP and mean BP based on the first 30 days of measurements were calculated. In all four cases they displayed a process in statistical control.

Figure 15.6a shows the EWMA chart of the body weight based on the first 30 measurements. All 65 measurements are depicted on the chart. It is noted that the body weight gets out of statistical control in that the EWMA drops below the lower control limit, indicating that the change in life style has had a beneficial effect on the body weight. Perhaps the vintage red wine was too tempting. At any rate, the weight seems to get back in statistical control, indicating that the beneficial effect on the body weight has not been sustained.

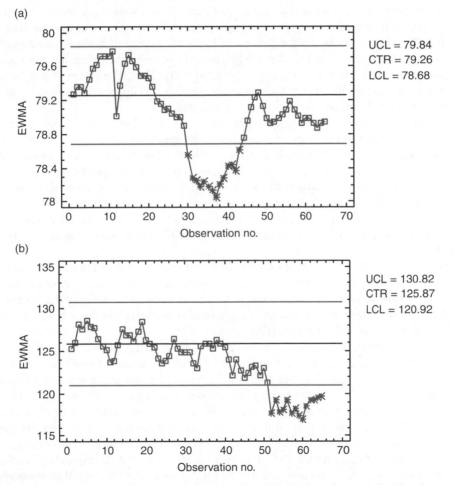

**Figure 15.6**  (a) EWMA chart for weight (kg). (b) EWMA chart for systolic blood pressure (mm Hg).

Figure 15.6b shows the corresponding EWMA chart of the systolic BP. After observation no. 50, the systolic BP drops below the lower control limit and stays there. The EWMA charts of diastolic and mean BP (not shown) show a similar pattern.

Of course nothing definite can be said about the causal relationship between BP and body weight or the magnitude of the temporal delay in response on this basis. Still control charts may be useful to study the temporal relationships between quantities in more controlled settings than those of the present experiment.

## 15.4    A cautionary note on the risk-adjustment of observational data

A process variable like a waiting time is straightforward to use for monitoring a single clinical process and for comparing several healthcare providers during a specified period. If the variable is an outcome measure in patients, however, risk-adjustment may be necessary to adjust for variation between the patients in terms of severity of disease, co-morbidities, and so on [8]. However, statistical risk-adjustment of observational data has the potential for generating results that may be very misleading [23]. Thus, great care should be taken when applying the results. The following study simulates a simple and intuitively obvious mechanism whereby misleading results may be produced.

Imagine two hospitals both receiving patients belonging to the same well-defined clinical entity and suffering from the same grave disease that requires major surgery. Assume that the same surgical procedure is used in both hospitals and that two patient factors influence these patients' risk of dying during operation: the presence of a specific genetic trait ($R_1$: 1 if the factor is present, otherwise 0) and the presence of infection of the organ to be operated on ($R_2$: 1 if present, otherwise 0). Patients with neither risk factor present have a 10% probability of dying during the procedure, regardless of which hospital they are admitted to. For patients with one factor present the probability is 30%, and for those with both factors present it is 60%.

We now conduct a simulation experiment based on these assumptions, simulating the experience of 2000 patients admitted to the two hospitals. To study the effect of patient case mix (the mixture of patients within a specified sample of patients) we vary the patient case mix between the hospitals. We examine the effect of risk-adjustment when both risk factors are known, and when only risk factor 2 is known.

Table 15.4 shows, for each of the above two hospitals, the case mix of 1000 patients admitted to the hospital and the results of the simulation experiments. These results have been analyzed under the assumption that both risk factors are known to the medical community (columns 5 and 6) and under the assumption that only one is known (columns 7 and 8). For example, the first row under hospital 1 shows the simulated probability of death in column 4. It is 0.100 because the patients of this category do not have either of the two risk factors present (see columns 2 and 3). The result of the simulation of 100 patients' experience is that 6 patients died (column 6). The next row (row 2) shows the corresponding results for patients with risk factor 1 present and risk factor 2 absent. Here the simulated probability of death is 0.300 and the result of the simulation that 62 of the 200 patients died, giving a simulated death rate of 0.310. Columns 8 through 10 show how the results would have been interpreted had risk factor 1 been unknown to the medical community. Notice that the two

**Table 15.4**  The results of a simulation study where the probability of death during a surgical procedure as a function of two risk factors (presence of a genetic trait and presence of infection of the organ operated on) was simulated. The probability of death, for given risk factor combination, is the same in the two hospitals, but the case mix differs between the hospitals.

| Hospital[a] | Genetic trait[b] | Infected organ[c] | Probability of death[d] | Result of simulation[e] | | | Genetic trait assumed unknown[f] | | |
|---|---|---|---|---|---|---|---|---|---|
| | | | | Mortality[g] | n | No. dead[h] | Mortality[i] | n | No. dead[i] |
| 1 | No | No | $p = 0.100$ | 0.060 | 100 | 6 | 0.227 | 300 | 68 |
| | Yes | No | $p = 0.300$ | 0.310 | 200 | 62 | | | |
| | No | Yes | $p = 0.300$ | 0.300 | 200 | 60 | 0.496 | 700 | 347 |
| | Yes | Yes | $p = 0.600$ | 0.574 | 500 | 287 | | | |
| 2 | No | No | $p = 0.100$ | 0.096 | 700 | 67 | 0.131 | 840 | 110 |
| | Yes | No | $p = 0.300$ | 0.307 | 140 | 43 | | | |
| | No | Yes | $p = 0.300$ | 0.233 | 120 | 28 | 0.381 | 160 | 61 |
| | Yes | Yes | $p = 0.600$ | 0.825 | 40 | 33 | | | |

[a]It is assumed that the quality of treatment and care is the same at the two hospitals.
[b]The presence of the genetic trait influences the probability of death (see parameters of simulation model in column 4).
[c]The presence of infection of the organ operated on influences the probability of death (see parameters of simulation model in column 4).
[d]The parameter value of the simulation model generating the data. For instance when the genetic trait is present and the organ is infected the probability of death is 0.600.
[e]Column 5, 6 and 7 show the result of the simulation for each combination of risk factors in each hospital.
[f]Column 8, 9 and 10 show how the results would have been classified had the information of the genetic trait been unknown to the medical community. For instance the results of the two first set of experiments would have been pooled and classified as data from patients without organ infection, and so on.
[g]The mortality observed in each of the 8 sets of simulation experiments. When compared to the value in column 4 one may appreciate the effect of the random variation.
[h]No. of dead is the number of fatal outcomes occurring during the $n$ simulations. $n$ is the number of independent simulations done for each type of patient in each hospital. $n$ has been varied between the hospitals to imitate difference between the case mix of the two hospitals.
[i]Using the same data that were generated by the simulation. For given value of 'infected organ' and given hospital, the data have been pooled imitating the situation where the risk factor 'genetic trait' is unknown to the medical community.

types of patients corresponding to rows 1 and 2 cannot be distinguished and we calculate the mortality for patients with risk factor 1 absent as $68/300 = 0.227$, and so on.

The mortality rates (hospital 1: 0.415 and hospital 2: 0.171 calculated from column 9 and 10) differ significantly between hospitals. However, we need to adjust for the difference in case mix. To do so, we perform a regression of risk factors and the hospital effect on $\mathrm{logit}(p_{ij})$ where $p_{ij}$ is the probability that patient $i$, treated at hospital $j$, dies. The independent variables include $R_1$, $R_2$, and $H_1$ (an indicator that is equal to 1 if the patient is treated at hospital 1 and

0 if treated at hospital 2). We have the model

$$\text{logit}(p_{ij}) = \alpha + \delta_1 H_1 + \beta_1 R_1 + \beta_2 R_2 + \varepsilon_{ij}.$$

Table 15.5 shows the result of the logistic regression analysis. The coefficients of both risk factors are highly significantly different from 0, while that of the hospital effect is not. This is no surprise to us because we conducted the experiment so that the hospitals only differed in terms of their case mixes.

Columns 9 and 10 of Table 15.4 show how the data resulting from the simulation would have been classified had the genetic trait been unknown. Patients with both risk factors present would not be distinguishable from patients with only risk factor 2 present, and patients with only risk factor 1 present would be classified as low-risk patients. The logistic regression model therefore becomes

$$\text{logit}(p_{ij}) = \alpha + \delta_1 H_1 + \beta_2 R_2 + \varepsilon_{ij}.$$

Table 15.5 (columns 6 through 9) shows that now the hospital coefficient is significantly different from 0, implying that the mortality rate of hospital no. 1 is higher than that of hospital no. 2 even if we adjust for case-mix differences. Thus, the presence of an unknown or unmeasured significant risk factor may bias the comparisons between healthcare providers.

Empirical studies [19] have demonstrated that statistical adjustment of observational data may fail to remove the main part of bias and occasionally dramatically increase systematic bias. This may, for example, result from omitted or unknown risk factors (as illustrated in the above example), misspecification of continuous variables (inappropriate conversion to binary variables or failure to recognize non-linear relationships), misclassification through the use of poor proxies for the proper covariate, measurement errors, and within-patient instability in covariate (e.g., because of circadian rhythms). As a minimum the following six points should be considered when statistical risk-adjustment of observational data is attempted.

1. Data should first be presented without adjustment.

2. Continuous variables such as age, weight, and so on should not be dichotomized since this throws away information and increases the likelihood of improper model specification.

3. The assumptions of the model building such as linearity, and so on should be checked [24].

4. When appropriate a hierarchical model should be used [25, 26].

5. The variation not accounted for by the risk-adjustment model should be measured and reported.

6. Observational data should be considered hypothesis-generating material, treated accordingly, and very explicitly presented as such.

Clearly the reporting of outcome data based on observational data cannot be avoided entirely, and in that case risk-adjustment is mandatory and the best we can do. Then one just has to proceed with caution.

**Table 15.5** The estimated coefficients of two logistic regressions of hospital $(H_1)^a$ and risk factors[b] $(R_1$ and $R_2)$ on logit$(p)$, where $p$ is the probability of dying during an operation. In the first regression analysis[c] both risk factors were known. In the second analysis[d] it was assumed that only one of the risk factors (factor 2) was known, imitating the situation where an important risk factor is unknown to the medical community.

| Parameter[e] | All risk factors known[c] | | | | One risk factor assumed unknown[d] | | | |
|---|---|---|---|---|---|---|---|---|
| | Estimate | SE[f] | p[g] | Estimated change in odds[h] | Estimate | SE | p | Estimated change in odds |
| $\beta_2$ | 1.30 | 0.127 | <0.00005 | 3.67 | 1.29 | 0.123 | <0.00005 | 3.63 |
| $\delta_1$ | −0.139 | 0.144 | 0.34 | 0.871 | 0.57 | 0.125 | <0.00005 | 1.77 |
| $\beta_1$ | 1.46 | 0.127 | <0.00005 | 4.32 | Factor assumed unknown | | | |

[a]$H_1$ is a binary variable that is 1 if the patient was operated on at hospital no.1 and 0 if he/she was operated on at hospital no. 2.

[b]Risk factor 1 $(R_1)$, 'presence of genetic trait'. R1 = 1 if trait is present, otherwise 0. Risk factor 2 $(R_2)$, 'presence of infection in organ operated on'. $R_2 = 1$ if infection is present, otherwise 0.

[c]logit$(p_{ij}) = \alpha + \beta_1 R_1 + \beta_2 R_2 + \delta_1 H_1 = -2.23 + 1.46R_1 + 1.30R_2 - 0.139H_1$.

[d]logit$(p_{ij}) = \alpha + \beta_2 R_2 + \delta_1 H_1 = -1.86 + 1.29R_1 + 0.57H_1$.

[e]$\alpha$ (the intercept) was estimated as $-2.23$ when both risk factors were assumed known, and as $-1.86$ when only one was assumed known.

[f]SE = standard error of estimate.

[g]p-value.

[h]$e$ estimate; for example, for the parameter $\beta_2$ we have $e^{1.30} = 3.67$.

## 15.5   Summary

In this chapter we discussed the difference between measures of quality that only depend on the quality of the output produced by a healthcare system and indicators of quality such as the result outcome survival that not only depend on the quality but also on other factors such as severity of the patient's disease, co-morbidity, and so on.

It was emphasized that result outcomes must be risk-adjusted to reflect the quality of care. By way of a simulated example we demonstrate how bias may lead to wrong conclusions if risk factors are not taken into consideration because they are unknown or unmeasured.

We recommend that structural data such as staffing levels and so on and process data that measures performance based on adherence to established clinical standards are preferred over result outcome data.

For illustrative purposes we show how control charts may be used to monitor healthcare systems using a throughput measure (waiting time) and the risk of infection as examples. The system monitored may also be an individual patient. The examples included comprise the monitoring of blood pressure in patients with hypertension and of peak flow rate in patients with asthma.

However, the techniques of industrial quality control may also be used for other purposes than monitoring and improving the quality of healthcare. Thus recently it has been recommended to use quality control charts for detection of temporal trends in cumulative meta-analysis [27].

## Appendix A

### 15.A.1   The EWMA chart

For a sequence of observations of $X_i$ with mean $\mu$ and variance $\sigma^2$, the EWMA statistic is defined as

$$Z_i = (1 - \lambda)Z_{i-1} + \lambda X_i \tag{A.1}$$

for $i = 1, 2, \ldots$; $\lambda$ is a parameter $(0 < \lambda \leq 1)$, and the starting value $Z_0 = \mu$, the process mean. It may be shown that

$$Z_i = \lambda \sum_{j=0}^{i-1} [(1 - \lambda)^j X_{i-j}] + (1 - \lambda)^i \mu. \tag{A.2}$$

Therefore, $Z_i$ is a weighted average of the $X_i$ $(j = 1, \ldots, i)$ and $\mu$, with the weights of $X_j$ decreasing exponentially. The weight of the current observation is $\lambda$; that of the previous one is $\lambda(1 - \lambda)$, and so on. The older the observation is, the smaller is the value $\lambda(1 - \lambda)^j$ with which it is weighted. It may be shown that the variance of $Z_i$ is

$$\left(\frac{\lambda}{2 - \lambda}\right) \left[1 - (1 - \lambda)^{2i}\right] \sigma^2. \tag{A.3}$$

When $i$ is large, an approximate variance is

$$\left(\frac{\lambda}{2-\lambda}\right)\sigma^2. \tag{A.4}$$

A EWMA chart can be established by plotting $Z_i$ with the center line at $\mu$ or a target value. The control limits are based on (A.3). We have

$$UCL_i = \mu + L\sigma\sqrt{\frac{\lambda}{2-\lambda}[1-(1-\lambda)^{2i}]} \tag{A.5}$$

$$\text{Center line} = \mu \tag{A.6}$$

$$LCL_i = \mu - L\sigma\sqrt{\frac{\lambda}{2-\lambda}[1-(1-\lambda)^{2i}]}, \tag{A.7}$$

where $L$ is a parameter. When $i > 10$, (A.4) may be used to obtain the control limits:

$$UCL = \mu + L\sigma\sqrt{\frac{\lambda}{2-\lambda}} \tag{A.8}$$

and

$$LCL = \mu - L\sigma\sqrt{\frac{\lambda}{2-\lambda}}. \tag{A.9}$$

Usually, $L = 3$ is used.

### 15.A.2 Logistic regression

Let $p_{ij}$ be the probability that patient $i$, treated by healthcare provider $j$, dies; logit($p_{ij}$) is the logarithm of the corresponding odds $p_{ij}/(1-p_{ij})$; $X_{vij}$ ($v = 1, \ldots, m$) is the $v$th risk factor that is measured in this patient and is related to the probability; and $H_h$ ($h = 1, \ldots, k-1$) is an indicator variable that is equal to 1 if the patient is treated by healthcare provider $j$, and 0 otherwise (provider no. $k$ of the $k$ providers serves as a reference, and $k > 1$). A logistic regression model is defined by

$$\text{logit}(p_{ij}) = \alpha + \sum_{h=1}^{k-1} \delta_h H_h + \sum_{v=1}^{m} \beta_v X_{vij} + \varepsilon_{ij} \tag{A.10}$$

where $\alpha$, $\beta_v$, and $\delta_h$ are the parameters of the regression equation and $\varepsilon_{ij}$ a random error. If $\beta_v$ is significantly different from 0, risk factor no. $v$ is significantly related to logit($p_{ij}$) and thereby to $p_{ij}$. An overall test may show that the parameters for providers, $\delta_h$, differ significantly. This fixed-effect model is adequate for the example discussed in this paper because there are only two providers and the values are statistically independent. When this is not the case, a hierarchical model is preferable [25, 26].

### 15.A.3   Autocovariance and autocorrelation

A time series $X_1, X_2, \ldots, X_n, \ldots$ or $\{X_t, t = 1, \ldots, n, \ldots\}$, comprising random variables with the same mean $\mu$ and standard deviation $\sigma$, is generated by a stationary process. For a stationary process, the covariance between $X_i$ and $X_j$, which are $\tau$ time units away, is defined as

$$\gamma(\tau) = \text{Cov}(X_i, X_j) = E\left[(X_i - \mu)(X_j - \mu)\right]$$

where $j = i + \tau$, $\mu$ is the mean of the stationary process, and $E$ is the expectation or mean value of a random variable. The equation applies to all pairs of random variables separated by $\tau$ time units; that is, for any $i$ and $\tau = 0, \pm 1, \pm 2, \ldots$; $\gamma(\tau)$ is called the autovariance of lag $\tau$. The autocorrelation of lag $\tau$ is defined as the correlation coefficient between $X_i$ and $X_j$. That is,

$$\rho(\tau) = \frac{\gamma(\tau)}{\sigma^2}.$$

For a sequence, $X_1, X_2, \ldots, X_n$, $\gamma(\tau)$ for $\tau = 0, 1, \ldots, n - 1$ can be estimated by

$$\hat{\gamma}(\tau) = \frac{\sum_{i=1}^{n-\tau} (X_i - \bar{X})(X_{i+\tau} - \bar{X})}{n - \tau},$$

where $\bar{X}$ is the average of $X_1, X_2, \ldots, X_n$. In particular, when $\tau = 0$, $\hat{\gamma}(0)$ is an estimator of the process variance. The corresponding estimator of the autocorrelation is given by

$$\hat{\rho}(\tau) = \frac{\hat{\gamma}(\tau)}{\hat{\gamma}(0)}.$$

## Acknowledgements

Our thanks are due to Christian Gluud and Will Guthrie for their thorough and constructive review.

## References

1. Montgomery, D.C. (2001) *Introduction to Statistical Quality Control*, 4th edn, John Wiley & Sons, Inc., New York.

2. Winkel, P. and Zhang, N.F. (2007) *Statistical Development of Quality in Medicine*, John Wiley & Sons, Ltd, Chichester.

3. Woodall, W. (2006) The use of control charts in health-care and public-health surveillance. *J Qual Technol*, **38**, 89–104.

4. Carey, R.G. (2003) *Improving Healthcare with Control Charts: Basic and Advanced SPC Methods and Case Studies*, ASQ Quality Press, Milwaukee, WI.

5. Hart, M.K. and Hart, R.F. (2002) *Statistical Process Control for Health Care*, Duxbury, Pacific Grove, CA.

6. Grigg, O. and Farewell, V. (2004) An overview of risk-adjusted charts. *J R Statist Soc A*, **167**, 523–539.

7. Cebul, R.D. (1991) Randomized, controlled trials using the metro firm system. *Med Care*, **29** (suppl), JS9–JS18.

8. Iezzoni, L.I. (1997) *Risk Adjustment for Measuring Healthcare Outcomes*, Health Administration Press, Chicago.

9. Rosenbaum, P.R. and Rubin, D.B. (1983) The central role of the propensity score in observational studies for causal effects. *Biometrika*, **70**, 41–55.

10. D'Agostino, R.B., Jr. (1998) Tutorial in biostatistics: propensity score methods for bias reduction in the comparison of a treatment to a non-randomized control group. *Stat Med*, **17**, 2265–2281.

11. Roberts, S.W. (1959) Control chart tests based on geometric moving averages. *Technometrics*, **1**, 239–251.

12. Zhang, N.F., Stenback, G.A., and Wardrop, D.M. (1990) Interval estimation of process capability index Cpk. *Commun Statist Meth*, **19**, 4455–4470.

13. Zhang, N.F. (1998) A statistical control chart for stationary process data. *Technometrics*, **40**, 24–28.

14. Zhang, N.F. (1998) Estimating process capability indexes for autocorrelated data. *J Appl Stat*, **25**, 559–74.

15. Aiken, L.H., Clarke, S.P., Sloane, D.M., *et al.* (2002) Hospital nurse staffing and patient mortality, nurse burnout, and job dissatisfaction. *JAMA*, **288**, 1984–1988.

16. Lilford, R., Mohammed, M.A., Spiegelhalter, D., and Thomsom R. (2004) Use and misuse of process and outcome data in managing performance of acute medical care: avoiding institutional stigma. *Lancet*, **363**, 1147–1154.

17. Benneyan, J.C. (1998) Statistical quality control methods in infection control and hospital epidemiology, Part 1: introduction and basic theory. *Infect Control Hosp Epidemiol*, **19**, 194–214.

18. Benneyan, J.C. (1998) Statistical quality control methods in infection control and hospital epidemiology, Part 2: chart use, statistical properties, and research issues. *Infect Control Hosp Epidemiol*, **19**, 265–277.

19. Finison, L.J., Finison, K.S., and Bliersbach, C.M. (1993) The use of control charts to improve healthcare quality. *J Healthc Qual*, **15**, 9–23.

20. Tennant, R., Mohammad, M.A., Coleman, J.J., and Martin U. (2007) Monitoring patients using control charts: a systematic review. *Int J Qual Health Care*, **19**, 187–194.

21. Glaszion, P., Irwig, L., and Mant D. (2005) Monitoring in chronic disease: a rational approach. *BMJ*, **330**, 644–648.

22. Boggs, P.B., Wheeler, D., Washburne, W.F., and Hayati F. (1998) Peak expiratory flow rate control chart in asthma care: chart construction and use in asthma care. *Ann Allergy Asthma Immunol*, **81**, 552–562.

23. Deeks, J.J., Dinnes, J., D'Amico, R., *et al.* (2003) Evaluating non-randomised intervention studies. *Health Technol Assess*, **7**, 1–186.

24. Bagley, S.C., White, H., and Golomb, B.A. (2001) Logistic regression in the medical literature: standards for use and reporting, with particular attention to one medical domain. *J Clin Epidemiol*, **54**, 979–985.

25. Greenland, S. (2000) Principles of multilevel modeling. *Int J Epidemiol*, **29**, 158–167.

26. Goldstein, H., Browne, W., and Rasbash, J. (2002) Tutorial in biostatistics: multilevel modeling of medical data. *Stat Med*, **21**, 3291–3315.

27. Kulinskaya, E. and Koricheva, J. (2011) Use of quality control charts for detection of outliers and temporal trends in cumulative meta-analysis. *Res Synth Meth*, **1**(3-4), 297–307.

# Part Four

# APPLICATIONS TO HEALTHCARE POLICY AND IMPLEMENTATION

# 16

# Modeling kidney allocation: A data-driven optimization approach

**Inbal Yahav**
*The Graduate School of Business, Department of Information Systems, Bar Ilan University, Israel*

## Synopsis

In the United States, more than 90 000 candidates are currently waiting for kidney transplantation, with an annual increase of about 20 000 candidates. The current allocation policy poorly matches donors with recipients. We present a two-phase allocation policy that combines an integer programming-based learning phase and a data-mining, real-time phase. Our policy outperforms the current system in multiple respects, such as increased life-year gained from kidney allocation and better match between organs and recipients.

## 16.1 Introduction

According to the US Scientific Registry of Transplant Recipients (SRTR) annual statistics, more than 90 000 candidates with kidney failure End Stage Renal Disease (ESRD[1]) are currently waiting for kidney transplantation, with an annual increase of about 20 000 candidates (see Figure 16.1).

---

[1] For more information see OPTN/UNOS (2008).

---

*Statistical Methods in Healthcare*, First Edition. Edited by Frederick W. Faltin, Ron S. Kenett and Fabrizio Ruggeri.
© 2012 John Wiley & Sons, Ltd. Published 2012 by John Wiley & Sons, Ltd.

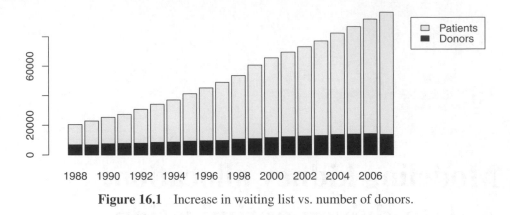

**Figure 16.1**    Increase in waiting list vs. number of donors.

The current allocation policy is based on a set of priority points. When an organ becomes available, each candidate registered on the Organ Procurement and Transplantation Network (OPTN) waiting list receives priority points according to a compatibility test between the patient and the donor, his/her waiting time and rank, and age (higher priority for younger and older populations). The compatibility test is a combined measure of tissue matching (also known as Human Leukocyte Antigen (HLA) matching) and the Panel Reactive Antibodies (PRA) test. PRA is a blood test that examines whether a candidate exhibits antibodies to the proteins of the donor. Priority points for compatibility are given with the objective of minimizing the rejection rate after transplant. Priority points for waiting time and age are given to compensate candidates with rare tissue types.

While giving priority points for waiting time is supposed to provide a sense of equity in access to transplantation, over the years those priority points have started to dominate the allocation system and have decreased the efficiency of allocations. The dominance of waiting time on priority points has transformed the system to a 'first come first transplant assignment' that disregards the potential afterlife of the transplanted kidney itself (OPTN/UNOS, 2008). As a result, the current system poorly matches the candidate and transplanted kidney expected life after transplant, resulting in death with a functioning kidney in many patients, and an increase in the need for retransplantation for many other patients. Moreover, the system also fails to achieve equity for several demographic groups with rare tissue types and high sensitization levels (Eggers, 1995).

According to OPTN/UNOS (2008), even with additional priority given to sensitized candidates (patients with PRA > 80%), highly matched kidneys, and children, the current system does not adequately balance equity and efficiency factors, as it utilizes only a few of the medical criteria that are now available to rank candidates. Furthermore, the PRA measure itself is known to be highly variable and inconsistent, as it is measured by different commercially available kits or locally procured cell panels, which often do not represent the entire donor population. The drawbacks of the current allocation policy have initiated an intensive debate and the need to consider alternative allocation policies (OPTN/UNOS, 2008). In 2004, the Kidney Allocation Review Subcommittee (KARS) was established with the goal of designing an allocation policy that maximizes the tradeoff between *equity* in access to transplantation and *efficiency*; that is, maximizing the aggregate health of the transplant candidate pool (Votruba, 2001). In 2008 the committee proposed four concepts that would together combine to determine a candidate's Kidney Allocation Score (KAS). The concepts are as follows.

LYFT **(Life Years From Transplant):** estimated survival duration in years that a recipient of a specific organ may expect to have, versus their remaining years on dialysis (at time of offer). LYFT is a function of the patient's profile (age, tissue type, etc.) as well as the donor's profile (age, cause of death, etc.).

DPI **(Donor Profile Index):** a continuous measure of organ quality based on clinical information. DPI increases individual matching by providing a better metric for deciding which organs are appropriate for which candidates.

DT **(Dialysis Time):** the length of time that the patient has been receiving dialysis at the time of the offer.

CPRA **(Calculated Panel Reactive Antibody):** measures the likelihood that the recipient and donor would be incompatible, based on HLA frequencies in donors. CPRA replaces the PRA measure in the current renal allocation system.

The formula for determining KAS provided by OPTN/UNOS (2008) is the following:

$$KAS = LYFT \times 0.8 \times (1 - DPI) + DT \times (0.8 \times DPI + 0.2) + (CPRA \times 0.04). \quad (16.1)$$

According to the proposed method, kidneys would be allocated to patients based on candidates' KAS, rather than priority points.

Compared to the current system, the new allocation policy is expected to increase the overall number of life years gained from the kidney allocation system by over 3000 years in its first year of operation. Additionally, transplantation rates for minority candidates (such as African-Americans), as well as candidates with high PRA levels, is expected to improve.

One of the main disadvantages of this allocation is that it does not account for future prospective donors and candidates' health condition degradation. In other words, the allocation decision is done in a *static* fashion, in which the decision is based only on the match between the *current arriving organ* and the candidates for the kidney. In this chapter we focus on the problem of designing a policy that balances the efficiency of the allocation with equity in access to transplantation. Despite the large dimensionality of the problem, the policy has to be computationally efficient. That is, making an allocation decision in a timely manner, and leaving sufficient time for tissue matching tests, organ shipping, and the actual transplant.

This chapter is organized as follows. In the reminder of this section we review the existing literature on the kidney allocation problem. We describe the kidney allocation problem in Section 16.2. In Section 16.3 we propose a two-phase policy that is composed of a learning phase and a knowledge-based deployment phase. In the learning phase we propose a stochastic optimization model that, on expectation, optimally allocates organs to candidates (given a specific allocation objective). As an input to the stochastic optimization problem we use the entire information of candidate and organ arrivals and a set probabilistic health condition and lifetime scenarios of candidates on the waiting list. We later use the knowledge gained from the learning phase to derive a knowledge-based, real-time allocation policy. The novelty of the two-phase method is that it incorporates the future uncertainty of allocations into the decision process, yet maintains computational feasibility regardless of the challenges that the large dimensionality of the problem presents.

In Section 16.4 we describe the analytical framework and briefly discuss the model estimation procedure. We deploy and evaluate our two-phase policy on the actual OPTN waiting list in Section 16.5.

Our results show a clear gap between the *efficiency* of our two-phase policy and that of the current priority point (PP) system and the proposed highest-KAS-first (HKF) policy. In particular, we find the following.

- Waiting time to transplantation is more than 0.5 years shorter (on average), according to our two-phase allocation policy.

- The match between organ and recipients improves, resulting in a lower organ rejection rate and a higher correlation between organs' survival years and recipient lifetime. A poor correlation between organ and recipient survival times increases the need for retransplantation on the one hand, and deaths with functioning organs on the other hand.

- Recipients' year-gain from transplanted kidneys increases by almost five months per recipient in the two-phase allocation, compared to HKF, and almost three years compared to the current PP system.

In terms of *equity*, we show that our allocation policy provides equal access to transplants for candidates of different races, ages, and tissue types.

Another important feature of our policy is that the variability of organ types offered to patients with similar health profiles is relatively small. That implies that the problem of patients' choice becomes less relevant. The reason is that patients have very low incentive to refuse organs: a patient who chooses to refuse an offer is most likely to be offered the same kidney quality all over again. We discuss these findings in Section 16.6.

### 16.1.1    Literature review

The organ allocation problem, and specifically cadaveric kidney (or *grafts* as they are called by the medical community) allocation, raises a very interesting operations research policy modeling problem that combines supply shortage with ever increasing demand. Unlike liver and lung allocation policies, in which the objective is to minimize the number of deaths on the list, kidney allocation is unique in that there exists the alternative of dialysis for candidates suffering from renal failure (OPTN/UNOS, 2008). This treatment option requires the allocation policy to be based upon many additional factors, such as post-transplant expected life, equity in access to transplantation, and so on. For the past two decades, operations research applications of organ transplantation have received great attention. Generally, the organ transplantation is modeled as a matching problem between donors and recipients with the goal of maximizing some reward function. Specifically, two perspectives of the problem have been addressed: the patient's perspective of deciding to accept or reject an organ offer, and the policy planner's perspective of designing an allocation decision model. Alagoz, Schaefer, and Roberts (2009) provide a comprehensive survey of operations research applications related to organ allocation in general. A specific survey of models for kidney allocation is provided by Zenios (2004). We next survey the key literature on kidney allocation models. We focus on the policy planner's problem and discuss the patient choice problem and the utility-maximizing *game* between the planner and the candidates. One of the most studied models for organ allocation is the sequential stochastic assignment problem introduced by Derman, Lieberman, and Ross (1972). In the Derman *et al.* model, as random jobs arrive, they must be assigned to workers. Rewards depend on the match between jobs and workers. Kidney allocation can be viewed as an application of Derman *et al.*'s model, where jobs are organs and workers are candidates for kidney allocation.

Righter (1989) and David and Yechiali (1995) propose Markov decision process (MDP) models for the sequential allocation of kidneys to patients, extending the results from Derman, Lieberman, and Ross (1972) to random environments. Randomness is reflected in graft arrival and candidate departure (death) rates. The authors raise the question of admission control and allocation of arriving organs, and discuss the threshold-based property of the expected optimal policy. The question of patient choice models in the context of kidney allocation has been repeatedly addressed in the literature of the last two decades. According to Zenios (2004), about 45% of the offered organs are rejected by the first patient who receives them (or by his/her physician). The rationale for a rejection is that, under the current allocation policy, once a candidate reaches the top of the list, s/he remains there until s/he accepts a graft.

Su and Zenios (2004, 2005, 2006) incorporate the patient choice question into the allocation problem. They consider a stylized model, in which the patients are homogeneous in their preferences. They model the allocation system as an $M/M/1$ queue where the queue is composed of patients, and the donors are 'service providers'. Here, the objective of the patients is to maximize their *individual* discounted quality of life (QoL) before and after transplant. The planner's objective is to maximize the *total* QoL. Similar to previous literature, the authors find that the optimal welfare (i.e., aggregated candidates' health) is achieved under a threshold-based policy, implying that it is optimal for the planner to reject organs under a certain quality. Su and Zenios (2005, 2006) extend the work to account for patient heterogeneity.

Su and Zenios (2005) present a stylized model that considers the sequential allocation of $n$ kidneys to $n$ patients. Each patient–kidney pair has its own type and rewards depending on the match between them. The planner's objective is to maximize the total expected reward. As noted earlier, the optimal policy is a threshold policy. Su and Zenios compare the optimal policy with and without patient choice, and demonstrate that patient choice may introduce significant inefficiencies. However, the authors also observe that minimizing the variability in the type of offers expected by each patient type reduces those losses. We will use this observation in our model to claim that policies that do not consider patient choice, yet yield minimum variability concerning the assigned kidney type to each group of patients, are consequently robust to patient choice.

For the more general and realistic representation, Zenios, Chertow, and Wein (2000) develop a fluid-based model that imitates the actual clinic environment. In this model the patient pool is divided into $K$ classes and the donors into $J$ classes. The division into classes is based on demographic, immunological, and physiological characteristics. The state of the system is defined as a vector of the number of patients in each class. Patients depart from the system through either death or transplant. Zenios *et al.* consider a control problem that combines three objective functions. The first objective is to maximize the quality of adjusted life which satisfies the efficiency criteria. Then, two equity criteria are considered: minimize inequity in (absolute) waiting time (first-come-first-serve), and minimize inequity in (relative) likelihood of transplantation. The authors develop a simulation-based study in which the distributions of the patients' and donors' characteristics, mortality rates, and arrival rates are estimated using data from UNOS (the United Network for Organ Sharing) 1995, the United States Renal Data System and the New England Organ Bank.

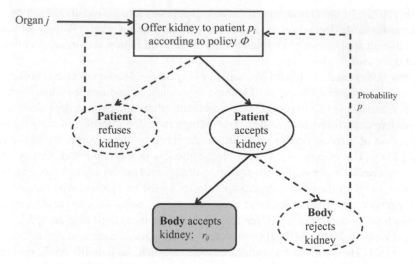

**Figure 16.2**    Schematic representation of kidney allocation.

## 16.2   Problem description

We consider the general problem of allocating kidneys to patients on the kidney waiting list. Organs are allocated upon arrival to patient $p_i$ according to some allocation policy $\Phi$. The patient then can either *accept* the kidney or *refuse* the kidney (seeking a better match). If the patient refuses the offered organ, the organ is re-allocated to another patient, according to the same policy $\Phi$. When a patient accepts the kidney, a transplant is performed. If a transplant is successful, the planner receives some reward $r_{ij}$. Otherwise, the organ is reallocated with some probability $p$, reflecting the probability that the organ is still qualified for retransplantation. Figure 16.2 illustrates the allocation scheme.

According to OPTN, most transplants are successful (approximately 95% of living-donor transplants are successful and more than 90% of deceased-donor transplants are successful, with increased success rate in recent years). We therefore assume that transplants are always successful. Additionally, we assume that patients always choose to accept offered kidneys (we later discuss the implications of this assumption on our model in Section 16.6). Our analyzed model based on these assumptions is marked with solid lines in Figure 16.2.

It is important to note that a kidney from a cadaver donor (approximately two-thirds of the transplants) can be preserved for up to 48 hours only (Hines and Marschall, 2008). Hence it is crucial to make an allocation decision in a timely manner, leaving sufficient time for tissue matching tests, organ shipping, and the actual transplant.

### 16.2.1   Notation

Let $P^t = \{p_1, p_2, \ldots\}$ be the pool of patients in the kidney waiting list at time $t$. Note that the patient pool changes over time, as patients may join the waiting list or depart from it (due to different reasons such as transplant, death, transplant in another country, etc.). We identify each patient by the tuple $(t_i, h^t_i, sp^t_i)$, representing respectively the date she/he was placed on the waiting list, his/her conditional health state information at time $t$ (e.g., age, dialysis time, weight to height ratio (BMI), sensitization level, etc.), given that she/he has not received a transplant until time $t$, and the probability that the patient has survived up to time $t$. The survival probability replaces the patient's departure time information, because the latter remains unknown until the actual departure event.

We use $O$ to denote the set of available organs for transplant, with $o_j = (t_j, d_j)$ being the $j$th organ, where $t_j$ is its arrival date, and $d_j$ is the profile of the donor who donated the organ. The donor profile includes information on his/her age, cause of death, whether or not she/he was diabetic, blood pressure at death time, and so on. The reward from allocating organ $o_j$ to patient $p_i$ at time $t$, given the patient's health state and expected mortality rate at time $t$ is given by $r_{ij}^t(h_i^t)$. Without loss of generality, we assume that the allocation decision time is negligible, and $t = t_j$. We therefore use an abbreviated notation: $r_{ij}^t$.

We define $x^\Phi$ to be the allocation decision under policy $\Phi$, with $x_{ij} = 1$ if organ $o_j$ is allocated to patient $p_i$ and $x_{ij} = 0$ otherwise. The objective is to find a policy that maximizes the total expected time-dependent reward, given by

$$TR^\Phi = \int r_t^{t'} x^\Phi \mathrm{d}t. \tag{16.2}$$

Note that $r_{ij}^{t_1}$ and $r_{ij}^{t_2}$ ($t_1 \neq t_2$) may take different values. We do not, however, restrict the *order* of these two values (i.e., $r_{ij}^{t_1}$ can be either greater than, equal to, or less than $r_{ij}^{t_2}$).

## 16.2.2   Choosing objectives

We are interested in obtaining the best attainable allocation of deceased donor kidneys to candidates.[2] Unlike liver and lung allocation policies, in which the objective is to reduce waiting list mortality and improve recipient survival during the first year following transplant, kidney failure is not an immediate cause of death and thus the allocation policy must be based upon different considerations such as quality of life (with and without a transplant), waiting time, sensitization level, and so on (OPTN/UNOS, 2008).

Following the KARS recommendation, we use the expected KAS (see equation (16.1)) as the allocation reward. The KAS metric is important in that it balances equity in access to transplantation and allocation efficiency factors (i.e., the aggregate health of the transplant candidate pool). However, we propose a dynamic allocation that utilizes the donors' and candidates' arrival distribution and candidates' expected health condition degradation and mortality rate. Given that, the reward function is given by:

$$r_{ij} = \begin{cases} KAS_{ij} & \text{if } p_i \in P^{t_j} \text{ (i.e. } t_i < t_j \text{ and patient } p_i \text{ has not departed by time } t_j) \\ 0 & \text{otherwise.} \end{cases} \tag{16.3}$$

As future departure events are unknown, we use the expected reward, denoted by the KAS value multiplied by the probability that the patients have not departed the waiting list by the time of the offer:

$$er_{ij} = KAS_{ij} sp_i^{t_j}. \tag{16.4}$$

---

[2] We disregard living-donor transplants, as those are allocated to family-related patients.

## 16.3    Proposed real-time dynamic allocation policy

We propose a two-phase allocation policy that provides real-time near optimal allocation under the critical constraint of making an allocation decision in a timely manner. The policy works as follows: (1) compute the expected optimal allocation of organs to candidates, based on the entire historical information available at hand, and (2) derive a knowledge-based allocation policy that utilizes the properties of the expected optimal allocation, and deploy this knowledge in real-time.

We next explain each of the two components in further detail.

### 16.3.1    Stochastic optimization formulation

We formulate the problem of allocating deceased kidneys to candidates in the OPTN waiting list as a stochastic optimization problem. Here, the entire input of kidneys and candidates (i.e., past and future arrivals) is available from the start. Whereas the information on kidney arrival times and donors profiles are complete, the available information on candidates' health conditions and lifetimes are only partial. The reason is that candidates who received a kidney under the current policy might not receive a kidney under any other policy. The health condition and lifetime of such candidates, had they not received a kidney, is unknown. We thus replace the missing information by a set of probabilistic scenarios.

Representing the allocation problem as a stochastic optimization problem serves two roles. First, it provides an upper bound on the best attainable expected performance by any real-time allocation scheme, *given a specific allocation objective* (e.g., expected KAS). Such upper bound will enable us to assess the performance of any real-time allocation policy. Second, it allows us to utilize the knowledge gained from the solution of the stochastic optimization problem, to derive a real-time knowledge-based allocation that generates a near-optimal allocation that is computationally fast.

Since allocation is a one-to-one mapping between kidneys and candidates, we can restate the allocation problem as a max-weighted matching problem on a bipartite graph (Edmonds, 1965). Specifically, consider a bipartite graph in which the organs constitute one set of nodes and the candidates constitute another. An edge between organ $j$ arriving at time $t_j$, and candidate $i$, is drawn if and only if $j$ arrives later than $i$ ($t_i \leq t_j$). The weight on this edge equals the expected reward of a successful transplant, $er_{ij}$. Note that the reward $er_{ij}$ is a function of the estimated health condition of candidate $i$ at time $t_j$ ($h_i^{t_j}$). A schematic representation of the stochastic optimization problem is given in Figure 16.3.

The objective is to maximize the overall allocation reward, denoted by the sum of edge weights:

$$
\begin{aligned}
\max \quad & \sum_{j \in O,\, i \in P} er_{ij}^t x_{ij} \\
\text{s.t.} \quad & \sum_{j \in O} x_{ij} \leq 1, \forall i \in P \\
& \sum_{i \in P} x_{ij} \leq 1, \forall j \in O \\
& x_{ij} \in \{0,\, 1\}.
\end{aligned}
\tag{16.5}
$$

The problem of finding the max-weighted matching is known to be NP-complete.

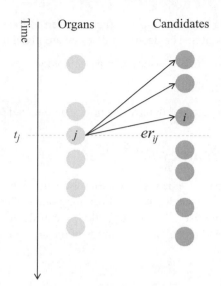

**Figure 16.3**   Schematic representation of the stochastic optimization problem.

From here on we refer to the solution of the above stochastic optimization problem as the *expected optimal allocation*.

## 16.3.2   Knowledge-based real-time allocation policy

The allocation proposed in Section 16.3.1 cannot be obtained in real time, as future kidney and candidate arrivals are unknown. One way of utilizing the stochastic optimization formulation is by repeatedly evaluating a reward of an assignment based on a probabilistic set of future scenarios ('stochastic dynamic allocation'). However, since the size of the problem is extremely large (more than 90 000 candidates are currently waiting for kidney transplantation, with an annual increase of about 20 000 candidates) and the stochastic optimization problem is NP-complete, such an approach would suffer from heavy computational requirements and thus may perform poorly in terms of solution time. Alternatively, we next propose a computationally efficient policy that can handle the dynamic and stochastic nature of the real-time problem.

We design a knowledge-based, robust allocation algorithm that meets the computational requirement and provides a near-optimal allocation (given KAS being the optimal objective). The algorithm operates in five steps.

1. Divide the dataset into training and holdout sets. The training set is used to construct and solve the stochastic optimization problem and determine the properties of the best attainable allocation. The holdout set is later used for performance evaluation (as is classically done in data mining).

2. Compute the expected optimal allocation, as given by problem (16.5), on the training set.

3. Let $A = a_1, \ldots, a_n$ be the set of paired allocations resulting from Step 2 ($a_1 = (p_1, o_1)$), and $S = s_1, \ldots, s_n$ be the profile of the donors and recipients in each

allocation. Derive a knowledge-based (herein referred to as KB) policy based on the common properties of $S$. The details of this step are given in Section 16.5.2.

4. Evaluate the performance of policy KB on the holdout set.

5. Deploy policy KB in real-time.

In the next section we evaluate and deploy this policy on the OPTN waiting list.

# 16.4     Analytical framework

In this section we describe the framework we used for conducting the stochastic optimization problem and deriving the knowledge-based allocation policy. The analysis in the section is based on the UNOS waiting list, as of August, 2008. We evaluate our policy on its equity in access to transplantation and its efficiency in terms of the allocation outcome.

## 16.4.1     Data

We consider a dataset of waiting list registrations and transplants of kidney and simultaneous kidney-pancreas[3] that have been listed or performed in the USA and reported to the OPTN between October 1, 1987 and August 15, 2008. The dataset includes records on both deceased and living-donor transplants. The data were exclusively provided by UNOS.

Preliminary analysis of the data exhibits a rapid increase in kidney donations over the last two decades. Hence, our analysis is based on the last five years only (January 1, 2004 – August 15, 2008), for which the data seem to have a stationary nature (e.g., the distributions of candidate and organ arrivals do not change significantly over time).[4] For the purposes of our study, we consider only deceased-donor transplants of kidneys and simultaneous kidney(s) and pancreas. For computational reasons, we apply the policies and evaluate them for a single geographic region. We randomly chose region no. 2 that contains the following states: Pennsylvania (PA), New Jersey (NJ), West Virginia (WV), Maryland (MD), Delaware (DE), and Washington DC (DC). The data contain a total of approximately 26 000 candidates, 3000 donors, and 5800 kidney donations.

## 16.4.2     Model estimation

An essential pre-step to designing any allocation policy is estimating candidates' health profile (current and prospective) and organ quality. In particular, the following properties are to be estimated: candidates' sensitization level (CPRA), year-gain from a given organ (LYFT) and survival probability, and organs' survival index (measured by DPI value).

These estimates can then be used in computing the KAS value for each candidate–organ pair.

The KAS score, along with the survival probability, is used to compute the expected KAS (also referred to as *expected reward*) and serves as an input to the stochastic optimization

---

[3] Simultaneous transplantation of the kidney and pancreas is performed for those who have kidney failure as a complication of insulin-dependent diabetes mellitus (also called Type I diabetes).

[4] Candidates that were placed in the OPTN waiting list before January 1, 2004 and are still on the waiting list as of that date are included in the study.

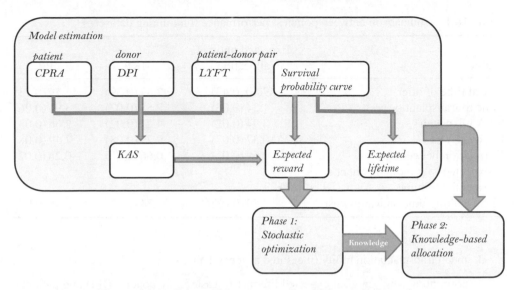

**Figure 16.4**   Schematic representation of the analytic study.

problem in equation (16.5). Finally, the allocation outcome of the stochastic optimization problem is used to derive our knowledge-based, real-time policy (KB).

A schematic representation of the model estimation procedure is provided in Figure 16.4. For brevity, we omit the details of this procedure from this chapter. A complete model estimation procedure is available in Yahav (2010).

## 16.5   Model deployment

We generate training and holdout sets by randomly assigning 10% of the patients and donors into the training set and another 10% into the holdout set. The reason for using only 10% in each dataset is due to the computational constraints of the software used (GAMS 23.2). The training set is used to build the model, and the holdout set is used for evaluating model performance. Each sample contains a random sample of patients (approximately 2500 patients) in the waiting list and a random sample of donors (approximately 300 donors). We repeat the analysis on the 10 different training and holdout samples, to estimate the performance error. For each set we estimate the model parameters, as discussed in Section 16.4.2.

In the next sections, we perform a stochastic optimization analysis and study the properties of the best attainable allocation, under the objective of maximizing the expected KAS score. We then derive a knowledge-based policy, based on these properties, and apply it in real-time settings.

We perform an evaluation study in which we compare our policy with the currect priority point (PP) system and KARS' proposed (HKF) policy. The performance of the policies is evaluated based on the following metrics:

1. mean time to transplantation

2. mean time on waiting list (of candidates who have not received a transplant)

**Table 16.1**  Comparison between policies' performance (on training dataset).

| Metric | Expected optimal allocation | HKF | PP |
|---|---|---|---|
| Age at time of offer | 47.40 (0.43) | 47.47 (0.39) | 46.79 (0.73) |
| Time to transplant (years) | 1.34 (0.05) | 2.58 (0.07) | 3.96 (0.06) |
| HLA mismatch | 3.94 (0.02) | 4.21 (0.02) | 2.66 (0.03) |
| Utility (LYFT) | 10.37 (0.07) | 9.79 (0.08) | 7.49 (0.08) |
| Correlation between graft expected lifetime and patient's expected lifetime | 0.69 (0.01) | 0.66 (0.01) | −0.28 (0.02) |
| Mean waiting time on waiting list | 3.59 (0.03) | 2.74 (0.03) | 2.45 (0.07) |

3. mean transplantation utility (measured as mean LYFT)

4. correlation between graft expected lifetime (measured by donor's DPI) and patient's expected lifetime

5. mortality rate.

## 16.5.1   Stochastic optimization analysis

We compute the expected optimal allocation (see equation (16.5)) of each training set, using GAMS 23.2 (www.gams.com/). The mean performance of the resulted allocation is summarized in Table 16.1 (column 2). In parentheses we report the standard error across different runs.

For a fair comparison between the expected optimal allocation and the current (PP) and proposed (by KARS (HKF)) allocation policies, we generated a computer program (in R 2.8.1, http://cran.r-project.org) that simulates a real-time environment, in which donors and patients arrive according to their actual arrival order in each replica, and depart (due to mortality) according to their lifetime distribution. We compute the performances of the allocation policies (HKF and PP) on these simulated datasets. We report their performances in Table 16.1 (columns 3 and 4).

Comparing the expected optimal allocation with the other two policies, we can see improvement in several respects. First, the mean time to transplantation of the expected optimal allocation is shorter compared to either of the other policies (1.34 years compared to 3.96 years and 2.58 years of the PP and HKF policies, respectively). Second, the mean HLA mismatch of the expected optimal allocation is improved compared to HKF, implying that the probability of successful transplantation is improved. Moreover, we find that approximately 65% of the patients that receive an organ under both HKF and the expected optimal allocation in our experiments had a better match with the organ they receive under the expected optimal allocation policy, compared to what they receive under HKF. The current (PP) policy has the lowest HLA mismatch, since priority points of an allocation are given based on the match between the donor and the patient. Comparing the utility from an allocation (or in other words, the year-gain from allocating kidneys to candidates), we find that the expected optimal allocation achieves the highest utility. On average, candidates that receive a transplant under the expected optimal allocation in our experiments are expected to live almost seven months longer than those who receive a kidney under the KAS policy, and almost three years longer than those who receive a kidney under the current PP policy. Finally, the expected optimal allocation better matches survival times of a transplanted kidney (measured by DPI, where low DPI corresponds to long expected organ survival) with expected lifespans of their recipient. This is a very important feature for two reasons. First, it decreases the probability that a patient would return to the waiting list after a transplanted graft failure. Second, it decreases the probability that a patient would die with a functioning graft, resulting in an increase in the graft utility. The actual waiting time of candidates in the waiting list increases under the expected optimal allocation by an average of approximately one year (compared to both PP and HKF policies). Although the increased waiting time may be considered a downside of the expected optimal allocation, it also implies that the expected optimal allocation does not operate as a 'first-come-first-transplant' policy. Instead, it gives higher weight to allocation and graft utility than to waiting time.

## 16.5.2  Knowledge-based real-time policy

We use the knowledge gained from the stochastic optimization model and the resulting expected optimal allocation and propose a knowledge-based policy that mimics the improvements that the expected optimal allocation suggests on the HKF policy. We consider improvement in the planes of *equity* and *efficiency*.

**Equity:** does the expected optimal allocation provide a sense of equity in access to transplantation, or are candidates prioritized based on their demographic and ethnic profile? Does the expected optimal allocation provide better or worse equity compared to HKF?

**Efficiency:** given that a candidate receives an organ allocation, what type of kidney would a recipient receive under the expected optimal allocation compared to HKF?

### 16.5.2.1  Equity

For the question of equity, we use the Kruskal–Wallis $\chi^2$ test (Kruskal and Wallis, 1952) to compare the median health profile of candidates (dialysis time, antigens, age, etc.) to those of organ recipients, according to the expected optimal allocation. Table 16.2 summarizes the test results.

We find that the expected optimal allocation gives high priority to candidates with high sensitization level (high CPRA value), diabetes, long dialysis time, and to those who are waiting for simultaneous kidney-pancreas transplant. This result is not surprising, considering the structure of the KAS score (equation (16.1)) that gives priority based on CPRA value (up to 4 'points'), dialysis time (between 0.2 and 1 point per year), and LYFT (between 0.2 and 1 point per additional years gained from the transplant), which increases with diabetes and the need for simultaneous kidney-pancreas transplant (Wolfe *et al.*, 2008). We also find that, unlike the current PP system, the expected optimal allocation does not prioritize based on candidates' antigens and, consequently, does not prioritize based on ethnicity (for the equity problem caused by candidates' antigens and tissue types, consider Eggers, 1995). To compare the equity of expected optimal allocation to that of the HKF policy, we perform a $\chi^2$ test on the two groups of organ recipients in our experiments. We find that the median is

**Table 16.2** Comparison between profile distribution of candidates and recipients under the expected optimal allocation (Kruskal–Wallis $\chi^2$ test).

| Metric | $\chi^2$ | $p$-value | Statistically equal? |
|---|---|---|---|
| CPRA | 77.46 | 0 | No |
| DIAB | 205.55 | 0 | No |
| KP | 16.05 | 0 | No |
| PrevTrans | 1.73 | 0.19 | Yes |
| DT | 171.51 | 0 | No |
| Age | 31.25 | 0.07 | Yes |
| A antigens | 0.09 | 0.77 | Yes |
| B antigens | 3.23 | 0.07 | Yes |
| DR antigens | 2.12 | 0.15 | Yes |
| BMI | 0.53 | 0.47 | Yes |
| Albumin | 8.58 | 0 | No |
| Ethnicity | 0.85 | 0.36 | Yes |

Metrics: DIAB – whether the patient has diabetes (1 = yes); KP – whether the patient is waiting for a simultaneous kidney-pancreas transplant (1 = yes); PrevTrans – number of previous transplants; A antigens – number of HLA-A antigens; B antigens – number of HLA-B antigens; DR antigens – number of HLA-DR antigens;

statistically equal at the 1% significance level on all the different metrics; implying that *the equity provided by both policies is statistically equal*. In fact, we find that the two recipient groups overlap by more than 70%. We conclude that the expected optimal allocation does improve the *equity* of the HKF policy.

### 16.5.2.2  Efficiency

To study the *efficiency* of the expected optimal allocation, we construct a regression tree on the allocation that maps organ types – that is, DPI values ( $y$ variable in the tree notation) – to recipients' health profile, such as Age, LYFT, CPRA, DT, Survival probability and their KAS value ( $x$ variable in the tree notation). In essence, the regression tree satisfies one main objective: it provides *knowledge* on what type of kidney is allocated to what type of candidates, in terms of their health-related and donor-patient-match-related properties. We later use this knowledge to develop our knowledge-based real-time policy. The resulting regression tree is given in Figure 16.5. On the regression tree, the patient pool is divided into six groups (six leaf nodes), based on their DT, Age, LYFT, and KAS value. The number in the leaf nodes represents the mean DPI assigned to each group.

Next, we study the actual distribution of organ quality, measured by the DPI value assigned to each patient type. We summarize the DPI distribution per group in Table 16.3. We also compare the distribution of organ types per patient group of the expected optimal allocation to that resulting from the HKF policy in Figure 16.6. The results are provided as side-by-side boxplots. In comparison, we find that the ranges of DPI values assigned to each group are smaller, implying that the match between donors and candidates is more accurate under the expected optimal policy. In other words, *the expected optimal allocation is more*

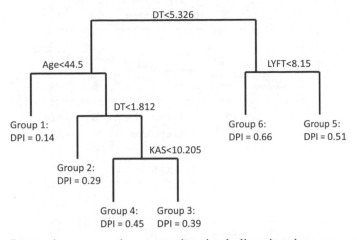

**Figure 16.5** Regression tree on the expected optimal allocation that maps organ types to recipients' health profiles and patient-donor matching information. Leaf nodes give mean DPI.

*efficient than the real-time HKF allocation* (for a discussion on the relationship between low kidney variance and patient choice consider Su and Zenios, 2005). We can backtrack to the efficiency insights of the expected optimal allocation to derive a knowledge-based real-time policy (KB): upon arrival of new organ $o_j$, with DPI value $dpi_j$, we consider patient groups $(g_k, k \in (1, 2, \ldots, 6))$ such that $dpi_j$ is to be within the [5%, 95%] percentile DPI range of these groups, according to Table 16.3. The organ is then allocated to the candidate with the highest KAS value within these groups. The policy is given in Algorithm 16.1.

Lastly, we compare the performance of the KB policy to that of PP and HKF on 10 different holdout sets. The results are summarized in Table 16.4. We find that KB significantly improves the performance of HKF and PP on three important planes: (1) decreased time to transplant, by an average of almost five months compared to HKF and two years compared to PP; (2) higher utility, by an average of almost five months compared to HKF and three years compared to PP; and (3) better match between graft expected lifetime and patient expected lifetime.

**Table 16.3**  Patient type and organ allocation.

| Group | Group properties | [5th, 50th, 95th] percentile DPI | Mean DPI |
|---|---|---|---|
| 1 | $DT < 5.326, Age < 44.5$ | [0.05, 0.14, 0.24] | 0.14 |
| 2 | $DT < 1.812, Age \geq 44.5$ | [0.18, 0.30, 0.44] | 0.29 |
| 3 | $DT \in [1.812, 5.326), Age \geq 44.5, KAS \geq 10.205$ | [0.24, 0.38, 0.51] | 0.39 |
| 4 | $DT \in [1.812, 5.326), Age \geq 44.5, KAS < 10.205$ | [0.31, 0.44, 0.55] | 0.45 |
| 5 | $DT \geq 5.326, LYFT \geq 8.15$ | [0.22, 0.54, 0.63] | 0.51 |
| 6 | $DT \geq 5.326, LYFT < 8.15$ | [0.53, 0.65, 0.81] | 0.66 |

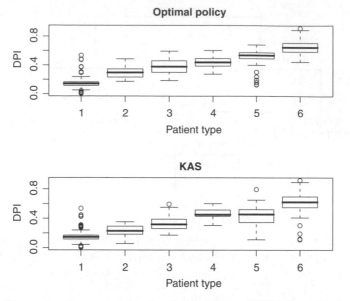

**Figure 16.6** Comparing the expected optimal allocation and HKF allocation in terms of DPI (smaller variance is better). The solid line represents the median DPI value, and the whiskers extend to the 5th and 95th percentiles.

## 16.6   Summary

In this work we discuss policies that allocate deceased donor kidneys to candidates with kidney failure. Following the OPTN report, we addressed the efficiency and equity in access to transplantation of the current allocation policy (Priority Points (PP)) and a new allocation policy, proposed by KARS in 2008 (Higher KAS First (HKF)). We then developed an alternative policy that is tailored to the properties of the kidney waiting list. Using a novel approach that combines data analytics and operations research methods, our allocation policy

**Table 16.4**   Real-time policies' performance (on holdout dataset).

| Metric | KB | HKF | PP |
| --- | --- | --- | --- |
| Age at time of offer | 46.89 (0.41) | 46.70 (0.42) | 46.16 (0.71) |
| Time to transplant (years) | 2.16 (0.05) | 2.57 (0.03) | 3.97 (0.06) |
| HLA mismatch | 4.29 (0.02) | 4.17 (0.02) | 2.61 (0.03) |
| Utility (LYFT) | 10.22 (0.06) | 9.80 (0.07) | 7.30 (0.08) |
| Correlation between graft expected lifetime and patient's expected lifetime | 0.68 (0.01) | 0.66 (0.01) | −0.29 (0.03) |
| Mean waiting time in waiting list | 2.85 (0.05) | 2.76 (0.04) | 2.45 (0.06) |
| Waiting list mortality | 15.92% (0.04) | 15.70% (0.05) | 16.05% (0.03) |

incorporates future prospect allocations into the decision making process, while accounting for dynamics in the queue, such as that of patients joining or leaving due to mortality.

**Algorithm 16.1 KB policy**

**On new organ $o_j$ arrival, with DPI value $= dpi_j$:**
$$G_j = \{g_k \mid dpi_j \in [5\%; 95\%] \text{ percentile DPI of group k}\}$$
$$P_j = \{p_i \in G_j\}$$
$$a = \{o_j \; ; p_i) \mid p_i \in G_j \text{ and } KAS_{ij} = \max_{pk \in Gj} \{KAS_{kj}\}.$$

Our work contributes to the kidney allocation field in both theoretical and applied aspects. In specific, we define a stochastic optimization problem that provides the best attainable allocation of organs to candidates in the OPTN waiting list, given a specific objective (e.g., expected KAS). The solution to the optimization problem serves as an upper bound to any real-time allocation policy that considers the same allocation objective. In addition, we use data mining tools to study this solution and mimic it in real time. In other words, we utilize the properties of the resulting allocation and derive a knowledge-based policy, which, combined with the HKF policy, yields a better allocation at both individual and social levels (compared to PP and HKF). As a by-product, we also numerically show the significant advantage of the proposed HKF policy over the existing PP system.

There are several directions for extending this work. First, in this work we focus on the planner problem, disregarding the patients' choice problem. However, literature shows that in practice about 45% of the offered kidneys are rejected by the first patient that receives them (or his/her physician). The rationale for such a decision is that once at the top of the list, it pays to wait for a better offer (Zenios, 2004; Su and Zenios, 2005). Patients' decisions might introduce inefficiencies into the system since transplants are delayed when patients reject offers. Understanding and modeling the patients' choice is hence a natural extension to our work.

Although we do not explicitly model patient choice, our analytical results show that, under the proposed policy, the types of kidneys offered to patients with the same health condition has a relatively small variation. Therefore, as suggested in Su and Zenios (2005), our proposed policy is expected to be robust to patient choice. The reason is that if a patient rejects an offer, she/he is most likely to receive a kidney of the same quality in the next offer.

Another possible extension of this work is evaluating recipients' lifespan and rejection rate after transplant. In this work, we show that our proposed method results in a better correlation between the lifetime of kidneys and patients, implying that the need for retransplantation decreases, as well as the rate of deaths with a functioning graft. On the other hand, we find that the actual tissue match (HLA match) degrades, compared to the other allocation policies, which may result in higher rejection rates.

On the methodological side, our stochastic optimization formulation can be extended to optimize the worst-case allocation rather than the expected performance (also referred to as minimax analysis or robust optimization). In the context of kidney allocation, the idea is to account for the uncertainty associated with the model estimation (such as mortality rate and organ quality) and to maximize the allocation outcome while minimizing the possible loss due to mortality. It is expected that worst-case optimization will yield a lower expected mortality rate compared to the current KB performance. To that end, the efficiency of the allocation is expected to increase. On the equity side, however, such a policy might give disproportionately high priority to the older population and to patients with more severe health conditions, leaving the less sick patients with low chance of receiving a transplant.

## Acknowledgement

This work was supported in part by Health Resources and Services Administration contract 234-2005-370011C. The content is the responsibility of the authors alone and does not necessarily reflect the views or policies of the Department of Health and Human Services, nor does mention of trade names, commercial products, or organizations imply endorsement by the US Government.

## References

Alagoz, O., Schaefer, A., and Roberts, M. (2009) Optimizing organ allocation and acceptance. In *Handbook of Optimization in Medicine* (eds P. Pardalos and E. Romeijn), Springer US, pp. 1–24.

David, I. and Yechiali, U. (1995) One-attribute sequential assignment match processes in discrete time. *Operations Research*, **43**(5), 879–884.

Derman, C., Lieberman, G., and Ross, S. (1972) A sequential stochastic assignment problem. *Management Science*, **18**(7), 349–355.

Edmonds, J. (1965) Paths, trees, and flowers. *Canadian Journal of Mathematics*, **17**(3), 449–467.

Eggers, P. (1995) Racial differences in access to kidney transplantation. *Health Care Financing Review*, **17**(2), 89–103.

Hines, R. and Marschall, K. (2008) *Stoelting's Anesthesia and Co-existing Disease*, 5th edn, Elsevier Health Sciences, New York.

Kruskal, W. and Wallis, W. (1952) Use of ranks in one-criterion variance analysis. *Journal of the American Statistical Association*, **47**(260), 583–621.

OPTN/UNOS (2008) Kidney Allocation Concepts: Request for Information. The OPTN/UNOS Kidney Transplantation Committee.

Righter, R. (1989) A resource allocation problem in a random environment. *Operations Research*, **37**(2), 329–338.

Su, X. and Zenios, S. (2004) Patient choice in kidney allocation: the role of the queueing discipline. *Manufacturing & Service Operations Management*, **6**(4), 280–301.

Su, X. and Zenios, S. (2005) Patient choice in kidney allocation: a sequential stochastic assignment model. *Operations Research*, **53**(3), 443–455.

Su, X. and Zenios, S. (2006) Recipient choice can address the efficiency-equity trade-off in kidney transplantation: a mechanism design model. *Management Science*, **52**(11), 1647–1660.

Votruba, M. (2001) Efficiency-equity tradeoffs in the allocation of cadaveric kidneys. Technical report, Working Paper, Princeton University.

Wolfe, R.A., McCullough, K.P., Schaubel, D.E. *et al.* (2008) Calculating life years from transplant (LYFT): methods for kidney and kidney-pancreas candidates. *American Journal of Transplantation*, **8**(4p2), 997–1011.

Yahav, I. (2010) A data analytical framework for improving real-time, decision support systems in healthcare. PhD thesis, Robert H. Smith School of Business, University of Maryland.

Zenios, S. (2004) Models for kidney allocation. In *Operations Research and Health Care: A Handbook of Methods and Applications* (eds M.L. Brandeau, F. Sainfort, and W.P. Pierskalla), Springer, pp. 537–554.

Zenios, S., Chertow, G., and Wein, L. (2000) Dynamic allocation of kidneys to candidates on the transplant waiting list. *Operations Research*, **48**(4), 549–569.

# 17

# Statistical issues in vaccine safety evaluation

## Patrick Musonda

*School of Medicine, Norwich Medical School, University of East Anglia, Norwich, UK.*
*Centre for Infectious Disease Research in Zambia (CIDRZ), Lusaka, Zambia*

## Synopsis

This chapter summarises some statistical issues in vaccine safety, in particular a detailed description of a popular method that is used in modelling adverse outcomes in vaccines, known as the self-controlled case series method, for which the author of this chapter spent three years developing and improving the method as part of his doctoral thesis (Musonda, 2006).

## 17.1 Background

The self-controlled case series method (SCCSM), or case series method for short, is a modified cohort method for estimating the relative incidence of specified events in a defined period after a point exposure. While the method was originally developed to investigate associations between vaccination and acute adverse events (Farrington, 1995; Farrington, Nash and Miller, 1996), it has subsequently been applied in other settings, for example in pharmacoepidemiology (Hubbard *et al.*, 2003; Hocine *et al.*, 2005). Becker, Li and Kelman (2004) have independently derived and applied the case series method in other areas of epidemiology. A step-by-step account of the theory, applications and modelling issues is given by Whitaker *et al.* (2006). The same paper by Whitaker *et al.* describes how the method

*Statistical Methods in Healthcare*, First Edition. Edited by Frederick W. Faltin, Ron S. Kenett and Fabrizio Ruggeri.
© 2012 John Wiley & Sons, Ltd. Published 2012 by John Wiley & Sons, Ltd.

can be implemented in various statistical software packages. The case series method in its semiparametric form (Farrington and Whitaker, 2006) can be applied to continuous exposures, but in this chapter we will consider point exposures only.

## 17.2    Motivation

The self-controlled case series model was developed in order to analyse vaccine-safety record-linkage data relating to measles, mumps and rubella (MMR) vaccination and aseptic meningitis (Farrington et al., 1995; Miller et al., 1993). For this study, episodes of aseptic meningitis arising in children aged 1–2 years over a defined calendar time period were obtained from laboratory and hospital records. The age and calendar time window determined by the period of event ascertainment defines an observation period for each child. From now onwards, the term 'case' refers to an individual who has experienced one or more events of interest over his or her observation period. Vaccination records were linked to cases, resulting in a combined data set that consisted of cases and their exposures. The difficulty with such data sets is that usually they do not comprise accurate denominators. Furthermore, it may not be wholly clear from which population the cases arise, and most likely the catchment areas of the hospitals from which the cases were obtained may not be clearly defined. Thus using methods such as cohort and case-control studies which are population-based methods would require ingenuity, especially since vaccine coverage in the population is unlikely to be uniform. If answers are required quickly about a possible association between an event of interest and the vaccine exposure, employing a cohort study may not be a good idea as it may take a long time, it would be very expensive to undertake and would require a large sample size. The self-controlled case series method was developed to deal with such difficulties. In the MMR and convulsions data set, a positive association between vaccination with the Urabe mumps strain and aseptic meningitis in the period 15–35 days post-vaccination was confirmed, and the composition of MMR vaccines used in the UK was changed (Farrington et al., 1995; Miller et al., 1993).

The self-controlled case series method is described in technical terms in the next section, but for other further details see Farrington (1995). Briefly, a retrospective Poisson cohort model is specified, and the case series model is derived from this by conditioning on the total number of events experienced by each individual in the observation period. A comparative evaluation of this method with case-control studies and cohort studies is demonstrated in the paper by Farrington, Nash and Miller (1996).

## 17.3    The self-controlled case series model

The self-controlled case series method is a conditional cohort method for estimating the relative incidence of specified events in a defined period after a point exposure. In this method, first an observation period is defined. Time within the observation period is classified as at risk or as control time in relation to point exposures that are regarded as fixed. We then condition on the number of events experienced by each individual over the observation period. The method allows valid inference about the relative incidence of events in risk periods relative to the control period, using data on cases only.

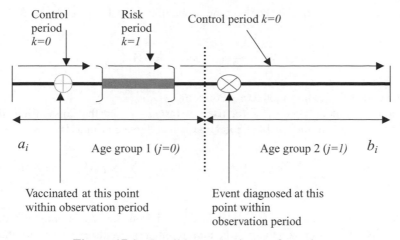

**Figure 17.1**   Possible case series configuration.

We now derive the general form of the likelihood of the self-controlled case series model. The pictorial configuration in Figure 17.1 will help to understand the general form of the likelihood described.

In Figure 17.1 we see a possible configuration in which an observation period $(a_i, b_i]$ is defined within which an individual $i$ was exposed (vaccinated) and a risk period (thick line) is defined shortly after the exposure. It is possible to have several risk periods depending on prior knowledge of which time intervals are important. For example Griffin *et al.* (1990) assumed that the effect of diphtheria, tetanus, pertussis (DTP) vaccine on febrile convulsions or encephalopathy had risk periods of 0–3, 4–7, 8–14, and 15–29 days after any dose of DTP. The observation period is further divided in age groups; in Figure 17.1 there are two age groups. As with risk periods, it is possible to define several age groups. The period outside the risk period is known as the control period. In Figure 17.1 it comprises of the period before vaccination, a period shortly after vaccination, and a period after the risk period. The event in this case was diagnosed some time after the risk period in age group 2, but could have occurred anywhere within the observation period. The observation period and the location of the risk period within it will generally vary between individuals.

In general, we assume that events arise within individuals as a non-homogeneous, age-dependent Poisson process. In what follows, a proportional incidence model is used to describe the relation between vaccination and the outcome of interest (Farrington, Nash and Miller, 1996).

Let individuals be indexed by $i = 1, 2, \ldots, N$, age groups be indexed by $j = 0, 1, \ldots, J - 1$ (0 denoting the reference age group) and the risk periods be indexed by $k = 0, 1, \ldots, K - 1$ (0 denoting the control period).

Further suppose we let the symbols $\lambda_{ijk}$, $e_{ijk}$, $n_{ijk}$ respectively denote incidence, length of time at risk, and number of events experienced by an individual $i$, in age group $j$ and risk period $k$ during the observation period $(a_i, b_i]$. The log-linear model $ln(\lambda_{ijk}) = \phi_i + \alpha_j + \beta_k$ is used to parameterise the incidence of an event for an individual effect $\phi_i$, age effect $\alpha_j$, and exposure effect $\beta_k$ (with $\alpha_0 = \beta_0 = 0$) . Thus the incidence function during the baseline period is simply $\lambda_{i00} = \exp(\phi_i)$. The Poisson probability model is given by:

$$\Pr[r] = \frac{e^{-\lambda} \times \lambda^r}{r!} \text{ where } r = 0, 1, 2, \ldots$$

and for the underlying cohort model, $n_{ijk}$ Poisson($\lambda_{ijk} \times e_{ijk}$).

For the cohort model, $\phi_i = x_i^T \gamma$ for fixed covariates $x_i$, and the Poisson log-likelihood kernel (which is equal to the log-likelihood up to an additive constant) is

$$\ell_{co}(\alpha, \beta, \gamma) = \sum_i \sum_{jk} n_{ijk}(x_i^T \gamma + \alpha_j + \beta_k) - \sum_i \sum_{jk} \exp(x_i^T \gamma + \alpha_j + \beta_k)e_{ijk}.$$

The self-controlled case series model is derived from the cohort model with the $\phi_i$ unrestricted by conditioning on the $n_{i..}$ (the total number of events experienced), thus giving a product multinomial distribution as described by McCullagh and Nelder (1989). So the log-likelihood kernel for the self-controlled case series model is

$$\ell(\alpha, \beta) = \sum_i \sum_{jk} n_{ijk} \log \left( \frac{\exp(\alpha_j + \beta_k)e_{ijk}}{\sum_{rs} \exp(\alpha_r + \beta_s)e_{irs}} \right).$$

We can see from above that the individual effects $\phi_i = x_i^T \gamma$ cancel out. This is because incidence rates are contrasted within the same individual's person-time; so that, in this sense, the method is self-controlled. Thus, provided the model is correct, inferences from a case series analysis cannot be confounded by fixed multiplicative individual effects, which might include genetic factors, location, socio-economic status, sex, underlying health status, individual frailty, and so on (Whitaker et al., 2006). Individual effects can nonetheless modify the exposure effect, but this can be modelled by including suitable interaction terms. Note that self-control applies to fixed covariates only and not age or time-dependent covariates.

In much of what follows we shall only need the log-likelihood in the following simplified situation. We suppose that there are no age effects, and that all individuals are observed over the same observation period, comprising two adjacent periods of duration $e_1$ (the risk period) and $e_0$ (the control period). Suppose that all individuals are vaccinated at the start of period $e_1$ and subsequently at increased risk during this period. Suppose that in a sample of $n$ events, $n_0$ occur in period $e_0$ and $n_1$ in period $e_1$ with $n = n_0 + n_1$. Let the ratio of the risk period to the observation period be $r$; that is,

$$r = \frac{e_1}{e_0 + e_1}.$$

Usually the risk period and the observation period will be specified in advance. However, only their ratio $r$ is required. Let $\rho$ be the relative incidence $e^\beta$ (so that $\beta = \log(\rho)$).

In this simple situation the log-likelihood kernel is equal to:

$$\ell(\beta) = n_1 \beta - n \log(e_1 e^\beta + e_0).$$

Note that this is the same log-likelihood kernel as for the binomial model

$$n_1 : B\,(n, p)$$

with

$$p = \frac{e^\beta e_1}{e^\beta e_1 + e_0}.$$

The maximum likelihood estimator $\hat{\beta}$ of $\beta$ is obtained by setting $\dfrac{\partial \ell}{\partial \beta} = 0$; that is,

$$\frac{\partial \ell}{\partial \beta} = n_1 - n\frac{e_1 e^\beta}{e_1 e^\beta + e_0} = 0,$$

giving

$$\hat{\beta} = \log\left(\frac{n_1/e_1}{n_0/e_0}\right) \quad \text{and} \quad \hat{\rho} = e^{\hat{\beta}} = \frac{n_1/e_1}{n_0/e_0}.$$

The likelihood ratio statistic for the test of $H_0 : \beta = 0$ for this simplified situation is then

$$D = 2[\ell(\hat{\beta}) - \ell(0)] = 2[n_1\hat{\beta} - n\{\log(e_1 e^{\hat{\beta}} + e_0) - \log(e_1 + e_0)\}],$$

where $\hat{\beta}$ is the maximum likelihood estimator.

## 17.4   Advantages and limitations

The following are the main advantages of the self-controlled case series method. The method uses cases only, and provides consistent estimates (as the number of cases becomes large) of the relative incidence. It controls implicitly for all fixed multiplicative confounders, that is, confounders that act multiplicatively on the baseline rates and do not vary (or do not vary much) with time over the observation period, such as variables relating to genetics, location, socio-economic status, gender, individual frailty, severity of underlying disease, and so on. Age or temporal variation in the baseline incidence is controlled for in the model. Further, under certain circumstances, the method has high efficiency relative to the retrospective cohort method from which it is derived by conditioning (Farrington, 1995). Assembling the required data is much more likely to be easier in the self-controlled case series method than cohort or case-control studies.

Like any other method, the self-controlled case series method has limitations, which we now give. The most restrictive limitation is that the method requires that the probability of exposure is not affected by the prior occurrence of an outcome; sometimes this condition may not be fulfilled. For non-recurrent events, the method works only when the event risk is small over the observation period. The method does not produce estimates of absolute incidence, only estimates of relative incidence. A further assumption is that the observation period is independent of the timing of events. A less severe limitation of the method is that it requires variability in the time or age of the event: if all events were to happen at exactly the same age, which is very unlikely but not impossible, then the method would fail.

## 17.5   Why use the self-controlled case series method

Investigations of suspected or hypothesised associations of adverse outcomes with transient exposures, such as vaccination, usually require epidemiological studies such as cohort studies and case-control studies. A disadvantage of a cohort study is that for rare events it has to be very large to achieve sufficient power. This may not be practical and can be very expensive. Sometimes researchers have got round this problem by reconstructing large retrospective cohorts (Ray and Griffin, 1989) using data sets assembled for other purposes. Case-control studies require smaller sample sizes. The main disadvantages with case-control studies are that they are more prone to selection bias, recall bias and ascertainment bias (Altman, 1991). Confounding by variables related both to avoidance of vaccination and to the outcome of interest is a major problem for both cohort and case-control studies, as noted by Farrington, Nash and Miller (1996). For example Fine and Chen (1992) found that parental education, ethnic group, age of the mother, maternal smoking, birth weight, evolving neurological disorders and conditions predisposing to seizures are related to both vaccination and to sudden infant death syndrome or encephalopathy and hence may be confounding factors. Both the cohort method and case-control method are data intensive, involving large cohorts or careful selection and matching of controls (Smeeth, Donnan and Cook, 2006). The self-controlled case series method aspires to control for fixed confounders by using cases only. This helps to reduce the data collection effort, and concentrates it on the cases.

Observations of clustering or troughs of events shortly after exposure lead to speculation about associations with exposure. There are several methodological difficulties involved in carrying out epidemiological studies to monitor such associations. Such studies are prone to many biases; for example, Fine and Chen (1992) found that there is often differential ascertainment of cases in recently vaccinated and unvaccinated individuals, and differential vaccination rates in individuals at higher or lower risk. Both would lead to bias in cohort and case-control studies; whereas case series studies may escape bias from the latter. The cohort method is based on comparisons of incidence rates for person-time aggregated both across and within individuals. But the self-controlled case series method removes the contribution of comparisons between individuals, focussing attention on event rates in different periods within each individual's observation time (Farrington, Nash and Miller, 1996). For this reason, individuals who experience no events contribute no information about the association between vaccination and outcome. Such individuals can be ignored without introducing any bias. On the other hand individuals who experience one or more events do contribute information on the risk period and age group in which the events occurred. The self-controlled case series method thus combines aspects of the case-control and cohort methods, using retrospectively ascertained vaccination histories in cases to estimate the relative incidence in different intervals after vaccination relative to a control period.

## 17.6   Other case-only methods

Looking at only cases to detect risk factors for diseases is not new. Various studies have been conducted in which only cases are used; for example, a Markov chain method using only cases was used by Aalen et al. (1980), and a similar method modified as survival analysis was used by Prentice, Vollmer and Kalbfleisch (1984). However, it has been argued (Farrington, 1995; Farrington and Whitaker, 2006) that the methods of Aalen et al. and Prentice et al.

give a valid test for no association but do not yield readily interpretable effect estimates. Another use of cases only can be seen in the case-crossover model developed by Maclure (1991). Maclure's method resembles a case-control method with referents selected from the case's own history. It has been argued (Vines and Farrington, 2001) that although the case-crossover method is self-matched, it only yields consistent estimates when the distribution of exposure in case and control time intervals is exchangeable, in particular implying stationarity of exposures. There are several variants of this method reviewed by Greenland (1996), and the case-crossover approach has been used in many settings (Maclure and Mittleman, 2000). Another method in which only cases are used is that of Feldmann (1993). In this method, a constant baseline incidence is assumed. Feldmann's method does give consistent estimates, though it is only approximately self-matched for rare events. The earlier approaches of using only cases have characteristics which the self-controlled case series method incorporates; in particular, it coincides with Feldmann's method when the disease is rare and the baseline incidence is constant. The self-controlled case series method is similar to Prentice's in that it also controls for age; it is similar to Maclure's in that it also controls for fixed confounders. The main difference between the case series method and the method of Maclure is that it is derived from the same statistical model as a cohort study design, and hence can handle non-exchangeable exposures and, in particular, controls for age effects. Furthermore in this method one does not need to specify the prior probabilities for exposure as required in some other case-crossover designs (Marshall and Jackson, 1993). Smeeth, Donnan and Cook (2006) describe the advantages and disadvantages of case-control and case-only study designs.

## 17.7   Where the self-controlled case series method has been used

This method has been used in various situations, but the main area it has been used is in modelling adverse events in vaccine studies. Table 17.1 was adapted from Whitaker *et al.* (2006), which documents published applications of the case series method. A review of applications to vaccine safety is given by Andrews (2002) and also by Farrington (2004). Independently, Navidi (1998) proposed what is essentially a case series method, with time-varying exposures, for application in studies of air pollution. This method is described as a bi-directional or ambidirectional case-crossover method. The case series version of this method is that in which the entire observation period is used as control. A similar approach has also been discussed by Lumley and Levy (2000). Farrington and Whitaker (2006) describe a generalisation of this approach, in which residual seasonality is controlled. Further, Farrington, Whitaker and Hocine (2007) describe a number of developments in modelling adverse outcomes that could be associated with vaccines.

A comparative evaluation of the self-controlled case series method has been undertaken by Farrington *et al.* (Farrington, Nash and Miller, 1996; Farrington, Whitaker and Hocine, 2007) and also by Glanz *et al.* (2006). In Farrington, Nash and Miller's (1996) comparisons, estimates of the relative incidence of febrile convulsions associated with MMR vaccine were obtained using the case series method, the case-control method and the cohort method. Theoretical arguments about the efficiency of the self-controlled case series method were presented. Overall the findings were that the self-controlled case series method produced results similar to the cohort method; whereas the 1–1 matched case-control estimates had

**Table 17.1**  Studies using the case series method.

| Exposure | Outcome | Reference |
|---|---|---|
| DTP vaccine | Febrile convulsion | Farrington *et al.*, 1995 |
| MMR vaccine | Febrile convulsion | Farrington *et al.*, 1995 |
| MMR vaccine | Idiopathic thrombocytopenic purpura | Farrington *et al.*, 1995; Miller *et al.*, 2001 |
| MMR vaccine | Aseptic meningitis | Farrington *et al.*, 1995; Dourado *et al.*, 2000 |
| MMR vaccine | Autism | Taylar *et al.*, 1999; Farrington, Miller and Taylor, 2001 |
| MMR vaccine | Invasive bacterial infection | Miller *et al.*, 2003 |
| MMR vaccine | Gait disturbance | Miller *et al.*, 2005 |
| Influenza vaccine | Asthma | Kramarz *et al.*, 2000; Tata *et al.*, 2003 |
| Influenza vaccine | Bell's palsy | Mutsch *et al.*, 2004 |
| Oral polio vaccine | Intussusception | Andrews *et al.*, 2001; Galindo *et al.*, 2001 |
| Oral rotavirus vaccine | Intussusception | Murphy *et al.*, 2001 |
| DTP, MMR, HBV, HIB, OPV vaccine | Wheezing | Mullooly *et al.*, 2002 |
| Antidepressants | Hip fracture | Hubbard *et al.*, 2003 |
| Antidepressants | Myocardial infarction | Tata *et al.*, 2005 |
| Long-haul air travel | Venous thromboembolism | Becker, Li and Kelman, 2004 |
| Influenza vaccine | Any medical visits | France *et al.*, 2004 |
| Common vaccines and infections | Myocardial infarction and stroke | Smeeth *et al.*, 2004 |

DTP = diphtheria, tetanus, pertussis; MMR = measles, mumps, rubella; HBV = hepatitis B vaccine; HIB = *Haemophilus influenzae* type B; OPV = oral polio vaccine.

wider confidence intervals, reflecting the lower power of the method for a given number of cases. In conclusion Farrington, Nash and Miller (1996) noted that the cohort study remains the 'ideal' design for the study of adverse reaction to vaccines, and should be used whenever feasible. However, for studies of rare adverse events or for routine surveillance purposes, large-scale cohort studies may be costly, impractical or prone to confounding. In such circumstances, the case series method provides a powerful and practical alternative to cohort and case-control studies.

## 17.8    Other issues that were explored in improving the SCCM

The self-controlled case series method is relatively new, and some statisticians and epidemiologists are naturally sceptical. This scepticism is a barrier to its use, in spite of its benefits, such as good power, reduced confounding and practicability. Testing-out and extension of the method was required to contribute to a better understanding of the method amongst the epidemiological community as a whole, including the pharmaceutical industry. The PhD thesis by Musonda (2006) explored the following issues.

- Further statistical properties of the method.

- Evaluation of its small-sample performance (Musonda *et al.*, 2008a).

- Improvement in the design of self-controlled case series studies by obtaining and validating sample size formulae (Musonda, Farrington and Whitaker, 2006).

- Extending the method's application to prospective surveillance (Hocine *et al.*, 2009; Musonda *et al.*, 2008b).

The case series method involves fitting a particular log-linear model using maximum likelihood. Thus, the asymptotic performance of the method is guaranteed by statistical theory. Expressions for the asymptotic bias, variance and the asymptotic mean square error of the estimate of relative incidence were derived. A graphical study of the bias, variance and asymptotic mean square error were given. Extensive simulations to study the validity of asymptotic results in finite samples under different situations were given. Results from the simulations were given, starting with what was called the standard scenario with varying number of cases and a range of true relative incidences. Further different risk periods, the effect of age, and different distributions of age at exposure were explored. Indefinite risk periods and the presence of unexposed cases were explored, and the effects of age, using several contrasting scenarios.

The estimation of sample sizes for case series studies was explored. Hitherto, there had been little work done on the design of self-controlled case series studies. Sample size formulae were developed and validated using simulations (Musonda, Farrington and Whitaker, 2006). The impacts of age effects on power and sample size were studied. An earlier published sample-size formula (Farrington, Nash and Miller, 1996) was validated. It was found that this formula is not accurate; hence, we investigated several alternative approaches. An extension of one successful approach of the sample size formula to take account of the effect of age (Musonda, Farrington and Whitaker, 2006) was derived.

Application of the self-controlled case series method in a prospective surveillance context was looked into. The issue of interest was how to apply the self-controlled case series method, which is a retrospective method, in a prospective way so that possible adverse outcomes with a new vaccine (or several vaccines in routine use) can be detected early so that remedial action can be taken. This constitutes a new application of the case series method. Following the Wald (1947) and Page (1954) method, we used the sequential probability ratio test (SPRT) and cumulative sum (CUSUM) based on the self-controlled case series method so as to apply the self-controlled case series method in a prospective situation. These approaches, along with extensive simulations to demonstrate their performance under different situations, were presented and published; see Hocine *et al.* (2009) and Musonda *et al.* (2008b). Sequential techniques are widely used to detect adverse outcomes using various approaches including Bayesian methods (Bate *et al.*, 1998).

Data on oral polio vaccine and intussusception, provided to us by GlaxoSmithKline Biologicals (Belgium) was analysed. This study was undertaken in preparation for field trials of a new oral rotavirus vaccine. These data required some ingenuity in how one applied the self-controlled case series method owing to censoring of exposure histories. A description of how to analyse such data was given. We went on to discuss how the findings of the thesis threw light on the results, and how they may inform the design of future studies and surveillance programmes based on the case series method.

## 17.9    Summary of the chapter

Overall, this chapter explores statistical issues in vaccine safety, in particular the self-controlled case series method. Largely, this has taken a descriptive form of this method. The interested reader can find thorough details in Musonda's thesis (2006) and in various references given in the thesis.

In conclusion, in terms of modelling adverse outcomes that may be associated with the exposure of vaccines, the author recommends use of the self-controlled case series method that is quicker to implement as compared to the cohort study, which may take a long time and be expensive. The case-control study has well-known problems of selection bias, recall bias and, in comparison to the self-controlled case series method, the estimates are not efficient.

## References

Aalen, O.O., Borgan, O., Keiding, N. and Thorman, J. (1980) Interaction between life history events: nonparametric analysis for prospective and retrospective data in the presence of censoring. *Scandinavian Journal of Statistics*, **7**, 161–171.

Altman, D.G. (1991) *Practical Statistics for Medical Research*, Chapman & Hall, London, pp. 93–94.

Andrews, N., Miller, E., Waight, P. *et al.* (2001) Does oral polio vaccine cause intussusception in infants? Evidence from a sequence of three self-controlled case series studies in the United Kingdom. *European Journal of Epidemiology*, **17**, 701–706.

Andrews, N.J. (2002) Statistical assessment of the association between vaccination and rare adverse events post licensure. *Vaccine*, **20**, S49–S53.

Bate, A., Linddquist, M., Edwards, I.R. *et al.* (1998) A Bayesian neural network method for adverse drug reaction signal generation. *European Journal of Clinical Pharmacology*, **54**, 315–321.

Becker, N.G., Li, Z. and Kelman, C.W. (2004) The effect of transient exposures on the risk of an acute illness with low hazard rate. *Biostastics*, **5**, 239–248.

Dourado, I., Cunha, S., Teixeira, M.D.G. *et al.* (2000) An outbreak of aseptic meningitis associated with a Urabe-containing MMR mass vaccination campaign: implications for immunisation programs. *American Journal of Epidemiology*, **151**, 524–530.

Farrington, C.P. (1995) Relative incidence estimation from case series for vaccine evaluation. *Biometrics*, **51**, 228–235.

Farrington, C.P. (2004) Control without separate controls: evaluation of vaccine safety using case-only methods. *Vaccine*, **22**, 2064–2070.

Farrington, C.P. and Whitaker, H.J. (2006) Semiparametric analysis of case series data. *Applied Statistics*, **55**(Part 5), 553–594.

Farrington, C.P., Nash, J. and Miller, E. (1996) Case series analysis of adverse reactions to vaccines: a comparative evaluation. *American Journal of Epidemiology*, **143**, 1165–1173; erratum **147**, 93 (1998).

Farrington, C.P., Miller, E. and Taylor, B. (2001) MMR and autism: further evidence against a causal association. *Vaccine*, **19**, 3632–3635.

Farrington, C.P., Pugh, S., Colville, A. *et al.* (1995) A new method for active surveillance of adverse events from diphtheria/tetanus/pertussis and measles/mumps/rubella vaccines. *Lancet*, **345**, 567–5699.

Farrington, C.P., Whitaker, H.J. and Hocine, M.N. (2007) Statistical issues in vaccine safety evaluation, in *Encyclopaedia of Statistics in Quality and Reliability* (eds F. Ruggeri, R.S. Kenett and F. Faltin), John Wiley & Sons, Ltd, Chichester, Example 3, pp. 2–3.

Feldmann, U. (1993) Epidemiologic assessment of risks of adverse reactions associated with intermittent exposure. *Biometrics*, **49**, 419–428.

Fine, P.E. and Chen, R.T. (1992) Confounding in studies of adverse reactions to vaccines. *American Journal of Epidemiology*, **136**, 121–135.

France, E.K., Glanz, J.M., Xu, S. *et al.* (2004) Safety of the trivalent inactivated influenza vaccine among children – a population based study. *Archives of Pediatrics and Adolescent Medicine*, **158**, 1031–1036.

Galindo Sardiñas, M.A., Zambrano Cárdenas, A., Coutin Marie, G. *et al.* (2001) Lack of association between intussusception among infants given an oral polio vaccine in Cuban children. *European Journal of Epidemiology*, **17**, 783–787.

Glanz, J.M., McClure, D.L., Xu, S. *et al.* (2006) Four different study designs to evaluate vaccine safety were equally validated with contrasting limitations. *Journal of Clinical Epidemiology*, **59**, 808–818.

Greenland, S. (1996) A unified approach to the analysis of case-distribution (case-only) studies. *Statistics in Medicine*, **18**, 1–15.

Griffin, M.R., Ray, W.A., Livengood, J.R. *et al.* (1990) Risk of seizures and encephalopathy after immunization with the Diphtheria Tetanus-Pertussis vaccine. *JAMA*, **263**, 1641–1645.

Hocine, M., Guillemot, D., Tubert-Bitter, P. and Moreau, T. (2005) Testing independence between two Poisson-generated multinomial variables in case series and cohort studies. *Statistics in Medicine*, **24**, 4035–4044.

Hocine, M.N., Musonda, P., Andrews, N.J. and Farrington, C.P. (2009) Sequential case series for pharmacovigilance. *Journal of the Royal Statistical Society Series A*, **172**, 213–236.

Hubbard, R., Farrington, C.P., Smith, C. *et al.* (2003) Exposure to tricyclic and selective serotonin inhibitor antidepressants and the risk of hip fracture. *American Journal of Epidemiology*, **158**, 77–84.

Kramarz, P., DeStefano, F., Gargiullo, P.M. *et al.* (2000) Does influenza vaccination exacerbate asthma? Analysis of a large cohort of children with asthma. *Archives of Family Medicine*, **9**, 617–623.

Lumley, T. and Levy, D. (2000) Bias in the case-crossover design: implications for studies of air pollution. *Environmetrics*, **11**, 689–704.

Maclure, M. (1991) The case-crossover design: a method for studying transient effects on the risk of acute events. *American Journal of Epidemiology*, **133**, 144–153.

Maclure, M. and Mittleman, M.A. (2000) Should we use a case-cross-over design? *Annual Review of Public Health*, **21**, 193–221.

Marshall, R.J. and Jackson, R.T. (1993) Analysis of case-crossover designs. *Statistics in Medicine*, **12**, 2333–2341.

McCullagh, P. and Nelder, J.A. (1989) *Generalized Linear Models*, 2nd edn, Chapman & Hall/CRC, p. 209.

Miller, E., Andrews, N., Waight, P. and Taylor, B. (2003) Bacterial infections, immune overload, and MMR vaccine. *Archives of Diseases in Childhood*, **88**, 222–223.

Miller, E., Andrews, N., Grant, A. *et al.* (2005) No evidence of an association between MMR vaccine and gait disturbance. *Archives of Diseases in Childhood*, **90**, 292–296.

Miller, E., Goldacre, M., Pugh, S. *et al.* (1993) Risk of aseptic meningitis after measles, mumps and rubella vaccine in UK children. *Lancet*, **341**, 979–982.

Miller, E., Waight, P., Stowe, J. and Taylar, B. (2001) Idiopathic thrombocytopenic purpura and MMR vaccine. *Archives of Diseases in Childhood*, **84**, 227–229.

Mullooly, J.P., Pearson, J., Drew, L. *et al.* (2002) Wheezing lower respiratory disease and vaccination of full-term infants. *Pharmacoepidemiology and Drug Safety*, **11**, 21–30.

Murphy, T.V., Garguillo, P.M., Massoudi, M.S. *et al.* (2001) Intussusception among infants given an oral rotavirus vaccine. *New England Journal of Medicine*, **344**, 564–572.

Musonda, P. (2006) The self-controlled case series method: performance and design in studies of vaccine safety. PhD thesis, The Open University.

Musonda, P., Farrington, C.P. and Whitaker, H.J. (2006) Sample sizes for self-controlled case series studies. *Statistics in Medicine*, **25**(15), 2618–2631.

Musonda, P., Hocine, M.N., Andrews, N.J. and Farrington, C.P. (2008b) Monitoring vaccine safety using case series CUSUM charts. *Vaccine*, **26**(42), 5358–5367.

Musonda, P., Hocine, M.N., Whitaker, H.J. and Farrington, C.P. (2008a) Self-controlled case series analyses: small sample performance. *Computational Statistics and Data Analysis*, **52**(4), 1942–1957.

Mutsch, M., Zhou, W., Rhodes, P. *et al.* (2004) Use of the inactivated intranasal influenza vaccine and the risk of Bell's palsy in Switzerland. *New England Journal of Medicine*, **350**, 896–903.

Navidi, W. (1998) Bidirectional case-cross-over designs for exposures with time trends. *Biometrics*, **54**(2), 596–605.

Page, E.S. (1954) Continuous inspection schemes. *Biometrika*, **41**, 100–115.

Prentice, R.L., Vollmer, W.M. and Kalbfleisch, J.D. (1984) On the use of case series to identify disease risk factors. *Biometrics*, **40**, 445–458.

Ray, W.A. and Griffin, M.R. (1989) Use of Medicaid data for pharmaco-epidemiology. *American Journal of Epidemiology*, **129**, 837–849.

Smeeth, L., Donnan, P.T. and Cook, D.G. (2006) The use of primary care databases: case-control and case-only designs. *Family Practice*, **23**, 597–604.

Smeeth, L., Thomas, S.L., Hall, A.J. *et al.* (2004) Risk of myocardial infarction and stroke after acute infection or vaccination. *New England Journal of Medicine*, **351**, 2611–2618.

Tata, L.J., West, J., Harrison, T. *et al.* (2003) Does influenza vaccination increase consultations, corticosteroid prescriptions or exacerbations in people with asthma or chronic obstructive pulmonary disease? *Thorax*, **58**, 835–839.

Tata, L.J., West, J., Smith, C. *et al.* (2005) General population based study of the impact of tricyclic and selective serotonin reuptake inhibitor antidepressants on the risk of acute myocardial infarction. *Heart*, **91**, 465–471.

Taylor, B., Miller, E., Farrington, C.P. *et al.* (1999) Autism and measles, mumps and rubella vaccine: no epidemiological evidence for a causal association. *Lancet*, **353**, 2026–2029.

Vines, S.K. and Farrington, C.P. (2001) Within-subject exposure dependency in case-crossover studies. *Statistics in Medicine*, **20**, 3039–3049.

Wald, A. (1947) *Sequential Analysis*, John Wiley & Sons, Inc., New York.

Whitaker, H.J., Farrington, C.P., Spiessens, B. and Musonda, P. (2006) Tutorial in biostatistics: the self-controlled case series method. *Statistics in Medicine*, **25**, 1768–1797.

# 18

# Statistical methods for healthcare economic evaluation

## Caterina Conigliani[1], Andrea Manca[2] and Andrea Tancredi[3]

[1]*Department of Economics, University of Roma Tre, Rome, Italy*
[2]*Centre for Health Economics, The University of York, York, UK*
[3]*Department of Methods and Models for Economics, Territory and Finance,
University of Rome 'La Sapienza', Rome, Italy*

## Synopsis

The increasing burden on the financial budgets of healthcare providers worldwide has emphasised the need to use healthcare resources as efficiently as possible. Healthcare economic evaluation has gained popularity in the last 20 years as a key tool to generate the information required by policy makers to achieve their goal. This chapter describes the statistical issues associated with the conduct of healthcare economic evaluation studies, considering both the analysis based on a single trial and the use of Bayesian comprehensive decision analytic models. Further issues such as the role of probabilistic sensitivity analysis and Bayesian evidence synthesis are also presented.

## 18.1   Introduction

Healthcare systems worldwide are under increasing financial pressure and, consequently, they need to use limited healthcare resources as efficiently as possible. This means (among other things) to invest in healthcare treatments that provide value for money. Healthcare economic evaluation (a particular form of which is known as *cost-effectiveness analysis*) is the vehicle through which evidence to inform the above decision can be produced. In fact, many countries

---

*Statistical Methods in Healthcare*, First Edition. Edited by Frederick W. Faltin, Ron S. Kenett and Fabrizio Ruggeri.
© 2012 John Wiley & Sons, Ltd. Published 2012 by John Wiley & Sons, Ltd.

have set up agencies whose role is to make recommendations as to which health technologies should be used.

Healthcare economic evaluation has been traditionally carried out using data collected alongside randomised controlled clinical trials (RCTs). Willan and Briggs (2006) focus on the role and methods of statistical inference in economic evaluation with data originating from RCTs. However, an increasingly important approach is to use the RCT data to develop an economic evaluation model to overcome some of the limitations of standard trial-based cost-effectiveness analysis (CEA) when this is used to inform funding decisions (Sculpher, Claxton and Drummond, 2006). This view is supported by the notion that single trials are often not the most appropriate vehicle to inform decision-making. Economic analyses based on single RCTs may in fact (1) be short in duration, (2) not be relevant to the jurisdiction of interest, (3) have not compared all the healthcare treatment strategies relevant to the decision-maker context, and (4) ignore the presence of other relevant evidence. In these cases it is more appropriate to use economic evaluation models to help address the above issues.

This chapter describes the statistical issues associated with healthcare economic evaluation, starting from a single trial-based analysis in Section 18.3, and moving on to the use of Bayesian comprehensive decision analytic models in Section 18.4. The standard tools for cost-effectiveness analysis are presented in Section 18.2, while the final section deals with further issues such as the role of probabilistic sensitivity analysis and Bayesian evidence synthesis.

# 18.2    Statistical analysis of cost-effectiveness

Health economic evaluation has been defined as 'the comparison of two or more alternative courses of action in terms of both their costs and consequences' (Drummond et al., 1997). Suppose, in particular, one needs to compare two treatments $T_1$ and $T_2$ in a set of new and existing technologies. Also suppose that under each treatment $T_j$ the population mean cost is $\gamma_j$ and the population mean efficacy is $\mu_j$ ($j = 1, 2$). Note that $\mu_j$ and $\gamma_j$ are computed over all patients with a given illness or condition that could be given treatment $T_j$, that is, over a finite population of patients, and in practical applications they are unknown and need to be estimated; this problem will be considered in detail in Section 18.3 and Section 18.4.

The key quantities in CEA are the mean health effect differential $\Delta_e = \mu_2 - \mu_1$ and the mean cost differential $\Delta_c = \gamma_2 - \gamma_1$. These outcomes are usually expressed using different *numeraire*, that is, monetary units for costs, and typically health outcomes – such as life-years gained or quality-adjusted life years (QALYs) – for the health effects.

## 18.2.1    Incremental cost-effectiveness plane, incremental cost-effectiveness ratio and incremental net benefit

A natural setting for presenting and comparing cost differentials and effect differentials is the incremental cost-effectiveness plane (see Black, 1999; O'Hagan, Stevens and Montmartin, 2000) shown in Figure 18.1; that is, the plane of possible pairs of values $(\Delta_e, \Delta_c)$ of the underlying true mean incremental effects and costs. In quadrant II, treatment $T_2$ is less effective and more expensive than treatment $T_1$, so it is unconditionally less acceptable; that

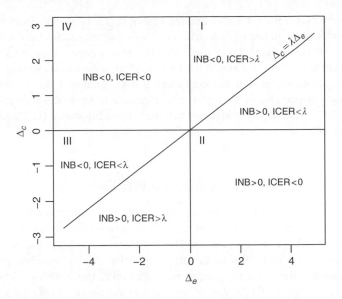

**Figure 18.1**  The incremental cost-effectiveness plane.

is, $T_1$ dominates $T_2$. Similarly, in quadrant IV, $T_2$ is both more effective and cheaper than $T_1$, and is therefore unconditionally preferred; that is, $T_2$ dominates $T_1$. In contrast, the comparison of the two treatments in quadrants I and III depends on the decision-maker's threshold value for a unit of effectiveness, which can be represented by a line of slope $\lambda$. That is, the quantity $\lambda$ represents the decision-maker's maximum willingness to pay to obtain one additional unit of effectiveness.

Notice that once we have a threshold value, the decision rule concerning what can be considered cost-effective is straightforward. Now, in quadrant I $T_2$ is both more effective and more costly than $T_1$, but below the line of slope $\lambda$ there is a sufficiently high increment in efficacy (relative to the increment in cost) for $T_2$ to be preferred. Analogously, in quadrant III $T_2$ is both less effective and cheaper than $T_1$, but below the line of slope $\lambda$ the reduction in cost is sufficiently high (relative to the reduction in efficacy) for $T_2$ to be preferred. It follows that the region of acceptability of treatment $T_2$ relative to $T_1$ is the portion of the plane below the line of slope $\lambda$.

Note that the region of acceptability of $T_2$ can be expressed in terms of what it is often considered to be the primary measure of the cost-effectiveness of a treatment, that is, the mean *incremental net benefit* (INB):

$$b_\lambda = \lambda \Delta_e - \Delta_c$$

(Stinnett and Mulahy, 1998), or in terms of the *incremental cost-effectiveness ratio* (ICER):

$$\rho = \Delta_c / \Delta_e.$$

However, while the definition in terms of the INB is quite straightforward, in that the region of acceptability simply equates to the INB being greater than zero, in terms of the

ICER it is necessary to consider both $\rho$ and the sign of $\Delta_e$ (as is obvious from Figure 18.1), so that $T_2$ is cost-effective relative to $T_1$ if, when $\Delta_e > 0$, $\rho < \lambda$ (i.e. if what the decision-maker is willing to pay for the achieved additional effectiveness is greater than the actual additional cost) or if , when $\Delta_e < 0$, $\rho > \lambda$ (i.e. if the loss in effectiveness is associated with negligible savings). Because of this, and due to the challenges associated with the statistical analysis of a ratio parameter (especially in the frequentist approach to statistical inference), basing the CEA on the INB is generally considered much more straightforward (O'Hagan, Stevens and Montmartin, 2000).

## 18.2.2    The cost-effectiveness acceptability curve

Notice that, since $\lambda$ is rarely unambiguously determined in practice, inference about the mean INB is generally presented by means of a *cost-effectiveness acceptability curve* (CEAC). This was introduced by van Hout, Al and Gordon (1994), and plots the probability that $T_2$ is cost-effective relative to $T_1$, that is, the probability that the net benefit is positive, against a range of possible values that the coefficient $\lambda$ can take. Equivalently, as pointed out for instance in Baio (2010), the CEAC can be seen as representing the area of the right tail of the distribution of the mean INB for a given value of $\lambda$.

It is interesting to note that, although the work of van Hout, Al and Gordon (1994) was apparently intended for a frequentist analysis of cost-effectiveness, the probability that the net benefit is positive does not exist nor have any meaning in the frequentist approach to statistical inference. In fact, as pointed out for instance in O'Hagan, Stevens and Montmartin (2000), in frequentist statistics unknown parameters are not random variables and do not have probability distributions. It is only in a Bayesian framework that parameters such as $\Delta_e$ and $\Delta_c$ are random variables, so that a probability such as $P(b_\lambda > 0)$ can be computed and interpreted.

In this sense, it is particularly interesting to consider the work by O'Hagan, Stevens and Montmartin (2000), where a frequentist interpretation of the CEAC is provided. In particular, it is shown that in some cases the CEAC coincides with 1 minus the classical frequentist $p$-value to test the null hypothesis that $T_2$ is not acceptable ($H_0 : \lambda\Delta_e - \Delta_c \leq 0$) against the alternative hypothesis that it is acceptable ($H_1 : \lambda\Delta_e - \Delta_c > 0$), although this correspondence applies only under some very strict conditions. In all other cases the CEAC does not really have a frequentist interpretation, which makes a Bayesian approach to CEA a particularly natural framework of analysis.

Indeed, the analytical framework outlined above should be placed in the context of the debate about the formal role of decision theory in health policy making (see, for instance, Claxton and Posnett, 1996; Claxton, 1999). In particular, supporters of its use argue that a maximised expected utility is the only criterion for choosing between two options, so that measures of significance are all irrelevant to clinical decision-making. When deciding between two treatments, assuming that the mean INB is the utility function, then maximising the expected utility means choosing $T_2$ over $T_1$ *iff* the expected mean INB is positive. At a given $\lambda$ value, the CEAC would then provide a measure of *decision uncertainty*, given the data available. As we will see in the final section, the extent to which the decision uncertainty associated with a given decision problem is too high given the cost associated with making the wrong decision becomes an empirical question that the policy maker can address using Value of Information Analysis techniques.

## 18.3    Inference for cost-effectiveness data from clinical trials

Consider the situation in which both cost and efficacy data are obtained on individual patients in a comparative RCT; that is, data consist of the effect $e_{js}$ and the cost $c_{js}$ of treatment $j$ on patient $s$ ($j = 1, 2; s = 1, 2, \ldots, n_j$). In order to assess if treatment $T_2$ is more cost-effective than treatment $T_1$, the analyst needs to compare the underlying true mean efficacy in each trial arm, $\mu_1$ and $\mu_2$, as well as the underlying true mean costs $\gamma_1$ and $\gamma_2$.

Note that cost-effectiveness analysis of RCT data relies on statistical models which describe the distribution of costs and effects and their interrelation across individuals in the trial. These, however, are rather difficult to determine, mainly because cost data obtained for individual patients in health economic studies typically exhibit highly skewed and heavy-tailed distributions, with a few patients incurring high costs because of complications or long treatments. Moreover, the distributions of cost data are often multimodal, for instance with a mass at zero. For a recent review on the statistical methods more widely used to handle cost data, and their ability to address these problems, see Mihaylova *et al.* (2011).

To illustrate this scenario, we present an example using the eVALuate trial (Sculpher *et al.*, 2004). This was a randomised controlled trial that compared laparoscopic assisted hysterectomy with standard hysterectomy. The latter was carried out via either abdominal or vaginal route, depending on the clinical characteristics of the patient. In the abdominal comparison, a total of 859 women with gynaecological symptoms were randomised (2 : 1 ratio) to either laparoscopic assisted hysterectomy ($T_2$) or standard abdominal hysterectomy ($T_1$). The trial had a median follow up of 52 weeks. The aim of the economic evaluation which was carried out alongside the eVALuate trial was to assess whether laparoscopic surgery offered value for money compared to the status quo at the time (i.e abdominal hysterectomy). During the study follow up, for each patient in the trial, the investigators collected healthcare resource utilisation and cost (in UK pounds). Health outcomes were measured in terms of QALYs at one-year follow up. For simplicity we use here the QALY at six weeks from hospital discharge. The data are shown in Figure 18.2, and clearly show that under both treatments the cost distribution is highly skewed and heavy tailed.

Note that a CEA for this kind of data can be performed both from a classical and a Bayesian point of view, and in both settings parametric and nonparametric techniques are in common use. In particular, a parametric analysis requires the introduction of a bivariate distribution for the data $(c_{js}, e_{js})$; one example that is often used as a baseline model is the bivariate normal distribution. Then representing this joint distribution as the product of the marginal distribution for costs and the conditional distribution for effects given costs, data like that in the eVALuate trial can be modelled as

$$c_{js} \sim f(c_{js} \mid \theta_j) \quad e_{js} \mid c_{js} \sim f(e_{js} \mid c_{js}, \phi_j).$$

so that the mean cost $\gamma_j$ depends on $\theta_j$, while the mean effect $\mu_j$ depends on both $\theta_j$ and $\phi_j$ ($j = 1, 2; s = 1, 2, \ldots, n_j$). This approach will be considered in detail in the next section from a Bayesian perspective. For the moment, remaining in the classical parametric framework, note that maximum likelihood methods can easily be used to estimate the model parameters $\theta_j$ and $\phi_j$, but do not generally provide satisfactory solutions in terms of evaluating the uncertainty about the ICER; see Willan and Briggs (2006) for a discussion on different methods for tackling this problem (such as approximated methods based on Taylor expansions, bootstrap simulations, Fieller method). Because of this, and given that the natural interpretation of

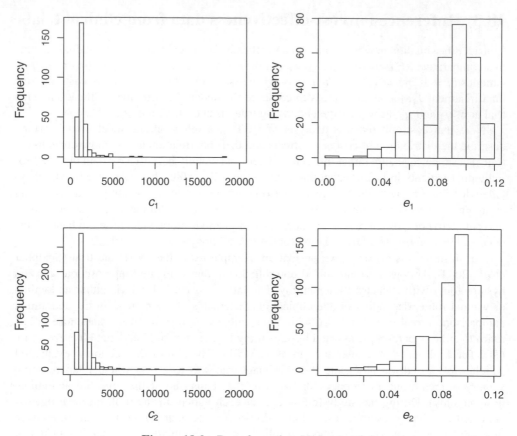

**Figure 18.2**    Data from the eVALuate trial.

the CEAC is only applicable in a Bayesian context, here we do not discuss any further the classical approach to CEA. Nonparametric methods that might be applied without specifying the underlying population distribution will be discussed in Section 18.3.2.

## 18.3.1    Bayesian parametric modelling

Bayesian parametric modelling has often been used in the context of cost-effectiveness analysis for both costs and efficacy data; in fact, at least in principle, it can lead to efficient inference (see, among others, O'Hagan and Stevens, 2001; O'Hagan and Stevens, 2002; Al and Van Hout, 2000; Fryback, Chinnis and Ulvila, 2001), and it easily allows inclusion of covariates in the analysis. To quote a few examples, O'Hagan and Stevens (2003) consider a lognormal distribution to model costs in a study where the efficacy outcome was binary; Thompson and Nixon (2005) compare modelling strategies for two commonly used distributions for cost data – the gamma and the lognormal distributions – in an example where the effects data are apparently adequately represented by a normal distribution. Using the same data set, Conigliani and Tancredi (2009) explore the behaviour of the generalised Pareto and the Weibull distributions, whereas Conigliani (2010) investigates also the use of the inverse Gaussian distribution.

One point emerges clearly from these parametric analyses: the conclusions in terms of cost-effectiveness are substantially sensitive to the assumptions made about the distributions of costs. This conclusion is also supported by simulation results published by Briggs *et al.* (2005). It might be argued that one should choose the parametric model that fits the data better, and rely on the corresponding conclusions. However the high skewness and kurtosis usually found in cost data implies that inference on costs will typically be very sensitive to the shape of the right tail of the fitted distribution beyond the range of the data, that is clearly very difficult to model accurately even when there is a substantial amount of data (Thompson and Nixon, 2005); for instance, Nixon and Thompson (2004) found that in their example data sets the different population mean estimates, obtained with different parametric models, were due almost entirely to possible costs more than twice the observed maximum cost. One consequence of this is that parametric models that fit the data equally well can produce very different answers, while in some cases models that fit badly can give similar results to those that fit well, so that better fit does not necessarily translate into more reliable conclusions.

To illustrate this point, consider again the eVALuate trial, and assume that under both treatments we model cost data with a lognormal, with a gamma, with a Weibull, or with a normal distribution; clearly we expect that in both arms of the trial the first three models fit the data much better than the normal distribution, but because it is hard to judge which of the lognormal, the gamma or the Weibull is better, the fit of each model to the data will be judged in terms of the deviance (minus twice log likelihood at the maximum likelihood estimate), in that a lower deviance indicates a better fit. Moreover, assume that under both treatments the conditional distribution for the effects is normal, and the potential correlation between costs and effects is modelled by assuming that $\mu_i$ is a linear function of $\gamma_i$ $(i = 1, 2)$. Weakly informative priors lead to the results in Table 18.1, Figures 18.3 and 18.4, and confirm the findings that the conclusions in terms of cost-effectiveness are substantially sensitive to the assumptions made about the distributions of costs. Moreover, by showing that the gamma and the normal distribution lead to very similar inferences, although the former has a much better fit than the latter, these results also confirm the finding that better fit does not necessarily lead to more reliable estimates.

**Table 18.1**  eVALuate trial: deviances of different parametric cost models and posterior summaries of cost and effect differentials.

| Model | Deviance | | $\hat{\Delta}_c$ | $PCI_{0.95}$ | $P$ $(\Delta_C > 0)$ | $\hat{\Delta}_e$ | $PCI_{0.95}$ | $P$ $(\Delta_e > 0)$ | ICER |
|---|---|---|---|---|---|---|---|---|---|
| | $T_1$ | $T_2$ | | | | | | | |
| Lognormal | 4402 | 9071 | 197 | 110 287 | 1.00 | 0.001 | −0.001 0.004 | 0.83 | 197000 |
| Gamma | 4527 | 9256 | 196 | 19 370 | 0.98 | 0.001 | −0.001 0.004 | 0.82 | 196000 |
| Weibull | 4658 | 9457 | 196 | 49 337 | 0.99 | 0.001 | −0.001 0.004 | 0.82 | 196000 |
| Normal | 4916 | 9873 | 193 | 19 369 | 0.98 | 0.001 | −0.001 0.004 | 0.82 | 193000 |

$PCI_{0.95}$ = 95% posterior credible interval.

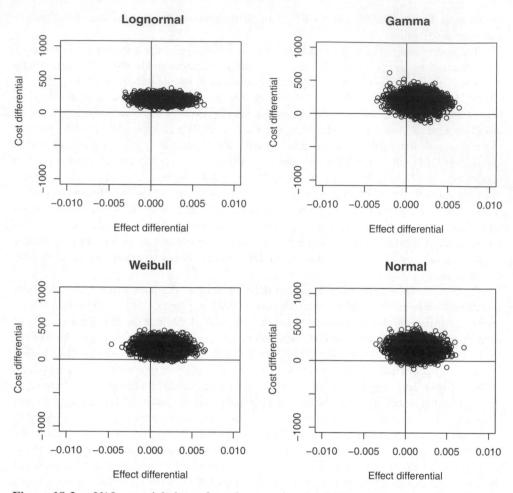

**Figure 18.3**  eVALuate trial: draws from the posterior distribution of $(\Delta_e, \Delta_c)$ under different cost models.

For these reasons, many authors (see, for instance, Nixon and Thompson, 2004; Thompson and Nixon, 2005; Mihaylova *et al.*, 2011) recommend that the sensitivity of conclusions to the choice of the model should always be investigated, so that model uncertainty becomes a crucial aspect of analysing cost-effectiveness data (although it is not obvious over what range of models the sensitivity analysis should be performed). Other authors (see, for instance, Nixon and Thompson, 2004; Thompson and Nixon, 2005), argue that since costs for individual patients must have some finite limits in practice, one could control the behaviour of the right tail by truncating a cost distribution at, say, twice the maximum observed cost (although ideally such a limit should be based on external prior information – for instance considering the maximum cost a provider could theoretically spend on an individual). Others advocate the use of formal model averaging techniques (Hoeting *et al.*, 1999) over a range of plausible models (see, for instance, Conigliani and Tancredi, 2009; Conigliani, 2010) or of models based on mixtures of parametric distributions (see, for instance, Atienza *et al.*, 2008), in order

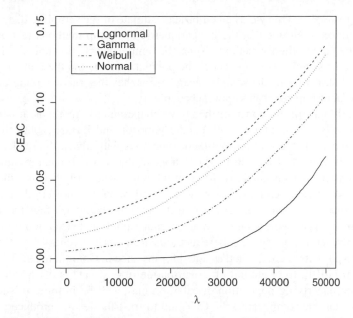

**Figure 18.4**  eVALuate trial: CEAC under different cost models.

to obtain flexible models able to accommodate excess zeros, overdispersion and heavy tails. While both approaches are data based, the problem here is the influence of the tail of the assumed distributions beyond the range of the data. Other authors (see, for instance, Nixon and Thompson, 2004; Bartkowiak and Sen, 1992; Willan, 2001) focus their attention on sample sizes, arguing that these must be large enough to enable sufficiently accurate modelling of the tail of the cost distribution. But by far the most common alternatives to parametric modelling in the context of cost-effectiveness analyses are nonparametric methods and transformation of the data, which will be considered in detail in the next sections.

## 18.3.2   Semiparametric modelling and nonparametric statistical methods

The difficulty of producing realistic probabilistic models for the underlying population distribution of costs has made very attractive (both in the literature and in practice) the possibility of considering nonparametric or semiparametric methods, which might be applied without specifying such a population distribution.

Two simple nonparametric methods are widely used in the context of cost-effectiveness analysis (O'Hagan and Stevens, 2002, 2003). The first one is based upon assuming that the sample mean follows a normal distribution. This assumption is justified by the Central Limit theorem (CLT), and the sample size needed for this approximation to be valid depends on the degree of non-normality in the distribution (although in practice 30 observations are usually enough even with the high degree of skewness encountered in the analysis of cost data). The second nonparametric method that is often used is the bootstrap. This entails randomly drawing a large number of *resamples* of size $n$ from the original sample (of size $n$) with replacement, and calculating the value of the parameter of interest for each of the corresponding samples. This yields an empirical estimate of the sampling distribution of the parameter of interest. Notice that the nonparametric bootstrap methods rest on asymptotic theory as do the normal-theory methods. Thus, the sample distribution tends to the population distribution as the sample size approaches the population size, and the bootstrap estimate of the sampling distribution of the sample mean approaches the true sampling distribution as the number of bootstrap replicates approaches infinity.

With regard to the performance of the above nonparametric methods, it is interesting to note the work of Briggs and Gray (1998) and Thompson and Barber (2000). In both papers the authors advocate the use of normal-theory methods, but advise the reader to check the validity of such methods by using the bootstrap, in that if the bootstrap and the normal-theory methods produce substantially different inferences (possibly because the sample size is small or the skewness is extreme), then the bootstrap should be preferred. In fact, what the bootstrap estimate of the sampling distribution shows is the extent to which the sample size is sufficiently large to justify the assumption of a normal sampling distribution for the parameter of interest. However, when applying these methods in cost-effectiveness data, the analyst will always have to pay extra care. In fact, as noted for instance in Conigliani and Tancredi (2005) and Conigliani (2010), the right tail of a distribution of cost data is often so heavy that the variance of the underlying population distribution may well be infinite. In such cases it is obviously not sensible to appeal to the CLT and to trust the results produced by statistical methods resulting from it. Moreover, as pointed out for instance in O'Hagan and Stevens (2003), even when (in sufficiently large samples) these simple nonparametric methods might strictly be valid, they may produce poor or misleading inferences. The reason is that, although in cost evaluations conceived to have an impact on medical policy the main interest is the total healthcare cost, so that it is inference on population mean costs that is informative, the sample mean is not necessarily a good basis for the inference. And this is because the sample mean is very sensitive to the kind of extreme sample values that are often encountered in cost data; it is unbiased, but it is not necessarily the most efficient estimator. It follows that nonparametric methods such as the normal-theory and the bootstrap, that are based on the sample mean, may be inappropriate in this setting, which warrants further examination of the nature of the underlying population distribution.

Another proposal by Conigliani and Tancredi (2005), which recognises the inability of standard parametric approaches to model the right tail of the cost distribution accurately, as well as the high influence of such tails in estimating the population mean, is to model the bulk of the data and the tails separately. In particular, Conigliani and Tancredi (2005) consider a distribution composed of a piecewise constant density up to an unknown endpoint and a generalised Pareto distribution for the remaining tail data. This mixture model, which is extremely flexible and able to fit data sets with very different shapes, allows the reporting of model-based inference for mean costs taking into account tail model uncertainty.

### 18.3.3    Transformation of the data

Another common approach that can be employed to handle cost data is to transform the data to a scale onto which it is reasonable to assume normality or another standard distributional form. In particular, approaches to find appropriate transformations have considered mainly the Box–Cox transformations (to achieve symmetry in error), with special attention devoted to log transformations (Mihaylova et al., 2011).

Note, however, that caution needs to be employed with such transformations, since mean values and confidence limits may be difficult to interpret on the transformed scales. In particular, the comparison of means on the transformed scale does not usually tell us much about the comparison of means on the original scale. Moreover, back-transformation onto the original scale is not always straightforward (see, for instance, Thompson and Barber, 2000; Briggs and Gray, 1998). Consider, for instance, a log transformation of the data. Estimating the population mean on the log scale using the sample mean of the log-transformed data, and back-transforming the latter to the original scale by taking its exponential, yields the geometric mean of the original data, not the arithmetic mean, which is what is needed for resource allocation decisions (Thompson and Barber, 2000).

In this respect, it is important to remember that the approaches for back transformation to the original scale are dictated by the nature of the error term on the transformed scale. If we assume for instance that the error term has a normal distribution with parameters $v$ and $\tau^2$ (i.e. that the original cost data follow a lognormal distribution), the mean on the original scale can be written in terms of $v$ and $\tau^2$ as $\gamma = \exp(v + \frac{\tau^2}{2})$. Then, letting $\hat{v}$ and $\hat{\tau}^2$ be the sample mean and the sample variance of log-costs, an obvious estimator of $\gamma$ would be $\hat{\gamma} = \exp(\hat{v} + \frac{\hat{\tau}^2}{2})$. Note that, unlike the sample mean, $\hat{\gamma}$ is a biased estimator of $\gamma$, but is naturally less affected by extreme observations, so that one can expect this to perform better in general. In this sense it is interesting to see the work of O'Hagan and Stevens (2003), where it is shown that $\hat{\gamma}$ is both asymptotically unbiased and asymptotically more efficient than the sample mean, and that in presence of outliers it leads to a much smaller estimate of $\gamma$ than the sample mean, so that it also appears to be much more accurate.

However the results in O'Hagan and Stevens (2003) are based upon assuming that cost data are exactly lognormally distributed, which of course is not in general true: the distribution of the error term on the transformed scale is usually unknown, and reliance on the assumption of normality or homoscedasticity can lead to inconsistent estimates (see, for instance, Mihaylova *et al.*, 2011; Conigliani and Tancredi, 2009). In this sense, it is interesting to cite the work by Royall and Tsou (2003), where, for the problem of the estimation of the mean, it is shown that while assuming, for instance, a gamma distribution, the object of inference continues to be the mean of the true generating process also when the model fails, if we assume the lognormal working model then what the likelihood represents evidence about when the model fails is not $E_f(c)$ but the quantity $\exp(E_f(\log(c)) + \frac{1}{2}\text{var}_f(\log(c)))$. In such cases it might be preferable to employ the sample mean rather than $\hat{\gamma}$, since at least for sufficiently large sample sizes the CLT can be invoked.

## 18.4  Complex decision analysis models

Parmigiani (2002) states 'Prediction models used in support of clinical and health policy decision-making often need to consider the course of a disease over an extended period of time, and draw evidence from a broad knowledge base, including epidemiologic cohort and case control studies, randomized clinical trials, expert opinions, and more.' This view is consistent with the notion that RCT evidence will always need to be integrated with other (possibly multiple) sources of evidence to estimate the parameters of interest in the decision problem. For instance, one may have several RCTs which assessed the effectiveness of a particular medication in a given clinical context. It would be erroneous to single out one of these studies and ignore the information provided by the rest of the evidence base. Similarly,

RCT evidence may need to be extrapolated over a longer time period than the study follow up. The study may have been conducted in a different jurisdiction (e.g. the USA), whereas the analyst needs to produce cost-effectiveness estimates to inform adoption decisions in the UK, and address issues like generalisability of the study results from the USA to the UK.

## 18.4.1   Markov models

The economic analysis of healthcare interventions does often involve some degree of modelling. Markov-type models, for instance, are very popular in health economics, given their ability to represent the long-term evolution of chronic diseases. Norris (1997) and Grimmet and Stirzaker (2001) represent two standard references providing complete accounts of the probabilistic aspects of these models, while Davison (2003) and Lindsay (2004) describe inference for them. An introduction to the practical aspects of Markov models from the health economics point of view can be found in Briggs and Sculpher (1998).

The basic idea underlying the use of these models for assessing the cost-effectiveness of a treatment is that each clinical state of the disease can be associated both with a measure of benefit, such as quality of life, and with a monetary measure of cost (e.g. medications, in-patient stay). Modelling the evolution of the disease allows one to predict the expected long-term costs and benefits of a medical treatment. In particular, discrete-time Markov models (also called Markov chains), with a discrete number of states, represent a natural and simple framework for representing a patient's health status over time. With these models the subject's history is divided into equally spaced intervals (days, months or years) with each interval representing a *cycle* in the model. During each cycle an individual can be in one of a finite set of health states. The essential feature of the Markov models is that during each cycle, given the entire past history of the subject, the transition probability from one health state to another depends only on the present state (i.e. 'Markovian assumption'). Loosely speaking, this means that in the simplest Markov model one assumes that the future is independent of the past given the present. This assumption can be relaxed using – where relevant – time-dependent transition probabilities (Hawkins, Sculpher and Epstein, 2005) or 'tunnel' states (Briggs and Sculpher, 1998).

In order to describe more formally the generic structure and the use of these models, we indicate with $t = 1, \ldots, T$ the cycle index, and we suppose that within each cycle $t$ a patient assumes one of $R$ states. In particular, during the first cycle each patient is assumed to be in one of the mutually exclusive $R$ states, according to a probability distribution represented by the row vector $\pi_1 = (\pi_{11}, \ldots, \pi_{1R})$. For each patient in state $r$ during cycle $t$ the probability of moving to state $s$ in the following cycle will be indicated with $p_{t+1,rs}$. These transition probabilities can be organised into the transition matrix $P_{t+1}$ comprising, for each row, the probability vector $(p_{t+1,r1}, \ldots, p_{t+1,rR})$. Hence, the marginal probability distribution $\pi_t$ for the patient state during cycle $t$ can be obtained through the recursive relationship

$$\pi_t = \pi_{t-1} P_t \ \ t = 2, \ldots T$$

Note that we are assuming that the transition probabilities of each state given the previous one may vary over time; that is, they depend on the cycle index $t$. Under this general assumption the Markov model is said to be non-homogeneous with respect to time. Matters simplify considerably, especially for the theoretical results concerning the limit behaviour of the Markov models, when the transition probabilities are the same in each cycle (i.e. homogeneous Markov model).

Long-term predictions of the parameters of interest (e.g. net benefit) can then be carried out by attaching costs and benefits to each possible health state in the model. For the moment, suppose that as a measure of health benefit we are interested in the expected number of cycles spent in a given health state. Let $T_r$ be the random variable indicating the total number of cycles spent by a patient in state $r$. Since $T_r$ is equal to $\sum_{t=1}^{T} X_{tr}$ where $X_{tr} = 1$ if the patient is in the state $r$ during the cycle $t$ and $X_{tr} = 0$ otherwise, we have that

$$E(T_r) = \sum_{t=1}^{T} \pi_{tr}.$$

A more general benefit measure can be obtained by considering a row vector $b$ comprising the benefits associated with spending one cycle in each state of the model. In fact, suppose that these benefits are discounted at the rate $\delta_b$ per cycle; then the total expected benefit for each patient is given by

$$m_e = \sum_{t=1}^{T} \frac{\pi_t b'}{(1 + \delta_b)^{t-1}}.$$

Note that by taking $\delta_b = 0$, $b_s = 0$ for each $s \neq r$, and $b_r = 1$, we have exactly the expression given above for the quantity $E(T_r)$. Moreover, if one of the states of the model corresponds to *death*, and one of the outputs we are interested in is patients' life expectancy (in terms of cycles), this can be simply obtained by taking a vector $b$ with all the elements equal to one but the death state which assumes the value 0. Weighting patients' survival by their health-related quality of life leads to the *quality-adjusted life years* (QALYs), the most popular measure of health benefit in use in health economic evaluation, which can easily be achieved by considering different values for elements of the vector $b$.

Similarly, suppose that the cost, at current prices, of spending a cycle in state $r$ is $C_r$, $r = 1, \ldots, R$. Let $C$ be the row vector $(C_1, \ldots, C_R)$ and let $C_0$ be a fixed entry cost. The total expected cost for each patient in the population is then given by

$$m_c = C_0 + \sum_{t=1}^{T} \frac{\pi_t C'}{(1 + \delta_c)^{t-1}},$$

where $\delta_c$ is a discount rate for future costs.

Note that in practical applications it is necessary to fix or to estimate the model parameters $\pi_1$ and $P_t$, and to propagate their uncertainty on the quantities $m_e$ and $m_c$.

Data sets from RCTs, hospital registers, population mortality statistics and observational studies may be used to inform the model. For example, to investigate the consequences concerning the choice of prosthesis in total hip replacement (THR), Fitzpatrick *et al.* (1998) (see also Spiegelhalter and Best, 2003) distinguish between patients suffering an operative death after a revision operation and patients dying for 'other causes'. For the transition probabilities to the operative death, a mortality rate estimated by previous clinical trials was assumed to increase linearly over time (expressed in years), while the national mortality rates published by the UK Office for National Statistics were employed to fix the transition probabilities for the other causes of death (e.g. competing risks).

In some cases, individual longitudinal data from RCTs may be used directly to estimate the transition probabilities to be used in the model (for one example see Henriksson *et al.*, 2008). For homogeneous chains, maximum likelihood estimates for the transition probabilities can be obtained by the row proportions of the one-cycle transition matrix $N$, whose generic elements $n_{rs}$ represent the number of times a transition from state $r$ to state $s$ occurred. Craig and Sendi (2002) discuss maximum likelihood estimation when the common observation interval and the desired cycle length do not coincide or when the observation intervals vary across the study.

In order to briefly illustrate a CEA based on Markov models, we consider the example illustrated in Simpson *et al.* (2008), where a transition model for HIV patients has been proposed. For each model cycle, the cohort of patients is distributed across 12 ordered health states plus death according to their CD4 cell count and viral load. The cost of treating AIDS events for each health status and a transition matrix, $P$, which has been estimated using hospital data for highly treatment-experienced HIV-1 patients, are reported in Simpson *et al.* (2004) and Simpson *et al.* (2008). Compared to the analyses presented in these papers, which consider a non-homogeneous model involving multiple therapeutic failures, here we assume that in both treatment groups patients do not change therapy. Patients in the control group will transit across health states according to the initial transition matrix $P$, while the transition matrix $Q$ of the cohort of patients receiving the new treatment has elements given by

$$q_{ij} = \begin{cases} (\alpha p_{ij}) \Big/ \left( \alpha \sum_{l=1}^{i} p_{il} + \beta \sum_{l>i} p_{il} \right) & j \leq i \\ (\beta p_{ij}) \Big/ \left( \alpha \sum_{l=1}^{i} p_{il} + \beta \sum_{l>i} p_{il} \right) & j > i \end{cases}$$

where $\alpha \geq 1$ and $0 \leq \beta \leq 1$. For a cohort of 10 000 simulated patients in the control group entering the study in the healthiest status, we obtained, without considering discounting rates, a mean lifetime survival of 13.2 years and a mean lifetime cost for the treatment of AIDS events of US\$12 347 253. Repeating the experiment for the new treatment group, letting $\alpha = 1.05$ and $\beta = 1$ in order to assume slightly higher probabilities of improving the health status than in the control group, we obtained a mean lifetime survival of 14.2 years and a mean lifetime cost of US\$12 978 433. The corresponding ICER was US\$631 180 per additional life year.

## 18.5   Further extensions

From a more general perspective, the problem of combining costs and benefits of a given intervention into a rational scheme for allocating resources can be formalised using a Bayesian decision-theoretic approach, in which rational decision-making is achieved through the comparison of expected utilities (Baio and Dawid, 2008). This approach has received increasing attention, in particular in the last couple of decades, when economic studies started to be aimed at specific decision-makers, and health systems all over the world have begun to use CEA as a formal input into decisions about treatments, interventions and programmes that should be funded from collective resources.

Specifically, let $u(y, T_j)$ be a utility function representing the value of applying treatment $T_j$ and obtaining the health economic outcome $y = (e, c)$; a common form of utility is the monetary net benefit $u(y, T_j) = \lambda e - c$. Also define the expected utility $U_j = E[u(Y, T_j)]$ as the expected value of the utility function obtained averaging out the uncertainty about both the population parameters and the individual variations. Then the most cost-effective treatment is the one which is associated with the maximum expected utility, $U^* = \max_j U_j$; that is, $T_2$ dominates $T_1$ if the expected incremental benefit $EIB = U_2 - U_1$ is positive (or if $U_2 > U_1$). Notice that when net benefit is used as the utility function, the expected incremental benefit reduces to $EIB = \lambda E(\Delta_e) - E(\Delta_c)$, that is, to the expectation over the distribution of the population parameters of the INB $b_\lambda$ defined in Section 18.2.1.

## 18.5.1    Probabilistic sensitivity analysis and value of information analysis

Note that since both individual variation and imperfect knowledge of the states of the world are integrated out, the analysis of the expected incremental benefit outlined above provides a rational scheme for allocating resources given the available evidence. A large part of the health economics literature suggests that the impact of this uncertainty (and in particular of the parameter uncertainty) in the final decision should be taken into account thoroughly, by means of a process known as Probabilistic Sensitivity Analysis (PSA; Parmigiani, 2002). PSA requires that all the inputs of a model (i.e. parameters for modelling RCT data or estimates plugged into an economic evaluation model) are considered as random variables, and explicitly analyses the uncertainty on these inputs by means of suitable indicators. In particular, the idea behind PSA is to compare the actual decision process, based on the analysis of EIB, to an ideal one, in which the uncertainty on the parameters is resolved, and it is typically conducted using a simulation approach (Doubilet *et al.*, 1985). Recently, as pointed out for instance by Claxton *et al.* (2005), most of the main agencies for health economic evaluation have updated their guidance for technology assessment, requiring the use of PSA as part of the cost-effectiveness models submitted for their consideration.

In order to briefly illustrate a PSA, consider again the Markov model for the HIV treatments described in Section 18.4.1, and in particular focus attention on the parameter $\alpha$, that controls the effectiveness of the new treatment with respect to the standard one. Here, instead of fixing a value for $\alpha$, we generate values for it from a uniform distribution in the interval $[1, 1.1]$. The results are shown in Figure 18.5, and point out that while the new treatment is almost always cost-effective at the threshold level of US\$750 000, with the lower threshold of US\$500 000 the probability of cost-effectiveness is only about 30%.

It is interesting to notice, as pointed out for instance in Claxton *et al.* (2005), that in health economic evaluations it is common to summarise the results of PSA by means of the CEAC, which has the form introduced in Section 18.2.2 provided the net benefit is used as a utility function. The CEAC, in fact, can be seen as the probability that a more precise knowledge of the distribution of the population parameters in the decision problem at hand would not change the optimal decision, and therefore can be used to represent the decision uncertainty surrounding the cost-effectiveness of a treatment (Baio and Dawid, 2008; Fenwick, Claxton and Schulpher, 2001).

Despite their wide use, some critical limitations of CEACs for presenting uncertainty have recently been brought up. Felli and Hazen (1999), for instance, point out that no explicit reference in the analysis of CEACs is made to the costs associated with a wrong decision; Koerkamp *et al.* (2007) show that very different distributions for the incremental net benefit

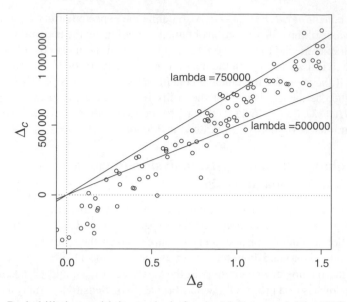

**Figure 18.5**  Probabilistic sensitivity analysis for the Markov model for HIV progression.

can produce the same CEAC, so that their interpretation is not always straightforward. For these reasons, a purely decision-theoretic approach to PSA based on the analysis of a standard tool in Bayesian decision theory, the *Expected Value of Distributional Information* (EVDI), is becoming increasingly popular in health economic evaluations (Felli and Hazen, 1999; Claxton *et al.*, 2001; Ades, Lu and Claxton, 2004; Baio and Dawid, 2008; Baio, 2010). In fact, by construction, the EVDI produces an indication of both how much we are likely to lose if we take the wrong decision, and how likely it is that we take it (Baio and Dawid, 2008). Moreover, regardless of the form of the utility function, the EVDI is defined as the expectation of the value of obtaining distributional information on the population parameters, that is, as the maximum amount that we would be willing to pay to obtain such information. In this sense, it also provides a more general answer to the question of whether it is economically efficient to make a decision given the data at hand, or if instead the consequences of making the wrong decision are too expensive (e.g. irreversibility, sunk costs), so that collection of further information is warranted. For further reading on this topic see the work by Claxton *et al.* (2001) and Claxton, Cohen and Neumann (2005).

## 18.5.2   The role of Bayesian evidence synthesis

Another area that is closely related to the analysis of the EVDI, and that is becoming increasingly popular in health economic evaluation, is that known as *quantitative evidence synthesis* (Sutton and Abrams, 2001; Ades *et al.*, 2006; Ades and Sutton, 2006) for decision-making. Since economic evaluations require a synthesis of all available evidence into probability distributions for the input parameters, evidence synthesis (e.g. meta-analysis and its extensions) provide a natural approach to quantify the value (and relevant uncertainty) of such parameters. Although the role of evidence synthesis can also be explored in clinical epidemiology, it is in a decision-making context that its fundamental role emerges, since typically decisions cannot be deferred and must be taken on the basis of all the information that is available. Specific advantages conferred by the Bayesian approach to this problem, which have been recognised for instance by the National Institute for Health and Clinical Excellence (NICE) in the UK, include the ability to include all pertinent information and full allowance for parameter uncertainty, as well as its coherent link to decision-making.

Specifically, there are different ways in which several items of information can be combined in the Bayesian setting for a CEA. In the simplest case, when each trial is assumed to provide an estimate of the same parameter, the data can be combined using a *fixed effects* meta-analysis, and the common pooled effect can be estimated with a weighted average of the individual study effects, the weights being inversely proportional to the within-study variances. If instead the aim is to combine information on items from the same type of study that are similar but not identical, then a random-effects meta-analysis can be employed. This represents a somehow intermediate position between assuming (as in the fixed-effects meta-analysis) that each observed effect size provides an estimate of the same underlying quantity, say $\theta$, and assuming at the other extreme that the true study-specific effects, say $\theta_i$, are totally unrelated; individual studies may not be estimating the same underlying effect, but in random-effects meta-analysis the unobserved $\theta_i$ are assumed to be similar, so that it is reasonable to consider them to have been drawn from a common underlying distribution. Note that this approach is particularly common especially in the Bayesian setting, due to the strong relationship between random effects and hierarchical modelling; in particular, the Bayesian notion of *exchangeability* provides a framework that includes most of the methods that have been proposed for evidence synthesis. Moreover, it is interesting to note that random-effects meta-analysis specifically allows for the existence of between-study heterogeneity (as well as the within-study variability), although it does not provide an explanation for it. However covariates can easily be included in the analysis, and regression-type models (often called *meta-regression models*) can be effectively employed to explain why study results may systematically differ and to identify associations between patient characteristics and outcome that might assist in individualising treatment regimes (Sutton and Abrams, 2001).

In recent years these simple forms of meta-analysis have been generalised and extended to increasingly complex data structures. These include combination of information from different study designs taking account of potential bias, mixed comparison, different follow-up periods, combination of evidence on multiple or surrogate end points, and combination of information on individual parameters with information on complex functions of the parameters. The aim of this section is to review some of the problems that arise in these multiparameter evidence syntheses, as well as some of the methods proposed for dealing with them. The need to check for consistency of evidence when using these methods is emphasised for instance in Ades and Sutton (2006).

Consider first the problem of combining studies that are heterogeneous with respect to the design and analysis. Much of initial work in this sense was carried out by Eddy, Hasselblad and Shachter (1992), who developed a general framework called the *confidence profile method* (CPM) that allows the explicit modelling of biases due to study design. Since this initial work, various methods for combining items of information in specific situations have been proposed in the literature. Muller *et al.* (1999), for instance, considered a hierarchical model to combine case-control and prospective studies; Li and Begg (1994) presented a model to estimate an overall treatment effect when some comparative studies are combined with non-comparative single-arm studies; Larose and Dey (1997) proposed a random-effects model to combine double-blind (closed) studies with open ones in which the investigator had knowledge of the treatment regime; Prevost, Abrams and Jones (2000) considered the problem of combining observational evidence with results from randomised trials. Although in some of these models (for instance Li and Begg, 1994; Larose and Dey, 1997) different study types estimate the same underlying mean effect, while in others (for instance Prevost, Abrams and Jones, 2000) different study types estimate different type-specific mean effects, one thing that all these methods have in common is that they produce a weighted average of the study-type-specific mean effects, with the weights determined by the model structure and the data, particularly the heterogeneity within each study type (Ades and Sutton, 2006). An alternative to this is to specify the weights explicitly; see for instance Spiegelhalter and Best (2003).

Another issue that often arises when combining several items of information for the purpose of CEA is that the evidence base is often fragmented, and the only way to consider all the evidence in a unified analytical framework is to conduct a *mixed treatment comparison* (Hasselblad, 1998). Indeed, in healthcare economic evaluation there is often absence of head-to-head trial evidence on all the options being compared, and past analyses have often been based on a series of trials making different pair-wise comparisons among the treatments of interest. Clearly these analyses cannot help to answer the real question that is of interest for decision-makers; that is, 'of all the possible courses of action which one is the most cost-effective?'; instead, mixed treatment comparison methods address exactly this problem. The basic idea is that in the absence of *direct evidence* comparing treatment $A$ and $B$, the relative treatment effect $\theta_{AB}$ can be estimated considering the information provided by studies which compared $A$ and $B$ with a third treatment $C$; using the terminology of CPM, $\theta_{AC}$ and $\theta_{BC}$ can be regarded as *basic* parameters, while $\theta_{AB} = \theta_{AC} - \theta_{BC}$ is effectively a functional parameter, that is, a function of the basic parameters. Ades and Sutton (2006) show how to generalise simple meta-analysis models to analyse mixed treatment comparisons, with the effect of reducing the parameter space to a set of basic parameters, assuming exchangeability of treatment effects holds over the entire ensemble of studies. For a particularly remarkable mixed treatment comparison analysis see for instance Dominici *et al.* (1999).

In Ades and Sutton (2006) a number of other issues related to evidence synthesis, as well as references to methods proposed for dealing with them, are considered. One point underlined by the authors and that we find particularly interesting is that the increasing use of formal decision analysis by bodies such as NICE is, among other things, imposing a new rationale for the use of evidence synthesis methods for decision-making. In fact, as we pointed out in the previous section, the realisation that resources for healthcare are limited and reliance on formal decision modelling are leading to substantial interest in expected value of information theory. Evidence synthesis is highly relevant in this context, since the ability to incorporate additional sources of evidence can have a considerable effect on the uncertainty surrounding the net benefit estimate and the EVDI; thus ignoring for instance indirect evidence may result in greater uncertainty. In this sense, the decision context clarifies the tasks that evidence synthesis might be required to do. Ades and Sutton (2006) conclude that it is reasonable to expect that more attention will be paid in the future to the assessment of uncertainty, and this will lead to a reconsideration of the way different types of evidence are combined for decision-making. In particular, special attention needs to be devoted to the problem of estimating the consistency of sources of evidence and, as there will often be insufficient evidence to determine this confidently, to the choice of reasonably informative priors on the degree of heterogeneity between different types of evidence.

## 18.6   Summary

Healthcare policy makers are required to use the limited resources as efficiently as possible, given the financial pressure under which many healthcare systems currently operate. One way to achieve allocative efficiency of healthcare resources is to identify which investment strategies (drugs, medical devices, diagnostics, etc.) provide value for money. Economic evaluation in healthcare (also known as cost-effectiveness analysis) generates the information required to address the above question. This chapter provided an overview of the statistical methods used in applied healthcare economic evaluation studies and the challenges faced by the analysts in dealing with the data, emphasising the emerging role that Bayesian statistical methods play in this context.

# References

Ades, A., Sculpher, M., Sutton, A. *et al.* (2006) Bayesian methods for evidence synthesis in cost-effectiveness analysis. *Pharmacoeconomics*, **24**, 1–19.

Ades, A.E. and Sutton, A.J. (2006) Multiparameter evidence synthesis in epidemiology and medical decision-making: current approaches. *Journal of the Royal Statistical Society Series A*, **169**, 5–35.

Ades, A.E., Lu, G. and Claxton, K. (2004) Expected value of sample information calculations in medical decision modeling. *Medical Decision Making*, **24**, 207–227.

Al, M.J. and van Hout, B.A. (2000) A Bayesian approach to economic analyses of clinical trials: the case of stenting versus balloon angioplasty. *Health Economics*, **7**, 599–609.

Atienza, N., Garcia-Heras, J., Munoz-Pichardo, J. and Villa, R. (2008) An application of mixture distributions in modelization of length of hospital stay. *Statistics in Medicine*, **27**, 1403–1420.

Baio, G. (2010) *Metodi Statistici per la Valutazione Economica in Sanit*, Aracne, Italy.

Baio, G. and Dawid, A. (2008) Probabilistic sensitivity analysis in health economics, Research Report 292/08, Department of Statistical Science, University College London.

Bartkowiak, A. and Sen, A.R. (1992) Minimum sample size ensuring validity of classical confidence intervals for means of skewed and platykurtic distributions. *Biomedical Journal*, **34**, 367–382.

Black, W. (1999) The ce plane: a graphic representation of cost-effectiveness. *Medical Decision Making*, **10**, 212–214.

Briggs, A. and Gray, A. (1998) The distribution of health care costs and their statistical analysis for economic evaluation. *Journal of Health Services Research and Policy*, **3**, 233–245.

Briggs, A. and Sculpher, M. (1998) An introduction to Markov modelling for economic evaluation. *Pharmacoeconomics*, **13**, 397–409.

Briggs, A., Nixon, R., Dixon, S. and Thompson, S. (2005) Parametric modelling of cost data: some simulation evidence. *Health Economics*, **14**(4), 421–428.

Claxton, K. (1999) The irrelevance of inference: a decision-making approach to the stochastic evaluation of healthcare technologies. *Journal of Health Economics*, **18**, 341–364.

Claxton, K. and Posnett, J. (1996) An economic approach to clinical trial design and research priority-setting. *Health Economics*, **5**, 513–521.

Claxton, K., Cohen, J. and Neumann, P. (2005) When is evidence sufficient? *Health Affairs*, **24**, 93–101.

Claxton, K., Neumann, P., Araki, S. and Weinstein, M. (2001) Bayesian value-of-information analysis. *International Journal of Technology Assessment in Health Care*, **17**, 38–55.

Claxton, K., Sculpher, M., McCabe, C. *et al.* (2005) Probabilistic sensitivity analysis for NICE technology assessment: not an optional extra. *Health Economics*, **14**, 339–347.

Conigliani, C. (2010) A Bayesian model averaging approach with non-informative priors for cost-effectiveness analyses. *Statistics in Medicine*, **29**, 1696–1709.

Conigliani, C. and Tancredi, A. (2005) Semi-parametric modelling for costs of healthcare technologies. *Statistics in Medicine*, **24**, 3171–3184.

Conigliani, C. and Tancredi, A. (2009) A Bayesian model averaging approach for cost-effectiveness analyses. *Health Economics*, **18**, 807–821.

Craig, B.A. and Sendi, P.P. (2002) Estimation of the transition matrix of a discrete-time Markov chain. *Health Economics*, **11**, 33–42.

Davison, A.C. (2003) *Statistical Models*, Cambridge University Press.

Dominici, F., Parmigiani, G., Wolpert, R. and Hasselblad, V. (1999) Meta-analysis of migraine headache treatments: combining information from heterogeneous designs. *Journal of the American Statistical Association*, **94**, 16–28.

Doubilet, P., Begg, C., Weinstein, M. *et al.* (1985) Probabilistic sensitivity analysis using Monte Carlo simulation. A practical approach. *Medical Decision Making*, **5**, 157–177.

Drummond, M., O'Brien, B., Stoddart, G. and Torrance, G. (1997) *Methods for the Economic Evaluation of Health Care Programmes*, Oxford University Press.

Eddy, D.M., Hasselblad, V. and Shachter, R. (1992) *Meta-analysis by the Confidence Profile Method*, Academic Press.

Felli, J. and Hazen, G. (1999) A Bayesian approach to sensitivity analysis. *Health Economics*, **8**, 263–268.

Fenwick, E., Claxton, K. and Schulpher, M. (2001) Representing uncertainty: the role of cost effectiveness acceptability curves. *Health Economics*, **10**, 779–787.

Fitzpatrick, R., Shortall, E., Sculpher, M. *et al.* (1998) Primary total hip replacement surgery: a systematic review of outcomes and modelling of cost-effectiveness associated with different prostheses. *Health Technology Assessment*, **2**(20), 1–64.

Fryback, D.G., Chinnis, J.O. Jr. and Ulvila, J.W. (2001) Bayesian cost-effectiveness analysis: an example using the GUSTO trial. *International Journal of Technology Assessment in Health Care*, **17**, 83–97.

Grimmet, G.R. and Stirzaker, D.R. (2001) *Probability and Random Processes*, 3rd edn, Clarendon Press.

Hasselblad, V. (1998) Meta-analysis of multi-treatment studies. *Medical Decision Making*, **18**, 37–43.

Hawkins, N., Sculpher, M. and Epstein, D. (2005) Cost-effectiveness analysis of treatments for chronic disease: using R to incorporate time dependency of treatment response. *Medical Decision Making*, **25**, 511–519.

Henriksson, M., Epstein, D.M., Palmer, S.J. *et al.* (2008) The cost-effectiveness of an early interventional strategy in non-st-elevation acute coronary syndrome based on the RITA 3 trial. *Heart*, **94**, 717–723.

Hoeting, J., Madigan, D., Raftery, A. and Volinsky, C. (1999) Bayesian model averaging: a tutorial (with discussion). *Statistical Science*, **14**(4), 382.

Koerkamp, B., Hunink, M., Stijnen, T. *et al.* (2007) Limitations of acceptability curves for presenting uncertainty in cost-effectiveness analyses. *Medical Decision Making*, **27**, 101–111.

Larose, D. and Dey, D. (1997) Grouped random effects models for Bayesian meta-analysis. *Statistics in Medicine*, **16**, 1817–1829.

Li, Z. and Begg, C. (1994) Random effects models for combining results from controlled and uncontrolled studies in meta-analysis. *Journal of the American Statistical Association*, **89**, 1523–1527.

Lindsay, J.K. (2004) *Statistical Analysis of Stochastic Processes in Time*, Cambridge University Press.

Mihaylova, B., Briggs, A., O'Hagan, A. and Thompson, S.G. (2011) Review of statistical methods for analysing healthcare resources and costs. *Health Economics*, **20**(8), 897–916.

Muller, P., Parmigiani, G., Schildkraut, J. and Tardella, L. (1999) A Bayesian hierarchical approach for combining case-control and prospective studies. *Biometrics*, **55**, 858–866.

Nixon, R.M. and Thompson, S.G. (2004) Parametric modelling of cost data in medical studies. *Statistics in Medicine*, **23**(8), 1311–1331.

Norris, J.R. (1997) *Markov Chains*, Cambridge University Press.

O'Hagan, A. and Stevens, J.W. (2001) A framework for cost-effectiveness analysis from clinical trial data. *Health Economics*, **10**, 303–315.

O'Hagan, A. and Stevens, J.W. (2002) Bayesian methods for design and analysis of cost-effectiveness trials in the evaluation of healthcare technologies. *Statistical Methods in Medical Research*, **11**, 469–490.

O'Hagan, A. and Stevens, J.W. (2003) Assessing and comparing cost: how robust are the bootstrap and methods based on asymptotic normality? *Health Economics*, **12**, 33–49.

O'Hagan, A., Stevens, J.W. and Montmartin, J. (2000) Inference for the cost-effectiveness acceptability curve and cost-effectiveness ratio. *Pharmacoeconomics*, **17**, 339–349.

Parmigiani, G. (2002) Measuring uncertainty in complex decision analysis models. *Statistical Methods in Medical Research*, **11**(6), 513–537.

Prevost, T., Abrams, K. and Jones, D. (2000) Hierarchical models in generalised synthesis of evidence: an example based on studies of breast cancer screening. *Statistics in Medicine*, **19**, 3359–3376.

Royall, R.M. and Tsou, T.-S. (2003) Interpreting statistical evidence using imperfect models: robust adjusted likelihood functions. *J Roy Stat Soc B*, **65**, 391–404.

Sculpher, M., Claxton, K., Drummond, M. and McCabe, C. (2006) Whither trial-based economic evaluation for healthcare decision making? *Health Economics*, **15**, 677–687.

Sculpher, M., Manca, A., Abbott, J. *et al.* (2004) Cost effectiveness analysis of laparoscopic hysterectomy compared with standard hysterectomy: results from a randomised trial. *British Medical Journal*, **328**(7432), 134–137.

Simpson, K.N., Luo, M.P., Churmey, E. *et al.* (2004) Cost-effectiveness of lopinavir/ritonavir versus nelfinavir as the first line highly active antiretroviral therapy regimen for HIV infection. *HIV Clinical Trials*, **5**, 294–304.

Simpson, K.N., Roberts, G., Hicks, C.B. and Finnern, H.W. (2008) Cost-effectiveness of tipranavir in treatment experienced HIV patients in the United States. *HIV Clinical Trials*, **9**, 225–237.

Spiegelhalter, D.J. and Best, N.G. (2003) Bayesian approaches to multiple sources of evidence and uncertainty in complex cost-effectiveness modelling. *Statistics in Medicine*, **22**, 3687–3709.

Stinnett, A.A. and Mulahy, J. (1998) Net health benefits: a new framework for the analysis of uncertainty in cost-effectiveness analysis. *Medical Decision Making*, **18**, 68–80.

Sutton, A. and Abrams, K. (2001) Bayesian methods in meta-analysis and evidence synthesis. *Statistical Methods in Medical Research*, **10**, 277–303.

Thompson, S.G. and Barber, J.A. (2000) How should cost data in pragmatic randomised trials be analysed? *British Medical Journal*, **320**, 1197–1200.

Thompson, S.G. and Nixon, R.M. (2005) How sensitive are cost-effectiveness analyses to choice of parametric distributions? *Medical Decision Making*, **25**, 416–423.

van Hout, B., Al, M. and Gordon, G. (1994) Costs, effects and c/e ratios alongside a clinical trial. *Health Economics*, **3**, 309–319.

Willan, A.R. (2001) Analysis, sample size, and power for estimating incremental net health benefit from clinical trial data. *Controlled Clinical Trials*, **22**, 228–237.

Willan, A.R. and Briggs, A. (2006) *Statistical Analysis of Cost-effectiveness Data*, John Wiley & Sons, Ltd.

# 19

# Costing and performance in healthcare management

**Rosanna Tarricone and Aleksandra Torbica**
*Department of Policy Analysis and Public Management, Centre for Research on Health and Social Care Management, CERGAS – Università Bocconi, Milan, Italy*

## Synopsis

This chapter describes and discusses the methods for cost analysis of healthcare services in order to assess and compare the economic value of health outputs at the level of healthcare organizations. The economic principles underpinning the assessment of the value of healthcare services – opportunity costs and shadow prices – are illustrated in Section 19.2; whereas the management accounting approach to cost services is described in Section 19.3. The key features of micro-costing and gross-costing are also discussed and their relevance explained according to the investigators' goals. The full costing is argued as the cost classification that better suits economic requirements for assessing the value of healthcare services. The technical phases that need to be taken to calculate full costs are also illustrated in Section 19.3. Section 19.4 discusses how costs and tariffs can be used to assess profitability of services delivery and benchmarking analysis across providers. The discussion of a case vignette helps in clarifying the use of costs and tariffs by decision-makers when actually applied to hospital services. The last section provides general conclusions and final recommendations on how management accounting principles can help translate economic paradigms in assessing and comparing the value of public productions in the healthcare sector for the decision-making process.

*Statistical Methods in Healthcare*, First Edition.  Edited by Frederick W. Faltin, Ron S. Kenett and Fabrizio Ruggeri.
© 2012 John Wiley & Sons, Ltd.  Published 2012 by John Wiley & Sons, Ltd.

# 19.1   Introduction

The issue of pricing and tariff setting in the public sector has been extensively investigated by both economic and management theory literature. The topic has frequently been used to underlie the conceptual differences in the objectives and methods adopted by these two disciplines. Microeconomics, a discipline that largely relies on simplifying assumptions and modelling in order to describe the general rules of behaviour, has provided several models for pricing public services, among which the marginal cost model appears dominant. Prices should equal marginal costs that accurately reflect the social opportunities foregone (opportunity costs) considering that the resources are drawn from alternative sources. The use of marginal costs in the public domain is however challenging, both from theoretical and from practical points of view, as illustrated in the following section. Management theory underpinning pricing of services in the public sector provides an attempt to overcome these limitations and adopts more relaxed assumptions in describing the actual behaviour of organizations, as illustrated in Section 19.4. Two basic approaches exist to determine prices and tariffs: (1) market-oriented pricing (competition and demand based), and (2) cost-based pricing. The underlying principle in the competition-oriented framework is that price and tariff level are decided based upon those applied by the competitors in the market. The competition-oriented model has gained importance in the public sector over the years, mainly due to full or partial liberalization taking place in many fields of public activity. The driving assumption is that the increased competition will improve, directly or indirectly through the incentives for innovation, the quality and the quantity of services provided in the market, which will benefit the society as a whole. While acknowledging the importance of both approaches, in this chapter the focus is extensively on the cost-based pricing, in line with the general focus of the book. More specifically, we extensively discuss the use of cost-based pricing for determining tariffs for reimbursement of hospital services and performance assessment.

# 19.2   Theoretical approaches to costing healthcare services: Opportunity cost and shadow price

Since economic resources are limited, any decision to undertake a healthcare programme will divert resources from an alternative use. Therefore there is an opportunity cost to carrying out the expenditure. This means that the benefits to be derived from the expenditure in question should be compared to the benefits that would have been obtained if the money had been used elsewhere. This is the concept of opportunity cost. If we put it the other way round, we essentially require a measure of the willingness-to-pay (WTP) for the forgone programme.

In essence what we have to measure when we are dealing with the costs of a healthcare programme is the opportunity cost of using a resource in the programme instead of its best alternative. This is valued by its shadow price. Shadow prices are identical to market prices under certain conditions; namely those of perfect competition where market prices equal marginal costs. However, the majority of markets depart from the ideal competitive model. There are, in addition, goods and services that are not sold on the market. Health and education are two typical examples. In all these cases market prices do not correspond to the value of the resources, or, just do not exist (Baumol and Blinder, 1994). This does not mean, however, that those resources do not have a price. If there is not an observable price, or the observable price is misleading, there is a shadow price, since each unit must have an opportunity cost in terms of some forgone alternative. The technical rule says that if a physical unit exists it must also be possible to find a shadow price that is the WTP of society for those resources (Mishan, 1988).

Shadow prices can be ascribed by using several strategies. Firstly, a consumer question-naire can be used. This relates to the method of using surveys to elicit consumers' WTP. Second, there may be markets for similar goods outside the public sector (e.g. private sector). Thirdly, the cost of providing a service could be used to indicate its social value. The assumption is that revenue costs, with the addition of capital costs and overheads, can serve as reasonable proxies of long-run marginal costs (Allen and Beecham, 1993). The first approach may be cumbersome to implement and the second one is not always feasible when healthcare services are the object of the analysis; therefore the assessment of production costs to provide healthcare services is the preferred option and the focus of the present work.

## 19.3   Costing healthcare services

Costing healthcare services requires one to identify all cost-generating components and attribute a monetary value to them.

Two methods can be used to cost services: the micro-costing and the gross-costing approach (Gold et al., 1996). With the first method, the cost of a service is assessed by summing up each single cost component (input) that has contributed to the provision of the service. If – for instance – the service to be evaluated is 'hospital admission', resources (personnel, medications, tests, meals etc.) used to produce the service need to be identified, measured and evaluated to be summed up. This means that the micro-costing is a 'bottom-up' approach; that is, the calculation of production (full) costs consists of transferring inputs to outputs. Conversely, with the gross-costing approach, the cost of a service (e.g. hospital admission) is assessed in a 'top-down' fashion, that is by dividing total costs of the service unit (e.g. hospital ward) by the total number of services (e.g. admissions) produced in a period of time. The two methods both aim at assessing unit costs of the services; however the level of precision attained by them is quite different. The result of the micro-costing approach is the 'actual' cost of the service; while the 'average' cost is the product of the gross-costing approach (Tarricone, 2006).

The micro-costing approach is very accurate and can in some ways be considered the 'gold standard' for cost assessment. Nevertheless, it is costly and time consuming, and its extensive use must be weighed against the benefits derived by such a detailed analysis. As a general rule, it can be stated that micro-costing is preferred because it spells out the production and cost functions related to the service under study and allows others to see how well the analysis matches their situation, where patterns of care may differ. Micro-costing is suggested when among the aims of the research analysis is that of highlighting the cost differences related to the service under consideration. Special attention must however be paid to the representativeness and comparability of such costs (Schulman et al., 1998; Raikou et al., 2000; Koopmanschap, Touw and Rutten, 2001) given that it is very likely that they differ across healthcare providers. Some relevant work has been aimed at ascertaining the transparency and comparability of costing data coming from either gross-costing (top-down) and micro-costing (bottom-up) approaches in multi-centre studies (Wordsworth et al., 2005). Findings reveal that, overall, the micro-costing approach provides greater consistency and transparency than the gross-costing since it details the cost components (Wordsworth *et al.*, 2005). Nevertheless, since the micro-costing approach is time consuming, it is important to evaluate when it is worth adopting. There are healthcare services whose main components are less sensitive to how budgets are formed and spread in healthcare centres. This means that micro- and gross-costing approaches would tend to similar results, thus not making a case for the micro-costing approach. Conversely, for services with a significant component of staff input and overheads, and significant sharing of staff or facilities between patient groups, a micro-costing approach is the best approach, since by detailing cost components it enhances comparability.

## 19.3.1    Measuring full costs of healthcare services

The question 'How much does the product cost?' is one of the most difficult to answer for any firm. Cost accountancy principles can help to respond to this question by measuring resources. A definition of cost accountancy is given by Maggert (1985): 'Cost accountancy is a system of accounting and engineering that identifies, to the lowest level of detail reasonably possible, all material and labour component costs of a product, and combines them with an allocation of applicable overhead costs to arrive at a total product costs' (Maggert, 1985).

While the assessment of the production costs for a single-product firm is fairly easy, the measurement of production costs for multi-product firms – as is the case for many healthcare providers – is much more complex since each product requires different quantities of resources and costs them differently. In general, the measurement of production costs consists of transferring inputs to outputs and involves the following steps (Anthony and Young, 2003; Mogyorosy and Smith, 2005):

1. definition of the cost object (output);

2. classification and evaluation of cost components (direct vs. non-direct costs);

3. selection of allocation methods;

4. calculation of full costs.

## 19.3.2    Definition of the cost object (output)

The definition of the output/activity is the first step in the measurement of production costs. Products cannot be defined easily in healthcare firms (Cleverley, 1987). The major dilemma arises in the area of patients versus products. The activity of a hospital, for instance, can be measured in bed days, or number of treated patients. A bed day can in its turn consist of other activities necessary to produce the final output (e.g. laboratory tests, meals). It can be stated, however, that a treated patient rather than an individual service provided in isolation generates revenue. This means that the wide range of services provided to patients, such as nursing, prescriptions and tests, should be viewed as intermediate products and not as final products. Although it can be generalised that patients are the final products of any healthcare provider, this does not prevent us from considering each single service (e.g. laboratory test, meal) as the object of our costing analysis. Whatever the cost object, a clear definition of the output and of all the activities necessary to produce it is relevant since it helps determine the product differences. The same output can be produced in different ways by combining a different number and types of intermediate activities. Looking at how intermediate services are produced and successively combined to treat the patient helps decision makers control the production process that is mainly managed by the physician. The lack of authority in this area is perhaps the greatest difference between healthcare firms and other business entities. Management at BMW can decide which automobiles will have factory-installed air conditioning and tinted glass. A hospital will find it very difficult to direct physicians to prescribe or not prescribe a given procedure when treating a patient.

Moreover, the clear definition of the cost object is important also for benchmarking analysis aimed at comparing the costs of single services (e.g. specialist visit) or treatment episodes (e.g. ambulatory rehabilitation) by different providers in a given time period or conversely by the same providers across different time periods (Finkler, 1994, 2001; Lucey, 2002).

### 19.3.3    Classification of cost components (direct vs. non-direct costs)

Inputs differ in two ways. They can be variable or fixed and direct or non-direct (Anthony and Young, 2003). Inputs are variable when there is a positive relationship with the output produced. Conversely, fixed costs remain constant as output increases. Inputs are direct when they can be attributed to the cost object directly. If a medical ward activity is the output to be measured, doctors represent an example of direct costs. If a treated patient is the output to be measured instead, doctors represent an example of direct and indirect costs as the cost of their time can be split into activities that are directly attributable to the patient's treatment and other activities that are only indirectly related to patients' treatment (e.g. training, co-ordinating a meeting).

Non-direct costs relate to inputs not directly attributed to a particular cost object, but need to be shared over a number of them. A further distinction is made between indirect costs and overheads or between supporting services and overhead activities (Goldschmidt and Gafni, 1990). Indirect resources are defined as resources that provide measurable services to other units/departments in an organisation so that there is a traceable, cause-and-effect relationship between the provider and user of the service. Examples are the laboratory and pharmacy in a hospital. Overhead 'activities', on the other hand, are those activities that contribute to the production of the final output but are not related in any way to the quantity or volume of the output; that is, they do not have a traceable, cause-and-effect relationship with other units/departments because there is no direct way to measure the consumption of the overhead activity's output. Management and Accounting, for instance, falls into this category.

### 19.3.4    Selection of allocation methods

Allocative methods and an allocative basis must be used to attribute non-direct costs (indirect costs and overheads) to the final output. The allocation of indirect costs stems from the need to know the full cost (e.g. variable and fixed direct costs plus variable and fixed non-direct costs) of providing a final product as opposed to the direct cost. A direct costing approach (variable and fixed direct costs) might, in some cases, suit short-term decisions; however in the long run such an approach leads to distorted decisions, since non-direct costs are ignored by decision makers. The rationale for considering non-direct costs is that all resources can be used in alternative ways in the long term and there is therefore an opportunity cost to using them. Furthermore, they may account for as much as 50% of total costs (Goldschmidt and Gafni, 1990) and excluding them from the calculus may lead decision makers to make inconsistent decisions and evaluations.

One of the major difficulties of allocating non-direct costs is that these costs are partially fixed with respect to changes in the level of service provided. It is stated that fixed costs – those that are held at a constant level, independent of the level of production – should be excluded from the analysis. Thus, costs should not be included for inputs or outputs that are unaffected by changes in the intensity or frequency of an intervention or are unaffected by decisions to do or not do the intervention (Gold et al., 1996). However, most input costs that are fixed in the short run will in fact be variable in the long run. For instance, the cost of the administrative staff of a hospital would be the same irrespective of the number of admissions per day. This happens for the cost of the facility as well. However, these costs are fixed in the short run but can be freed and re-allocated to alternative uses in the long run. Given this perspective, short-term variable cost is an insufficient measure of production cost (Cooper and Kaplan, 1987). Thus, a full costing approach which includes fixed non-direct costs is the method here suggested in the cost estimation of health inputs.

Different methods have been developed to allocate indirect costs and overheads (Karmarkar and Pitbladdo, 1993).

The simplest method among those reviewed by Drummond et al. (2005) concerns the direct allocation to the final activity based on suitable measures of consumption. The direct allocation ignores interaction of overhead departments; that is each overhead is allocated directly to final cost centres (e.g. clinical wards). More sophisticated methods go from a step-down allocation with or without iterations to a simultaneous allocation (Drummond et al., 2005). These last methods do consider interaction of overhead departments.

Conventionally, indirect costs are allocated to the users in proportion to the level of consumption. Practically, this can be seen as dividing indirect costs by the allocation base (measure of usage) to arrive at a per-unit allocation rate. The major problem in using the allocation rate for charging the indirect costs to users is that the allocation rate depends upon both the efficiency level of the provider and the activity volume of other users (Goldschmidt and Gafni, 1990). The efficiency level of the provider affects the total cost of the service, and the activity volume of other users affects the per-unit cost. This allocation method can be misleading and highly distortive. Managers of user units are frustrated by conventional allocations as they are charged with categories of cost over which they have no control or accountability (that is why they often prefer the direct costing approach). Overhead providers on the other hand do not have any incentive to increase efficiency since the cost of their activity is borne by other units. They all address the problem of 'who consumes' but do not take much into account 'how much' is consumed. A classic example is the cost of security services apportioned by floor area; a pharmacy manager, with a small floor area who places a high value on having dangerous drugs protected, pays less than the canteen manager who is unfortunate enough to require a large floor area for production. In an attempt to move away from these measures, Goldschmidt and Gafni (1990) suggested that: (1) the fixed costs of a supporting service should be charged to the factor that creates the demand for the service, using the dual-rate-charging method; and (2) the overhead costs should be charged to the binding constraint of the organisation (the bottleneck to increasing output).

The dual-rate-charging method is commonly used by many electric and gas providers in USA as well as in other countries like Italy. Users are basically billed for two charges: (1) a charge for the right to use the service, based on the fixed costs; and (2) a charge for the actual use, based on the variable costs. Some healthcare organisations may be characterised by a seasonal demand which represents the bottleneck. This happens for instance to many district hospitals in Italy that are located in small tourist cities, whose population increases 10 times during the summer. In this case the peak season is where the bottleneck falls, because in other periods there is idle capacity. If we were to allocate for instance the fixed costs of the radiology equipment, the usage of equipment in the peak season can be used as the allocation base for capacity costs. The suggested method of allocating overheads is that of finding the binding constraint, that is, the bottleneck in the production process, and to use it as an allocative base.

The method suggested by Goldschmidt and Gafni goes someway in the same direction traced by activity-based costing (ABC), a methodology that has gained importance and that emphasises the identification of the activities that drive the final cost of a service (Cooper, 1988; Goldschmidt and Gafni, 1990). ABC basically tries to overcome the distortions introduced by conventional cost systems that use volume-related allocation bases (e.g. direct labour hours, direct costs) alone to trace costs to products also when some of the product-related activities are unrelated to volume.

### 19.3.5    Calculation of full costs

Once one has identified the object of the cost analysis, measured direct costs and allocated non-direct costs, the production cost is given by summing up each cost component, as better illustrated in the following sections where the measurement of full costs of healthcare services is clarified by using a concrete example.

## 19.4    Costing for decision making: Tariff setting in healthcare

Prices and tariffs in the public sector are meant to satisfy numerous, frequently contrasting aims, and they are adopted in the presence of several constraints (political, ethical, administrative and technical) (Bean and Hussey, 1996). The two terms (prices and tariffs) are sometimes used interchangeably since tariffs may be understood as a special case of 'prices' where pricing levels are not determined by market forces, but are centrally set or negotiated.

In general, prices and tariffs in the public sector are used for two main objectives:

1. to cover the production costs of services providers (cost recovery)

2. to orient behaviour of consumers and service providers.

The two objectives can be pursued with different intensity; that is, one may be more important than the other according to current health policy agenda. In some cases, the public entity may decide to forego one of these two objectives. This is the case for public goods and services with negative demand, for which free-of-charge provision is the only way to incentivise the consumption (e.g. vaccination). In other situations, tariffs may be set above the production costs so as to generate additional revenues (surplus). This can be justified by public entities in order to generate revenues to subsidize other services that are provided either below cost or free at the point of consumption.

Following this short general overview, we focus on one specific application of a cost-based model for tariff setting in the healthcare field: the definition of tariffs for hospital reimbursement under a prospective payments scheme. We choose this example to illustrate advantages but also possible risks in using a cost-based approach in determining tariffs. Finally, this example allows us to discuss how costing methods and tariffs may be used to measure and compare one particular aspect of hospitals' performance, as illustrated below.

## 19.4.1    General features of cost-based pricing and tariff setting

In general, a cost-oriented approach implies that prices/tariffs of goods and services are based predominantly on the production costs, while the issues relating to market forces (competition or demand) are neglected or not considered at all. The rationale for tariff setting is cost recovery. Under this approach, it is argued that all the relevant costs must be included in the cost calculation, because in the long run no service is sustainable if all costs are not covered. This is defined as *full cost pricing* and is based on full absorption costing (Finkler, 1994).

In principle, setting prices or tariffs on the basis of full costs should ensure that revenues cover production costs, thus allowing public organizations to pursue long-run economic equilibrium. Second, it should be based on objective data, straightforward and easy to monitor (audit). For these reasons, the full costing approach to tariff setting has been and continues to be widely used in the public sector. Although widely used, full cost pricing has been extensively challenged both from the theoretical (conceptual) and practical (implementation) points of view.

From the conceptual viewpoint, full cost pricing was first criticized for its intrinsic inequality. Vertical inequality cannot be avoided if all consumers are required to pay the same tariff for certain services. The level of sacrifice associated with the tariff will vary greatly across various groups of consumers based on their income, among other factors. This objection has often resulted in introducing multiple tariffs, the application of which does undermine, however, the rationale behind the full cost principle. Second, full cost pricing was accused of incentivising inefficiencies, especially if applied to services produced in non-competitive markets (e.g. monopolies). In these cases, it is necessary to control for costs' increase, to analyze the reasons for that increase and decide whether it should result in an increase in tariffs. Third, by introducing full cost pricing, public organizations renounce the pursuit of the 'behavioural effect' of tariff application. In this model, in fact, prices are simply a function of costs.

From the practical point of view, the main problem with full cost pricing is how to define and calculate full costs of the service under consideration, as already explained in Section 19.3.

Further problems in setting tariffs for specific goods and services on the basis of full cost estimation refer to economies of scope and scale. Economies of scope occur when the full cost of joint production is less than the cost of producing the individual products. In other words, the cost of a particular product or service can be affected by the production of other products or the delivery of other services. Economies of scope exist whenever the costs of providing two or more services jointly by the same organization are less than the costs of providing them separately. This is relevant for healthcare services that are normally delivered by multi-product organizations. Economies of scale, on the other hand, refer to reductions in unit cost as the size of the facility and the usage levels of other inputs increase. For example, a hospital that achieves economies of scale lowers the average cost per 'hospital admission' through increased volume of activity since fixed costs (that normally represent a significant share of hospital costs) are shared over an increased number of products.

## 19.4.2    Cost-based tariff setting in practice: Prospective payments system for hospital services reimbursement

In this section we describe one concrete application of costing for decision making in healthcare: the definition of tariffs for hospital reimbursement. In general, tariffs exchanged between payers and providers of healthcare services may have different forms and can aim at remunerating either single procedures (i.e. fee for service) or cases (Langenbrunner and Wiley, 2002). The most widely used payment system is based on diagnosis-related group (DRG) classification. Development of DRGs began in the late sixties at Yale University in order to create an effective framework for monitoring utilization of services in a hospital setting. The DRG system was originally developed as a system for describing hospital production (Fetter, Freeman and Mullin, 1985; Fetter, 1991, 1999). DRGs operationally define the hospital product in terms of classes of patients with similar expected patterns of resource use.

A few decades after its original inception, DRG classification was used by the US Federal Government for defining a prospective payment system in order to fund hospital care for Medicare patients (Fetter, 1992). In this most well-known application of a DRG system, each group is assigned a specific 'value' (tariff) reflecting the intensity of resource consumption needed to treat patients assigned to that group. In this way, hospitals are being reimbursed a fixed amount based on the diseases and procedures of a patient, regardless of what services have actually been delivered to treat the patient. Thus, hospitals may sustain losses if their accrual costs exceed the tariff, or enjoy profits if their costs are below. In this way, the role of DRGs as a payment mechanism is not only aimed at reimbursing providers, but also encouraging efficient delivery and discouraging provision of unnecessary services. A plethora of studies investigated to what extent the DRG-based reimbursement system succeeded in achieving these objectives.[1]

After its adoption in the USA, the approach eventually migrated to most healthcare systems in affluent countries, both social-insurance and National Health Service based. Over the past 20 years, most European countries have introduced DRGs or similar grouping systems as instruments for hospital services reimbursement (Schreyogg et al., 2006).

Consistently with the incentives created by the new funding arrangements, public and private hospitals have developed cost accounting systems to understand the impact of the new funding mechanisms on economic performance and to exert more control on their organizational units. In general, following the introduction of DRGs, hospitals regularly perform cost accounting exercises to evaluate performance of their units, to make service production decisions (e.g. expanding volume of care in particular areas) and to make simulations about revenues and costs (e.g. break-even analysis). Thus, it became evident that using appropriate costing methodologies is of paramount importance, since different methods would inevitably lead to different results.

Although costing is an essential part of DRG tariff determination in all countries, further elements influencing the tariff setting should be mentioned. These elements stem from the important objective of the tariff-based funding to steer providers' behaviour, and sometimes are called 'adjustment factors' (Schreyogg et al., 2006). For example, DRG tariffs may be used to provide incentives for the provision of specific services (i.e. higher reimbursement for services provided in day hospital regime) or to correct undesired outcomes of the funding

---

[1] For a recent review on the topic see: EuroDRG project at http://www.eurodrg.eu.

system (selection of patients). In these cases, cost analysis underpinning the definition of a tariff is important but not sufficient to define its final value. These considerations must be taken into account when using a DRG-based system as a framework for evaluation of profitability or benchmarking analysis.

## 19.5    Costing, tariffs and performance evaluation

Beyond pricing and tariff setting, the information on full costs of carrying out a particular service may be used for two additional aims: (1) profitability assessment (by comparing costs with tariffs), and (2) comparative analysis (i.e. benchmarking by comparing costs across providers) (Anthony and Young, 2003). As to profitability assessment, full costing estimation is essential to assess whether a particular service or programme is making or losing money. This information is fundamental to pursue financial viability, the cornerstone principle for all types of organizations, even non-profit institutions that must recover the full costs of providing services to remain financially viable over the long run. Full cost information may also assist in undertaking a cost comparison across different organizations that deliver similar products or services. In short, the information on full costs of healthcare services is important in performance evaluation no matter whether the comparison is being done across different time periods of the same hospital or across different hospitals.

For completeness, it is important to clarify how we define performance, considering it is a very wide term. Propper and Wilson (2006) discuss a variety of forms of performance measurement at different levels. At the hospital level of performance they distinguish between measures of outcome and measures of process (Propper and Wilson, 2006). While acknowledging the importance of both, they recognize that outcome measures (for example inpatient mortality) are often the result of factors outside the control of the healthcare system and consequently cannot always provide useful guidelines to the decision makers on what to do to improve the performance. On the other hand, process measures can provide insights on the production function and inform about possible improvements to achieve the same level of output (i.e. efficiency).

Following this line of reasoning, in this chapter we define performance in terms of process measurement and we illustrate a concrete example of how costing analysis together with information on DRG tariffs can be used for hospitals' performance evaluation and benchmarking.[2]

The study was conducted in five hospitals in three Regions in Italy, and the final aim was (1) to analyze differences in the costs of hospital services and (2) to assess the profitability of hospital services vis-à-vis regional tariffs.

In order to achieve these objectives, we adopted a novel approach, developed within the EU HealthBasket project, termed 'case vignette' (Busse, Schreyogg and Smith, 2008). In essence, case vignettes are defined as reasonably detailed descriptions of different episodes of care. The case vignettes depict 'typical patients' including age, gender and relevant co-morbidity. In this way, the potential differences due to patient mix are standardized, and observed variations in costs are investigated in relation to other explanatory variables. In other words,

---

[2] The empirical analysis presented in this chapter was conducted within a wider research project, HealthBasket, aimed at identifying and developing methodology for cost comparison between nine EU countries. For further information on the HealthBasket project, please refer to: www.ehma.org/index.php?q=node/81).

the estimates obtained are sensitive to clinical decisions regarding treatment patterns and unit costs of resources used, thus providing an adequate framework for performance evaluation. Detailed description of the method and its advantages and limitations in comparative cost assessment study has already been published (Busse, Schreyogg and Smith, 2008).

The cost assessment was performed following the phases adopted by the accounting approach as described in Section 19.3:

1. definition of final cost object (output);

2. classification and evaluation of cost components (direct vs. non-direct costs);

3. Selection of allocative methods and allocative basis;

4. calculation of the full costs.

## 19.5.1    Definition of final cost object

The precise definition of the final cost object is of fundamental importance in cost comparison studies. In our example, the final cost object was a patient hospitalized with acute myocardial infarction as described by the case vignette (Box 19.1). The choice of this acute myocardial infarction (AMI) was driven by the following main reasons. First, AMI is a very common disease that, together with other heart-related disorders, represents a major cause of overall mortality and morbidity in adults. Consequently, it is a frequently treated condition in hospitals. Second, the number of treatment and diagnostic strategies has been significantly enriched in recent years due to important technological advancements in cardiology. Thus, AMI represents a suitable case study for investigating different choices and associated costs in comparative cross-provider analysis (Tiemann, 2008).

**Box 19.1**    Case vignette on acute myocardial infarction (AMI)

Healthy male, 50–60 yrs old, without relevant comorbidities developed a sudden acute chest pain. An ambulance is called and transports the patient within 2 hours since the onset of symptoms to hospital. The patient shows typical ECG alterations and is admitted and treated for AMI. The patient is diagnosed and treated according to adopted clinical practice in the hospital. No significant complications occur and progress is as expected for patient age group. At the end of hospitalization period, patient is discharged to rehabilitative institution or home.

(Tiemann, 2008)

## 19.5.2    Classification and evaluation of cost components

In order to assess the full cost of the cost object defined in the previous step, it is necessary to identify and evaluate all inputs necessary to produce it. The inputs were classified as direct or non-direct according to a standard framework (see Section 19.3.3).

The direct cost components were assessed through a micro-costing, bottom-up approach, and the process consisted of two distinct phases: (1) measurement of the quantities and (2) monetary evaluation of resources used.

Data on quantity of resources used for treating the AMI patient were gathered using ad-hoc designed questionnaires administered to clinicians and administrative staff. A questionnaire was developed to allow accurate documentation of the services that the patient of the case vignette would have received. In order to facilitate the identification of resources used, each episode of care was articulated in different phases following the temporal axis (admission, hospital stay, discharge). These methods are deemed appropriate in cases where patients use a wide range of services over a particular period. An observer-based questionnaire and/or interview is argued to be more accurate if compared to a self-reported questionnaire, but it can be time consuming and costly to administer (Johnston *et al.*, 2001).

The quantity of the following resource items (direct costs) was measured: personnel time (time spent directly for the patient); drugs; medical devices; diagnostic, imaging and lab tests; disposables and procedure time (time spent in the operating room). The unit costs for all direct cost components were estimated on the basis of information provided by the hospital Accounting Department.

Non-direct costs components included indirect costs and hospital overheads. In short, *indirect costs* referred to resources attributed to the Service Unit (e.g. personnel time, cleaning, supervision time, meals, maintenance) that are not attributed to individual patients and thus need to be indirectly allocated to patients. *Hospital overheads* referred to costs that are not directly associable to final activities for the patients but that contribute anyway to the overall functioning of the hospital. These include the cost for the administration (personnel, accounting etc.), commercial costs, janitorial activities, central health activities (e.g. prevention of infections) and costs of other resources that are not traced to individual wards or intermediate organisation units.

As to the costs of personnel, the direct and indirect components were determined by asking staff members to estimate the proportion of time spent in caring for patients and carrying out those activities (e.g. co-ordinating a meeting) that are not directly attributable to single patients. Based on staff estimation, we assumed that 50% of the time of personnel is spent on direct patient care. The remaining 50% was therefore part of indirect costs and allocated to each case using direct allocation methods as described below.

### 19.5.3    Selection of allocative methods and allocative basis

The overheads allocation process requires two inputs: the amount of costs to be allocated and criteria for allocation (allocation base). In the present example, ward overheads, hospital overheads and the personnel indirect care costs (as defined above) were allocated to the final cost object (case vignette) using the direct allocation method. The basis for allocation was total number of hospital days (length of stay; LOS). More precisely, total non-direct costs (indirect and overheads) were divided by the total number of days, and the resulting rate was multiplied by the average length of stay (ALOS) of the vignette case as reported by the clinician.

### 19.5.4    Calculation of the full costs

Having identified the object of the cost analysis, measured and evaluated direct costs and allocated indirect costs and overheads, the cost of output is given by summing up each cost component.

Full costs of output = Direct costs for treated patient + Share of Service Unit indirect costs
+ Share of hospital overheads.

## 19.5.5  Results

The final results of the cost analysis in the five hospitals are presented in Table 19.1. In all hospitals, the treatment of choice for the patients fitting the description of the case vignette was percutaneous transluminal coronary angioplasty (PTCA) with coronary stents. The duration of the procedure is similar across hospitals. However, there are great differences as to type of stents employed in the procedure. With the exception of hospital H5 that uses the more costly drug eluting stents (DES) for 90% of AMI patients, other providers use the less innovative bare metal stents (BMS) for the majority of cases (80% in H2 and H3; 70% in H1). BMS are used in all cases treated in H4.

After the procedure, patients are treated in intensive care coronary care units (CCUs) and then transferred to the cardiology ward. While this practice is in some ways standard and

**Table 19.1**  Resource use and costs for an acute myocardial infarction patient in five hospitals (H1–H5).

| | H1 | H2 | H3 | H4 | H5 | Mean | Standard deviation |
|---|---|---|---|---|---|---|---|
| **Resources** | | | | | | | |
| ALOS (days) | | | | | | | |
|    Coronary care unit | 3 | 2 | 2 | 1.5 | 2 | **2.1** | **0.5** |
|    Cardiology ward | 7 | 3.5 | 4 | 3 | 8[a] | **4.4** | **1.8** |
|    Total | 10 | 5.5 | 6 | 4.5 | 10 | **7.2** | **2.6** |
| Duration of PTCA | 60 | 90 | 90 | 60 | 60 | **72** | **16.4** |
|    procedure (min) | | | | | | | |
| Drug eluting stents (%) | 30 | 20 | 20 | 0 | 90 | **32** | **34** |
| Personnel time (min/day) | | | | | | | |
|    Cardiologist | 30–60 | 20–30 | 45–60 | 20–60 | 20–60 | **40** | |
|    Nurses | 45–180 | 90–165 | 60–120 | 40–75 | 40–120 | **94** | |
| **Direct costs** | | | | | | | |
|    Personnel | 853 | 653 | 869 | 333 | 1557 | 853 | 449 |
|    Drugs | 1051 | 923 | 578 | 650 | 342 | 709 | 282 |
|    Exams (lab and | 586 | 556 | 499 | 242 | 463 | 469 | 136 |
|    diagnostic) | | | | | | | |
|    Devices | 1153 | 1067 | 1244 | 590 | 1900 | 1958 | 470 |
|    Disposables | 1589 | 880 | 927 | 784 | 440 | | |
| **Total direct cost** | **5232** | **4079** | **4117** | **2598** | **4703** | **4298** | **986** |
| **Personnel indirect costs** | **1752** | **1291** | **909** | **731** | **1992** | **1335** | **537** |
| **Non-direct costs** | | | | | | | |
|    Service Unit (ward) | 737 | 1222 | 773 | 404 | 1286 | 423 | 367 |
|    Hospital | 1168 | 1284 | 1158 | 652 | 637 | 980 | 310 |
| **Total** | **1904** | **2505** | **1931** | **1055** | **1922** | **1864** | **518** |
| **Grand total** | **8888** | **7875** | **6958** | **4385** | **8616** | **7344** | **1816** |
| **Regional tariff** | **7878** | **7878** | **7878** | **7216** | **7437** | | |

[a]Out of which, 6 days in semi-intensive care unit.

implemented by all hospitals, significant differences are observed in patients' length of stay, which ranged from 4.5 days in H4 to 10 days in H1 and H5. The differences were particularly evident in the number of days spent in the cardiology ward (ranging from 3 days in H4 to 8 days in H5), while the length of stay in CCUs appears rather similar.

As to personnel time dedicated to patient care, estimates appear similar across hospitals. On average, physicians dedicate approximately 60 and 30 minutes a day to patient care in CCU and cardiology ward, respectively. Nurses, on the other hand, spend 132 and 55 minutes a day in the two settings respectively.

The average total costs for treating the AMI patient (as described in the case vignette) were €7344, ranging from a minimum of €4385 in H4 to €8888 in H1. The reasons for these significant differences in total costs can be explained by looking at the different cost components.

One of the cost components presenting significant differences was personnel. Across all phases of AMI treatment, from emergency room to discharge, these costs range from €333 (H4) to €1557 (H5) and reflect both the different length of stay and the different amount of time spent by physicians and nurses to treat the case illustrated in the vignette. The H5 employs a higher amount of personnel resources for a longer period of time due to the presence of a semi-intensive care unit where patients' monitoring is more intense than in a normal ward. This type of Unit is present exclusively in H5. H4 has a much lower value for direct personnel costs because of a much shorter length of stay.

Considering that all five providers adopt PTCA with stents as the treatment of choice, this is reflected in high costs for hemodynamic laboratory and devices. All but H4 spend about €2000 for medical devices and disposables used during the procedure. Cost variability is due to the type of devices used to perform PTCAs, and in part to their unit cost. More specifically, unit costs for DES varied from €1920 to €2350 and for BMS from €590 to €1100. The BMS is used in all cases treated in H4, and consequently the device costs result is significantly lower for this provider.

As underlined above, the use of CCUs appears more homogeneous than the use of the Cardiology ward. While, for the former, data show a variation from 1.5 to 3 days, for the latter, the range goes from 2 to 8 days. These differences explain the different amount of overheads attributed in the five hospitals given that overheads are allocated according to the direct allocation method with the allocative basis being the length of stay (i.e. overheads are calculated per day of stay and then multiplied by the number of days reported for the case of interest). Therefore, large variations in LOS should have resulted in large variations of overheads across the five hospitals. Instead, overheads are relatively similar. This similarity is much more evident if H4, somehow the outlier for this vignette, is excluded: overheads per case vary from €1904 to €2505. This is because hospitals with longer LOS have lower overheads per day.

Given these findings, it is important to identify key issues that can help correctly interpret the estimates. We strongly believe that direct costs are more appropriate to analyze and compare how the five hospitals manage AMI patients. For example, despite all providers adopting the same procedure for AMI patients (i.e. PTCA), LOS greatly differs and this probably indicates different clinical attitudes and different intensity in the use of hospital resources. In addition, choice of medical technology varies greatly across the five hospitals, reflecting different clinical patterns and propensities of clinicians to use innovative technologies vs. traditional ones.

The allocation of overheads is significantly more problematic. From one side this allocation is important because modern medicine involves complex organizations, many very important activities that aim to make direct care safe and effective, and relevant administrative costs. This means that decisions regarding the estimates of total overheads and, more importantly, the system to allocate them to 'cost objectives' have a relevant impact on cost estimates. Our results show that overheads are a driver of cost variability across providers. We do think that an important source of variation in the overheads is due to the way they are estimated and apportioned. Given the lack of precise and standardized rules across providers, there is the risk that differences are due to different accounting decisions. For this reason we urge caution when comparing overheads across providers. In addition, we suggest thinking about the possibility of standardizing the way overhead costs are apportioned to services, while we are aware that consensus on the basic scientific principles will not be enough to ensure meaningful comparability.

As to profitability assessment, cost estimates are very close to reimbursement tariffs. If we exclude H4, hospitals have total costs, inclusive of overheads, ranging from €6958 to €8888. This interval is relatively narrow (about 20% of the mean value) and close to the reimbursement fees that stay in the €7000–8000 range. However, it is important to underline that reimbursement tariffs vary slightly among the three geographical Regions represented in the sample. Thus, in our sample, it is difficult to reach any definitive conclusion on the possible impact of tariffs on providers' behaviour. However, it may be noticed that tariffs do not seem to be sufficient to cover costs when more innovative and more costly technologies are used. In the case of H5, where DES are used in 90% of patients, the difference between the total costs and the tariff is around 14% of the total costs. This may be a potential obstacle for a wider use of innovative technologies, although recent evidence showed that tariff values have no significant impact on the diffusion of DES in Italy (Cappellaro, Ghislandi, and Anessi-Pessina, 2011).

## 19.6   Discussion

Cost assessment of hospital services provides valuable information to managers for numerous decision problems. For example, the cost analysis may be used to compare costs of providing services with the revenues obtained through reimbursement tariffs (i.e. profitability assessment), to allow managers to define areas where cross subsidization is required to ensure financial viability of the organization as a whole. Furthermore, cost assessment may be used to perform cost comparison among different healthcare providers and allow managers to identify the most efficient combination of inputs for producing defined outputs. Different decision problems will require different costing methodologies (Anthony and Young, 2003).

With particular focus on hospital services, the following were identified as the main explanatory variables of cost variation across providers: patient mix, diagnostic and treatment (use of technologies, resource intensity) strategies, unit costs for personnel and technologies, and the cost calculation method (Street et al., 2010). From this, it emerges that, for comparative cost analysis, it is fundamental to describe the particular service, including the case mix of the target population and the organizational settings. In addition, cost comparison can be meaningful only if costs are measured in the same way (using standardized costing methodology and reasonably good compliance to it) (Hakkinen and Joumard, 2007; Busse, Schreyogg and Smith, 2008).

The empirical study presented in this chapter provides a valuable contribution in this respect. It sheds light on the important issues to be considered in evaluating and comparing costs of hospital services. While acknowledging theoretical contributions from both economic and accounting literature, it puts major emphasis on challenges faced when applying those principles in practice.

Results of our analysis should also be interpreted in the light of a wider discussion on the use and impact of healthcare performance reports. Bevan (2007) discusses the impact of reporting health system performance on four different stakeholders: third-party payers, patients, physicians and providers (Bevan, 2007). It is argued that providers are the most sensitive of the four groups to performance assessment reports. Bevan further states that outcome measures (for example, hospital mortality) must be closely related to process of care that can be manipulated. In our analysis we focus on the latter by exploring the different combination of inputs across hospitals adopted to treat patients with the same characteristics.

Several limitations of our empirical study must be mentioned. Using case vignettes as the final cost object clearly oversimplifies the clinical reality where resources and costs needed to treat AMI patients may vary substantially. Thus, we cannot state that the cost estimates obtained represent the average costs for treating AMI in Italy. Conversely, they are likely to underestimate the true average costs since they refer to a relatively simple clinical case.

A second limitation, and probably the most important one given the focus of the book, regards the small sample of providers (five hospitals in three regions). This prevented us from using any meaningful statistical tool to further elaborate on our results. We can only state that, if we had more observations, multi-level models would be most appropriate to be able to account for the hierarchical structure of the data and provide more accurate estimates of region-, hospital- and patient-level effects in explaining the cost differences (Tiemann, 2008). While acknowledging this limitation, we must underline that the main focus of our analysis is on the costing of healthcare services and the potential use of this information for evaluating providers' performance in terms of efficiency.

A third limitation concerns the different ability of hospitals included in the study to provide precise estimates of costing data needed for the analysis. None of the five hospitals had readily available costs at patient level. This is mainly because the nature of accounting systems in Italian hospitals takes the ward and not the patient as the principal 'cost object' (Fattore and Torbica, 2006). Italian clinicians are held accountable for the whole functioning of the ward; that is, for the costs they incur and the relationship between costs, volume of care and case mix of the patients. Additional indicators of clinicians' performance include quality and appropriateness of care delivered by the organizational unit under their responsibility. This brings us to the final limitation of the present study. It should be noted that we discussed performance and benchmarking evaluation across hospitals based upon costs assessment only. Examining the quality of services provided, and patients' health outcomes after the hospital treatment, was beyond the focus of the present study. On the basis of our results, we cannot say much on whether the patients treated at H4 (with lowest costs and with lowest adoption rate of innovative technologies) were better or worse than those treated with more costly and innovative technologies, for instance. Thus, to fully evaluate hospital performance, data on health outcomes and not only costs would need to be gathered and compared. Regarding this, it is worth pointing out that Chapter 10 in this volume brings in the different perspective on the performance of hospitals by using the AMI survival rate as the main output measure. In that chapter, the reader may appreciate a more sophisticated statistical analysis (i.e. a hierarchical Bayesian model) to quantify the variations across healthcare providers and to explain the variations with hospital- and patient-level characteristics (see Chapter 10).

## 19.7   Summary

Cost analysis has seldom been of concern for economic analysts in the healthcare field because economists are keen to explain the theoretical framework within which economic evaluation would need to be performed, but they seldom combine theory with practical applications. As regards prices and charges in the healthcare sector, many economists have warned analysts to use them with no adjustments (Mishan, 1988), but few of them have shown how to cost services whenever prices do not reflect the opportunity costs. Most studies use market prices unadjusted, and it has often been remarked that health economists recognise that market imperfections exist in healthcare, unless they are undertaking an economic evaluation (Drummond *et al.*, 2005). While for some cost categories like drugs, medical devices and rehabilitation items (eyeglasses, hearing aids, speech devices etc.), there is a market and prices can be taken as indicative of the marginal costs, in many other cases (hospitalisation, outpatient care, tests, primary care etc.) market values do not reflect the marginal costs as markets do not operate perfectly or do not have a reasonable level of competition. Against this background it is difficult to talk of opportunity cost in the pure sense of welfare economics. Opportunity costs of healthcare alternatives can be proxied by an analysis of the resources employed in production. This means that a separate analysis would need to be performed in order to assess the economic value (full cost) of these services that do not have a market price, or whose price is not deemed representative of the opportunity costs of resources used. The full cost concept is the one that approximates the long-run marginal cost and is therefore put forward as the correct measure for assessing services (Allen and Beecham, 1993; McCrone *et al.*, 1998).

Management accounting principles can serve this purpose and should be used to measure the costs of providing healthcare services. The choice between what has been defined by Gold *et al.* (1996) as gross-costing (that is, gross approaches such as dividing total costs of the service unit by the total number of services) and micro-costing (the direct enumeration and costing-out of every input consumed) must balance the needs of the analysis with the difficulty and expense of obtaining a cost estimate (Gold *et al.*, 1996).

As a general rule it can be stated that micro-costing is preferred because it spells out the production and cost functions related to the service under study and allows others to see how well the analysis matches their situation, where patterns of care may differ. Micro-costing is compulsory when among the aims of the research analysis is that of highlighting the cost differences related to the service under consideration.

In conclusion, it must be underlined that, undoubtedly, the traditional health economics framework provided significant contributions to development of methods for costing health-care services. We argue, however, that in developing guidelines to compare costs across providers and/or against reimbursement tariffs, the cost accounting principles stemming from the management theory should be given greater importance than has been done so far. Given their greater ability to capture important issues at organizational level, we would advise researchers to adopt methodologies more in line with a management approach to costing.

# References

Allen, C. and Beecham, J. (1993) Costing services: ideals and reality, in *Costing Community Care* (eds A. Netten and J. Beecham), Ashgate, p. 25.

Anthony, R.N. and Young, D.W. (2003) *Management Control in Nonprofit Organizations*, McGraw-Hill, New York.

Baumol, W.J. and Blinder, A.S. (1994) *Economics. Principles and Policy*, The Dryden Press, Forth Worth.

Bean, J. and Hussey, L. (1996) *Costing and Pricing Public Sector Services. Essential Skills for the Public Sector*, HB Publications, London.

Bevan, R.G. (2007) Healthcare performance reports, in *Encyclopedia of Statistics in Quality and Reliability* (eds F. Ruggeri, R.S. Kenett and F. Faltin), John Wiley & Sons, Ltd, Chichester, pp. 1–6

Busse, R., Schreyogg, J. and Smith, P.C. (2008) Variability in healthcare treatment costs amongst nine EU countries – results from the HealthBasket project. *Health Econ*, **17**(1 Suppl), S1–S8.

Cappellaro, G., Ghislandi, S. and Anessi-Pessina, E. (2011) Diffusion of medical technology: the role of financing. *Health Policy*, **100**(1), 51–59.

Cleverley, W.O. (1987) Product costing for health care firms. *Health Care Manage Rev*, **12**(4), 39–48.

Cooper, R. (1988) The rise of activity-based costing – Part One: what is an activity-based cost system? *J Cost Manag*, **2**(2), 45–54.

Cooper, R. and Kaplan, R.S. (1987) How cost accounting systematically distorts product costs, in *Accounting & Management* (eds W. Bruns and R. Kaplan), Harvard Business School Press, Boston, MA, pp. 204–229.

Drummond, M.F., Sculpher, M.J., Torrance, G.W., O'Brien, B.J. and Stoddart, G.L. (2005) *Methods for the Economic Evaluation of Health Care Programmes*, Oxford University Press, Oxford.

Fattore, G. and Torbica, A. (2006) Inpatient reimbursement system in Italy: how do tariffs relate to costs? *Health Care Manag Sci*, **9**(3), 251–258.

Fetter, R.B. (1991) Diagnosis related groups: understanding hospital performance. *Interfaces*, **21**(1), 6–26.

Fetter, R.B. (1992) Hospital payment based on diagnosis-related groups. *J Soc Health Syst*, **3**(4), 4–15.

Fetter, R.B. (1999) Casemix classification systems. *Aust Health Rev*, **22**(2), 16–34; discussion 35–18.

Fetter, R.B., Freeman, J.L. and Mullin, R.L. (1985) DRGs: how they evolved and are changing the way hospitals are managed. *Pathologist*, **39**(6), 17–21.

Finkler, S.A. (1994) *Essentials of Cost Accounting for Healthcare Organizations*, AN Aspen Pubblications, Maryland, USA.

Finkler, S.A. (2001) *Budgeting Concepts for Nurse Managers*, WB Saunders, New York, USA.

Gold, M.R., Siegel, J.E., Russell, L.B. and Weinstein, M.C. (1996) *Cost Effectiveness in Health and Medicine*, Oxford University Press, New York.

Goldschmidt, Y. and Gafni, A. (1990) A managerial approach to allocating indirect fixed costs in healthcare organizations. *Health Care Manag Rev*, **15**(2), 43–51.

Hakkinen, U. and Joumard, I. (2007) Cross-country analysis of efficiency in OECD healthcare sectors: options for research. OECD Economics Department Working Papers no. 554, Paris.

Johnston, K., Buxton, M. , Jones, D. and Fitzpatrick, R. (2001) Collecting resource use data for costing clinical trials, in *The Advanced Handbook of Methods in Evidence-Based Healthcare* (eds A. Stevens, K. Abrams, J. Brazier, R. Fitzpatrick and R. Lilford), SAGE Publications, London, pp. 215–231.

Karmarkar, U. and Pitbladdo, R. (1993) Internal pricing and cost allocation in a model of multiproduct competition with finite capacity increments. *Manag Sci*, **39**(9), 1039–1053.

Koopmanschap, M.A., Touw, K.C. and Rutten, F.F. (2001) Analysis of costs and cost-effectiveness in multinational trials. *Health Policy*, **58**(2), 175–186.

Langenbrunner, J.C. and Wiley, M.M. (2002) Hospital payment mechanisms: theory and practice in transition countries, in *Hospitals in a Changing Europe* (eds M. McKee and J. Healy), European Observatory on Health Care Systems, pp. 150–170.

Lucey, T. (2002) *Costing*, Thompson Learning.

Maggert, T.A. (1985) *Cost Accounting: a Health Care Management Tool*, Healthcare Financial Management Asociation, Illinois.

McCrone, P., Thornicroft, G., Phelan, M. *et al.* (1998) Utilisation and costs of community mental health services. PRiSM Psychosis Study. 5. *Br J Psychiatry*, **173**, 391–398.

Mishan, E.J. (1988) *Cost-Benefit Analysis*, Routledge, London.

Mogyorosy, Z. and Smith, P. (2005) The main methodological issues in costing healthcare services. A literature review. CHE Research Papers, The University of York.

Propper C. and Wilson D. (2006) The use of performance measures in health care systems, in *The Elgar Companion of Health Economics* (ed. A. Jones), Edward Elgar Publishing Limited, Cheltenham, pp. 326–334.

Raikou, M., Briggs, A., Gray, A. and McGuire, A. (2000) Centre-specific or average unit costs in multi-centre studies? Some theory and simulation. *Health Econ*, **9**(3), 191–198.

Schreyogg, J., Stargardt, T., Tiemann, O. and Busse, R. (2006) Methods to determine reimbursement rates for diagnosis related groups (DRG), a comparison of nine European countries. *Health Care Manag Sci*, **9**(3), 215–223.

Schulman, K., Burke, J., Drummond, M. *et al.* (1998) Resource costing for multinational neurologic clinical trials: methods and results. *Health Econ*, **7**(7), 629–638.

Street, A., Scheller-Kreinsen, D., Geissler, A. and Busse, R. (2010) *Determinants of Hospital Costs and Performance Variation: Methods, Models and Variables for the EuroDRG Project*. Working Papers in Health Policy and Management, Vol. **3**, Department of Health Care Management, TUB Berlin.

Tarricone, R. (2006) Cost-of-illness analysis. What room in health economics? *Health Policy*, **77**(1), 51–63.

Tiemann, O. (2008) Variations in hospitalisation costs for acute myocardial infarction – a comparison across Europe. *Health Econ*, **17**(1 Suppl), S33–S45.

Wordsworth, S., Ludbrook, A., Caskey, F. and Macleod, A. (2005) Collecting unit cost data in multi-centre studies. Creating comparable methods. *Eur J Health Econ*, **6**(1), 38–44.

# Part Five

# APPLICATIONS TO HEALTHCARE MANAGEMENT

# 20

# Statistical issues in healthcare facilities management

## Daniel P. O'Neill[1] and Anja Drescher[2]

[1] Jones Lang LaSalle Americas, Inc., Chicago, IL, USA
[2] Jones Lang LaSalle, Minnetonka, MN, USA

## Synopsis

The Healthcare System is understandably driven by a constant need to innovate and to become more efficient in order to survive. As those demands intensify, the effects that were historically felt primarily by teams in the operating rooms are extending to those teams in, of all places, the boiler rooms! Innovative management of health systems' facilities and capital repair and replacement spending is becoming increasingly important to achieving system-wide efficiency and cost reduction objectives. As a result of this growing attention and sophistication, the list of interdependent issues facing these teams is exploding. Facilities Management teams are increasingly required to understand how technology and tools like statistics and Six Sigma can be used to measure and improve quality throughout the physical environment of care, while decreasing the costs to deliver facilities-related services. Additionally, the capital that is allocated to repairing and replacing many aging facilities has never been more scarce; requiring these same teams to provide substantive metrics and objective analysis to support capital funding requests.

## 20.1   Introduction

The healthcare industry has historically considered Facilities Management (FM) operations to be a simple support function and a relatively minor part of its supply chain. But as the

*Statistical Methods in Healthcare*, First Edition.  Edited by Frederick W. Faltin, Ron S. Kenett and Fabrizio Ruggeri.

healthcare business continues to evolve, FM teams are undergoing intense levels of scrutiny and are experiencing an evolution in performance expectations and reporting responsibilities. These changes have resulted in facilities teams developing an understanding of the value and the commensurate challenge of collecting and measuring meaningful statistical healthcare facilities data. The interpretation and translation of that data into outcomes that are valued by key decision-makers is also proving to be especially critical.

As healthcare systems evolve and begin to operate more proactively, the intensity and focus on innovation and change is rightly spreading from the operating table to some of the non-core functions and practices within the system, including FM. It is crucial for facilities teams to understand the tools and systems available to quickly and effectively manage these changes and expectations.

Hospitals and healthcare systems are facing unprecedented pressures to find efficiencies throughout their businesses. This mandate has never been more intense due, in large part, to healthcare reform. The ever-increasing system complexities driven by reporting requirements and information and technology improvements are compelling healthcare businesses to seek creative methods to:

1. reduce operating costs throughout the labor and supply chain;

2. objectively illustrate the need for capital and establish a credible methodology to prioritize projects and allocate these resources; and,

3. define and measure facilities-related service performance wherever it affects the patient experience.

The pressures on the system-wide financial equation are numerous and complex: patient revenue is down and will only experience further pressure as government-sponsored programs alter reimbursement payments and payment structures for various procedures and aspects of care. This top-line revenue dilemma has necessarily garnered much of the leadership focus from hospital executive teams who have the unique talents and aptitude to proactively drive necessary change in the industry.

While many functions and practices are fully represented at the healthcare business planning table, invariably, real estate is not one of them. The average hospital systems' real-estate-related expenses ranks third behind only personnel and supplies, and the average balance sheet is loaded with real-estate-related opportunities that can provide a new source of cost savings for hospital leadership teams. This emerging understanding presents both tremendous opportunity and incredible challenge for a business imbued with so many complex interdependencies.

Administrators and hospital executives have historically viewed their real estate in a strictly tactical manner – as a support function – and one that can be most efficiently managed in a decentralized, local environment. However, some innovative organizations are beginning to take an approach to real estate and asset management that rips a page right out of Corporate America's recent experience. By incorporating subject-matter experts side-by-side with its best business minds, healthcare systems are benefitting from world-class real-estate practices and operational efficiencies that are rooted in a centralized approach, and ones that bring the systems and tools necessary to quickly and efficiently assess multiple functions embedded in the real estate and facilities spectrum. Gathered in an objective and well-planned manner, statistical data can provide hospital system leaders the information necessary to accentuate strategic change mandates, and pave the way for dramatic process improvement. The challenge in the healthcare industry is not unique: there is a growing understanding that real estate is not a core competency for healthcare providers/managers, and that hospital executive teams can benefit from experiences and work produced outside the industry.

Additionally, for nearly every system, merger and acquisition (M&A) as a core financial strategy – whether it be for growth or for survival – is unveiling further incredible opportunities to harness the benefits of size and scale and to deal with the difficulties of integrating disparate processes and geographies and teams. M&A can be messy – sometimes even disastrous – and further highlights the opportunity for healthcare to learn from experiences and comparisons within other industries. By seeking outside real-estate expertise during the due diligence process, systems are seeing the inherent value in centralizing real estate facilities and functions across the system.

Acquisition as a catalyst for driving change and decision-making cannot be overstated. As an example, after nearly 18 months of considering various options to manage an already geographically diverse portfolio of hospitals, one system recently engaged outside consulting assistance to develop a customized database and provide subsequent recommendations to harness the power of the system's newfound scale (its portfolio grew by almost 50%). In doing so, the system was exposed to the potential financial savings and quality improvements available from an integrated facilities and capital projects management model. By customizing the processes for the specific complexities and needs seen only in hospitals, while at the same time imparting the benefits derived from multiple experiences during similarly complex life sciences and financial corporate client acquisitions, the system saw itself on the leading edge of an industry phenomenon whose benefits may become integral to health systems across the globe.

The inherently disparate environments created by M&A highlights the real value of systems' partnering to manage their non-core professional services; a method that significantly reduces business risk while exploiting knowledge and opportunities gained by infusing subject-matter experts' broad access to multiple industry models and iterations. This 'governance' approach to managing non-core services serves the collaborative corporate governance decision-making model very efficiently.

This chapter will introduce a series of practical statistical issues facing FM teams in healthcare systems, and will describe ideas for 'next' practices that could be deployed by most FM teams with appropriate resources. These next practices attempt to exhibit a value proposition that is straight-forward and simple in order to quickly gain the necessary attention from healthcare decision-makers and influencers.

## 20.2    Healthcare facilities management

### 20.2.1    Description

**Definition**

> Facilities Management is the process of planning, managing, maintaining, rationalizing, and accounting for facilities and associated services, while simultaneously seeking to reduce the associated costs. The primary focus of facilities management is to provide the optimum level of facility [quality] for the least financial outlay.
>
> —(Glossary of Building Terms from Standards Australia (SAA HB50-1994))

*Facilities Management*, at the macro level, is all about strategic planning, asset life-cycle evaluation and integration and management of the multiple sources of information and data involved at the hospital system level. At the micro level, FM is maintenance and operations of individual assets, it is management of routine capital projects, and it is managing the daily services that affect the connected environment of patient care. This comprehensive view of responsibilities creates a continuous life-cycle loop for managing the healthcare systems' integrated real-estate services and needs. This loop, while seemingly efficient, is often difficult for individual facilities teams to navigate on their own (Mercury Computer Systems, 1994).

Satisfying multiple stakeholders with wide-ranging operational and financially focused goals provides a daily dose of dichotomy for FM teams that truly necessitates disciplined, repeatable practices and decision-making in order to provide the consistency and efficiency that is expected.

Critical clinical operational priorities for FM teams are generally characterized (Mercury Computer Systems, 1994) by the need for:

- compliance with regulatory requirements
- flexible, timely availability of space
- minimal disruptions in the physical environment of care
- a consistent, clean and safe environment for patients and staff
- an efficient response to facility concerns

. . . while fiduciary responsibilities drive a competing level of priorities including:

- proactive maintenance of asset and building systems
- maintaining a return on assets and invested capital
- efficiently deploying operating dollars
- coherent capital planning and spending.

## 20.2.2   Relevant data

> In order to improve something you have to be able to change it. In order to change it you have to be able to understand it. In order to understand it you have to be able to measure it. – An expert
>
> —(Lichiello and Turnock, 1999).

'FM/RE [Facilities Management/Real Estate] has parted from the perception of real property as a purely tangible asset and is considering its value as an immaterial asset with long-term earnings expectations. This shift necessitates the development of metrics to highlight the strategic value of FM/RE, along with its impact on the financial statement' (Keith, Atkin and Bröchner, 2005).

Relevant data is essential to demonstrating value to the organization and to gaining the respect necessary to command an appropriate allocation of system resources. Validated metrics, aligned with organization-specific operational priorities, are the foundation for performance measurement, for benchmarking, for identifying areas for improvement and for exhibiting transparency throughout operations.

Data also need to be properly defined and standardized to ensure consistency, repeatability and scalability across the organization. Accuracy (rate of error), completeness (reporting of data as required) and currency (age of data relative to time of collection and collection frequency) will achieve the desired data quality level (Beschen *et al.*, 2001).

Historical data from existing systems can be used, but may deliver inconsistent comparisons with future data-collection efforts.

These statistical challenges require FM teams to determine how well past data represent desired metrics and performance going forward and how reproducible the information is.

Following Nelson (2006), FM is confronted with both tangible (continuous and discrete) and intangible (discrete only) measurements. Intangibles differentiate FM from many management disciplines in the patient care environment and thus contribute to the potential value. The primary challenge facing facilities managers is quantifying services that do not normally have numeric outcomes. This leads to significant subjectivity permeating most data.

'*Performance Measurement* is the regular collection and reporting of data to track work produced and results achieved' (Lichiello and Turnock, 1999). It is vital to multiple intangible aspects of FM outcomes.

Three essential aspects of performance often surface during tactical discussions on Performance Measurement (see, for example, Alexander (1996); Williams (1996)). As defined in Sapri and Pitt (2005):

- **'physical performance** relates to the behaviour of the building's fabric and embraces physical properties such as structural integrity, heating, lighting, energy efficiency, maintainability, durability etc.'

- **'functional performance** concerns the relationship of the building with its occupiers and embraces issues such as space, layout, ergonomics, image, ambience, communication, health and safety and flexibility, etc.'

- **'financial performance** arises from the physical and functional performances of the building and comprises capital and recurrent (life-cycle) expenditures, depreciation and efficiency of use etc.'

Utilizing an objective Six Sigma tool, it is possible to identify a *ranking of importance of performance measures* by placing Patient and Executive Requirements (the 'Voice of the Customer', or VOC) and the three main components of FM measurements into a Quality Functional Deployment (QFD) matrix (Table 20.1).[1]

The results present a clear dominance of financial performance metrics followed by the functional measurements throughout the environment of care.

Translating the analysis into actionable key performance indicators produces three paramount objectives for facilities teams to focus on.

  I. Streamline operations and create real, substantive operating savings.

 II. Provide objective measurements to influence the allocation of capital to facility infrastructure improvements.

III. Quantify the quality of the patient care experience wherever it is touched by facilities-related responsibilities and work.

---

[1] For information on this and other basic statistical and Six Sigma tools in this chapter, see Ruggeri, Kenett and Faltin (2007).

**Table 20.1**   QFD – Performance Measurement – weight.

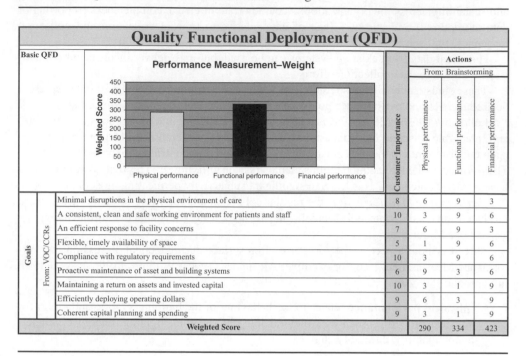

| | | | Customer Importance | Physical performance | Functional performance | Financial performance |
|---|---|---|:---:|:---:|:---:|:---:|
| **Goals** | **From: VOC/CCRs** | Minimal disruptions in the physical environment of care | 8 | 6 | 9 | 3 |
| | | A consistent, clean and safe working environment for patients and staff | 10 | 3 | 9 | 6 |
| | | An efficient response to facility concerns | 7 | 6 | 9 | 3 |
| | | Flexible, timely availability of space | 5 | 1 | 9 | 6 |
| | | Compliance with regulatory requirements | 10 | 3 | 9 | 6 |
| | | Proactive maintenance of asset and building systems | 6 | 9 | 3 | 6 |
| | | Maintaining a return on assets and invested capital | 10 | 3 | 1 | 9 |
| | | Efficiently deploying operating dollars | 9 | 6 | 3 | 9 |
| | | Coherent capital planning and spending | 9 | 3 | 1 | 9 |
| **Weighted Score** | | | | 290 | 334 | 423 |

CCR – Critical Customer Requirement; VOC – Voice of the Customer.

## 20.3   Operating expenses and the cost savings opportunities dilemma

With operating margins for most US healthcare systems being meager at best, true operational savings can be a huge lever in a system's financial equation. It may seem obvious, but bears repeating: if a 2% operating margin is assumed, in order for the system to increase its operating margin by $1 000 000, the system can either find an additional $50 000 000 in revenue, or it could remove $1 000 000 in system operational inefficiencies. This simple restatement often gets the innovative wheels turning for hospital and clinical teams whose direct impact on revenue growth is negligible, but whose impact on a hospital's efficiencies is broad and deep.

Most participants in the healthcare system hope for a panacea someday where costs to consumers decrease or at least hold steady over time. For this endeavor to be taken seriously, every aspect of the supply chain included in the delivery-of-care spectrum must innovate and find new ways to keep quality high while controlling expenses. It is reasonable to assume that *all* expenses throughout the healthcare system must be on the table for review and resetting.

This may sound like a logical foundational to start a cost-cutting discussion. But the healthcare industry has tremendous competing pressure to provide best-in-class quality patient experiences, not unlike the high-end hospitality industry, where service level expectations can be extraordinary, and produce situations where high-touch service is a critical and influential profitability metric.

This service dilemma often leads consensus-driven hospital executives to take a risk-averse approach to facilities operations, which in turn leads to some of the most inefficient facilities operations in any industry. In fact, in our experience, even among hospitals within the same geography and system, the decentralized silos and decision-making regarding facilities can create an environment where sharing of facilities best practices is almost non-existent. The use of standard industry facilities best practices to deliver operating cost efficiencies and savings, while keeping quality of service high, is ubiquitous in nearly every other industry – including the hospitality industry – and healthcare, however reluctantly, seems to be catching on.

The real estate services apparatus has a history of diving headlong into the deep end of seemingly very murky pools, expanding its influence into myriad new industries with practical, logical roadmaps. By starting slowly, executing low-risk, high-reward solutions first, facilities teams can establish the credibility necessary to implement more sophisticated programs that use objective metrics to not only minimize concerns about service quality, but actually show improvements over time. The results often speak for themselves, and by partnering to merge multiple, seemingly conflicting goals, facilities operations can lead hospital systems in driving innovative quality improvements and cost controls that are valued by patients and the demanding financial influences alike.

## 20.4   The case for baselining

The absence of a sophisticated peer grouping and relevant iterations of operational data creates an inherent problem in the healthcare facilities world. In order to decipher where to begin in the march to efficiency nirvana, determining baseline operating expenses and categorizing them properly is a vital step. Hospital systems' default accounting practices, while perfectly suited for the business of providing care for and billing patients and insurance companies, are ill-fitted for its real estate and properties functions. The absence of an industry-tested real-estate chart of accounts and inadequate site-level accounting transparency causes significant issues when FM teams are tasked with mining their operations for inefficiencies. When teams don't know what they don't know, meaningful operating savings may be very difficult or impossible to achieve.

As anecdotal evidence of this – during operating reviews of numerous hospital systems' financial accounting data, using simple stratifications of known data through proven comparative lenses used in many other industries – a credible efficiency table can be quickly developed to compare one hospital facility to another. This often leads to the development of 'quick wins' for facilities teams to achieve with appropriate allocation of system resources.

The industry has historically not needed to use a specific real-estate chart of accounts, due to the view that real estate and facilities are support functions. Nor has there been much of an attempt to categorize operating expenses in a consistent manner and form as is available for real-estate uses in other industries. A relatively simple operating expense comparison between healthcare facilities and complex office buildings may provide valuable insight for healthcare facilities to use as industry develops a relevant database of its own. While it may seem like a feeble comparison due to the different primary uses, by utilizing the iterative parsing techniques practiced by buildings that have to collect and allocate expenses from multiple different users, healthcare facilities could learn some valuable lessons.

The office building industry is one that is built on benchmarking, and this has led to tremendous innovation and copy-catting within certain geographies, producing valid data comparisons demanded by sophisticated rent-paying tenants with multiple options for space. Hospitals and health systems face a tremendous challenge in figuring out how to integrate real-estate accounting into their already complex financial systems. One option that is getting some traction in the industry is to use some reverse engineering to back into an expense budget for a system's real estate, utilizing previous full year histories and an actual real-estate industry standard chart of accounts. This helps to establish a baseline for an important parallel activity of re-categorizing expenses on a site-by-site basis – attempting to allocate costs by 'how and where' they are used. With this baseline, future iterations of coding expenses and budget preparation can be completed with better accuracy and more consistency.

Attributes of best-in-class 'next' accounting practices will include electronic invoice presentment programs to eliminate all paper coding of invoices, and outsourcing the entire real-estate accounting function to third parties who will accept all the risk associated with the operating expense spend and be able to formulate reporting that integrates easily into the healthcare industry general ledger.

The real-estate management industry has survived a variety of financial challenges by creating a sense of cooperation and sharing of accurate information across peer organizations to create a competitive, cost-conscious culture that breeds innovation and a 'tinkering' mentality, producing multiple industry-specific solutions based on solid baseline comparisons. Property-based accounting tools are sophisticated enough to allow for different types of uses within the same complex, or building, or even room, which will provide ample bandwidth for the myriad uses of space in healthcare locations. Inherent in the more sophisticated real-estate accounting systems are options to slice up and compare, side-by-side, expenses in core hospital functional space uses, doctor office uses, $24 \times 7$ urgent care uses, labs and research areas, medical office complexes, and computer and related facilities areas, to name just a few. Eventually, the healthcare industry operating expenses will be better understood and will produce a peer information sharing network for the collective benefit of the entire industry. The sharing of this data may seem a little foreign in a world where data privacy is paramount, but the innocuous make-up of this data will truly serve to revolutionize the practice.

## 20.5    Facilities capital . . . is it *really* necessary?

### 20.5.1    Facilities capital management

Management and deployment of a hospital system's capital budget is an extraordinarily opaque endeavor. While systems have historically allocated tens of millions of dollars to various projects annually, hospital executives frequently lack confidence that its approach to deploying capital is methodical and based on rigorous objective priorities. In addition to this transparency and prioritization gap, competing opportunities to spend system capital dollars on income-producing technology and equipment regularly leave facilities and infrastructure further underfunded.

Add the political tension of competing to hire the best hospital specialists who demand the newest technology to ply their trade . . . and many healthcare organizations are not surprisingly left with aging physical assets and unsustainable building conditions. This often evolves into inevitable surprise capital requirements and a sense of anxiety that building a sustainable infrastructure investment program is hopeless. Facilities teams must continue to be disciplined and create sound, effective and compelling business cases of their own to compete in this sophisticated, and sometimes not-so-logical arena.

Healthcare executives and administration would be well served by beginning a discussion on capital by thinking about how it would answer any or all of the following questions.

1. Does the Hospital System have visibility and transparency into the capital spend necessary for its real estate and facilities infrastructure?

2. If so, are the projects prioritized – and how are they prioritized?

3. Is each of the core business groups/practices involved in capital forecasting? Are they aware of the process? Should they be?

4. How are capital expenditures for the system approved? Do these processes/approvals have the correct exposure to system leadership?

5. Is the system and each major hospital or clinic able to forecast capital annually, quarterly? How accurate are the forecasts? What would an ideal reporting cadence and threshold look like?

6. Are the business/practices' requirements met through the current process?

7. Is funding for System-wide initiatives planned strategically? Are these processes well communicated so functional business leaders have the visibility they need to be confident that the organization is making the correct investments?

8. Is the system able to logically and objectively compare one project to another?

Compounding these complexities are the surprises that unnerve Chief Financial Officers. Imagine a 4-million dollar Emergency Department (ED) improvement project being revised upward to 7.5 million dollars due to a shortage of equipment with 12-month lead times that had to be shipped in from abroad to avoid shutting the facility down. In various versions, this is the kind of real-life challenge routinely heard in conversations with hospital system executives.

And with aging buildings and infrastructure systems, many hospitals continue to roll the dice hoping that they can delay operational improvements – 'just one more year' – seeking a new source of funds to allocate to these needs. This theory leads to infrastructure systems that run to failure, dictating emergency replacement at a significantly higher, unbudgeted cost. With appropriate tools, the practice of allocating hospital system capital can be much more effectively managed and understood.

The statistical issues with facilities' capital can be broken down into three primary challenges: (1) collecting comprehensive data on each potential 'opportunity' to spend it; (2) providing a deliberate, objective set of attributes to measure how important competing projects are; and (3) applying a repeatable, disciplined approach to managing each and every project to complete it on time and on budget.

## 20.5.2   A census of opportunities

In order to capture each of the potential 'opportunities' to deploy capital, it is essential that a single source of truth be developed to capture attributes and data points in an easily accessible

**Table 20.2**    Asset inventory: example of metrics.

| ASSET INFORMATION | | SCHEDULES | |
|---|---|---|---|
| Asset Name: | Property/Room: | 25 ton heat pump - HVAC | |
| Asset no.: | Serial no.: | **LOCATION INFORMATION** | |
| Asset Class: | Asset Rank: | Property: | Space: |
| Manufacturer: | Model: | Employee: | Room/Area: |
| In-Service Date: | Vendor: | Quantity Available: | |
| Asset Status: | Status Comments: | Asset Comments: | Status: |
| Asset Description: | | **WARRANTY INFORMATION** | |
| Asset Safety | | Warranty Contract no. | |
| Comment: | | Effective Date: | Expiration Date: |
| | | Expiration Contact: | Expir. Contact Phone: |
| | | Maint. Contract no.: | Maintenance Vendor: |
| | | Contract Exp. Date: | No. of Days Notif. Exp.: |
| | | **PURCHASE INFORMATION** | |
| | | Purchase Date: | Purchase Amount: |
| | | Cost Center: | Purchase Order no.: |
| | | Estimated Life(yrs): | Estimated Life(hrs): |
| | | Annual Runtime(hrs): | Capital Repair Cost: |
| | | Est. Repl. Cost: | Life Expectancy Date: |
| | | **ASSET CLASS DETAILS** | |
| | | Compressor Volt:: | Compressor Amps:: |
| | | Fan Motor Volts:: | Fan Motor Amps:: |
| | | Type of Condenser: | If Air Cooled: Condenser Fan Motor Volts: |
| | | If Air Cooled: Condenser Fan Motor Amps: | If Air Cooled: Condenser Fan Motor HP: |
| | | Refrigerant Type: | Refrigerant Quantity: |
| | | Lbs/Oz Refrig. Cirt. 1: | Lbs/Oz Refrig. Cirt. 2: |

format insuring that the playing field is level – at least at the start of the game! This single source might consist of a database with consistent fields to be completed by each requestor, it might be a spreadsheet built to be sorted by like items and like fields, or it could be a sophisticated tool that provides very comprehensive capabilities to sort and compare projects in myriad ways.

Managing assets and equipment based on a statistically known life cycle insures that capital and operating expenses are deployed on a straight-line basis to avoid ugly spikes in spend that result from poor proactive planning and a known aversion to spending dollars at all on 'non-revenue-generating stuff.'

Another hallmark of best-in-class programs is a census tool used to track every single piece of equipment in the system. The program is intended to inventory, track and document the maintenance of, track the useful life of, and estimate the replacement cost of all assets included in a building envelope. The uses for the census tool are multiple. It establishes a probable baseline capital plan that extends well beyond a usual 5-year plan. In fact, if done in a comprehensive manner, it is possible to project capital needs for a facility for 20 years and beyond. See Table 20.2.

### 20.5.3    Prioritization and efficiency factors

In order to effectively spend the 'next' capital dollar that is made available as a resource to a facilities team, it is critical to insure that these opportunities are measured objectively and prioritized in a manner that is credible in the eyes of the executive management team.

It is also critical that these objective factors provide hospital executive teams a simple way to understand when equipment is reaching a critical replacement stage and when

**Table 20.3**  Capital investment prioritization metrics: examples.

| Quality | Asset | Prioritization and Efficiency |
|---|---|---|
| **Regulatory Employee Health Safety** | **Operational** | **Factors** |
| Security upgrades (e.g. cameras, badge-readers) | Roofing | Core/Critical Site |
| Fire (sprinklers, detection equip.) | Parking (e.g. resurfacing) | Payback Period |
| Regulatory/Fire Life Safety | Window Seals | Functionality |
| | Foundation/concrete | Redline |
| **Workplace Quality** | HVAC | Obsolete |
| Single-trade carpet and paint | EMS | Customer Facing |
| Jobs | Control systems that manage HVAC (VAV systems) | End of Useful Life |
| Landscaping | Control systems that manage electrical systems | Not Applicable |
| Improvements/Repair | Electrical panel upgrades (switch gears) | Lease End Date / Site Longevity |
| | Boilers | |
| | Plumbing upgrades | |
| | Elevators | |
| | Backup Supply (UPS/Generators) | |
| | Recycling | |
| | Water conservation | |
| | Energy conservation | |

HVAC – Heating , Venting and Air Conditioning; EMS – Energy Management System; VAV – Variable Air Volume (System); UPS – Uninterruptible Power Supply.

equipment has fallen into a critical state of disrepair leading to failure and expensive emergency replacements.

Examples of factors that might be considered include the following.

- **Core/criticality of the site** – not all types of buildings or spaces within a building have the same criticality, and some are extensively patient-facing, or consumer-facing, and others are primarily back office.

- **Payback period** – some projects, especially those relating to energy or utility cost reduction will have a simple payback on the invested capital that should enter into the equation.

- **Functionality** – what stage of life is the asset in? Is it already broken? Is it obsolete technology or no longer able to be fixed? Is it at the end of its useful life – denoting a measure of inefficiency and a baseline for replacement?

- **Lease end date/site longevity** – an objective categorization, measured in years, of how long the building is expected to remain in the system's portfolio.

See Table 20.3.

## 20.5.4  Project management

A third aspect of an effective capital deployment program is comprised of the execution and management of the projects themselves. While it would be possible to write an entire chapter on effective real-estate project management, a summary of aspects of a quality delivery model would include the use of:

- widely integrated and accessible technology to manage and update projects' progress;

- integrated systems to pay invoices;

- sound, repeatable and simple bidding process;

- consistent, objective contract for all goods and services.

Sound, fundamental project management starts with adequate comprehensive planning and an understanding that proper planning is the simplest way to insure that capital is efficiently deployed. This is often easier said than done, as it requires an up-front commitment to spending dollars now . . . to avoid having to spend two or three times those dollars later when the options are limited.

Given the sheer size of the dollars spent, and given the experiential evolution of project management in the corporate space, most healthcare systems would see significant cost avoidance and a more efficient deployment of capital by understanding and accessing the systems, tools and processes available throughout the construction and project management trades within the industry.

## 20.6    Defining clean, orderly and in good repair

### 20.6.1    Customer focus

Delighting patients with high standards for hospital cleanliness, neatness and orderliness is important. And providing a high quality, physical environment that is commensurate with the high-touch level of medical care they expect to receive is becoming an increasingly important quality metric in a hospital's reimbursement equation. While 'new' may not be a sustainable standard for FM teams to strive for, it is a statistical benchmark that provides an objective starting point as facilities teams evaluate maintenance and attempt to objectively recommend areas to focus on and improve, and where to prioritize operating expense and capital dollars.

The gradual, intentional or unintentional deferral of expenses is oftentimes barely noticeable in the first few years following 'new construction' or the opening of a facility. It is assumed that spaces need less attention and money when new. But eventually, depending on the life-cycle of the asset in question – whether that asset is a chair, or flooring or temperature control within a room – obsolescence, dating, or wear-and-tear will potentially lead to an unacceptable condition for patients, and could require an incredible amount of money to resolve.

This can be an especially daunting situation when hospitals merge. It accentuates the differing prioritizations and philosophies concerning the need for replacement of basic furniture, fixtures and facility equipment. This lack of consistency can paralyze FM teams due to the inability to quantify the extent of the defects and the cumulative effect of aging facilities.

Disparate conditions throughout the environment affecting the patient care experience cause:

- interdependent operational difficulties

- decreased patient satisfaction

- underutilization of space

- disagreement on an acceptable standard baseline for what is clean, orderly and in good repair

- an overall environment of poor prioritization and unnecessary spending.

Creating baseline metrics for overall facilities performance along a variety of functional areas is becoming more and more critical to bottom-line operations. By statistically measuring and obtaining an appropriate baseline for facilities conditions, the FM team can establish a credible long-term infrastructure management program that can garner its share of annual expense and capital spending.

By using Six Sigma methodologies we can create a scalable, repeatable and measurable process around defined standards of what a *clean, orderly and in-repair* workplace looks like, to establish a facilities condition index and then track it over time. Eventually, these results will create an experience history with multiple data points to more effectively prioritize non-recurring operating expense projects and routine facilities capital spend to the opportunities that will have shown to produce the most value to the organization.

## 20.6.2   Metrics and methods

Objectively defining 'clean, orderly and in good repair' is a tremendous statistical struggle for many FM teams: is the bathroom clean enough when there is water on the counter? When there is only one newspaper left in the stall? When there are smudges on only one of three mirrors? And how does one differentiate between worn carpeting in the waiting room of the lobby versus worn carpeting under a desk in the back office? And should you specifically detail differences between 'faults' that have the potential to affect business continuity and ones that don't? An example of this type of fault would be a simple exit light out – on one hand this is a very routine fault in an office environment that could be fixed in the normal course of business, but if it is an emergency center, this may be important to a regulatory accreditation inspection and subject the organization to a much stiffer penalty if not noticed and fixed in a timely manner. A facility condition and inspection system that allows for prioritization of such work could be a valuable tool to help measure efficiency.

'I'll know it when I see it' the old adage goes. This statement goes a long way in helping define quality in a facilities environment. Or maybe it might be better stated as, 'I'll know it when I *don't* see it.' If, upon inspection, one finds no faults with an object or some other physical thing, then it is often considered the highest condition standard. Think 'new.'

Using a new car as an example might be good imagery. Over time the car can be driven and used. It may still be visibly 'new' to the driver and the public as long as the newer versions of the car do not include a body style change – if the body style is changed it may alter the thoughts of 'newness' even though the car may have no visible defects. The new body style may alter the buying decisions of the public. As scratches and rips and tears and smudges become more visible, the cumulative effect of these 'defects' could also be evident and affect buying decisions. In these two cases though, fixing the smudges and rips and tears would appear to be cheaper than buying a new model – although both choices would appear to provide the same outcome – a 'new' car. And for cars in use, a car that is absent of noticeable defects is worth more than one that is full of defects.

The reason this discussion is germane to healthcare facilities is that the public is increasingly being asked quality questions about the patient care experience from well-respected surveying agencies. And if a patient has a choice between riding in a 'newer' looking car – all else being equal – they will likely choose it. If that 'newer car' is Hospital A, it will have a happy, paying customer. If that 'older' car is Hospital B – it may wonder what factor caused the customer to make the buying decision to go elsewhere.

And it is even more critical when those defects are either seen regularly or are more visible to more people – a rip in the driver's seat is not the same as a rip in the carpeting in the trunk. A scratch on the front windshield is more important than one on the back window. And the transmission under the hood . . . who cares, right? It is not visible and only marginally affects the experience of the driver and potential passengers – until it breaks and the car is down for unanticipated repairs that can be very stressful and expensive for myriad reasons. How a facilities team triages and fixes (or chooses to not fix or replace due to limited resources) equipment affecting the environment of patient care can be an effective tool in increasing patient satisfaction scoring – ultimately affecting the bottom line as the patient experience becomes more and more relevant to reimbursements from government-sponsored programs.

An important consideration in this theory is that is it relevant, and statistically important, for a facilities team to show that they are first completing the easy, inexpensive opportunities to deploy their labor and operating expense dollar – and to show that they are prioritizing the remaining opportunities to spend money and time.

## 20.7    A potential objective solution

An equation that could determine relative cleanliness, orderliness and state of repair of any facility appears to be a good place to start. Having worked extensively with Six Sigma to assess processes in a real-estate environment, the authors put forth a quality quotient of facility condition that will be determined by the Six Sigma calculation of 'defects per million opportunities' as its objective measuring stick. But how does one translate the numerator and the denominator into valid measures for healthcare facilities? A process flow might be developed as follows.

- The basic unit of measure is the *pro-active work order* – a description of work required that has been identified by a member of the facilities team during regularly scheduled inspections.

- Pro-active work orders identify 'defects' as opportunities to either fix something or render some repair or replacement to bring it back into 'new' condition.

- A defect might then be multiplied by an assigned 'weighting' based on the specific requirements of the entity; these may include severity or criticality of the work or cost to complete the task. This produces a repeatable definition for 'defect' for the organization to scale across multiple sites.

- The Space or square feet (SF) is the denominator into the equation over which the defects are to be detected.

The guiding measurement is now defined as the number of *Defects/Square Feet* and can be scaled depending on the ratio of defects acceptable to an organization. It is possible to then use appropriate mathematical equations to get a comparable level of sigma efficiency. Where a site is unlikely to attain a '6' on the efficiency scale due to the diverse regulatory and operational checklists facilities teams face, improvement from a baseline and holding up certain sites as the standard should lead to a roadmap for improvement for every site and

**Table 20.4**   Six Sigma scale – allowable defects.

| Allowable defects per 5000 SF Six Sigma scale 3.0–6.0 | | |
|---|---|---|
| Defects /million SF | Allowable defects per 5000 SF | Equals to Six Sigma score |
| 0 | 0 | 6.00 |
| 233 | 1 | 5.00 |
| 337 | 2 | 4.90 |
| 687 | 3 | 4.70 |
| 968 | 5 | 4.60 |
| 1350 | 7 | 4.50 |
| 1866 | 9 | 4.40 |
| 2555 | 13 | 4.30 |
| 3467 | 17 | 4.20 |
| 4661 | 23 | 4.10 |
| 6210 | 31 | 4.00 |
| 8198 | 41 | 3.90 |
| 10725 | 54 | 3.80 |
| 13903 | 70 | 3.70 |
| 17864 | 89 | 3.60 |
| 22750 | 114 | 3.50 |
| 28716 | 144 | 3.40 |
| 35930 | 180 | 3.30 |
| 44565 | 223 | 3.20 |
| 54799 | 274 | 3.10 |
| 66807 | 334 | 3.00 |

every team. It is also highly unlikely to reach a 3.0 sigma level due to an incredibly high number of defects this scale shows.

By creating a baseline or lower limit (3.0) and a target or upper limit (5.0), the results can be monitored using a simplified control chart.

In order to have the same level of measurement and results, a space is divided into partitions of 'X' SF each that allow 1 defect / X SF as an equal scale for different-sized buildings.

Table 20.4 shows an example for 5000 SF partitions. Now a Hospital with 15 000 SF is allowed 3 defects to reach Sigma Level 5.0, where a building with 150 000SF is allowed 30 defects.

From our earlier discussion, the performance measurements of facilities fall into the three components – physical, functional and financial – and based on those criteria, pro-active work orders could be categorized as

- Business continuity/accreditation (financial)
- Customer facing (functional)
- Building critical (physical).

**Table 20.5**  Prioritization of work orders.

| Prioritization Model | | Cost | |
| --- | --- | --- | --- |
| Client Priorities | Customer Importance Rating | Work Order | Capital |
| Business Continuity/Accreditation (Financial) | 6 | 9 | 3 |
| Customer Facing (Functional) | 3 | 9 | 3 |
| Building Critical (Physical) | 1 | 9 | 3 |

| Work Order Categories | Prioritization | Work Order Weight = Cost Measure × Customer Importance Rating |
| --- | --- | --- |
| Business Continuity/accreditation - Work Order | 1 | 54 |
| Customer Facing - Work Order | 2 | 27 |
| Business Continuity/accreditation - Capital | 3 | 18 |
| Building Critical - Work Order | 4 | 9 |
| Customer Facing - Capital | 5 | 9 |
| Building Critical - Capital | 6 | 3 |

By multiplying assigned measures based on customer importance and cost to cure the defects, an automatic prioritization and identification of the most critical work is defined.

The QFD *'Performance Measurement – weight'* (Table 20.1) shows that financial and functional performance are the top client priorities, shown as the *customer importance* rating.

Work orders focusing on quick, low-cost completions will be assigned a higher value than high-cost capital tasks (Table 20.5).

The pro-active work order with the highest weight result (business continuity/accreditation), representing the defect, shows the highest value opportunity.

This flexible model can be visually reported in a Site Condition Scorecard (Table 20.6). The Scorecard offers a comprehensive and objective overview of the weighted issues that contribute to the overall site condition. It identifies cost-effective *quick wins* that touch on all three components of facility measurements, and provides a disciplined road map for deployment of operating expenses. Site condition improvement over time is then tracked through a representative control chart.

Completing high-value work orders or defects results in more appealing facility conditions and, consequently, better site condition scores.

The identified higher-cost work (lowest weighted defects) is included in the census of opportunities identified earlier in this chapter. This census becomes a resource and a single source of truth to compare one project to another. Over time, this process allows for prioritization of operating and capital dollars.

The scorecard provides a foundation to deliver results that are congruent with why we measure.

**Table 20.6**  Scorecard example.

## SITE CONDITION - SCORECARD

| Date of Inspection | Country | Region | State | City | Address | Total Lease RSF | Facilities Manager | Current SITECON Score |
|---|---|---|---|---|---|---|---|---|
| 28-Dec-10 | USA | E | MN | City | 1234 Address | 150,000 | Jane Doe | **5.00** |

| | |
|---|---|
| Lease - Rentable Square Footage | 150,000 |
| no. of 5000 SF Units | 30 |
| Current no. of Total Actual Work Orders | 3 |
| Current no. of Defects (weighted work orders) | 39 |
| Current no. of Defects per 5000 SF | 1 |

| 1  Unsatisfactory | Need Improvement | Satisfactory | Excellent |
|---|---|---|---|
| 1.00 - 3.90 | 4.0 - 4.40 | 4.50 - 4.90 | 5.00 - 6.00 |

Building Condition Control Chart

Legend: SITECON Score, Target, Satisfactory, Needs Improvement, Unsatisfactory, Upper Limit, Lower Limit

WO = Work Orders
Total Open WO = Open WO Previous Qrt + New WO
no. of Defects = Weighted WO

| Importance of Work Order | Combination of Criticality and Cost | Weight of Work Order | YTD Total Work Orders | YTD Work Order Complete | 1st Quarter — Status Date: 31-Mar-10 | | | | | 2nd Quarter — Status Date: 30-Jun-10 | | | | | 3rd Quarter — Status Date: 30-Sep-10 | | | | | 4th Quarter — Status Date: | | | | |
|---|---|---|---|---|---|---|---|---|---|---|---|---|---|---|---|---|---|---|---|---|---|---|---|---|
| | | | | | no. Completed WO | no. OPEN WO | NEW WO | no. TOTAL Open WO | no. of Defects | no. Completed WO | NEW WO | no. TOTAL Open WO | no. of Defects | no. Completed WO | NEW WO | no. TOTAL Open WO | no. of Defects | no. Completed WO | NEW WO | no. TOTAL Open WO | no. of Defects | | |
| 1 | Business Continuity/Accreditation - Work Order | 54 | 33 | 43 | 0 0 | 10 | 23 | 33 | 1782 | 30 1620 | 6 | 9 | 486 | 12 ## | 4 | 1 | 54 | 1 54 | 0 | 0 | 0 | | |
| 2 | Customer Facing - Work Order | 27 | 18 | 17 | 0 0 | 0 | 10 | 10 | 270 | 9 0 | 3 | 3 | 81 | 4 0 | 2 | 1 | 27 | 4 0 | 1 | 1 | 27 | | |
| 3 | Business Continuity/Accreditation - Capital | 18 | 19 | 19 | 2 36 | 0 | 9 | 7 | 126 | 5 90 | 5 | 6 | 108 | 5 90 | 1 | 2 | 36 | 7 126 | 5 | 0 | 0 | | |
| 4 | Building Critical - Work Order | 9 | 9 | 8 | 0 0 | 0 | 2 | 2 | 18 | 2 18 | 2 | 5 | 45 | 4 36 | 1 | 2 | 18 | 2 18 | 1 | 0 | 9 | | |
| 5 | Customer Facing - Capital | 9 | 13 | 18 | 0 0 | 5 | 7 | 12 | 108 | 10 90 | 5 | 5 | 45 | 5 45 | 1 | 1 | 9 | 3 27 | 2 | 0 | 0 | | |
| 6 | Building Critical - Capital | 3 | 4 | 3 | 0 0 | 0 | 1 | 3 | | 1 3 | 2 | 2 | 6 | 1 3 | 0 | 1 | 3 | 1 3 | 1 | 1 | 3 | | |
| **TOTAL** | | 96 | 108 | | 2 36 | 15 | | 65 | 2307 | 57 1821 | 22 | 30 | 771 | 31 # | 9 | 8 | 147 | 18 228 | 13 | 3 | 39 | | |
| no. of Defects / 5000 SF | | | | | | | | | 77 | | | | 26 | | | | 5 | | | | 1 | | |
| SITECON Score | | | | | | | | | 3.60 | | | | 4.00 | | | | 4.60 | | | | 5.00 | | |

RSF – Rentable Square Footage.

We measure to:

1. control variation

2. assess our processes

3. assess continuous improvements

4. manage improvements to meet the established objectives.

Translating the measurements into outputs and simple reports often helps FM teams produce compelling arguments.

By delivering succinct and meaningful output, healthcare FM teams will not only be more credible with decision makers and influencers, but will also benefit from a clearer voice at the table when competing for operating expense and capital dollars.

## 20.8   Summary

Facilities Management operations within the healthcare industry are maturing quickly. This business within the business has always had a significant impact on the environment of patient care and is one that is woven into the fabric of the daily patient care experience – an aspect of the enterprise financial equation that has a growing impact on profitability. Myriad pressures: the speed at which hospital and health systems have needed to change, to cut costs while enhancing the quality of operations, to integrate disparate systems as the result of merger out of necessity, not of choice, have produced a set of challenges requiring an overhaul of the existing FM paradigm.

Hospital systems are developing an understanding that Real Estate is an untapped resource – one that can be exploited to drive out operational inefficiencies, to drive sustainable cost savings across the portfolio of properties, to help reveal the need for and better assess the prioritization and management of a significant annual capital plan. And also, to more objectively describe and maintain the physical locations where patient care is delivered insuring that the voice of the patient is driving how value is described – and how it is objectively measured.

Taking this paradigm a step further, leading edge organizations are already taking advantage of groups of practices developed both within the healthcare sphere but  – most importantly – also adapted from industries operating outside the walls of the hospital. Techniques that have been developed on factory assembly lines, in state-of-the-art communications facilities and in data-intensive banking industries can bridge the operational gap that has developed in many hospital facilities' systems.

Data integrity is a crucial underlying theme woven into nearly every statistical challenge facing healthcare FM and real-estate teams. And in order to successfully integrate these statistical FM business issues into the healthcare executive's lexicon, teams will need to define well what data needs to be collected and measured. Analyzing that data to insure that the output is both relevant and easily understood is also a logical step in the process. Creating a continuous improvement model to access newer ideas and having the ability to institute new practices without undue pressure from executive leadership is also important to sustain early successes. And, lastly, turning the page in the healthcare industry to boldly take the actions and imbue the processes necessary to embrace the tremendous changes both current and future will help develop the flexibility needed for this tumultuous business to thrive.

# References

Alexander, K. (1996) *A Strategy for Facilities Management; Theory and Practice*, E & FN Spon, London.

Beschen, D., Day R., Jordan, G. and Rohm, H. (2001) The Performance-Based Management Handbook, Volume 4, Collecting Data to Assess Performance. The Performance-Based Management Special Interest Group, www.orau.gov/pbm/pbmhandbook/Volume%204.pdf (accessed April 12, 2012).

Keith, A., Atkin, B. and Bröchner, J. (eds) (2005) *Facilities Management/Innovation and Performance*, Spon Press, New York.

Lichiello, P. and Turnock, B.J. (1999) The Turning Point Guidebook for Performance Measurement, Turning Point National Program Office at the University of Washington, www.rwjf.org/publichealth/product.jsp?id=14384 (accessed April 12, 2012).

Mercury Computer Systems (1994) BEIMS. White Paper: Facilities Management, Brief Overview, Mercury Computer Systems (Aust) Pty Ltd, Melbourne, http://www.whitepapersdb.com/whitepaper/10435/facilities-management (accessed April 19, 2012).

Nelson, M.-M. (2006) Measuring FM Performance, pfm Magazine Online (August 15), www.pfmonthenet.net/featuresarchive/article.aspx?ArticleID=9302 (accessed April 12, 2012).

Ruggeri, F., Kenett, R.S. and Faltin, F.W. (2007) *Encyclopedia of Statistics in Quality and Reliability*, John Wiley & Sons, Ltd, Chichester.

Sapri, M. and Pitt, M. (2005) Performance measurement in facilities management; state of knowledge, in *21st Annual ARCOM Conference, 7–9 September 2005, SOAS, University of London*, Vol. **1** (ed. F. Khosrowshahi), Association of Researchers in Construction Management, pp. 431–440. Available at: www.arcom.ac.uk/publications/procs/ar2005-0431 0440_Sapri_and_Pitt.pdf.

Williams, B. (1996) Cost-effective facilities management: a practical approach. *Facilities*, **14** (5/6), 26–38.

# 21

# Simulation for improving healthcare service management

**Anne Shade**

*Good Decision Partnership, Dingwall, Scotland, UK*

## Synopsis

Emphasis on improving the timeliness of service and of other performance measures in healthcare systems is driving the need to anticipate the impact of process changes before they are put into effect. There is a decision component to such situations, as well, since in many cases a number of improvement alternatives are proposed, and must be compared to assess the potential of each, as well as any unintended consequences. The impracticality of actually trying all – or perhaps any – of the proposed changes before a final decision can be made, places a premium on techniques which can implement and observe the changes in a virtual world first. Simulation tools provide such capabilities. These range from basic spreadsheet models which are purely calculational in nature, to advanced stochastic methods which can create, operate and compile a virtual history of proposed future systems. This chapter presents and compares a number of such techniques, discussing the merits and limitations of each. We then proceed to discuss several case studies of real-world problems where the methodologies have been used to good effect.

## 21.1 Introduction

Managers who turn to simulation models are often motivated by some special challenge, perhaps a major expansion (into a new hospital or factory, for example), or a requirement to make substantial performance improvements (to meet an imposed target, or to outdo

*Statistical Methods in Healthcare*, First Edition. Edited by Frederick W. Faltin, Ron S. Kenett and Fabrizio Ruggeri.
© 2012 John Wiley & Sons, Ltd. Published 2012 by John Wiley & Sons, Ltd.

competition). There is generally a need to understand how a new or altered process would perform, and to be sufficiently convinced of a successful outcome in order to make the relevant decisions to proceed.

Targets requiring major performance improvements have been imposed on the National Health Service (NHS) in the UK in recent years, and this has encouraged the use of process simulations to help explore new options. Historically patients have had to wait for months, sometimes even years, for both out-patient and in-patient treatment through the NHS. In the 1990s, according to a (now replaced) NHS site (www.18weeks.nhs.uk), 'waits of more than six months for a first out-patient appointment were not uncommon, and tens of thousands of people waited more than two years for an operation.' As a result of many improvement initiatives, the NHS is now in a position to state that 'the longest you should wait after being referred by your GP [general practitioner] until you start your treatment is 18 weeks – that is, unless you choose to delay treatment or there is a clinical reason why you should wait longer. Wherever possible, you will wait less than this, with the average wait being around eight weeks. Any hospital appointments, tests, scans or other procedures that you may need before being treated will all happen within this maximum time limit.'

Achieving and maintaining these reduced waiting times has necessitated a 'fundamental service transformation' with patients experiencing 'dramatically shorter overall pathways, as there is a shift from stages of treatment to whole pathways, and from small service-focused improvement to whole pathway transformation across organisational boundaries'.

Clearly in an organisation as large as the NHS (in 2004 the NHS employed 1.3 million people, making it one of the top five employers in the world), one cannot sensibly experiment with change on the scale envisioned, not least because of the risk that such experiments would have an adverse effect on patient care. However, highly graphical and animated simulation models have helped (and are continuing to help) managers visualise how a transformed process could operate. The construction and refinement of such models can provide a highly productive focus for discussions of strengths and weaknesses of both existing and proposed systems.

This chapter will cover various aspects of simulation ranging from talk-though and walk-through simulations and spreadsheet modelling, through to discrete event simulation and system dynamics. Used appropriately, they all have a useful role to play in providing insights and solutions to a wide variety of healthcare problems, but the focus of the chapter will be on discrete event simulation with several examples from models created using a software package called SIMUL8.

## 21.2 Talk-through and walk-through simulations

A straight-forward talk-through or walk-through simulation of a process can often identify areas for improvement. By taking time to step, literally or metaphorically, through the key stages in a process, those involved can focus their attention on selected areas while not losing sight of the bigger picture. In this way problems amenable to simple and immediate solutions may well be identified without recourse to more intensive and expensive studies. Post-it notes can be used to facilitate walk-through or talk-through discussions by displaying work centres, storage and queues in the order in which they are encountered by a patient, or any other item of interest such as a lab sample or report as it moves through the system. However, talk-through and walk-through simulations should only be used in relatively uncomplicated situations in which modest amounts of data can provide a reliable guide for corrective actions and process improvements. For example, it was noted that donors attending blood donor clinics in the UK have long complained about the apparently unnecessary amount of time they are kept waiting, with the result that many donors gave blood once but never returned. By carrying out a walk-through simulation of the process from start to finish, it was quickly seen that there were opportunities to streamline the process by placing certain key pieces of equipment in alternative locations, thus leading to a significant reduction in wait times (personal communication, 2010, Mike Brittain Business Analyst, NHSBT (NHS Blood and Transplant)). This technique of capturing the stages of a process in a simple display along with readily available data is widely used in the process improvement methodology known as 'Lean', where it is referred to as *value-stream analysis* or *value-stream mapping*.

## 21.3   Spreadsheet modelling

Simple spreadsheet modelling can provide information on, for example, the cost implications of making changes to a process. With just basic skills in Excel, a series of formulae can be used to link various input figures such as the number of patients likely to require surgery and the cost of conducting an operation. In this way it is possible to quickly run through a variety of scenarios with the formulae automatically computing sets of numerical results.

The word 'simple' is important here. Users who are expert in programming (in Visual Basic for example) can create very sophisticated models which are ostensibly spreadsheets. However, here we use the term 'spreadsheet modelling' to refer to the more commonplace use of the menu options within programs such as Excel to create linked computations involving values in the cells.

Like talk-through and walk-through modelling, spreadsheet modelling is not well suited to complex situations. Because of the simplistic relationship between the input parameters, the results can only provide a snapshot view of a process. In addition, it is difficult to make allowances for factors such as seasonal changes in admission figures or variability in a patient's Length of Stay (LoS), for example. Furthermore, the results produced by a spreadsheet model give no indication of the changing pattern of patient waiting times and queue lengths over time, or the impact that a problem in one section of a process might have on another, apparently unrelated, process. Nonetheless, since healthcare planners and analysts are generally familiar with spreadsheets, they provide a tool which can be quickly and readily used for superficial examination of the relationships amongst several input values.

By creating macros and adding additional programming, one can make a spreadsheet simulation more flexible, but for the same expenditure of time and effort one is likely to get more useful insights by using a discrete event simulation package such as SIMUL8 or ExtendSim, or a system dynamics package such as IThink. These can not only compute various snapshot results, but also provide a dynamic visualisation of what is going on in the process over a period of time. In addition, the risks associated with creating brand-new code to handle something complex are avoided. Off-the-shelf simulation software typically has many years of testing behind it, and many thousands of users to provide some reassurance that the core functions are working properly, and that any new errors introduced by version updates will have a wide exposure and therefore an increased chance of being detected and corrected. By custom-building code in a spreadsheet to handle the core, non-application-specific functions of a simulation package, one risks not only re-inventing the wheel, but worse: failing to re-invent it correctly.

## 21.4    System dynamics

System dynamics is a high-level methodology for studying and managing complex interactions and feedback systems over extended periods of time. It is often used when modelling ecological, economic and population systems, and, as such, it can be a useful planning tool in healthcare when considering the introduction of, for example, a new type of screening for a population cohort with a view to providing early intervention for any detected health problems. Because the focus is on the flow of many thousands, perhaps even millions of individuals, through a system, it is not possible to distinguish individual patients. This restricts the usefulness of this type of software to planning at a national level where the aim is, for example, to gauge the number of interventions, treatments sessions or doses of vaccine that might be needed annually.

## 21.5    Discrete event simulation

Although it is possible to develop approximations to continuous-flow (system dynamics) models in some discrete event simulation packages, their core strength lies in being able to look at, and react to, an individual's characteristics. And since most administrators and planners are involved with the day-to-day management of hospitals and clinics, rather than with high-level policy planning, their attention tends to be focused on finding ways to ensure the smooth flow of patients through a system with the minimum of unnecessary queuing or waiting time. For this reason, this chapter will concentrate on discussing the benefits that can be gained from modelling at this more granular, or event-based, level. In general, little theoretical knowledge is required of what goes on within processes – they are merely characterised by estimates of the resources required (including inputs, people and time) for each task to be completed. This empirical knowledge is often available, or capable of being readily collected.

Whether the intention is to map out-patient and in-patient pathways with a view to finding ways to treat more people more quickly, or to determine the best locations for fast response emergency vehicles, or to identify the number of beds required in a pandemic, healthcare planners can use simulations to quickly investigate alternative ways of dealing with these sorts of issues without causing inconvenience to staff and patients, or putting lives at risk. Discrete event simulation (DES) provides the ideal tool: a variety of scenarios can be explored in order to find effective, workable and affordable solutions given the specific constraints in the system, whilst simultaneously maximising or minimising certain key performance indicators.

One of the great advantages that both DES and system dynamics modelling have over spreadsheet modelling is that the input parameters can vary over time. Some of these input parameters will show relatively predictable variation at some level of aggregation (admissions of elderly patients suffering from influenza ('flu') usually peak in the winter, and children tend to suffer more broken limbs in the summer holidays than at other times of year, while attendances at A&E fluctuate by time of day, day of the week, and by season). In parallel,

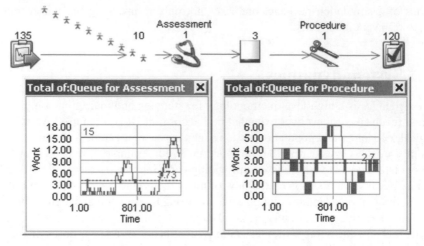

**Figure 21.1**  Numerical, graphical and visual displays of data in a SIMUL8 model.

unexpected events such as a major terrorist attack or an explosion at a chemical works can also be triggered at random intervals to determine where the bottlenecks would be if a hospital was faced with a sudden influx of patients, and to investigate how the new and existing patients could best be handled in view of the constraints existing in the system.

Results related to the passage of time may simply be displayed as numerical and graphical outputs, but some software packages also provide a visual representation of how a process is behaving, as can be seen in Figure 21.1, where the number of patients queuing for treatment is displayed in various ways.

Let us now look at some aspects of DES in a little more detail. Discrete event simulation is generally used to model the progress of entities through a series of often complex and inter-related procedures such as those involved in a cardiac, orthopaedic, or cancer patient pathway, where the entities are most often patients, but may also be, for example, blood or tissue samples. Each entity, whether it be a patient or a tissue sample, can be assigned a set of characteristics based on statistical distributions or probability profiles created specifically to correspond to the demographics of a particular population. To take a simple example, patients are often classified according to the severity of their condition and, as such, may be regarded as Urgent (an emergency), Routine or Elective (pre-booked appointment). Historical medical records can be analysed to find out the likelihood of an individual arriving at an Accident and Emergency department (A&E) requiring urgent, life-saving treatment, and the equivalent proportion of entities in the simulation can then be similarly classified. Rules built into the simulation will then ensure that emergency patients will receive the appropriate medical interventions ahead of routine or elective patients, just as one would expect to see in reality. Furthermore, each patient may be assigned a number of additional characteristics sampled from probability distributions based on historical patient data, since their route through the patient pathway is likely to depend not only on the severity of their illness but on characteristics like age, sex, presenting symptoms, outcome of tests and so on; while other characteristics may be used to determine the length of time required for each stage in the individual's treatment or diagnosis. See Figures 21.2 and 21.3.

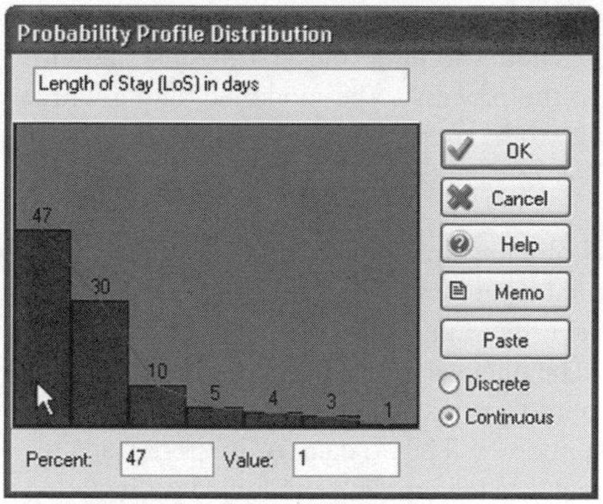

**Figure 21.2** Example of probability function for the LoS for a patient ranging between one and seven days.

## 21.6 Creating a discrete event simulation

Regardless of the process to be modelled, or the software to be used, the approach to building a simulation should be the same. Begin by ensuring that the reason for developing the model has been clearly defined, since this will help to identify the type of results that need to be extracted, which in turn will determine the nature and detail of the input data. During preliminary discussions, it is also important to identify the key procedures in the process, and their sequence. This may appear to be self-evident, but sometimes participants discover gaps or disagreements in their knowledge of a process, or have difficulty in agreeing which procedures or steps are 'key'. Restricting the detail to an appropriate level can be the hardest

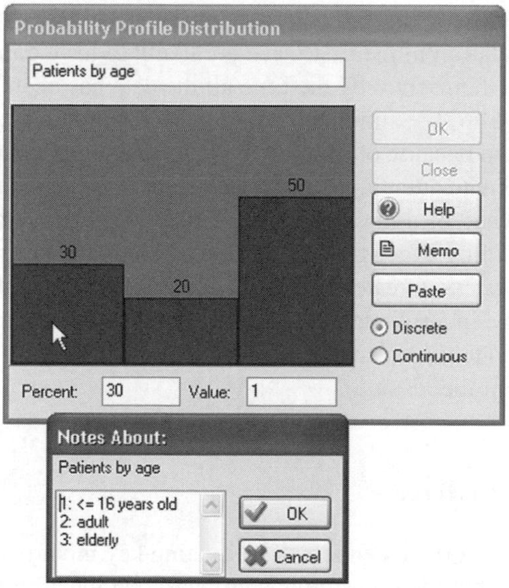

**Figure 21.3** Example of probability function for a patient falling into a particular age band.

part of developing a simulation. However, once this stage is complete it is generally a relatively straightforward matter to build the first model. The most important requirements are a clear description of the process to be modelled, along with a high level of familiarity with the software package to be used, in order to construct a credible representation of how the different activities link to each other. This helps to identify priorities for data collection and analysis.

Many of the benefits of using simulation models to support discussions of processes can be obtained by trying 'what if' analyses, and some of these need not have extensive, or indeed any, historical data to back them up (although every opportunity to obtain new data to test model predictions should be pursued). For example, what might happen in our process if some proportion of a key resource (people, or equipment, say) was suddenly reduced? If this has not happened in the past, there will be no data for it. Or perhaps we do not have detailed data for the spread of times required to complete a specific task included in the model. The analyst can still proceed by making a guess (and documenting it as such). He or she is then able to say that 'if the spread is like this, then we get the following results', or perhaps 'it does not seem to matter much what the spread is here – the range of plausible vaues we have tried all lead to much the same result'. It should be noted that a precise replication of observed results is generally not a requirement for a useful simulation model. Generally, getting in the right vicinity can suffice. It must not be forgotten that the real world has many more effects and factors than can be sensibly captured in a model. The aim is to capture what we believe to be the most important, and then see if credible outputs are obtained under a range of conditions. Seeking to incorporate masses of data and detail is to fail to understand the limitations of modelling (a model is a simplification of a process), of process knowledge (not always complete), and of the data itself (which may contain errors, omissions, or be poorly defined).

The utility of informed guesses (subjective estimates) for some model parameter settings (e.g. a triangular distribution of a task duration) should not be underestimated. The aim of most practical simulations is to produce a timely and workable solution to a problem. To spend months tracking down and analysing data sets in order to create a very accurate model is generally self-defeating. If the lead-time in producing a model is too long, those who commissioned the simulation in the first place are likely to have come up with some sort of solution to the problem themselves by the time all the data has been analysed and the model developed. In the long run, the simulated solution might indicate a more effective way of dealing with the issue, but because of its tardiness it is of negligible value if key decisions have been made and management attention is now elsewhere. If, on the other hand, a first-iteration model is built in the space of a few hours, using plausible estimates of volumes and cycle times, it is already providing a focus for discussion and may well provide useful insights into ways to improve the process. Greater accuracy, in the form of statistical distributions based on historical data, can be incorporated into subsequent iterations, but even then detailed data analysis can be restricted to those distributions where minor changes to their shape and spread have a marked impact on the results.

## 21.7    Data difficulties

Let us look more closely at three benefits of estimating key input parameters.

First of all, the fact that there is so much emphasis on meeting target times in the NHS means it can be difficult to find historical data relating to activity times. In general, the type of data that is routinely collected is intended to help answer target-related questions. As a result, it may be impossible to find documented information on the length of time it takes to carry out a particular procedure.

Furthermore, hospital managers may argue that there is no need to record cycle times, as they know, for example, that eight people are routinely booked into each four-hour clinic session. The assumption therefore is that this equates to 30 minutes of contact time between patient and clinician. However, by talking to the clinician one may discover that the actual contact time is on average just 25 minutes. If so, the throughput of the clinic is being artificially constrained because of the appointment booking system. In reality, there is the potential to handle 9.6 patients per clinic session. And indeed there is even the potential to handle 10 patients by simply increasing the time of the clinic session by 10 minutes. This is a classic example of how easily cause and effect can be confused.

Collecting good quality data is a non-trivial task, requiring both careful planning and very careful execution. In particular, care must be taken to avoid alienating staff by imposing intrusive observers; for example, the proverbial 'stranger with a clipboard and stopwatch' appearing out of the blue. The preferred approach is for those involved in the process to be engaged with the modelling, and conduct the data collection themselves under supervision. When time is short, a brief visit to a process to capture a snapshot of data (e.g. number of people in each waiting area) can be useful to anchor the initial modelling with real data. But to capture the process variability (including unexpected disruptions) requires data collection spread over sufficient time to expose the process to its main sources of variation (e.g. shift changes, absent staff, equipment failures, administrative delays, supply chain variation, differences in diagnostic skills, and so on).

Secondly, Professor George Box's famous phrase, 'all models are wrong but some models are useful' (Box, 1979) is just as true in healthcare simulations as in any other field of science. Models provide a simplified view of reality, and as such they enable non-experts to quickly get an understanding of very complex systems. Sometimes knowing the actual number of patients being admitted over a week, or the actual cycle times for a set of medical procedures, will not add greatly to the benefits to be gained, particularly in the early stages of developing a model. Indeed, developing a simulation commonly acts as a catalyst to bring together a disparate group of professionals who may not meet in the normal course of events. The ensuing debates, which generally focus on how the model is not telling the whole, complicated story of a particular process, tend to expose any areas where the group has a sketchy or incomplete understanding of the way the process functions and often leads to startling and unexpected insights – simply because the group have allowed themselves time to think through the process in detail. In other words, the simulation provides a vehicle for rational and measured discussion with the knowledge that, if necessary, a very detailed simulation can eventually be developed complete with statistical distributions to model variability in the input parameters.

Thirdly, some input data will always have to be estimated. Certain factors, such as the time required for a medical procedure, are measurable and can be controlled to a certain extent. For example, it may be possible to reduce the average time by introducing new or better equipment, and variation around this average may be reduced by ensuring that everyone involved follows standardised procedures. However, other factors are uncontrollable: the number of patients requiring hospitalisation during a flu pandemic; the number of women becoming pregnant in a given year; the number of obese or diabetic patients who will need medical intervention in 10 years' time. Regardless of the sophistication of your forecasting techniques, these types of inputs to a simulation will always be estimates.

Consequently, at least in the initial stages of developing a simulation, there is a great deal to be gained by estimating the input data so that the model can immediately start to produce benefits by acting as a focus for discussion. Where reasonably realistic figures are required, it is quicker, and much less hassle, to ask individuals who are actually involved in carrying out a procedure to provide an estimate based on their experience. When asked, 'How long does this job take on average? What's the shortest time you need to do this task? And how long will it take you on a bad day?', staff will be able to respond immediately with an approximate minimum, mode and maximum time: exactly what you need to set up a simple triangular distribution which will provide a reasonable, if crude, representation of the central values, spread, and skew of the timings.

A similar approach works well when estimating other variables such as daily, monthly, seasonal or annual patient admissions, or the proportion of patients falling into various categories.

A sensitivity analysis can be conducted in due course to find out which, if any, of these simple triangular distributions have a marked impact on the results when their parameters are varied slightly. In this way it is easy to avoid devoting excessive amounts of time and effort to unnecessary data analysis, and to concentrate instead on providing a speedy response. Alternatively, a statistician can work on the necessary data analysis at the same time as the model developer works on the simulation. But it cannot be emphasised enough that the simulation itself is such a useful tool, that one should not be tempted to defer starting on the simulation until all the relevant data has been gathered.

It is worth bearing in mind that specifying a distribution implies a degree of stability. Care should be taken when attempting to simulate a process where, for instance, the average cycle time in one time period is very different from the average cycle time in another time period. This type of changing behaviour in a system can be handled in various ways, including using different distributions depending on the time of day or the day of the week. The important thing is not to assume that a single distribution will always suffice. Furthermore, one ought to bear in mind that statistical distributions are themselves 'models', and as such are only approximations to some aspects of the observed data, or real process parameter. The common ground between the statistician and the simulation expert is their tentative creation of models, and their use of them to encourage deeper discussion with subject-matter experts who may wish to compare the simulated results with past performance, or to make testable forecasts of what might happen under various specified circumstances.

# 21.8    Complex or simple?

Simulations are useful for answering well-focused questions and looking for solutions to specific problems. Therefore, it is usually better to have a suite of simple models which may superficially look the same, but which can be used to answer a number of completely different questions, each with their own assumptions built-in, than to attempt to create a 'super-model' which can be interrogated to find the solution to all problems. In addition to the inordinate effort required to build and validate such a model, one invariably finds that there are circumstances where the input parameters are not flexible enough to investigate solutions to issues which were not anticipated at the time the model was created. So immediately one is forced to either adapt the existing model, or create a new one. Simple but very useful models can frequently be developed and checked for accuracy in just a few hours, while a

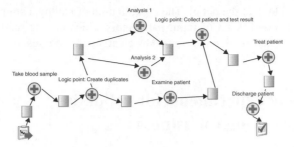

**Figure 21.4**   An example of a simulation under development where all decision points are visible.

complex one might well take months. What is better? Ten simple, well-focused models? Or one unwieldy monster that doesn't really answer any question properly?

Simplification is also necessary when looking at the potential capacity of a system. Imagine developing a model that is to be used to predict the maximum numbers of patients that could potentially be treated in a perfectly ordered world; that is, where there are sufficient staff available, no artificial waiting times are built into the system, equipment does not break down, and all patients arrive on time for their appointments. The only constraints that should be incorporated into the simulation are those relating to the minimum time it ought to take for a patient to be treated at each staging point in their pathway. The results from a model like this demonstrate the theoretical physical capacity of the system which then acts as a reference point from which planners can investigate, for example, what would happen if a new appointments system is introduced that leads to a reduction in DNAs (patients who Did Not Attend). A baseline model of this type is deterministic but can subsequently be readily adapted to show the impact in the real world of adding variability to treatment times, patient arrival rates, staff numbers, and unexpected breakdowns in equipment, through the use of appropriate statistical distributions.

On a similar note, it is always worth making a model look tidy and simple. Most models will include building blocks which have been incorporated as decision-points to facilitate functionality, but once a model is complete, it is advisable to hide these to aid understanding, for example by reducing clutter in order to highlight key features (see Figures 21.4 and 21.5). Furthermore, it is worth customising the graphics of the remaining visible building blocks, so the intended audience can quickly make sense of what they see. As the old aphorism says, 'a picture paints a thousand words'. The same applies to the underlying data and rules controlling the behaviour of the simulation, and numerical results. Everything should be presented clearly, in spreadsheet and graphical formats, so it quickly makes sense to

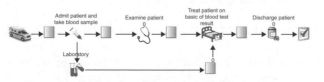

**Figure 21.5**   Customising graphics, and hiding unnecessary building blocks, highlights the key processes.

anyone who needs to look at the detail. The combination of having a simple visual depiction of a situation coupled with a set of input parameters which can be readily edited to allow testing of 'what-if' scenarios, all underpinned by clearly defined rules, makes simulation very powerful.

## 21.9    Design of experiments for validation, and for testing robustness

Many people who develop and use simulations are planners and analysts, rather than statisticians. Whilst they may be building simulations quickly in order to clarify ideas and assumptions, and to get a better understanding of the interactions between the factors under investigation, they want to have the confidence that the underlying methodology, and hence the results generated by simulations, are based on sound statistical theory. But regardless of whether a simulation is a rough approximation or a highly detailed representation of a process, it is important to verify that the model works in the manner intended.

One way to carry out these sorts of quality checks is to run the simulation using a historical data set for which the outcomes are already known. Alternatively the simulation may be run a number of times, varying the input parameters each time, and using common sense to check the credibility of the ensuing results. However, depending on the number of variables in the system, there may be many hundreds of possible permutations remaining even after implausible or impossible combinations of factors have been eliminated. Even if the testing process can be automated, running a simulation so many times can be unwieldy and time consuming. But, using a technique called *Design of Experiments* in conjunction with the careful selection of both controllable (e.g. number of staff) and uncontrollable (e.g. number of patients requiring operations) factors and their settings, provides the tester with a very powerful method of checking whether the results under a variety of conditions all appear sensible. If some conditions produce questionable results the developer is in a position to quickly identify the main contributing factor, or factors, which caused them.

In a simple designed experiment, the number of runs can be restricted by only using two values for each of the input parameters. Imagine one has three simulation parameters of interest, for example the number of nurses (denoted by parameter $X_1$), operating theatres ($X_2$), and patients requiring operations ($X_3$) in a hospital. By running the simulation with just a low ($-$) and a high ($+$) setting for each of these variables, there will be eight different combinations of settings (see Table 21.1). For each one, a set of outcomes, or response variables ($Y$), which might include the total number of operations that can be carried out per week, and the utilisation of the operating theatres and nurses, can be captured from the model for subsequent analysis.

The effect of a factor, such as $X_3$, say, is estimated by subtracting the mean value of $Y$ at the low level of $X_3$ from that at the high level; that is,

$$\text{Effect of } X_3 \text{ is defined as } (Y_5 + Y_6 + Y_7 + Y_8)/4 - (Y_1 + Y_2 + Y_3 + Y_4)/4.$$

Furthermore the interactions of these factors may also be estimated from the data. This allows the analyst to investigate the extent to which the impact of $X_3$, say, depends on the settings of $X_1$ and/or $X_2$. Details can be found in any elementary book on designed

**Table 21.1**   Design for a three-factor experiment.

| Simulation run | $X_1$ | $X_2$ | $X_3$ | Outcome |
|:---:|:---:|:---:|:---:|:---:|
| 1 | – | – | – | $Y_1$ |
| 2 | + | – | – | $Y_2$ |
| 3 | – | + | – | $Y_3$ |
| 4 | + | + | – | $Y_4$ |
| 5 | – | – | + | $Y_5$ |
| 6 | + | – | + | $Y_6$ |
| 7 | – | + | + | $Y_7$ |
| 8 | + | + | + | $Y_8$ |

experiments. The book by Daniel Sloan (1997) is particularly accessible, and is devoted to healthcare examples.

The number of possible combinations of settings grows very rapidly as more factors are included. However, a careful selection of a balanced fraction of these possible combinations can provide sufficient insight in many situations. This technique is known as 'fractional factorial design', and it has been widely used in science and industry over the past 70 years or so. It is described in Sloan's (1997) book and at a more advanced technical level in a wide range of statistical texts, for example Kenett and Zacks (1998), or, more recently, the chapter on industrial experiments in Coleman *et al.* (2008) provides a concise introduction. This can allow large numbers of factors to be explored using relatively few simulation runs. The fewer the runs, the more ambiguity in the results, but sometimes a coarse analysis is enough to identify major features. Follow-up designs can be used to resolve specific ambiguities that seem important or interesting.

In addition to using designed experiments for basic error checking in a model, they provide a very powerful way to investigate the robustness of a system to changes in both controllable and uncontrollable factors, and thereby to help identify the most favourable combinations of factor settings for given performance goals or criteria. Certain factors, such as the number of hospital beds, the number of available staff, and the admission of elective patients, are usually prescribed with fixed values. On the other hand the rate of arrival of emergency patients and their LoS are largely stochastic and obviously cannot be determined by planners, although they can be estimated. The methodology makes it perfectly feasible to tease out interaction effects amongst controllable factors, or between controllable factors and uncontrollable factors. And by manipulating the controllable factors one can look for one or more scenarios in which the system is robust enough to handle the workload even when faced with variation in the uncontrollable factors.

These very simple designs and associated analyses have been widely used in industry to great effect. More sophisticated designs have also been found useful, and these ideas are spreading into healthcare simulation. For example, Dehlendorff *et al.* (2010) studied the impact of controlled and uncontrolled factors on the larger end of the range of orthopaedic waiting times in a Danish hospital.

Whether or not one decides to carry out designed experiments on a simulation, the choice of response variable ($Y$; also known as key performance indicator (KPI)) is important: your choice of $Y$ will be largely dictated by the areas of concern in the process. Nevertheless, the software will usually generate a host of additional $Y$s, thus providing the opportunity to study other aspects of the process should the need arise.

It is possible to optimise simulations in other ways; for example the optimisation software, OptQuest (http://www.opttek.com), is claimed by the developers to be integrated into over 95% of simulation software products on the market and uses algorithms such as tabu search, neural networks and scatter search. Taking into account any constraints on decision variables such as minimum and maximum staff numbers specified by the user, the software can be programmed to search for combinations of $X$s that will enable certain specified $Y$s such as profit or throughput to be maximised at the same time as minimising other $Y$s such as costs. Many trials are then run using various combinations of the $X$s which are intelligently varied in response to the resulting $Y$s, making it easy to identify strategies which are likely to provide good outcomes. This is a less elegant and informative method than using designed experiments, but it can provide some suggestions for improvement with relatively little effort on the part of the programmer.

## 21.10    Other issues

Certain aspects of simulations are the subject of much ongoing debate. These relate to warm-up periods, the length of simulated time that a model should run for, and the number of runs there should be in a trial (a trial being a set of runs).

Should a simulation be primed with work-in-progress (WIP)? A good example of this being patients already on waiting lists for treatment. Or is it better to include a warm-up period equivalent to some weeks, months or years to allow the simulation to be populated with a representative WIP? And if so, how long should the warm-up period be? Or should a combination of both predetermined WIP and warm-up be used?

How long should a run last? Is it better to set a simulation up to run for a long period of time? Or is it better to have many shorter runs where different values are sampled from the distributions each time? Whatever the run length, it is clearly not wise to base changes to a process on the results from a single run, since these may be atypical. By running a trial composed of multiple runs, one can get a more accurate indication of typical averages for the results of interest, along with confidence limits for these averages. But what is the best number of runs to have in a trial? Should the number of runs vary depending on the number of decision factors?

More discussion of these topics is available on a website at Warwick University.[1] A very useful review of technical aspects of discrete event simulation, with many pointers to recent literature, is given in the chapter on simulation in industrial statistics in Coleman *et al.* (2008).

---

[1] http://www2.warwick.ac.uk/fac/soc/wbs/projects/autosimoa/.

## 21.11    Case study no. 1: Simulation for capacity planning

Case study provided by Kirstin Dickson, Head of Health Economics: Policy, Planning and Performance, NHS Ayrshire and Arran, in 2010.

As part of a major review of services, a health board in Scotland wanted to investigate the impact of changing the way elective and emergency services were provided at two district general hospitals situated some 10 miles apart. Both hospitals provided Accident and Emergency services (A&E) and, aside from a few small specialties,[2] all major specialties such as Trauma, Orthopaedics, and Gynaecology were duplicated across both sites. This duplication was a driving factor for seeking to change the delivery of care and to separate elective referrals and emergency admissions.

The first simulation to be developed modelled the existing situation. Key inputs were the number of patients being admitted each day to each specialty (via the two A&E departments as well as via GP referrals), and their LoS. Historical data were used to determine the number of elective referrals each day, and the frequency of patients presenting at A&E. In addition, the historical records enabled probability profiles to be created to determine the proportions of patients being admitted to each specialty from each of the two A&E departments and, for each individual entering a specialty, the likelihood of their remaining there for a given time period before discharge; in other words, their LoS.

The purpose of the study was to compare current bed requirements with bed requirements if various major changes in patient pathways were implemented. Amongst the proposals being discussed, it was suggested that it would be more efficient to end the duplication of specialties, and simultaneously to restrict one of the A&E departments to treating relatively minor injuries and illness, while the other would specialise in handling major trauma cases. In parallel with this, it was planned to set up a short-stay Combined Assessment Unit close to A&E, with both surgical and medical input, where A&E patients could stay briefly while a decision was made about whether they were to be admitted or discharged in order to avoid 'inappropriate admissions'. At that time, patients were often admitted to a ward while lab work was carried out. Although these patients needed to be monitored until their test results came through, their state of health did not merit their occupying a bed in a specialty ward.

A second, related, model was subsequently developed to demonstrate the impact of the proposed structural changes to patient pathways. Modelling the effect of dealing with patients at one or other of the A&E departments depending on the severity of their condition was relatively straightforward since the probability of a patient suffering from a minor injury as opposed to major trauma could be determined by analysing existing medical records.

In comparison, modelling the impact of introducing a combined assessment unit was more difficult, as similar short-stay units were only beginning to be introduced in the UK; meaning little or no historical data was available for daily, weekly or annual patient numbers, LoS and so on. Instead, input parameters were initially estimated, then varied systematically to ascertain the impact of changes in demand on the number of beds required.

The models were deliberately kept simple and the LoS for patients in each specialty encompassed, where appropriate, theatre time, ICU (intensive care unit) time and ward stay time (see Figure 21.6).

---

[2] The American word 'specialty' seems to have displaced 'speciality' in UK healthcare circles, and so is used here.

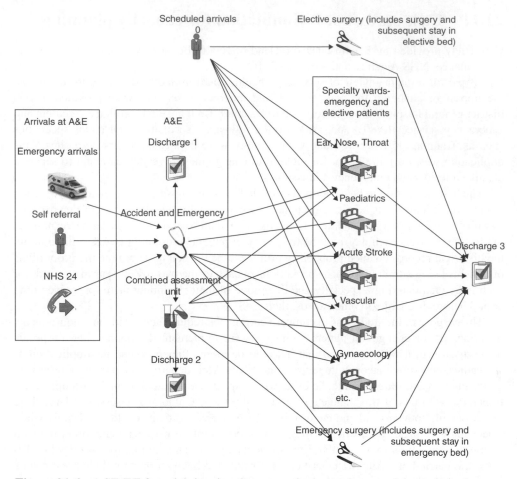

**Figure 21.6** A SIMUL8 model showing the way patients may be routed through the process.

A large number of professionals were involved in the review. Of these, a few were familiar with SIMUL8, but many were initially dubious about its usefulness. Interestingly, this actually worked to the SIMUL8 developers' advantage as many of the sceptics created their own Excel models of sections of the overall process and found, sometimes to their surprise, that their results supported the findings of the main model.

With models developed in both SIMUL8 and Excel to support their case, the NHS Board ultimately received approval from the Scottish Government for their proposed changes to the delivery of elective and emergency services.

## 21.12   Case study no. 2: Screening for vascular disease

Case study provided by Marianne Scholes, Principal Operational Research Analyst, NHS Medical Directorate, Department of Health, in 2010.

In March 2009, the Department of Health introduced a five-yearly screening programme, NHS Health Check, for all 40–74 year-olds in England in an effort to reduce the incidence of vascular disease, namely coronary heart disease, stroke, diabetes and kidney disease.

Due to the scale of the project, it was essential to assess the anticipated costs, and expected benefits, before implementing the programme. Although Excel was used initially to estimate the number of staff required, the number of tests that would have to be carried out annually, and their cost, it soon became evident that a spreadsheet was not versatile enough to readily handle the complexity of the system and, additionally, lacked the facility to produce the results in a visual manner which was easy to interpret. Being faced at this point with the choice of developing a system-dynamics model or a discrete event simulation, the policy team opted for DES because it allowed them to model the progress of individual members of the population through the five-yearly cycle of screening. System dynamics was rejected because a model functioning at population level would not have contained enough detail to generate the required outcomes. With DES, on the other hand, each member of the population cohort being modelled was treated as an individual. Of these, some would not suffer from any risk factors at the time of screening and therefore would not need any tests or treatment, while those exhibiting high blood pressure, high cholesterol, high BMI, or a combination of these, would subsequently undergo factor-specific tests and receive medical interventions and life-style advice; all of which could be clearly costed.

This study was able to use anonymised patient-level data for 1.4 million people, taken from 472 local doctors' practices (GP practices). A model was created consisting of 50 practices designed to be typical of the practice areas found in the complete set of 472. For each model run, the number of patients in each age group to be invited for screening each year was specified. A patient entering the model was assigned the characteristics of a patient randomly sampled from the correct age group within the 1.4 million. The ensuing results were extrapolated to provide information on how many staff would be required nationwide to carry out screenings, the laboratory facilities and staff required to analyse blood samples, the number of resulting prescriptions for statins and other drugs, the number of staff required to run clinics giving advice on smoking cessation, weight loss, diet, exercise and so on, as well as the associated costs. Furthermore, the model provided information on the potential savings to be made by the NHS by comparing the costs of these interventions against the long-term costs of treating people once they had developed vascular disease.

This simulation proved to be an extremely useful tool at the planning stage, and continues to be used to check the implications of further proposed policy changes. Not only does it provide the numerical information required, but the visual nature of the display makes it easy to interpret at a glance.


## 21.13    Case study no. 3: Meeting waiting time targets in orthopaedic care

Case study provided by Catriona Sked, Senior Information Analyst, 18 Weeks RTT Collaborative, Business Intelligence Department, NHS Ayrshire and Arran, in 2010.

In 2004 the NHS announced a plan to reduce the time a patient would have to wait for non-emergency hospital treatment to a maximum of 18 weeks. To achieve this, hospital managers typically had to solve two problems; in the short term, they needed to take steps to clear the existing backlog of patients, while, in the longer term, they needed to find reliable ways to maintain the required rate of flow of patients through the pathway so as to consistently meet the 18-week target.

Simulation was quickly identified as a tool which could be used to explore the impact on waiting times of a range of proposed improvement initiatives, and many hospitals and health boards across the UK adopted the discrete event package, SIMUL8, because of its ability to model pathways at patient level, and because of its relative ease of use.

For example, the planners at a hospital in the west of Scotland had identified a variety of possible ways to reduce the orthopaedic waiting list and then used SIMUL8 to test the impact these changes would have on the waiting list and how long it would take for orthopaedics to comply with the 18-week target under a variety of different circumstances. A high-level model of the patient pathway was built over four days. This incorporated an Excel front end containing all the input variables so as to make it easy for non-SIMUL8 users to create and test alternative scenarios. Having identified the areas in the pathway where changes were required, staff subsequently embarked on a programme of improvements using a variety of Lean methodologies in order to streamline these. This process is ongoing, but the simulation will be validated once the improvements have been implemented by incorporating revised data for treatment times, allocation and availability of staff, and so on, along with distributions to model referral rates based on current GP practices, and up-to-date waiting-list data.

Since the overall patient pathway is expected to remain essentially the same and because the model was built at a macro rather than a micro level, the simulation contains sufficient flexibility to be useful over a number of years. For example, meeting the 18-week target may well be just the first step in a continuing cycle of improvement; it is highly likely that the government will demand even shorter waiting times in the future. Consequently, the simulation can be used again and again to identify new pinch points in the system when waiting time targets are reduced further, if referral rates increase, or to demonstrate how many extra procedures can be carried out annually if additional theatre time becomes available, or if improved techniques and equipment result in a reduction in the time required to carry out certain operations. What's more, there is no requirement to alter just one variable at a time; multiple input parameters can be altered simultaneously.

## 21.14    Case Study no. 4: Bed Capacity Implications Model (BECIM)

Case study provided by David Bensley, Operational Research Programme Manager, Department of Health, in 2010.

Simulation models in the Department of Health (DH) are developed to meet national strategic objectives as opposed, for example, to tactical models generated directly for the NHS.

The Bed Capacity Implications Model (BECIM) was originally developed to explore the 'price', in terms of levels of bed occupancy, of responding to emergency and elective demand while maintaining a low risk of cancelling elective operations. It has been a notable success and has since been used for a wide range of strategic applications such as the capacity implications of introducing booked appointments systems for elective surgery, and of introducing dedicated stroke units. In addition, it has been used to simulate capacity requirements for dealing with

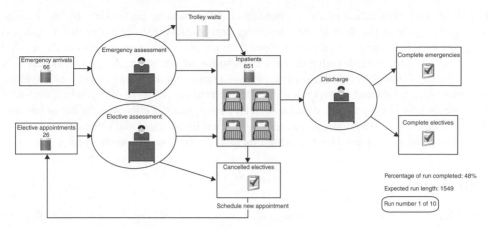

**Figure 21.7**    Bed Capacity Implications Model (BECIM) with customised graphics.

unpredictable or unforeseen events such as the arrival of planeloads of military casualties from Iraq. (See Figure 21.7.)

BECIM was developed by the Economics and Operational Research Division (EOR) of DH using SIMUL8, with an interactive, user-friendly front-end, written in Excel, used for data input and collecting simulation results. It is a generic simulation model which enables the exploration of relationships between admission rates, trolley waits, bed occupancy, LoS for emergency and elective operations, last minute cancellations and delayed discharges.

In addition to its use for strategic applications in the DH, it has also been made available to NHS hospital trust managers as a learning tool to assist with medium- to long-term planning, as opposed, for example, to day-to-day organisation on the wards.

Clearly a generic, high-level model such as BECIM has limitations: the simulation is based upon the structure of a typical trust and cannot model the resource details, pathway structures or dynamics between different specialties of any given trust. Furthermore, no attempt is made to directly model seasonal variations in patient admissions, although this could be addressed if necessary. However, it is clear that much can be gained in terms of overall understanding by modelling an approximation of the reality within a trust.

The model has been presented at national and international conferences and a paper is in preparation.

## 21.15    Summary

In summary, simulation provides a very powerful and flexible tool for investigating and testing a variety of scenarios, without immediate operational risk and at modest financial cost. The links to statistical methods and thinking are many, and indeed the interaction of the modeller with the client can be very similar to that of the statistician and client. In each case, there is a sounding-out of client requirements, level of knowledge, availability of data, identification of performance measures and influencing factors. This is followed by the creation of tentative models to facilitate further discussion and the exploration of ideas, as well as the identification of areas where more data would be particularly useful. Finally, for a given cycle or iteration of the modelling process, forecasts based on the model can be produced which can be used to guide practical actions. The client wants clarity, a sense that good and proper methodologies have been followed, the strengths and weaknesses of which are familiar to the modeller/statistician, and a sense that the client's needs and expertise have been recognised and incorporated. Modern simulation software, like modern statistical software, is now so easy to use at an introductory level, that the client can be his or her own modeller/statistician after some initial training to familiarise them with the software and to raise their awareness of any pitfalls and risks which would call for specialist help.

# References

Box, G.E.P. (1979) Robustness in the strategy of scientific model building, in *Robustness in Statistics* (eds R.L. Launer and G.N. Wilkinson), Academic Press, New York.

Coleman, S., Greenfield, T., Stewardson, D. and Montgomery, D.C. (eds) (2008) *Statistical Practice in Business and Industry*, John Wiley & Sons, Ltd, Chichester.

Dehlendorff, C., Kulahci, M., Merser, S. and Andersen, K.K. (2010) Conditional value at risk as a measure for waiting time in simulations of hospital units. *Quality Technology & Quantitative Management*, 7(3), 321–336.

Kenett, R.S. and Zacks, S. (1998) *Modern Industrial Statistics*, Duxbury Press, Pacific Grove, California.

Sloan, D.M. (1997) *Using Designed Experiments to Shrink Health Care Costs*, ASQC, Quality Press.

# 22

# Statistical issues in insurance/payor processes

## Melissa Popkoski

*Pharmacy Administrative Services, Horizon Blue Cross Blue Shield of New Jersey, Newark, NJ, USA*

## Synopsis

Payment of healthcare providers is one of the developed world's most widespread processes – one which is handled in vastly different ways across different societies. One common issue is the complexity involved in trying to assure that payments are accurate and timely, while at the same time taking precautions to avoid waste and fraud. In the United States, private and public entities and systems must interact in the attainment of these goals. As a part of this picture, Medicare Part D, which supports the cost of prescription medications to seniors and the disabled, is one of largest pharmaceutical reimbursement programs in the world. This chapter discusses the many types of information that must come together from various sources, for patients to receive their medication and for payors and providers to be fairly compensated. A case study of one payor's process improvement efforts is discussed in detail.

## 22.1   Introduction

In healthcare reimbursement processes, there are a number of data elements that need to be aligned in order for a claim to be processed and paid correctly. 'Correctly' in this case means paying at the specified level of benefits, as agreed to in the member or group contract, using the appropriate eligibility information for the member, to the correct party – doctor, hospital, pharmacy, lab, and so on – for the intended services, and at the contracted rates provided on the given date.

*Statistical Methods in Healthcare*, First Edition.  Edited by Frederick W. Faltin, Ron S. Kenett and Fabrizio Ruggeri.
© 2012 John Wiley & Sons, Ltd.  Published 2012 by John Wiley & Sons, Ltd.

Examples of data elements associated with member's eligibility include:

- subscriber identification number

- subscriber address

- relationship of the member to the contract holder; for example, self or dependent, spouse or child

- age

- status of the member within the group; for example, active or retiree.

Generally, the source for this information is either the employer group with whom the primary card holder is a current or retired employee, or the member themselves. In the United States, those senior citizens covered by Medicare Part C and Part D have an additional entity providing this information to the insurers offering health coverage; namely, the Center for Medicare and Medicaid Services (CMS), an agency of the US federal government.

For this particular group of members more granular levels of eligibility status are held.

- HICN – the number assigned by the Social Security Administration to an individual identifying him/her as a Medicare beneficiary.

- Contract – the alphanumeric five-byte field identifying the Part C or Part D plan.

- PBP – the three-byte code identifying the specific Plan Benefit Package within the contract.

- LICS level – identifies Low Income Subsidy (LIS) members to whom low income cost sharing (LICS) is available.

If a Medicare beneficiary's income and resources fall within federal poverty guidelines as published by the Social Security Administration, he or she is eligible for a subsidy which will assist in payment of monthly premiums, reduce co-payments for brand and generic drugs and eliminate the coverage gap. The data field specifically tied to LIS members is a three-byte numeric value indicating the level of assistance for which the member is eligible.

This chapter will focus on the complexities and statistical variations that exist within the payment processes for submission and reimbursement of prescription drug claims under the Part D program.

## 22.2    Prescription drug claim processing and payment

### 22.2.1    General process: High-level outline

When a prescription claim is submitted to a payor there are several algorithms performed in claims processing systems to ensure that the claim processes for the correct line of eligibility, for the appropriate member, on the date the drug was dispensed. Generally speaking, after some initial checks to ensure the member has coverage and is eligible to receive the specific drug and quantity on the given date, a claim is submitted.

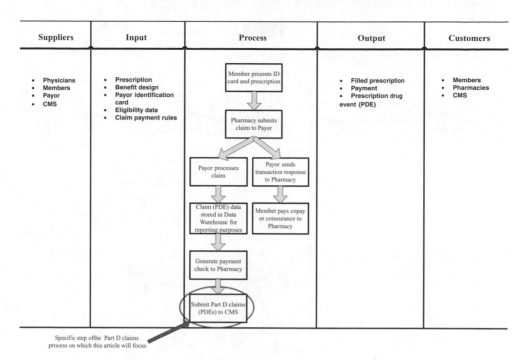

| Suppliers | Input | Process | Output | Customers |
|---|---|---|---|---|

**Figure 22.1**   Prescription drug event submission and payment.

Figure 22.1 provides a schematic representation of prescription drug claim processing and payment.[1]

## 22.2.2   Prescription drug plan Part D claims payment process

The US federal healthcare program offers prescription drugs to the aged and disabled under the Prescription Drug Program, Part D, which is administered by private insurance plans and subsidized by the Center for Medicare and Medicaid Services (CMS). As compared with a typical private payor individual or group health insurance policy, this program has an added layer of complexity in the reimbursement/payment process of prescription claims.

Specifically, for Part D claims, the process and payment of prescription claims have a few more steps. Pharmacies submit claims and payors process and pay them as outlined above. Additionally, since Medicare subsidizes premiums and reimburses a portion of the claims payment, and CMS maintains eligibility information for all Medicare beneficiaries, all Part D (and, for that matter, Part C) claims must be submitted to CMS at a very detailed level for reimbursement to the payor (see Figure 22.2).

Once a Part D claim, or PDE, has been paid by the payor, which could be done through a delegated Pharmacy Benefit Manager (PBM), claims are aggregated and systemically

---

[1] For information on this and the other continuous improvement tools used throughout this chapter, see Ruggeri, Kenett and Faltin (2007).

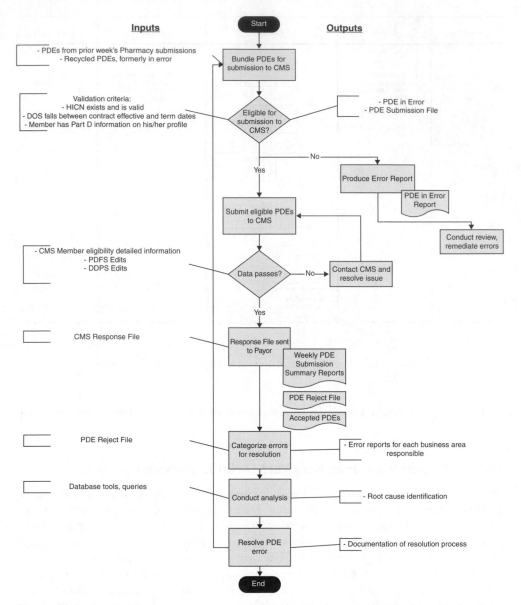

**Figure 22.2**   Part D PDE process – submission to finalized status. PDFS – Prescription Drug Front End System; DDPS – Drug Data Processing System.

submitted to CMS on a regular (for example, weekly) basis. CMS takes these claims, aligns each one to eligibility information maintained by their internal systems, using systemic algorithms, and identifies either accepted or rejected PDEs based on a number of factors determined to isolate PDEs that are appropriate for reimbursement.

A brief description of Pharmacy Benefit Managers (PBMs): it is fairly common in the USA for health insurers to outsource components of the pharmacy business to PBMs due to the complexity of the pharmacy benefits, claim adjudication and payment and negotiations with pharmaceutical companies and retail pharmacy networks. There are great economies of scale by having an entity handle the pharmacy business for several payors, since in-sourcing this function would require significant staff along with organizational and technological infrastructure.

One set of factors CMS uses to isolate PDEs appropriate for reimbursement centers around eligibility. If a PDE contains data elements in the eligibility criteria that do not match CMS' system, the claim will be rejected and the payor will not receive reimbursement for the claim in question, even though the claim has already been paid to the pharmacy by the payor at the point of sale. As such, it must be that the payor, PBM and CMS' systems have identical eligibility information for Part D members in order for 100% of the claims submitted to CMS to be accepted for reimbursement.

PDE Rejects fall into several categories with error codes that identify the field on the claim record that is in error, according to CMS. There are over 120 unique error codes, of which approximately 23 are related to eligibility.

Table 22.1 depicts the quantity of CMS-defined errors for each data element, or combination thereof, related to eligibility information.

**Table 22.1**   CMS Part D eligibility error codes.

| Data element(s) edited relating to eligibility | Count of PDE reject codes |
| --- | --- |
| Date of Service (DOS) | 5 |
| Date of Service (DOS) and Contract and Drug Coverage Status Code | 3 |
| Date of Service (DOS) and Contract and Plan Benefit Package | 1 |
| HICN | 2 |
| Low Income Cost-sharing Subsidy Amount (LICS) and Date of Service | 1 |
| Low Income Cost-sharing Subsidy Amount (LICS) and Drug Coverage Status Code and Date of Service | 1 |
| Patient Date of Birth (DOB) | 1 |
| Patient Gender | 1 |
| Patient Pay Amount and Other TrOOP Amount and PLRO and Pricing Exception Code | 5 |
| Patient Pay Amount and Other TrOOP Amount and Pricing Exception Code | 1 |
| Submitting Contract and Contract of Record | 1 |
| Submitting Contract and PBP and Date of Service | 1 |
| Grand total | 23 |

TrOOP – true out of pocket; PLRO – patient liability reduction due to other payor amount.

To further explain, the five errors that could occur on the Date of Service (DOS) transpire based on the systemic comparisons CMS performs, comparing the data on the PDE file submitted by the payor or its delegate (typically a PBM) to that which is maintained on CMS' own internal systems. A more robust description is best understood with an example; for date of service in particular there are several details that could signal information is out of sync between CMS and the payor, including but not limited to:

- the date of service is later than the date of death

- the beneficiary is not enrolled in Part D on the date of service

- the beneficiary must be enrolled in this contract (as stated on the PDE) on the date of service.

For the last point, since Part D beneficiaries can change Part D plans, it is possible a beneficiary was enrolled in a Part D contract with another payor, is indicated as such on CMS' system, yet the prescription was filled (the date of service occurred) with the benefits, and therefore contract, he/she thought they were enrolled in at that time.

The focus of the work in the case study which follows centered on decreasing the volume of PDE Rejects related to eligibility. The goal was to maximize the acceptance rate of PDEs, thereby correctly receiving reimbursement from CMS for claims that were paid at the point of sale, but for which at that time, or subsequently, the payor did not have eligibility information that was in sync with CMS.

## 22.3   Case study: Maximizing Part D prescription drug claim reimbursement

A process improvement approach was taken to analyze current processes and procedures in place as performed by the payor, and its PBM, to manage the Part D PDEs rejected for reimbursement from CMS. The improvement effort began at the end of 2009, with the focus being to resolve rejected PDEs for dates of service in calendar year 2009. The reject data for 2008 were used as a benchmark.

Table 22.2 depicts the total PDE rejects by category for calendar years 2008 and 2009 as of February 2010.

In addition to collecting and summarizing data by reject category, a root-cause analysis was performed on both a qualitative and quantitative basis, to identify the causes for the high

**Table 22.2**   Frequency of PDE rejects.

| Edit category | 2008 rejects | 2009 rejects |
|---|---|---|
| Eligibility | 33 825 | 33 205 |
| LICS | 11 968 | 6 764 |
| Cost | 11 225 | 6 215 |
| Missing/invalid data elements | 628 | 56 |
| Misc | 544 | 936 |
| Catastrophic coverage | 534 | 4 046 |
| Non-covered drug | 173 | 25 |
| NDC | 143 | 640 |
| Adj/Del | 74 | — |
| | 59 114 | 51 887 |

NDC – national drug code; Adj/Del – adjustments/deletions.

volume of PDE rejects. The results of the analysis are depicted in the fishbone diagram in Figure 22.3. Critical root causes are circled.

The critical root causes with the most significant contribution to the high volume of PDE errors circled on the figure are the following.

1. No procedure to proactively identify claims for adjustment due to retro LICS and/or retro member ID changes.

2. Retro status changes from CMS are the norm and can date back several years.

3. Ownership for all components of error correction workflows within and between payor and PBM is not clearly defined.

4. Confirmation bias and polarization tendencies inhibit effective problem solving.

The first two root causes center around the ability to effectively handle retro-activity. A retroactive enrollment change is defined as a change that occurs on a member's eligibility detail with an effective date that is prior to the date that the change was made. As an example, suppose that on 1/1/09, member Jane is enrolled in contract ABC, and that on 2/1/09 a notification is received terminating her enrollment in ABC with an effective date of 1/1/09 and enrolling her in contract DEF.

Retroactive eligibility changes are further complicated when prescriptions have been filled, in other words claims have been incurred and paid, during the time period to which the retroactivity applies. Furthermore, for the Part D population, CMS dictates much of the retroactive changes as part of the day-to-day exchange of eligibility files with payors. The subset of the Part D population with frequent retroactivity for which changes often date back several years are the members who are eligible for LIS as identified by the Social Security Administration. There are several levels of cost sharing, known as LICS levels, available to those who qualify, depending on the beneficiaries' income as assessed by the US Government. Another example: member Jane fills a prescription on 1/1/09. At that time all systems – payor, PBM and CMS – have her as LICS Level 1. On 3/31/09 CMS sends an enrollment transaction update on member Jane, changing her LICS level from 1 to 2 with an effective date of 1/1/09. Subsequently, her claims must be adjusted to now pay under the updated appropriate line of eligibility.

The challenge for the payor conducting the study was that there was no way to proactively identify those claims that need to be adjusted, or moved, to the appropriate, updated, line of eligibility – in the example above, to the line with LICS level 2. To solve this problem in the short term, a program was developed to compare PDE rejects with eligibility reject codes to the current lines of eligibility in the payor's system. Those PDEs which fell into a new line of eligibility were queued for claims adjustment, triggering a resubmission of the PDE under the now-current and in-sync line of eligibility, matching that which CMS has.

A longer term option of investing in changing the configuration of the enrollment and claims system and how data is exchanged, on Part D members in particular, is also being pursued.

The third and fourth critical root causes focus on how the work is performed within the payor's organization. At the onset of this improvement process, there was very limited documentation in the form of workflows and procedures or data to drive action to reduce PDE rejects. Multiple parties, with different organizational reporting relationships, have a stake in maximizing the acceptance rate of PDEs – Operations, Pharmacy Management, Finance, Actuarial, Medicare Compliance – and there was a lack of clarity on who owned what, with

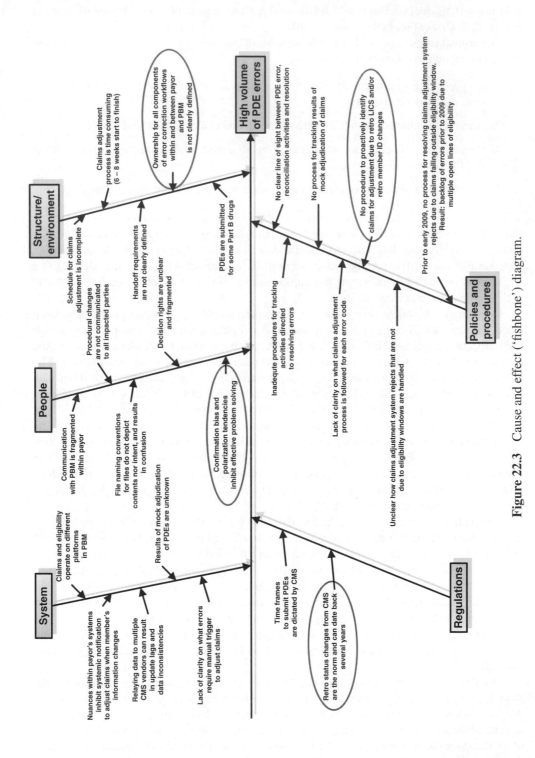

**Figure 22.3**  Cause and effect ('fishbone') diagram.

no one group responsible for the end-to-end process. Additionally, there were limited data and reporting that was published to drive action and assess the effectiveness of activities taken to reduce PDE rejects. To solve these problems, workflows and procedures were documented, and documents outlining roles and responsibilities were created and vetted with all parties. Most importantly, a bi-weekly report summarizing the PDE rejects by responsible party was produced, and results-based goals, as reported on bi-weekly reports, were shared across departments.

The last root cause touches on the softer side of this effort and tendencies that exist with groups of people when problem solving. Confirmation bias occurs when an individual has a hypothesis and collects and interprets all related information to prove his/her hypothesis correct. Polarization occurs when one individual has an opinion and another individual has a separate opinion, and for reasons personal or otherwise the first individual does everything they can to prove the other wrong. To handle this, in group sessions, the facilitator of the group informed them that this was behavior that was occurring and counterproductive to solving the problem. This approach, combined with the solutions to the first two root causes addressed the behavior that was prevalent before the improvement effort began. In addition, the joint review of data subdued debates, and perceptions were adjusted to match reality in a more objective and less emotional problem-solving environment.

Once the team had grounded itself with the data, and gained clarity on the root causes driving the high volume of PDE rejects, the improvement efforts began. As a first step, workflows and procedure documents were developed and implemented to work the PDE reject categories. Developing the workflows provided the needed clarity on ownership. The reject resolution work began in earnest in March 2010 with intense focus through June 2010 to meet the CMS deadline for PDE submission. Subsequently, 2008 was revisited once the deadline for 2009 was met.

Figure 22.4 depicts the PDE rejects for calendar year 2009 dates of service, before and after the implementation of the improvement efforts.

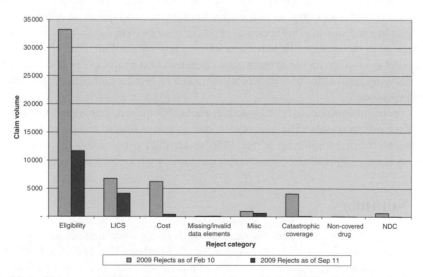

**Figure 22.4** Volume of PDE rejects for dates of service in 2009 – before and after implementation of improvement effort.

**Table 22.3**   PDE quality metrics.

|  | PDE acceptance rate(%) As of Feb 10 | PDE acceptance rate(%) As of Sep 11 |
|---|---|---|
| 2008 | 97.97 | 98.63 |
| 2009 | 97.90 | 99.35 |
| 2010 | n/a | 99.38 |

|  | PDE rejects As of Feb 10 | PDE rejects As of Sep 11 |
|---|---|---|
| 2008 | 59114 | 43253 |
| 2009 | 51887 | 17004 |
| 2010 | n/a | 15478 |

Payors and CMS alike use the PDE acceptance rate as a measure for quality over the process, which is calculated as the total accepted PDEs divided by total submitted PDEs. The payor for this case study submitted approximately 2 500 000 PDEs for Part D beneficiaries for each calendar year 2008 and 2009.

Table 22.3 depicts the PDE acceptance rate and reject count by calendar year before and after the implementation of the improvement effort. Over the period reflected in the table, 2009 rejections dropped by two-thirds.

## 22.4   Looking ahead

Adopting a mindset of continuous improvement is important when dealing with any complex process, such as Part D prescription drug claim reimbursement, to ensure the improvements are incorporated and maintained as part of day-to-day work and not as an ephemeral project with a beginning and an end. This is critical, especially since PDE data will be of even greater significance with the changes Health Care Reform has on the Part D product. The payor on which this case study focuses continues to examine best practices, perform cost–benefit analysis for long term solutions, and look for ways to reduce complexity and streamline payment processes.

PDE reject data continues to be reviewed on a detailed basis and funneled to the responsible parties to remediate rejects. The acceptance rate is a key metric in assessing continuous improvement efforts. Monitoring of the PDE reject data over time will provide another opportunity for the application of basic statistical tools, such as control charts.

## 22.5   Summary

In this chapter, we have considered the various kinds of data that must come together from pharmacies, insurers, and government in order for US Medicare Part D claims to be properly paid and reimbursed. The time-varying nature of this information poses a great challenge to timely processing and payment, as the information in payor and government agency databases must be 100% in agreement for all of the pieces to come together. We have looked at a typical payor process flow for paying Part D claims, and at a case study of the process improvement efforts one payor organization conducted in order to expedite its receipt of full reimbursement for qualified payments.

# Reference

Ruggeri, F., Kenett, R.S., and Faltin, F.W. (eds) (2007) *Encyclopedia of Statistics in Quality and Reliability*, John Wiley & Sons, Ltd.

# 23

# Quality of electronic medical records

## Dario Gregori[1] and Paola Berchialla[2]

[1]*Unit of Biostatistics, Epidemiology and Public Health, Department of Cardiac, Thoracic and Vascular Sciences University of Padova, Padua, Italy*
[2]*Department of Public Health and Microbiology, University of Torino, Turin, Italy*

## Synopsis

Electronic Medical Records are an essential component of today's administration of healthcare. Besides their main purposes – that is, to facilitate the planning, organization, administration and evaluation of healthcare provision – electronic data also play a crucial role in fostering research progression in the medical field.

Electronic data nevertheless suffer from major drawbacks, regarding their suitability for the research purposes in terms, in particular, of accuracy and precision, and in general of quality. This chapter first reviews the main sources and uses of electronic data in the medical field. Then, a systematic description of the issues emerging regarding data quality, along with the possible remedial actions, is provided.

## 23.1   Introduction

With the huge growth of individual health and medical data there is a need for electronic tools to manage the quality, timeliness and origination of such data, which may come from several systems: admission, discharge and transfer, laboratory, computerized physician order

*Statistical Methods in Healthcare*, First Edition. Edited by Frederick W. Faltin, Ron S. Kenett and Fabrizio Ruggeri.
© 2012 John Wiley & Sons, Ltd. Published 2012 by John Wiley & Sons, Ltd.

entry, pharmacy, diagnostic imaging, radiology information systems, emergency departments and so on. An Electronic Medical Record (EMR) is commonly defined as a medical record in an electronic format. According to the International Organization for Standardization (ISO) definition (ISO/DTR 20514 (ISO, 2004)), EMRs designate a repository of patient data in digital form, stored and exchanged securely, and accessible by multiple authorized users. They contain retrospective, concurrent and prospective information, and their primary purpose is to support continuing, efficient and high-quality integrated healthcare.

Electronic Medical Records are the core of any computerized health information system. Their importance in healthcare delivery has been recognized for a long time. One of the earliest examples of EMR implementation was at the Regenstrief Institute of Indianapolis in the 1970s. McDonald (1976) pointed out that physicians were often unable to detect critical abnormalities in the patients' records due to the great amount of data it would had been necessary to process; concluding that 'It is very likely that the physicians [. . .] were simply unable to detect all the multitudinous conditions specified by the standards'. Thus, using the Medical Record System of the Institute, McDonald showed that the use of computer-generated reminders based on patient-specific laboratory data reduced physician errors in the detection of life-threatening events.

Ideally, EMRs should be an environment composed of the clinical data repository, clinical decision support system, computerized provider order entry, and should provide tools for maintaining secondary healthcare activities such as administration, quality assurance, research and epidemiology (Tang and MacDonald, 2001; Garets and Davis, 2005). To achieve these aims, EMR systems should add information-management tools in order to provide clinical alerts, linkage with sources of medical knowledge for healthcare decision monitoring and support, and analysis of aggregate data both for outcomes research and management of the healthcare delivery system. This implies that an EMR system should contain three basic components: order entry system (computerized orders for prescriptions and computerized orders for tests), reporting system of test results, and patients' medical documentation. Depending on the healthcare institution's established information technology (IT) infrastructures, EMRs are comprised of two kinds of records: (1) older records, which are usually scanned and stored in graphic format or pdf format and include physicians' notes and laboratory tests (for example x-rays or other test results such as ultrasounds or MRIs); and (2) records that are electronically native.

As shown in Figure 23.1, beyond patients' medical records data, a comprehensive EMR system should include also a clinical data research repository. However, it is not yet common, for example, to use clinical data repositories for the support of clinical trials and thus enhance clinical research (Kahn *et al.*, 2007). The problem is relevant when considering secondary use of electronic medical records. So far, IT infrastructures have been developed with the aim of supporting clinical trials management (Payne, Greaves and Kipps, 2003). They have been focused mainly on the data management system, such as web-based remote data entry or electronic data capture systems (Higgins *et al.*, 1995; Wubbelt, Fernandez and Heymer, 2000; Brandt *et al.*, 2003; Meadows, 2003), without considering the need for integration with other electronic medical records system components. As an example, there is an increasing number of bioinformatics databases with genomics and proteomics data (Lee *et al.*, 2006), which are usually kept completely separate from other medical record systems, also as a consequence of security requirements that must be met.

Data warehousing (Figure 23.1) is a function that is relatively new for healthcare institutions. In many hospitals and healthcare organizations, the integration of data within data

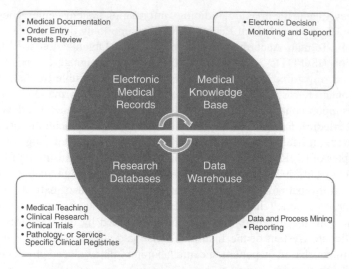

**Figure 23.1** A representation of an Electronic Medical Records system. Adapted from Prokosch and Ganslandt (2009).

warehouses is still limited to administrative data sources. While the aim of data warehousing is to integrate data from a population of original databases into one comprehensive platform, clinical data warehousing up to this point has been limited more to manipulating data records (Johnson and Chatziantoniou, 1999) or visualizing data warehouse contents in an interactive view (Bito *et al.*, 2001), or still to supporting disease management programs (Ramick, 2001) or cost analysis (Muranaga, Kumamoto and Uto, 2007).

In terms of a formal definition, often Electronic Medical Records, Electronic Health Records (EHRs) and Electronic Patient Records (EPRs) are used interchangeably or generically to refer to electronic or digital records, although specific differences between them have been defined. For example, an EHR is generally intended as a longitudinal record of a patient's care carried out across different institutions and sectors, in contrast to EMRs, which belong to a system which is established locally; while an EPR is usually defined as encapsulating a record of care provided by a single site. However, such differentiations are not consistently reflected in the use of the terms (Habib, 2010).

The 2003 Institute of Medicine Patient Safety Report describes an EMR system as encompassing 'a longitudinal collection of electronic health information for and about persons; [timeless] electronic access to person- and population-level information by authorized users; provision of knowledge and decision-support systems [. . .] and support for efficient processes for healthcare delivery' with the aim of enhancing the quality, safety, and efficiency of patient care (Institute of Medicine, 2003). According to Yamamoto *et al.* (Yamamoto and Khan, 2006), the advantages of EMRs can be summarized as 'optimizing the documentation of patient encounters, improving communication of information to physicians, improving access to patient medical information, reduction of errors, optimizing billing and improving reimbursement for services, forming a data repository for research and quality improvement and reduction of paper'.

The multidisciplinary computerized medical record, however, has not yet become a reality in many countries. Up to now, electronic information systems have not achieved the same degree of penetration in healthcare as observed in other sectors, showing furthermore a wide variation from country to country and from medicine specialty to medicine specialty. In many cases, in fact, EMR adoption has evolved around local systems designed for local use.

In the early 2000s, national penetration of EMRs had reached over 90% in primary care practices in Northern European countries (Norway, Sweden and Denmark) but was limited to 17% of physician office practices in the USA (Burt and Sisk, 2005). On the other hand, those EMR systems that have been implemented served mainly for administrative rather than clinical purposes. Over the past decade, the attitude towards the computerization process that considers EMRs as a necessary tool for improving quality of healthcare has become stronger in almost all western countries. Evidence has increasingly shown that current systems are not delivering sufficiently safe, high-quality, efficient and cost-effective healthcare (Coiera, 2003). The responses to this have been at national level. Governments in many countries, such as Australia, Canada, Denmark, Finland, France, New Zealand, the UK, the USA and others, have announced implementation of plans to build integrated computer-based national healthcare infrastructures based around the deployment of interoperable electronic medical record systems. As a result, many of these countries aim to have EMR systems deployed for their populations within the next 10 years (Health Information Strategy Steering Committee, 2005; Stroetmann et al., 2006; UK Department of Health, 2008).

As healthcare systems are going to implement EMRs, there are as yet no common standards. Intentionally, the World Health Organization (WHO) does not contribute to an internationally standardized view of medical records nor to personal health records, even if it contributes to a minimum requirements definition for developing countries (World Health Organization. Regional Office for the Western Pacific, 2006). However, the International Organization for Standardization (ISO) has settled on standards in the scope of the HL7 platform for healthcare informatics. HL7 is a messaging standard that is widely used in messaging across healthcare applications to send structured, encoded data from one application, for example the laboratory system, to another one, such as the EMR. Today there are in use two major versions of HL7. One is HL7 v. 2x, which is commonly used by the existing applications, and the other one is HL7 v. 3, the Reference Information Model (RIM), which provides a more robust ability to represent complex relationships. The Certification Commission for Healthcare Information was established to certify that software producers have implemented HL7 and other standards in order to ensure that the resulting applications can exchange data. Respective standards are available with ISO/HL7 10781:2009 Electronic Health Record-System Functional Model, Release 1.1.

## 23.2 Quality of electronic data collections

An electronic record may be created for each service a patient receives; it could be a radiology or a laboratory test, a pharmacy prescription or the result of an administrative action.

Data quality can be viewed as the 'totality of features and characteristics of a data set that bear on its ability to satisfy the needs that result from the intended use of the data' (Arts, De Keizer and Scheffer, 2002). A data quality problem occurs when there is a violation on one or more of the quality dimensions that makes data unfit for use. Incorrect spellings of person names, wrong date of birth and even untimely or not up-to-date data are examples of quality issues that can impact on the usability of the electronic medical records.

Data accuracy, that is, the correctness of the content of the data, which is often the concern when discussing quality of data, is only one of the 'foundational features' or dimensions that contribute to data quality. In Health Informatics, data quality concerns: (1) the accuracy, (2) the completeness, (3) the relevance, (4) the timeliness, and (5) the accessibility that make data appropriate for use (D'Onofrio and Gendrom, 2001; Kerr, Norris and Stockdale, 2008).

Accuracy is the extent to which data correctly report the 'real world' values they are intended to represent. Completeness is the extent to which all the required information is available; for example data values are not missing, or recorded in an unfeasible way. In some cases, missing data is irrelevant, but when the information that is missing is critical to a specific objective, completeness becomes an issue. Relevance refers to the extent to which the data meet the needs of users. Timeliness of data refers to the extent to which data are collected within a reasonable time period and are available within a reasonable timeframe. Ideally, data should be made available in near real time, for example to support decision making. Finally, accessibility refers to how easily data can be accessed and to the awareness of what type of healthcare information is being collected and where it is stored.

Other quality dimensions concern the comparability, the duplication, the integrity and the consistency of data. Comparability is the extent to which data values conform to specified formats. Maintaining conformance to specific formats is important in data representation, presentation, aggregate reporting, searching and for establishing key relationships. Duplication is a measure of unwanted multiple, unnecessary representations of the same medical record. Integrity is the extent to which data is missing important relationship linkages. The inability to link related records together may actually introduce duplication across the systems. Consistency or coherence is the extent to which distinct instances do not provide conflicting information about the same data object. It is important that values are consistent across data sets and interdependent attributes reflect their expected consistency.

Understanding the key quality dimensions is the first step to improving data quality. Equally important when developing a strategy to enhance data quality is the identification of the underlying causes of what is called 'dirty data' or, in other words, the presence of errors within data. Roughly, two categories of errors can be distinguished: (1) systematic errors and (2) random errors. Among the sources of systematic errors that can be cited are: programming mistakes; bad definitions for data format; violations of the rules established for data gathering; and also poor training of operators involved in data collection. On the other hand, random errors can be caused for example by typing errors, data transcription problems due to illegible data source or hardware breakdown, mistakes or ultimately deliberately misleading statements of patients or others providing primary information. It could be noted that data entry is the data collection task which is responsible of the majority of errors, across sectors and settings (according to the Data Warehousing Institute, data entry is responsible for 76% of the errors). This fact points out the critical role played by humans and the likelihood of human errors.

To establish data quality within a healthcare setting and to prevent data quality issues in the system or at least limit their consequences, it is important to develop comprehensive strategies, which include both automated and manual procedures. Solutions for improving data quality (Teperi, 1993; AHIMA Coding Products and Services Team, 2003; Porcheret *et al.*, 2004; Koppel *et al.*, 2005) should be aimed at: (1) standardizing data entry fields and instructions for entering data; (2) implementing real-time quality feedback procedures; (3) designing data elements, such as the user interface, to avoid errors (using, for example, checking rules in the fields where manual entry is involved); (4) developing and adhering to guidelines for documenting the healthcare services that were provided to the patient; (5) building human capacity – that is, the most important training.

Many researchers point out that data quality is an issue that needs to be assessed from the data users' perspective. In the context of medical records, data quality can be defined as 'the totality of features and characteristics of a data set, that bear on its ability to satisfy the requirements stated in a particular specification, which reflects the implied needs of the user' (Abate, Diegert and Allen, 1998). Thus, the challenge in implementing EMR systems is bringing together all the data that will be available for each patient. Data can be collected from different sources, including medical records, patient surveys or administrative databases. Each of these sources has its primary purposes – for example administrative database are used to pay bills or to manage healthcare services – and thus each of them complies with different levels of quality.

A high-quality electronic medical record system should be serving also as an evidence-based decision-making tool. EMRs can have a positive impact on quality of care, patient safety and efficiencies; however, without accurate and appropriate content in a usable and accessible form, these benefits will not be realized. As recognized by the Connecting for Health Common Framework, 'data problems represent the dark side of the tremendous potential offered by the adoption of health IT systems'. (Connecting for Health Common Framework, 2006).

Following is a brief summary of the principal data quality issues which affect the principal source of medical data classified as administrative databases, health surveys, patients medical records, clinical trials and clinical epidemiology studies.

## 23.2.1   Administrative databases

In the course of providing their services, healthcare institutions gather administrative data usually at the level of individual users. Data is mainly collected from claims and healthcare providers' systems. Common elements include the type of clinical service that has been provided, the diagnosis and the procedure codes, the prescriptions that have been filled, the location of the service, the amount billed and eventually the amount reimbursed.

Due to their specific purposes, administrative databases are available electronically and are less expensive to acquire than other medical record data. They encompass the entire population of patients and share uniform coding systems and practices across institutions.

However, they face challenges due to the fact that, except for demographic data, they contain limited clinical information. Furthermore, since their primary purpose is billing, they lack accuracy for public reporting, allowing limited insight into the quality and the appropriateness of care, and typically one does not encounter completeness and timeliness of data.

## 23.2.2   Health surveys

Surveys are a data collection tool to gather self-reported information from patients. Common questions addressed concern reports on the healthcare services provided, the treatment received and the perceptions of the outcomes. Among the advantages they present, it is worth mentioning that there exist well-established methods for survey design and administration. On the other hand, survey administration could be costly and there is the possibility of misleading results if questions are poorly worded or they favor one response over another (response bias), administration procedures are not standardized and the sampled population is not representative of the population as a whole (sampling bias).

### 23.2.3   Patient medical records

Medical records document patients' medical history. Typically they include deep clinical detail and thus they entail the cost, complexity, and time required for compilation. Difficulties in the data entry process are posed when patients receive clinical services across different sites, if a different record format for storing information is used. The routine task of electronic data entry itself can be a possible source of errors.

### 23.2.4   Clinical trials

Clinical trials can produce very high-quality data. Data can be collected from several sources such as interviews, questionnaires, participant or laboratory examinations, and many countermeasures can be adopted during the planning phase to ensure the collection of high-quality data. Typically, data collected include demographic/baseline patient information, measures of adherence to the study treatment, concomitant treatments, adverse events, and primary and secondary response variables aimed at answering questions about benefit/risk of the treatment being tested. With the rise of internet technologies, IT has been broadly applied in the management of clinical trials databases. In particular, web-based remote data entry systems have been developed. On the other hand, the reverse side of high-quality data is that they may not address all topics of interest. However, the convergence of online clinical trials data management with EMRs has the potential to improve the management of clinical research data and physician management of their clinical research operations.

### 23.2.5   Clinical epidemiology studies

A number of criteria relate to the quality of epidemiological data: (1) nature of the data; that is, whether the data are from case registries, physicians' records, general population surveys or hospital and clinical cases; (2) the availability of data; that is, whether data are available from government and research organizations (for example some organizations perturb data before they are released in order to protect the privacy of individuals); (3) the completeness of population coverage; that is, representativeness, and the inclusion of subclinical cases, or thoroughness; (4) the utility of the data for various types of epidemiological research, such as studies of incidence or prevalence, studies of mortality, and so on.

## 23.3   Data quality issues in electronic medical records

Maintaining the quality of medical records is a critical issue for effective healthcare, and it is widely acknowledged as problematic. Though EMR quality is often considered only within the narrow aim of data verification and validation, it should also concern the equally critical issues of assuring that EMR data are appropriate for their use (D'Onofrio and Gendrom, 2001).

Inappropriate use of data comprises: inadequate structures for ensuring accurate, complete and timely data management; inadequate training and procedural guidelines given to the staff involved in data collection; failures due to fragmentation and inconsistencies among the tasks carried out to provide data collection services (Gendrom and D'Onofrio, 2001; Connecting for Health Common Framework, 2006).

Specific data quality attributes have been widely considered (Brown and Sonksen, 2000; Miller and Sim, 2004). They form a set of requirements, which can be summarized as follows (Gendrom and D'Onofrio, 2001; Orfanidis, Bamidis and Eaglestone, 2004).

1. **Accessibility and availability:** EMR data should be available for authorized users only, and access should be fast via easy-to-use interfaces. Privacy should be strictly maintained and overriding of authorization constraints should be recorded along with documented reasons.

2. **Security and confidentiality**.

3. **Usability:** EMRs should be accessible in different data formats for ease of retrieval, allowing for interoperability between different operating systems.

4. **Provenience:** that is, the EMRs should be linked to metadata that identify the context in which they were created.

5. **Data validation:** the status of the EMR data should be provided, indicating whether data are pending, and by metadata on times of entry and retention.

6. **Integrity:** standards should be established for new data, and inconsistency and duplication should be removed.

7. **Accuracy and timeliness:** that is, the content of EMRs should be as near real-time as possible.

8. **Completeness:** that is, the existence of further data should be indicated, possibly with links to other data.

9. **Consistency:** that is, there should be consistency between items of multiple data from multiple sources. EMRs should comply with the existing relevant standards, such as security, data protection and communication standards.

Such quality attributes point out the difficulty of treating electronic medical records as structured data, at least in a conventional manner, since EMRs can be comprised of different sources of data. Another important issue related to quality is ensuring that data are fit for their purpose. For example, the requirement for data consistency as well as non-duplication may not always be completely appropriate. Inconsistencies and duplication may have significance if they reflect differences in medical opinion, erroneously recorded, or multiple diagnostic tests. Identifying such anomalies is important, since it could reveal inappropriate recording of outcomes or misunderstandings in data definitions, database shortcomings and poor user training which has resulted in poor data quality (Boyle and Cunningham, 2002).

The quality of electronic medical records also affects the quality care of healthcare institutions (Porcheret et al., 2004). Healthcare quality standards can not be prescinded from the implementation of documentation guidelines and data standards practices. The quality of the documentation in the EMRs is reliant upon the information entered by those involved in the patients' care. As already pointed out, documentation and data content within EMRs have to be accurate, complete, and accessible and usable by authorized users.

Documentation must substantiate the quality of care assessments provided against specific standards by integrating them into documentation guidelines. It is critical that structured and unstructured data stored meet standards of quality and adhere to documentation guidelines not only for internal but also for secondary healthcare purposes.

The documentation within the medical record system must be comprehensive enough not only to fulfill administrative functions and legal issues but also for supporting healthcare quality standard and research activities (Williams, 2006; World Health Organization. Regional Office for the Western Pacific, 2006). In fact, documentation that a visit has occurred or a diagnostic test or a medical procedure has been undertaken is required to support the payment process (the billing for the patient and the payment of claims). At the same time, the documentation is indispensable for protecting the legal interest of patients and physicians, as well as the healthcare organization, in the presence of medical malpractices cases. Medical record documentation is important also for physicians when making decisions about medical staff reappointment.

Documentation must enable the support of decision making to provide the most cost-efficient healthcare benefits, since analysis of trustworthy data can be helpful in identifying problems and suggesting solutions for improving the quality of care. Data completeness and accuracy allow healthcare providers to plan for services and administration. Documentation is central to allow for continuity between those caring for the patients currently and those who will take care of them in the time to come. Effective health information exchange (Shapiro *et al.*, 2011) can reduce or eliminate duplication or redundancy of diagnostic tests and the risk of treatment errors, facilitate investigation of public health agencies in indentifying threats to public health and improve the efficacy of public health reporting.

Documentation is important also because it provides the information necessary for research studies. A standard of data quality is necessary, for example, for clinical trials. But medical records could also be used by registries to identify the most effective treatment modalities or to identify epidemiological causes for disease.

The quality of documentation guidelines and data standards depends on the obligations of privacy and security. Levels of security, limited access to information that patients contribute to caregivers, and audit trails are integral to maintaining the confidentiality of the electronic medical record (Williams, 2006). In addition legislative and regulatory aspects become essential for developing a documentation quality plan: it is essential, for example, to address standards for health information exchange, including technical standards to enable different healthcare network computer systems to communicate and safely transfer data. Integrated sharing of clinical information among numerous stakeholders surely benefits from reporting quality and performance indicators to government and private organizations sponsoring quality initiatives (Stroetmann *et al.*, 2006). Also worthy of mention is e-discovery – that is, discovery of data created or maintained in electronic format – which is becoming a crucial part of gathering and using evidence in legal proceedings, complementing traditional methods such as photocopies or printouts of patient medical records (American Health Information Management Association, 2006; Williams, 2006).

## 23.4    Procedure to enhance data quality

In order to enhance data quality and thus to improve the quality of care, some best practices are widely recommended (Ware and Gandek, 1998; Williams, 2006; World Health Organization.

Regional Office for the Western Pacific, 2006). Among them, it is important to cite the access permissions to the data, which must be clearly defined. Clear policies on who can document and update data in the EMR systems are essential to set up a workflow and contribute to the quality and timeliness of the data itself. Also, lack of standards and common terminologies among different EMR systems are some of the reasons for poor data quality when different data sources have to be integrated, as pointed out by Harris, Ruggieri and Chute (2003): 'Electronic patient records today are highly idiosyncratic, vendor-specific realizations of patient record subsets. They adopt few, if any, health information standards, and very rarely accommodate controlled terminologies where they might be sensible. The reason for this epidemic of incompatible data has more to do with the limitations of available information standards and machine able vocabularies than with any fundamental unwillingness to adopt standards. A compelling business case, for system vendors or patient providers, simply has not emerged to foster standards adoption and systems integration'.

Standardized formats of data are a key tool for ensuring data consistency. EMR systems must meet privacy and security standards requirements. Three main authorities/organizations are in charge of defining standards for EMRs: the Health Level Seven (HL7) organization, the Comité Européen de Normalization – Technical Committee (CEN TC) 215, and the American Society for Testing and Materials (ASTM) E31. The HL7 organization, which operates in the United States and is accredited by the American National Standards Institute (ANSI), develops the most widely used healthcare-related electronic data exchange standards in North America. CEN TC 215 is the preeminent healthcare IT standards developing organization in Europe. Both HL7 and the CEN collaborate with the ASTM. The HL7 version 3 Reference Information Model (RIM) provides an object model of clinical data that can be extended to other biomedical fields such as genomics, for example. This is not without difficulty. The RIM provides a representation of the semantic and lexical connections that exist between the information carried in HL7 standard report messages. This may work well for one specialty area, such as pathology, but may not be useful for other clinical users, for example internists, who need different views of the same data. Thus, tools are needed to navigate across different vocabularies and ensure interoperability across different clinical domains.

Data integrity policies and procedures, to be followed in order to protect the integrity of the data for all information entered into the EMR, are also recommended. To this end, it is important to have individuals who are trained to monitor the EMR system and are dedicated to the audit process.

Finally, using established data dictionaries is important to provide standard data definitions for fields which have to be entered. The use of structured data and standard clinical vocabularies greatly enhances the interoperability of electronic medical systems. To create interoperable EMRs for sharing information, standards are needed for: (1) clinical vocabularies; (2) healthcare message exchanges, in which one system exchanges messages with another; (3) EMR ontologies (i.e., standard representation of knowledge domains across different fields). Much attention has been paid to the effort of data integration by means of definition of ontologies (Yu, 2006; Liu, Hogan and Crowley, 2011) and mapping multiple standards in the same domain; for example a unified medical language system (UMLS) (Bodenreider, 2004) for Systematized Nomenclature of Medicine (SNOMED) and International Classification of Disease (ICD). However, mapping concepts between different ontologies in the same domain or different versions within the same ontology requires good mapping references, which on the other hand can often be inadequate; this is usually the case for cancer registries (Edge *et al.*, 2010)

### 23.4.1   Clinical vocabularies

Clinicians use several terms to designate the same medical concept. In the absence of structured vocabularies, an automated system is not able to recognize different terms as being equivalent. Thus, vocabularies are a key factor for accessing electronic medical records.

Typically, vocabularies are used to search knowledge resources or identify appropriate resources, for example using key words, and to support quality improvement and data integration. Vocabularies are a key component also for data exchange and analyses within and across different domains or clinical fields, and they are required for all secondary uses of clinical data.

When a clinician evaluates a patient, the documentation usually comprises unstructured information (free text), such as history and physical findings, and allows for controlling inconsistencies when data is captured at the point of care, for example in an emergency department. Following the clinician evaluation process, the unstructured information is transformed into more coded data, which are primarily used for billing and reimbursement purposes, but could be useful also for analytical and research purposes and cost analysis. These claims-related structured data sets include primarily Current Procedural Terminology codes and Diagnosis Related Groups (DRGs) which classify medical, surgical and diagnostic services provided by the healthcare organization.

Among clinical vocabularies, the most widely adopted ones are the International Classification of Disease (ICD) and the Systematized Nomenclature of Medicine (SNOMED) and the Logical Observation Identifiers, Names, and Codes (LOINC).

The ICD is primarily used to classify morbidity and mortality data for identifying the disease for which the patient was treated. The ninth and tenth revisions of ICD are the most commonly used versions.

SNOMED is developed by SNOMED International, which is a division of the College of American Pathologists, and it is designed to be a comprehensive, multi-axial, controlled terminology, created for the indexing of the entire medical record. SNOMED-CT (Clinical Terms) is aimed at specifying the core file structure of SNOMED Clinical Terms. It is a collaborative terminology developed jointly by the National Health Service in the United Kingdom and the College of American Pathologists, integrating the British system of Read Codes and SNOMED-RT (Reference Terminology), the latest version of SNOMED.

The Logical Observation Identifiers, Names, and Codes (LOINC) is most widely used in laboratory systems. It is a set of codes used primarily to identify individual laboratory results, clinical observations and diagnostic study observations.

### 23.4.2   Ontologies

Ontology is a representational vocabulary for a shared domain of knowledge. It provides definitions of classes, relations, functions and other objects (Musen, 2000; Schulz and Stenzhorn, 2007; Smith and Scheuermann, 2011). Generally, ontologies are used to specify *classes* that represent concepts in the domains of interest and the relationships that can exist among them. They encode knowledge in a domain and also knowledge that spans across domains, making ontology useful where there is a compelling need for sharing domain information.

Obviously, different ontologies may represent the same concepts with different entities and relationships, modeling information in multiple ways. Even if a degree of interoperability among different healthcare institutions and domains is guaranteed by ontology extensions, there is however the need to integrate different ontologies; that is, to define core relationships and definitions (also called *primitives*) that allow ontologies to map terms to their equivalents in other ontologies (Dinakarpandian, Tong and Lee, 2007).

### 23.4.3    Potential technical challenges for EMR data quality

Among the issues to consider when discussing data quality processes and the strategies to improve the data quality dimensions, the Master Patient Index (MPI) is one of the most technically complex and challenging (Baldwin, 2001; Williams, Robinson and Toth, 2006; Wheatley, 2008).

Healthcare institutions should ensure the EMR system will identify and correct errors that may interfere with establishing the identity of each individual patient. It is absolutely critical to make sure that each patient has a unique identifier, called the Master Patient Index, to link all health facts (Littlejohns, Wyatt and Garvican, 2003). Errors in the MPI not only compromise the integrity of the data but can also endanger patients' safety, inducing caregivers to make treatment decisions based on incomplete or inaccurate data. Whenever patients are admitted to a hospital or a healthcare facility, they are typically assigned a unique medical record number that is used by clinicians and for administrative purposes to identify, track and cross-reference the medical records. However, it is not very common that MPIs share a unique identifier for a patient across records, thus resulting in patient medical record duplications and overlays. Furthermore, small errors in MPI due to incomplete or inaccurate data can themselves originate duplications and overlays. Errors in the MPI can be caused by a discrepancy in patient identification attributes such as misspellings of names, use of aliases or a variation in other identifying attributes such as address and phone numbers that change over time. Also, limitations of search capabilities (many search algorithms are based on exact matching, which cannot recognize typographical errors for example) can lead to similar problems.

Given the aforementioned criticalities, EMR systems face a significant challenge in ensuring that data errors do not occur and duplicate or split records are not created. It is generally accepted that the potential for an adverse impact on patient care is substantial when more than 1 in 10 medical records has only part of the patient's information within the hospital's system, and there is also an upward trend in error rates as record numbers increase. At the same time, it has been shown that for success in providing accurate data, the MPI error rate should not exceed 2% (Fernandes, 2008), and some organizations are even using a target of 1%.

To address the challenges that an effective MPI management imposes, technology solutions, which include human intervention, and the re-engineering of the patient registration processes, are required. Alternative solutions should be based on the use of data profiling software tools, which allow for the identification of common patterns of data errors (erroneous data entry, in the majority of cases of errors in the MPI). It should also be ensured that patient identification systems do not rely uniquely on exact matching systems but include advanced strategies such as probabilistic matching.

One should not underestimate the fact that, if data are being maintained in more than one electronic medical system, they must be cleaned up in all systems, so that bad data do not propagate across the systems. If healthcare institution policies are determined in order to optimize standardization towards assurance of data quality, it is important to consider whether current systems allow for supporting an optimal level of quality, and the maintenance of true quality data may require the replacement of obsolete or non-supportive technologies.

Another issue to face when considering the challenge posed by the quality of EMRs is the general systems' lack of consideration for the research process. Since inefficiencies in clinical trial data collection cause delays, increase of costs and may reduce clinician participation in medical research, EMRs have often been cited as a significant new tool for advancing clinical trial capabilities into standard clinical practice (Kahn *et al.*, 2007). Indeed, EMRs are designed to mainly support healthcare provision rather than assist clinical researchers. This has led to the implementation of systems by healthcare organizations' information technology departments that affect the use of EMR data for clinical research. This is strictly associated with the fact that much of the information contained in electronic records, for example, is entered as unstructured free text, which is useful for the individual communication but unsuitable for quantitative analyses. In addition, few data standards are widely implemented, really limiting the ability to conduct analysis across health institutions and even across departments; thus limiting the use of EMRs for secondary purposes (Prokosch and Ganslandt, 2009; Terry *et al.*, 2010).

The problem of using established EMRs for secondary purposes is linked also to the problem of data integration. Data integration between different sources into a unified database with consistent description and logical organization itself poses an obstacle to the quality of EMR systems (Bernstein and Haas, 2008; Agrawal *et al.*, 2009). In order to extract meaningful information from two different data sources, for example to link recorded patients' history from medical surveys with recorded dates of a disease, it is necessary to have these data distinguishably aligned to individual persons. However, even if dealing with a small number of patients, linking data together often fails due to data inconsistencies (different date format, missing values) and data fragmentation (multiple medical record numbers for the same patient) (Mercer *et al.*, 1995). Biomedical data are in general heterogeneous, inconsistent and fragmented. Combining electronic medical records from different repositories maintaining the integrity of the original data frequently requires tackling four distinct problems.

The first problem encountered is due to heterogeneity. Data elements and/or schemes for the same domain are designed by independent parties and usually they are semantically different. To further complicate matters, data sources are subject to periodical update in all their aspects, including data structures, ontology standards and instance data coding methods. Often, these sources do not provide metadata or mapping references between older and newer dataset versions.

The second problem concerns data inconsistencies. Many biomedical domains do not have established ontologies; while others have more than one set of standard taxonomies. For example, there are three official taxonomies for describing cancers: SNOMED (Wingert, 1985; Ceusters, 2011), the International Classification of Disease (Cimino *et al.*, 2009) and the NCI-thesaurus (de Coronado *et al.*, 2004).

The third problem is due to data fragmentation. Most data sources are kept completely isolated, such as a genomic database. Such data sources typically do not have the primary identifiers of a person created in other data sources, so often require manually repetitive entry of the same records into different sources. This practice increases the risk of human error.

Finally, the fourth problem is due to low interoperability. The majority of clinical data sources are neither programmatically accessible (syntactic interoperability) nor have metadata available for the source data (semantic interoperability). As a consequence, data cannot be utilized until they are cleaned, unified, standardized and integrated.

Beyond common record architectures, integration of different data sources requires communication protocols ensuring security and confidentiality of information, which are linked to the ethical and legal issues of privacy and access rights. Furthermore, the purpose of data integration is to deliver integrated, high-quality data. This purpose can be realized choosing between different information integration approaches, such as data warehousing, view integration, or data mash-up systems, which use the Internet to aggregate information from multiple providers (Halevy, 2001; Goble and Stevens, 2008).

In the following we focus on data warehousing, which appears to provide a better solution to ensure data integration (Kimball *et al.*, 1998).

### 23.4.4    Data warehousing

A warehouse delivers integrated information by organizing and storing data from different sources within a physical scheme so that integrated data can be reused for a variety of applications and purposes (Louie *et al.*, 2007).

Since a warehouse is thus focused on a multidimensional database, which requires data availability, it appears to be more flexible with regard to the original data source than other solutions, which all require data sources to be interoperable and accessible. For this property, warehousing is generally considered more suitable for historical data accumulation, quality data integration, and post-integration data and annotation (Halevy *et al.*, 2005). For example, in biomedical informatics, the warehousing approach is the preferred solution for personalized biomedical data integration (Wang *et al.*, 2009).

The major limitation of the warehousing approach is its association with stale data and the resource-consuming nature of system maintenance, which point to data supply issues as the major obstacle to data integration, and point out the need for a data extraction-transformation-loading process that determines the quality and freshness of integrated data (Lowe and Ferris, 2009).

Three distinct conceptual modeling methods are often employed for database design: the Entity-Relationship model; the Entity-Attribute-Value representation with classes and relationships model; and the Object-Oriented Database (OODB) (Chen, 1976; Trujillo and Palomar, 2001; Dinu and Nadkarni, 2007; Lowe and Ferris, 2009).

Often, the Entity-Relationship model is preferred due to technical advantages, such as a solid mathematical foundation, data structure semantic clarity and data presentation transparency. These features support satisfactory query performance at the user-application interface and, as a function of the semantic clarity and consistency for each attribute element during cross-source data processing, the delivery of useful data and consumable information is better ensured (Dinu and Nadkarni, 2007).

At the implementation level, it is suggested that a data warehouse has a single large table along with many smaller-dimension tables, to improve performance by reducing the time-consumption of the process, that is, the answering of a query.

## 23.5    Form design and on-entry procedures

Very early attempts were made to provide tailored form design suitable for data on-entry procedures in biomedical research and EMR systems (Hanley, 1978). Structured data entry entails information being entered directly in the coded format needed by the EMR. Thus, well-designed user interfaces are required in order to minimize the time and effort for entry procedures. To this end a consistent use of standards in medical terminologies is recommended, along with the use of medical knowledge to anticipate the categories used to capture information, and design input screens to locate them immediately. The addition of basic edit checks, for example only allowing entry of numeric information in numeric fields and forcing all text comments to be entered, would improve the quality of EMRs and the usability of clinical data. Simple range checks, for example a message warning if a clinical parameter is outside the physiological range, can simplify correct entering.

The timely and accurate transfer of patient information into the computer is the most difficult and labor-intensive and time-consuming step in the maintenance of an EMR system. Responsibility for data entry involves many health professionals. The transfer of data from its source to an EMR requires two separate procedures: data capture and data input.

### 23.5.1    Data capture

If the aim of the medical record is restricted to containing information about variables under the control of the healthcare institution maintaining the EMR system, data capture is straightforward, although it requires time and resources to interface the data source with the EMRs.

Capture of comparable information across a patient's hospitalization, for example an admission to the emergency department or a visit to a consulting physician, could turn out to be complicated. In fact, relevant information may go unnoticed or even lost, or it might not have sufficient detail. Restricting the scope of the medical record to information that is only the medical record that is returned to the practice can limit the system capability to provide feedback about patient care. For example, an EMR system in a medical clinic cannot make accurate recommendations about the need for a certain diagnostic test if this test is requested by, and returned to, an external laboratory that provides the service. In fact, in this case the healthcare institution would need to develop special procedures in order to get copies of the test results for data entry into the medical system. Similarly, inpatient EMR systems are limited in their ability if data collected in one department are not accessible to other departments.

However, it seems that the trend toward larger, integrated and self-contained healthcare systems will tend to reduce the problem of data capture. Nevertheless, the standards required to transfer data faithfully and automatically from data source systems to EMRs is still a significant issue which affects the quality of the EMR system. It has been warned that the transition from paper-and-pencil data collection to electronic medical record throughout electronic data capture systems is not without risks, mostly in specific fields such as that of clinical trials, which presents challenges that, if not appropriately dealt with, can lead to expensive mistakes (Schmier, Kane and Halpern, 2005).

### 23.5.2    Data input

Data may be entered in free-text or coded form or in a form that combines both free text and codes. Since data are classified and standardized, using coding facilitates selective retrieval of patient data or administrative functions such as billing and reimbursements. When there are only a few codes, a selection list can simplify the data input. The most important disadvantage of coding consists in the cost of translating the source text into valid codes. There is also the potential for errors when coding, which, in contrast to errors in free-text entry, are difficult to identify, because of the lack of the internal redundancy of text.

Immediate coding by physicians (for example through menu selection) yields codes that the EMR can use to guide physicians' data input and decisions. If menus are carefully designed, their use will be more accurate than coding by other personnel. However, the use of trained coders to input data could have the advantage of yielding more uniform coding.

Various digital sources of coded data exist in healthcare settings. For example laboratory and pharmacy systems, or electrocardiogram charts. Data from these systems can communicate with an EMR system through standard protocols, such as HL7, thus establishing an automated procedure of data input.

### 23.5.3    Error prevention

In order to prevent transcription errors when clinical information is entered, EMR systems must apply internal validity checks. Several different methods can be implemented to detect erroneous data entered.

The simpler method consists in enrolling two independent persons who enter medical records producing two distinct databases. Where inconsistencies are detected, there is a clear indication of data-entry errors that must be checked and re-entered (ISO/DTR 20514; Schumock, Hutchinson and Bilek, 1992; Abate, Diegert and Allen, 1998; Smith *et al.*, 1998; Williams, 2006).

Automated check procedures at data entry could also be performed (Schumock, Hutchinson and Bilek, 1992; Wagner and Hogan, 1996; Schriger *et al.*, 1997; Makoul, Curry and Tang, 2001). In brief, they can be summarized as: range checks, which can detect or prevent entry of values that are out of range; pattern checks, which identify specific patterns in data (for example, the digit pattern of a telephone number); verifying that values have the correct mathematical relationship (for example numbers expressed as a percentage that must add up to 100); consistency checks, for example, checking that medical records with prostate cancer diagnosis are related to male patients); warning of unlikely differences between values recorded at different times (for example the results of two or more laboratory tests); spelling checks, which verify the spelling of single words.

However, not all data errors can be detected through automated-procedure data checks; for example data errors that are still within the range of correct values are unlikely to be discovered. In addition to the automated routines, a visual check of the entered data is usually recommended (Brender, Nohr and McNair, 2000). Analyses of the data, for example by simple cross tabulation, could help to uncover anomalies (Schriger *et al.*, 1997). The coordinating center of a registry can control data quality by visiting the participating centers and performing data audits, comparing data recorded with the original data source (for example paper patient record) (Makoul, Curry and Tang, 2001).

### 23.5.4    Physician-entered data

Physician-gathered patient information poses the most difficult challenge to data validation of EMR systems. Physicians record four kinds of information: (1) patient histories; (2) findings from the physical examination; (3) interpretation of the patient's findings; (4) physician's diagnostic and treatment plans. Physicians' notes can be entered into the EMR trough transcription of dictated or written notes. Dictation and transcription is a common option for data entry of textual information. If physicians dictate their reports using standard formats, then the transcriptionist maintains their structure in the transcribed document. Furthermore, digital voice dictation itself can also be stored in the EMR and retrieved without transcription, perhaps with the aid of existing data compression algorithms. However, even if recorded notes can be played back in real time, clinicians cannot look for specific information. Furthermore, the transcription is associated with delays before the notes are available, and carries the requirement that the author reviews, corrects and signs their content.

A second data-entry method consists of using a structured non-electronic encounter form. Then physicians' notes are transcribed and encoded by trained personnel. Up to now, this approach has been revealed as the most successful.

Finally, as a third alternative, physicians can enter data directly into electronic medical records. Direct data entry can be simplified by using custom selection menus that contain lists of coded information for specific problems. To be useful, however, selection menus must neither contain too many codes, nor impose a rigid hierarchy (Kuhn, 1996).

It is not at all clear and undisputed that electronic record keeping saves time. Maintaining EMRs can slow physicians' workflow since it is time consuming learning how to use them effectively (Boonstra and Broekhuis, 2010). However, it must also be considered that using EMR systems improves the overall quality and functionality of data documentation (Hayrinen, Saranto and Nykänen, 2008; McAlearney *et al.*, 2010).

## 23.6    Quality of data evaluation

The quality of data recorded in EMRs is extremely important since the success of EMRs depends on the quality of the information available to healthcare professionals who are involved in decision making about patient treatments and in communication with other healthcare givers. It is important therefore to assess the quality of information entered in electronic systems. Data quality assurance comprises all the planned and systematic actions required to provide confidence that data meet the standard requirements.

Actually, standardized methods for assessing the quality of data in EMR systems are still lacking. Quality data assessment should make use of markers of quality which comprise internal reference standards based on objective and diagnostic EMR elements, for example through triangulation procedures with multiple data sources, such as prescription data, diagnosis and also notes (Thiru, Hassey and Sullivan, 2003).

The data included in paper-based patient records have often provided the gold standard against which the reliability of EMRs has been assessed. Chan, Fowles and Weiner (2010) provided an overview of the current state of the literature about the quality of medical records from the perspective of quality measurement. Even if they warn that many of the articles they analyzed described research conducted in large and often academically affiliated hospitals, while smaller healthcare institutions are not well represented, the results suggest some of the most relevant problems which affect the quality of medical records.

An increasing number of research studies are focusing on the many features or dimensions which define data quality. Increasingly, data quality of medical records is associated with healthcare quality (Moczygemba and Hewitt, 2001). In determining health data quality, the type of disease which is reported plays a role: for example, documentation of chronic disease appears to be more accurate than documentation for other acute conditions (Chan, 2008; Chan *et al.*, 2008). Greater data completeness is observed with manual rather than electronic data collection, because automated data entry usually relies on structured fields and it is characterized by missing data in free-text fields, whereas paper-based data have many different options for documentation, from structured fields to free-text notes. This suggests the need of new data documentation and entry procedures for EMRs, which can minimize variability in data completeness. It is interesting to note that the reliability of free-text data extraction programs seems to be quite good, even if the generalization of the finding is sensitive to the specific data extraction strategy adopted.

The assessment of the quality requires the definition of a gold standard as reference. In the absence of a gold standard, manual charts, surveys or interviews can be used to evaluate data quality. Many studies have evaluated multiple dimensions of data quality. Quality dimensions addressed were accuracy, completeness, comparability across study sites or data systems, and validity. Few studies explicitly addressed granularity, that is, the correct level of detail of data, or timeliness (Neil and Nerenz, 2003).

When considering data completeness, a certain degree of vulnerability was observed among the examined data sources. Data quality was poor within medication lists. Data capture which includes automatic population of the data source through electronic linkage with outside sources, and manual entry into structured or free-text data fields, and data extraction, significantly affect data completeness.

Data completeness for different data elements, such as clinical status, laboratory results and clinical procedures, was most often reported as varying widely among examined studies. The electronic medical data sources for these elements were often not clearly specified.

Across studies, data completeness varied substantially, ranging between 0.1 and 51% for blood pressure and 10 and 38% for smoking status assessment. Clinical relevance could be an important contributor to data completeness, according to previous findings (Persell *et al.*, 2006; McGinnis *et al.*, 2009). It is interesting to note that, where a health condition documented in a problem list varies by condition, chronic conditions are more likely to be documented than acute conditions, probably because the former are automatically linked as a consequence of clinical actions. On the other hand, the laboratory results field likely requires manual entry and this fact contributes thus to missing data. A substantial variability in missing data was observed across different clinical departments. Studies reporting that the same clinical content can be found in different or multiple locations within the EHR suggest that the variation in data completeness reflects differences in documentation practices or different methods implemented for data capture. These results suggest that if data are not extracted from the appropriate locations or if data are regularly recorded in a free-text field, automatic extraction techniques very likely lead to having higher missing-data rates.

There is evidence that order entry may provide better data than entered laboratory results for determining clinician performance (Benin *et al.*, 2005). Order entry is an electronic process by which clinicians directly enter medication orders and laboratory tests and procedures. The system then transmits the order directly to the pharmacy. Order entry systems have become increasingly common in the inpatient setting as a strategy to reduce medication errors at the ordering and transcribing stages, since they ensure standardized, legible and complete orders.

Automated extraction of structured electronic medical record performs reasonably well across different types of data. In particular, Tang *et al.* (2007) found that automated electronic medical record data extraction identified 97% of patients with diabetes, compared with expert review as standard reference. Rosenman *et al.* (2008) found that laboratory reports in the electronic medical records identified 99% of a prenatal syphilis screen, and Baker *et al.* (2007) found that automated extraction identified 94.6% of congestive heart failure patients with left ventricular ejection factor data, and between 70 and 94% of appropriate prescriptions, when compared with hybrid review (automated extraction empowered by manual review of electronic notes).

However, automated extraction techniques can miss important data. Manual review of free-text fields showed increased data completeness by between 1.9 and 23.2% among congestive heart failure patients (Baker *et al.*, 2007). Other studies (Goulet *et al.*, 2007) showed lower data completeness when comparing automated electronic medical record data abstraction with manual electronic medical record data entry. Perhaps surprisingly, completeness for data elements electronically abstracted from the same electronic medical record system can vary. A comparative study of HIV-related data elements found that absolute differences in the percentage of documented values were between 2% and 35% in two data repositories from the same EMR system (McGinnis *et al.*, 2009). Goulet *et al.* (Goulet *et al.*, 2007; McGinnis *et al.*, 2009; Chan, Fowles and Weiner, 2010) agree that these findings point out the influence of both data extraction methods and documentation practices on data completeness.

Although data accuracy is rarely assessed as a dimension of data quality, emerging evidence highlights the potential of free-text data abstraction programs for accurately extracting data. Laboratory results as a data category exhibit greater data accuracy (Teperi, 1993; Staes *et al.*, 2006; Goulet *et al.*, 2007; McGinnis *et al.*, 2009). On the other hand, medication lists are reported to propagate significant errors, mainly observed in concomitance of retention of discontinued medication (Kaboli *et al.*, 2004; Staroselsky *et al.*, 2008). Also prescriptions of medications are not without errors. However, it has been showed that most errors do not have clinically important consequences (only 0.3% of them are classified as serious) (Varkey, Cunningham and Bisping, 2007), even if they may have more important effects from a quality measurement point of view.

Regarding data accuracy, automated abstraction of structured electronic medical records generally accurately produces laboratory test data and identifies medications and the right candidates for therapy (Persell *et al.*, 2006; Baker *et al.*, 2007; Goulet *et al.*, 2007). Even in this case, the high level of accuracy of data reflects their clinical value.

Important clinical information is often recorded within free-text sections of the EMR. Assessing free-text data extraction programs, such as natural language processing algorithms, provides evidence of accurate data about patient clinical status (Hazlehurst *et al.*, 2005; Baldwin, 2008; Pakhomov *et al.*, 2008; Murff *et al.*, 2011).

Indeed, natural language processing programs function effectively for variables that are narrowly and consistently defined (Thielke, Hammond and Helbig, 2007). Beyond natural language processing programs, which are very common, data abstraction using search-term methods also performed reasonably well, as showed by Benin *et al.* (2005), who evaluated such methods for identifying cases of pharyngitis, showing that performance rates were very similar using the search-term strategy and the reference manual EHR review, with only a 3% difference. As for the other quality dimensions, these findings also point out the role of documentation in the accuracy of data.

Data comparability is usually regarded as a secondary feature for data quality. However, studies focused on it showed a substantial variation in data content and documentation across clinical locations and data systems. In particular, many studies reported a high degree of variation in missing data by clinical locations (Goulet *et al.*, 2007).

In a fairly recent paper (de Lusignan *et al.*, 2004) it is shown that simply having different codes used to label patients of similar clinical status led to data unreliability across institutions. Systematic differences in missing data by institution are very common, and data extraction problems appeared to contribute to these problems (McGinnis *et al.*, 2009). Ricciardi *et al.*

(2005) showed that terminology standardization efforts on list entries, led to a substantial variability. Even within the same organization, data comparability is not assured (Hicken, Thornton and Rocha, 2004; Gold and Wang, 2007; Linder, Kaleba and Kmetik, 2009). Local naming conventions and locally developed glossaries also appear to contribute to the lack of data comparability across institutions or clinical locations (Linder, Kaleba and Kmetik, 2009; McGinnis *et al.*, 2009). The use of free-text fields can negatively affect measure validity by making it difficult to correctly identify eligible cases or appropriate exclusions. For example, Persell *et al.* (2006) examined cases of quality failures for coronary heart disease measures, which were calculated in an automated form using structured electronic medical records. Through manual review of free-text notes, Persell *et al.* (2006) found that 15 to 81% of cases identified as quality failures actually satisfied the performance measure or met appropriate exclusion criteria. Other studies in literature (Baker *et al.*, 2007) confirm such evidence and suggest that appropriate exclusions are often missed when automated extraction methods based on data from structured fields are used.

## 23.7   Summary

From a broad point of view, poor data comparability is an important limitation to the use of electronic medical record for quality reporting. To enhance data comparability, healthcare institutions need to pay attention to the data source for quality measurement, improvement of standardized data documentation and extraction procedures, and to implementing effective programs in order to facilitate data harmonization across institutions.

One of the major issues, confirmed by relevant scientific literature, still is represented by the very basic observation that poor documentation practices and inadequate EMR design can compromise measure validity and, in the very final extent, it can affect data usefulness and quality.

## References

Abate, M., Diegert, K. and Allen, H. (1998) A hierarchical approach to improving data quality. *Data Qual J*, **33**(4), 365–369.

Agrawal, R., Garcia-Molina, H., Gehrke, J. *et al.* (2009) The Claremont report on database research. *Commun ACM*, **52**(6), 56–65.

AHIMA Coding Products and Services Team (2003) Practice brief. Managing and improving data quality (updated). *J AHIMA*, **74**(7), 64A–64C.

American Health Information Management Association (2006) The new electronic discovery civil rule. *J AHIMA*, **77**(8), 68A-68H.

Arts, D.G., De Keizer, N.F. and Scheffer, G.J. (2002) Defining and improving data quality in medical registries: a literature review, case study, and generic framework. *J Am Med Inform Assoc*, **9**(6), 600–611.

Baker, D.W., Persell, S.D., Thompson, J.A. *et al.* (2007) Automated review of electronic health records to assess quality of care for outpatients with heart failure. *Ann Intern Med*, **146**(4), 270–277.

Baldwin, F.D. (2001) Once is enough. An enterprise-wide master patient index can eliminate duplicate entries and overlays with unique patient identifiers. *Healthc Inform*, **18**(7), 30–33.

Baldwin, K.B. (2008) Evaluating healthcare quality using natural language processing. *J Healthc Qual*, **30**(4), 24–29.

Benin, A.L., Vitkauskas, G., Thornquist, E. *et al.* (2005) Validity of using an electronic medical record for assessing quality of care in an outpatient setting. *Med Care*, **43**, 691–698.

Bernstein, P.A. and Haas, L. (2008) Information integration in the enterprise. *Commun ACM*, **51**, 72–79.

Bito, Y., Kero, R., Matsuo, H., Shintani, Y. and Silver, M. (2001) Interactively visualizing data warehouses. *J Healthc Inf Manag*, **15**(2), 133–142.

Bodenreider, O. (2004) The Unified Medical Language System (UMLS), integrating biomedical terminology. *Nucleic Acids Res*, **32** (Database issue), D267–D270.

Boonstra, A. and Broekhuis, M. (2010) Barriers to the acceptance of electronic medical records by physicians from systematic review to taxonomy and interventions. *BMC Health Serv Res*, **10**, 231.

Boyle, D. and Cunningham, S. (2002) Resolving fundamental quality issues in linked datasets for clinical care. *Health Inform J*, **8**(2), 73–77.

Brandt, C.A., Deshpande, A.M., Lu, C. *et al.* (2003) TrialDB: a web-based Clinical Study Data Management System. *AMIA Annu Symp Proc*, **2003**, 794.

Brender, J., Nohr, C. and McNair, P. (2000) Research needs and priorities in health informatics. *Int J Med Inform*, **58-59**, 257–289.

Brown, P.J. and Sonksen, P. (2000) Evaluation of the quality of information retrieval of clinical findings from a computerized patient database using a semantic terminological model. *J Am Med Inform Assoc*, **7**(4), 392–403.

Burt, C.W. and Sisk, J.E. (2005) Which physicians and practices are using electronic medical records? *Health Affairs*, **24**(5), 1334–1343.

Ceusters, W. (2011) SNOMED CT's RF2: is the future bright? *Stud Health Technol Inform*, **169**, 829–833.

Chan, K.S., Fowles, J.B. and Weiner, J.P. (2010) Review: electronic health records and the reliability and validity of quality measures: a review of the literature. *Med Care Res Rev*, **67**(5), 503–527.

Chan, S. (2008) Factors associated with the use of electronic information systems for drug dispensing and medication administration records in nursing homes. *J Am Med Dir Assoc*, **9**(6), 414–421.

Chan, W.C., Wright, C., Tobias, M., Mann, S. and Jackson, R. (2008) Explaining trends in coronary heart disease hospitalisations in New Zealand: trend for admissions and incidence can be in opposite directions. *Heart*, **94**(12), 1589–1593.

Chen, P. (1976) The entity-relationship model – toward a unified view of data. *ACM TODS*, **1**(1), 9–36.

Cimino, J.J., Hayamizu, T.F., Bodenreider, O. *et al.* (2009) The caBIG terminology review process. *J Biomed Inform*, **42**(3), 571–580.

Coiera, E. (2003) The electronic medical record, in *A Guide to Health Informatics*, 2nd edn, Arnold, London, pp. 111–123.

Connecting for Health Common Framework (2006) Background Issues on Data Quality. Available online at: www.connectingforhealth.org/commonframework/docs/T5_Background_Issues_Data.pdf (accessed April 14, 2012).

D'Onofrio, M. and Gendrom, M. (2001) Data quality in the healthcare industry. *J Data Qual*, **7**(1), 87–93.

de Coronado, S., Haber, M.W., Sioutos, N., Tuttle, M.S. and Wright, L.W. (2004) NCI Thesaurus: using science-based terminology to integrate cancer research results. *Stud Health Technol Inform*, **107** (Pt 1), 33–37.

de Lusignan, S., Hague, N., Brown, A. and Majeed, A. (2004) An educational intervention to improve data recording in the management of ischaemic heart disease in primary care. *J Public Health (Oxf)*, **26**(1), 34–37.

Dinakarpandian, D., Tong, T. and Lee, Y. (2007) A pragmatic approach to mapping the open biomedical ontologies. *Int J Bioinform Res Appl*, **3**(3), 341–365.

Dinu, V. and Nadkarni, P.M. (2007) Guidelines for the effective use of entity-attribute-value modeling for biomedical databases. *Int J Med Inform*, **76**(11–12), 769–779.

Edge, S.B., Byrd, D.R., Compton, C.C. *et al.* (2010) *AJCC Cancer Staging Handbook*, 7th edn, Springer.

Fernandes, L. (2008) Clean data: the path to electronic medical records. *J Clin Eng*, **33**(3), 151–153.

Garets, D. and Davis, M. (2005). Electronic Patient Records, EMRs and EHRs: Concepts as different as apples and oranges at least deserve separate names. Healthcare Informatics Online, McGraw-Hill.

Gendrom, M. and D'Onofrio, M. (2001) Data quality in the healthcare industry. *Data Quality*, **7**(1).

Goble, C. and Stevens, R. (2008) Data curation + process curation = data integration + science. *Brief Bioinform*, **9**(6), 506–517.

Gold, J.A. and Wang, J. (2007) Implementing electronic health records in physician offices: lessons learned. *WMJ*, **106**(3), 163–164.

Goulet, J.L., Erdos, J., Kancir, S. *et al.* (2007) Measuring performance directly using the veterans health administration electronic medical record: a comparison with external peer review. *Med Care*, **45**(1), 73–79.

Habib, J.L. (2010) EHRs, meaningful use, and a model EMR. *Drug Benef Trends*, **22**(4), 99–101.

Halevy, A.Y. (2001) Answering queries using views: A survey. *VLDB J*, **10**(4), 270–294.

Halevy, A., Ashish, N., Bitton, D. *et al.* (2005) Enterprise information integration: successes, challenges and controversies. Proceedings of the 2005 ACM SIGMOD International Conference on Management of Data, Baltimore, Maryland 2005, pp. 778–787.

Hanley, J.A. (1978) A language for computer generation of medical data forms. *Biometrics*, **34**, 288–297.

Harris, M.R., Ruggieri, A.P. and Chute, C.G. (2003) From clinical records to regulatory reporting: formal terminologies as foundation. *Healthc Financ Rev*, **24**(3), 103–120.

Hayrinen, K., Saranto, K. and Nykänen, P. (2008) Definition, structure, content, use and impacts of electronic health records: a review of the research literature. *Int J Med Inform*, **77**(5), 291–304.

Hazlehurst, B., Sittig, D.F., Stevens, V.J. *et al.* (2005) Natural language processing in the electronic medical record: assessing clinician adherence to tobacco treatment guidelines. *Am J Prev Med*, **29**(5), 434–439.

Health Information Strategy Steering Committee (2005) *Health Information Strategy for New Zealand*, Ministry of Health, Wellington.

Hicken, V.N., Thornton, S.N. and Rocha, R.A. (2004) Integration challenges of clinical information systems developed without a shared data dictionary. *Stud Health Technol Inform*, **107**, 1053–1057.

Higgins, S.B., Jiang, K., Plummer, W.D. Jr. *et al.* (1995) Pivot/Remote: a distributed database for remote data entry in multi-center clinical trials. *Medinfo*, **8** (Pt 2), 1097.

Institute of Medicine (2003) *Patient Safety: Achieving a New Standard of Care*, National Academy Press, Washington, DC.

ISO (2004) ISO/DTR 20514 *Health Informatics – Electronic Health Record – Definition, Scope, and Context*, International Organization for Standardization.

Johnson, S.B. and Chatziantoniou, D. (1999) Extended SQL for manipulating clinical warehouse data. *Proc AMIA Symp*, **1999**, 819–823.

Kaboli, P.J., McClimon, B.J., Hoth, A.B. and Barnett, M.J. (2004) Assessing the accuracy of computerized medication histories. *Am J Manag Care*, **10**(11 Pt 2), 872–877.

Kahn, M.G., Kaplan, D., Sokol, R.J. and DiLaura, R.P. (2007) Configuration challenges: implementing translational research policies in electronic medical records. *Acad Med*, **82**(7), 661–669.

Kerr, K.A., Norris, T. and Stockdale, R. (2008) The strategic management of data quality in healthcare. *Health Inform J*, **14**(4), 259–266.

Kimball, R., Reeves, L., Ross, M. and Thornthwaite, W. (1998) *The Data Warehouse Lifecycle Toolkit: Expert Methods for Designing, Developing and Deploying Data Warehouses*, John Wiley & Sons, Inc.

Koppel, R., Metlay, J.P., Cohen, A. *et al.* (2005) Role of computerized physician order entry systems in facilitating medication errors. *JAMA*, **293**(10), 1197–1203.

Kuhn, K. (1996) [Electronic documentation of findings and image in ultrasound diagnosis]. *Radiologe*, **36**(1), 47–50.

Lee, T.J., Pouliot, Y., Wagner, V. *et al.* (2006) BioWarehouse: a bioinformatics database warehouse toolkit. *BMC Bioinform*, **7**, 170.

Linder, J.A., Kaleba, E.O. and Kmetik, K.S. (2009) Using electronic health records to measure physician performance for acute conditions in primary care: empirical evaluation of the community-acquired pneumonia clinical quality measure set. *Med Care*, **47**(2), 208–216.

Littlejohns, P., Wyatt, J.C. and Garvican, L. (2003) Evaluating computerised health information systems: hard lessons still to be learnt. *BMJ*, **326**(7394), 860–863.

Liu, K., Hogan, W.R. and Crowley, R.S. (2011) Natural Language Processing methods and systems for biomedical ontology learning. *J Biomed Inform*, **44**(1), 163–179.

Louie, B., Mork, P., Martin-Sanchez, F., Halevy, A. and Tarczy-Hornoch, P. (2007) Data integration and genomic medicine. *J Biomed Inform*, **40**(1), 5–16.

Lowe, H.J. and Ferris, T.A. (2009) STRIDE – an integrated standards-based translational research informatics platform. *AMIA Annu Symp Proc*, **2009**(5), 391–395.

Makoul, G., Curry, R.H. and Tang, P.C. (2001) The use of electronic medical records: communication patterns in outpatient encounters. *J Am Med Inform Assoc*, **8**(6), 610–615.

McAlearney, A.S., Robbins, J., Hirsch, A., Jorina, M. and Harrop, J.P. (2010) Perceived efficiency impacts following electronic health record implementation: an exploratory study of an urban community health center network. *Int J Med Inform*, **79**(12), 807–816.

McDonald, C.J. (1976) Protocol-based computer reminders, the quality of care and the non-perfectability of man. *N Engl J Med*, **295**(24), 1351–1355.

McGinnis, K.A., Skanderson, M., Levin, F.L. *et al.* (2009) Comparison of two VA laboratory data repositories indicates that missing data vary despite originating from the same source. *Med Care*, **47**(1), 121–124.

Meadows, B.J. (2003) Eliciting remote data entry system requirements for the collection of cancer clinical trial data. *Comput Inform Nurs*, **21**(5), 234–240.

Mercer, L., Widmer, J., Prada, J., Grogan, K. and Tresnan, L. (1995) The registration function as a critical dependency in a lifetime clinical record (LCR). *Medinfo*, **8** (Pt 1), 461.

Miller, R.H. and Sim, I. (2004) Physicians' use of electronic medical records: barriers and solutions. *Health Affairs*, **23**(2), 116–126.

Moczygemba, J. and Hewitt, B. (2001) Managing clinical data in an electronic environment. *Health Care Manag (Frederick)*, **19**(4), 33–38.

Muranaga, F., Kumamoto, I. and Uto, Y. (2007) Development of hospital data warehouse for cost analysis of DPC based on medical costs. *Methods Inf Med*, **46**(6), 679–685.

Murff, H.J., FitzHenry, F., Matheny, M.E. *et al.* (2011) Automated identification of postoperative complications within an electronic medical record using natural language processing. *JAMA*, **306**(8), 848–855.

Musen, M.A. (2000) Design and use of clinical ontologies: curricular goals for the education of health-telematics professionals. *Stud Health Technol Inform*, **72**, 40–47.

Neil, N. and Nerenz, D. (2003) Learning to leverage existing information systems: Part 1. *Principles*. Jt Comm J Qual Saf, **29**(10), 523–530.

Orfanidis, L., Bamidis, P. and Eaglestone, B.M. (2004) Data quality issues in electronic health records: an adaptation framework for the Greek Health System. *Health Inform J*, **10**(1), 23–36.

Pakhomov, S.V., Jacobsen, S.J., Chute, C.G. and Roger, V.L. (2008) Agreement between patient-reported symptoms and their documentation in the medical record. *Am J Manag Care*, **14**(8), 530–539.

Payne, P.R., Greaves, A.W. and Kipps, T.J. (2003) CRC Clinical Trials Management System (CTMS): an integrated information management solution for collaborative clinical research. *AMIA Annu Symp Proc*, **2003**, 967.

Persell, S.D., Wright, J.M., Thompson, J.A., Kmetik, K.S. and Baker, D.W. (2006) Assessing the validity of national quality measures for coronary artery disease using an electronic health record. *Arch Intern Med*, **166**(20), 2272–2277.

Porcheret, M., Hughes, R., Evans, D. *et al.* (2004) Data quality of general practice electronic health records: the impact of a program of assessments, feedback, and training. *J Am Med Inform Assoc*, **11**(1), 78–86.

Prokosch, H.U. and Ganslandt, T. (2009) Perspectives for medical informatics. Reusing the electronic medical record for clinical research. *Methods Inf Med*, **48**(1), 38–44.

Ramick, D.C. (2001) Data warehousing in disease management programs. *J Healthc Inf Manag*, **15**(2), 99–105.

Ricciardi, T.N., Lieberman, M.I., Kahn, M.G. and Masarie, F.E. Jr. (2005) Clinical terminology support for a national ambulatory practice outcomes research network. *AMIA Annu Symp Proc*, **2005**, 629–633.

Rosenman, M.B., Tao, G., Szucs, K.A. *et al.* (2008) Prenatal syphilis screening rates measured using Medicaid claims and electronic medical records. *Sex Transm Dis*, **35**(4), 387–392.

Schmier, J.K., Kane, D.W. and Halpern, M.T. (2005) Practical applications of usability theory to electronic data collection for clinical trials. *Contemp Clin Trials*, **26**(3), 376–385.

Schriger, D.L., Baraff, L.J., Rogers, W.H. and Cretin, S. (1997) Implementation of clinical guidelines using a computer charting system. Effect on the initial care of health care workers exposed to body fluids. *JAMA*, **278**(19), 1585–1590.

Schulz, S. and Stenzhorn, H. (2007) Ten theses on clinical ontologies. *Stud Health Technol Inform*, **127**, 268–275.

Schumock, G.T., Hutchinson, R.A. and Bilek, B.A. (1992) Comparison of two systems for documenting pharmacist interventions in patient care. *Am J Hosp Pharm*, **49**(9), 2211–2214.

Shapiro, J.S., Mostashari, F., Hripcsak, G., Soulakis, N. and Kuperman, G. (2011) Using health information exchange to improve public health. *Am J Public Health*, **101**(4), 616–623.

Smith, B. and Scheuermann, R.H. (2011) Ontologies for clinical and translational research: introduction. *J Biomed Inform*, **44**(1), 3–7.

Smith, S.A., Murphy, M.E., Huschka, T.R. *et al.* (1998) Impact of a diabetes electronic management system on the care of patients seen in a subspecialty diabetes clinic. *Diabetes Care*, **21**(6), 972–976.

Staes, C.J., Bennett, S.T., Evans, R.S. *et al.* (2006) A case for manual entry of structured, coded laboratory data from multiple sources into an ambulatory electronic health record. *J Am Med Inform Assoc*, **13**(1), 12–15.

Staroselsky, M., Volk, L.A., Tsurikova, R. *et al.* (2008) An effort to improve electronic health record medication list accuracy between visits: patients' and physicians' response. *Int J Med Inform*, **77**(3), 153–160.

Stroetmann, K.A., Jones, T., Dobrev, A. and Stroetmann, V.N. (2006) *eHealth is Worth it. The Economic Benefits of Implemented eHealth Solutions at Ten European Sites* (eHealth IMPACT project study supported by the European Commission Information Society and Media Directorate-General), Office for Official Publications of the European Communities, Luxembourg.

Tang, P.C. and MacDonald, C.J. (2001). Computer based patient record systems, in *Medical Informatics: Computer Applications in Health Care and Biomedicine* (eds E.H. Shortliffe and L.E. Perrault), Springer, New York.

Tang, P.C., Ralston, M., Arrigotti, M.F., Qureshi, L. and Graham, J. (2007) Comparison of methodologies for calculating quality measures based on administrative data versus clinical data from an electronic health record system: implications for performance measures. *J Am Med Inform Assoc*, **14**(1), 10–15.

Teperi, J. (1993) Multi method approach to the assessment of data quality in the Finnish Medical Birth Registry. *J Epidemiol Comm Health*, **47**(3), 242–247.

Terry, A.L., Chevendra, V., Thind, A. *et al.* (2010) Using your electronic medical record for research: a primer for avoiding pitfalls. *Fam Pract*, **27**(1), 121–126.

Thielke, S., Hammond, K. and Helbig, S. (2007) Copying and pasting of examinations within the electronic medical record. *Int J Med Inform*, **76** (Suppl 1), S122–S128.

Thiru, K., Hassey, A. and Sullivan, F. (2003) Systematic review of scope and quality of electronic patient record data in primary care. *BMJ*, **326**(7398), 1070.

Trujillo, J. and Palomar, M. (2001) Designing data warehouses with OO conceptual models. *Computer*, **34**(12), 66–75.

UK Department of Health (2008) Health Informatics Review: Report, DH Publications.

Varkey, P., Cunningham, J. and Bisping, D.S. (2007) Improving medication reconciliation in the outpatient setting. *Jt Comm J Qual Patient Saf*, **33**(5), 286–292.

Wagner, M.M. and Hogan, W.R. (1996) The accuracy of medication data in an outpatient electronic medical record. *J Am Med Inform Assoc*, **3**(3), 234–244.

Wang, X., Liu, L., Fackenthal, J. *et al.* (2009) Translational integrity and continuity: personalized biomedical data integration. *J Biomed Inform*, **42**(1), 100–112.

Ware, J.E. Jr. and Gandek, B. (1998) Methods for testing data quality, scaling assumptions, and reliability: the IQOLA Project approach. International Quality of Life Assessment. *J Clin Epidemiol*, **51**(11), 945–952.

Wheatley, V. (2008) Quality impact of the master patient index. *J AHIMA*, **79**(10), 78–79.

Williams, A. (2006) Design for better data: how software and users interact onscreen matters to data quality. *J AHIMA*, **77**(2), 56–60.

Williams, K., Robinson, K. and Toth, A. (2006) Data quality maintenance of the Patient Master Index (PMI), a 'snap-shot' of public healthcare facility PMI data quality and linkage activities. *HIM J*, **35**(1), 10–26.

Wingert, F. (1985) Automated indexing based on SNOMED. *Methods Inf Med*, **24**(1), 27–34.

World Health Organization. Regional Office for the Western Pacific (2006) *Medical Records Manual: A Guide for Developing Countries*, World Health Organization, Geneva.

Wubbelt, P., Fernandez, G. and Heymer, J. (2000) Clinical trial management and remote data entry on the Internet based on XML case report forms. *Stud Health Technol Inform*, **77**, 333–337.

Yamamoto, L.G. and Khan, A.N. (2006) Challenges of electronic medical record implementation in the emergency department. *Pediatr Emerg Care*, **22**(3), 184–191; quiz 192.

Yu, A.C. (2006) Methods in biomedical ontology. *J Biomed Inform*, **39**(3), 252–266.

# Index

activity-based costing (ABC), 392
acute myocardial infarction, 187, 204,
    219–21, 225, 227, 306, 360, 396, 398
active pharmaceutical ingredient (API), 163
adaptive design, 5, 10, 16–18, 22, 43,
    50–52, 80, 99–100, 103–5, 110,
    112–13, 116, 161–2
adverse event, 7, 23–4, 40, 42, 122–7, 131,
    140, 142, 146, 150, 152, 160, 254,
    256–7, 261, 264, 278, 280, 290, 353,
    359–62, 462, 467
age dependence, 355–6
age group, 30, 33, 42, 45, 191, 355, 358,
    396, 431, 441
allocation, 10, 29–31, 52, 104, 113–14,
    116–17, 119–20, 186–7, 202, 313,
    335–51, 375, 389–92, 397, 399,
    410–11, 413, 442
area profiling, 207
area under curve (AUC), 60
areal data, 188–9, 191–2, 196, 210
association, 33, 41, 125, 196–7, 203–7, 231,
    246, 353–4, 358–9, 381
autocorrelation, 204–5, 209, 262, 309, 312,
    318, 320–22, 330
autocovariance, 330
average run length (ARL), 263, 269–70,
    273–4, 278, 284
Aviation Safety Reporting System (ASRS),
    123, 125

Bayesian analysis, 19, 22, 48–52, 65–7, 99,
    104, 107–10, 127–8, 132, 137, 152,
    173–4, 182, 185–6, 193, 197–200, 204,
    206, 209, 220–23, 225, 243, 361,
    365–6, 368–70, 378, 380–81
Bayesian evidence synthesis, 365,
    380–82
Bayesian hierarchical model, 36, 49, 66,
    185–6, 189, 192–4, 200, 204–6, 207–9,
    221, 326, 381, 401
Bayesian networks, 132–3, 135,
    137–9
belt,
    black, 298–303
    green, 298, 300–303
    master black, 263, 299
    yellow, 298, 300, 302–3
benchmarking, 386, 390, 395, 401, 410,
    414, 418, 450
beneficiary, 446, 450
Besag–York–Mollié model, 192–5,
    197–200, 202, 206, 210
bias, 15, 24, 29–32, 36–40, 46–8, 52–3, 75,
    92, 94, 105–7, 112–15, 124, 135, 160,
    169–82, 186–8, 196, 198, 205–6, 223,
    231–2, 237, 240, 243, 245–7, 262, 314,
    326, 328, 358, 361–2, 374–5, 381,
    451–3, 462
black swan, 128, 130–31
blinding, 9, 29, 31–2, 53, 113, 232

*Statistical Methods in Healthcare*, First Edition. Edited by Frederick W. Faltin, Ron S. Kenett and Fabrizio Ruggeri.
© 2012 John Wiley & Sons, Ltd. Published 2012 by John Wiley & Sons, Ltd.